Proteins in Pathology and Physiology

Proteins in Pathology and Physiology

Editor: Camille Finlay

AMERICAN
MEDICAL PUBLISHERS
www.americanmedicalpublishers.com

AMERICAN
MEDICAL PUBLISHERS
www.americanmedicalpublishers.com

Cataloging-in-Publication Data

Proteins in pathology and physiology / edited by Camille Finlay.
p. cm.
Includes bibliographical references and index.
ISBN 979-8-88740-401-1
1. Proteins. 2. Proteins--Pathophysiology. 3. Proteins--Metabolism--Disorders.
4. Proteins--Physiological effect. I. Finlay, Camille.
RC632.P7 P76 2023
616.399 5--dc23

American Medical Publishers,
41 Flatbush Avenue,
1st Floor, New York,
NY 11217, USA

ISBN 979-8-88740-401-1 (Hardback)

Contents

Preface

The purpose of the book is to provide a glimpse into the dynamics and to present opinions and studies of some of the scientists engaged in the development of new ideas in the field from very different standpoints. This book will prove useful to students and researchers owing to its high content quality.

Proteins are biopolymeric structures that are made up of amino acids. They are essential for the body as they are an important constituent of cells. Proteins are also involved in important physiological and biochemical processes such as biochemical reactions, hormonal signalling, cell-receptor interactions, apoptosis, etc. Proteins are characterized based on their structures. There are four structural levels, namely, primary, secondary, tertiary and quaternary. The primary structure of proteins is made up of linear order of amino acid residues that are connected via peptide bonds. Secondary protein structure consists of alpha helix, beta-pleated sheet, and beta-turn, and these shapes are stabilized by hydrogen bonds. The tertiary protein structure consists of a 3D shape and it is formed by the interaction of the polypeptide chain backbone with an aqueous environment. Quarternary protein structure is formed from multiple polypeptide chains called subunits. Body requires proteins for growth and maintenance of cells and tissues. They are involved in various functions such as supporting the regulation and expression of the DNA and RNA, moving essential molecules in the body, supporting muscle contraction and movement, etc. The aim of this book is to present researches on the physiological and pathological aspects of proteins. Its extensive content provides the readers with a thorough understanding of the subject.

At the end, I would like to appreciate all the efforts made by the authors in completing their chapters professionally. I express my deepest gratitude to all of them for contributing to this book by sharing their valuable works. A special thanks to my family and friends for their constant support in this journey.

Editor

1

Tau Phosphorylation in a Mouse Model of Temporal Lobe Epilepsy

*Marianna Alves†, Aidan Kenny†, Gioacchino de Leo, Edward H. Beamer and Tobias Engel**

Department of Physiology and Medical Physics, Royal College of Surgeons in Ireland, Dublin, Ireland

***Correspondence:**
Tobias Engel
tengel@rcsi.ie

†These authors have contributed equally to this work

Hyperphosphorylation of the microtubule-associated protein tau and its resultant aggregation into neurofibrillary tangles (NFT) is a pathological characteristic of neurodegenerative disorders known as tauopathies. Tau is a neuronal protein involved in the stabilization of microtubule structures of the axon and the aberrant phosphorylation of tau is associated with several neurotoxic effects. The discovery of tau pathology and aggregates in the cortex of Temporal lobe epilepsy (TLE) patients has focused interest on hyperphosphorylation of tau as a potential mechanism contributing to increased states of hyperexcitability and cognitive decline. Previous studies using animal models of status epilepticus and tissue from patients with TLE have shown increased tau phosphorylation in the brain following acute seizures and during epilepsy, with tau phosphorylation correlating with cognitive deficits in patients. Suggesting a functional role of tau during epilepsy, studies in tau-deficient and tau-overexpressing mice have demonstrated a causal role of tau during seizure generation. Previous studies, analyzing the impact of seizures on tau hyperphosphorylation, have mainly used animal models of acute seizures. These models, however, do not replicate all aspects of chronic epilepsy. In this study, we investigated the effects of acute seizures (status epilepticus) and chronic epilepsy upon the expression and phosphorylation of tau using the intra-amygdala kainic acid (KA)-induced status epilepticus mouse model. Status epilepticus resulted in an immediate increase in total tau levels in the hippocampus, in particular, the dentate gyrus, and phosphorylation of the AT8 epitope (Ser202, Thr205), with phosphorylated tau mainly localizing to the mossy fibers of the dentate gyrus. During epilepsy, abnormal phosphorylation of tau was detected again at the AT8 epitope with lower total tau levels in the CA3 and CA1 subfields of the hippocampus. Chronic epilepsy in mice also resulted in a strong localization of AT8 phospho-tau to microglia, indicating a distinct pattern of tau hyperphosphorylation during chronic epilepsy compared to status epilepticus. Our results reaffirm previous observations of tau phosphorylation post-status epilepticus, but also elaborate on tau alterations in epileptic mice which more faithfully mimic TLE. Our results confirm seizures affect tau hyperphosphorylation, however, suggest epitope-specific phosphorylation of tau and differences in cell-specific localization according to disease progression.

Keywords: tau phosphorylation, AT8, status epilepticus, epilepsy, mouse models

INTRODUCTION

Tauopathies are a diverse group of neurodegenerative disorders characterized by misfolded, aggregated and aberrant forms of the microtubule-associated protein tau (Götz et al., 2019). These tauopathies have been traditionally limited to diseases in which tau was a primary pathology feature such as Alzheimer's Disease, Pick's Disease, progressive supranuclear palsy and chronic traumatic encephalopathy (Götz et al., 2019). Recent studies are identifying, however, an increasing number of disorders with tau pathology. These new tau-associated disorders include the neurodegenerative disorders Huntington's and Parkinson's Disease as well as Temporal lobe epilepsy (TLE; Fernández-Nogales et al., 2014; Tai et al., 2016, p. 4; Cisbani et al., 2017, p. 3). TLE is the most common form of acquired epilepsy in adults and particularly prone to pharmacoresistance (Schmidt and Löscher, 2005) and, although not defined as a neurodegenerative disease, tau-based aggregates which directly correlate with cognitive decline have been identified in TLE patient brain (Thom et al., 2011; Tai et al., 2016, p. 4).

Tau is a microtubule-associated protein, primarily found in neurons and located in axons (Janning et al., 2014). Although tau can be targeted by numerous kinases *in vivo*, this is limited to a small group of well-characterized kinases which includes Glycogen synthase kinase-3β (GSK-3β), Cyclin-dependent kinase 5 (CDK5) and Microtubule-affinity-regulating kinase (MARK; Martin et al., 2013b). These kinases work in tandem with a group of phosphatases [Protein phosphatase-1, -2 and -5 (PP1/2/5)] to curate the modifications and thereby the function of tau in the cell (Martin et al., 2013a). This cycle of phosphorylation is ultimately the mechanism by which abnormal forms of tau are typically generated with imbalances in kinase/phosphatase activity resulting in hyperphosphorylation of tau, leading to misfolding and aggregation (Götz et al., 2019). The primary mechanism by which these aberrant modifications induce neurodegeneration in cells is heavily debated and can be loosely divided into two groups including a loss-of-function, where hyperphosphorylation of tau blocks its interaction and stabilization of microtubule structures possibly impacting on axonal transport and synaptic transmission (Feinstein and Wilson, 2005), or a toxic-gain-of function where hyperphosphorylation of tau drives aberrant interactions such as disruption of the trafficking and anchoring of receptors in dendritic compartments or negatively affecting mitochondrial function (Hoover et al., 2010; Lasagna-Reeves et al., 2011).

Tau is well known to have a significant influence on neuronal activity and seizures. Several studies have shown tau to be integral to hyperactivity in mouse models of status epilepticus where knock-down of tau is neuroprotective and ameliorates seizure activity (Holth et al., 2013), while tau overexpression models have been shown to result in hyperexcitability and seizures (García-Cabrero et al., 2013). These findings are, however, at odds with conflicting studies where tau hyperphosphorylation and overexpression have been shown to dampen neuronal excitability (Angulo et al., 2017; Busche et al., 2019). The mechanism behind this bi-directional effect in which both aberrant increases and decreases in tau induce a synaptic dampening and reduction in excitatory activity remains unexplained and requires further investigation of the underlying molecular processes.

Studies in experimental seizure models have identified a wave of increased kinase activity in neurons resulting from seizure activity which includes several kinases which all putatively act on tau phosphorylation: GSK-3β, CDK5, extracellular signal-regulated kinase (ERK) and protein kinase A (PKA; Liang et al., 2009; Gangarossa et al., 2015). The induction of seizures in mice has also been shown to cause long-term downregulation of the phosphatase PP2A, potentially compounding the imbalance of tau hyperphosphorylation (Liang et al., 2009). Previous investigations of seizure-induced changes in tau phosphorylation have been limited to the induction of convulsive status epilepticus *via* a systemic injection of kainic acid (KA) which produces inconsistent pathology and hippocampal epileptogenesis (Sloviter et al., 2007). The processes and cellular responses of the periodic and less severe seizure activity in chronic epilepsy are, however, distinct from the initial intense excitation of status epilepticus.

In this present study, we investigated the impact of status epilepticus and chronic epilepsy on the phosphorylation and localization of tau using the intra-amygdala KA mouse model of status epilepticus (Mouri et al., 2008). The intra-amygdala KA mouse model is a refined model for the focalized induction of status epilepticus and reliable stimulation of epileptogenesis (Henshall et al., 2000; Mouri et al., 2008) and, therefore, the study of tau phosphorylation in this model may help to shed further light on tau pathology seen in TLE patients.

MATERIALS AND METHODS

Animals Model of Status Epilepticus

All animal experiments were performed in accordance with the principles of the European Communities Council Directive (2010/63/EU). Procedures were reviewed and approved by the Research Ethics Committee of the Royal College of Surgeons in Ireland (REC 1322) and the Irish Health Products Regulatory Authority (AE19127/P038). All efforts were maximized to reduce the number of animals used in this study. Mice used in our experiments were 8- to 12-week-old male C57BL/6 mice, obtained from the Biomedical Research Facility, Royal College of Surgeons in Ireland (Dublin, Ireland). Animals were housed in a controlled biomedical facility on a 12 h light/dark cycle at 22 ± 1°C and humidity of 40–60% with food and water provided *ad libitum*. Status epilepticus was induced by a unilateral stereotaxic microinjection of KA (Sigma-Aldrich, Arklow, Ireland) into the amygdala, as described (Brennan et al., 2013). A guide cannula was affixed over the dura (coordinates from Bregma: AP = −0.94; L = −2.85 mm) and the entire skull assembly fixed in place with dental cement. Then a 31-gauge internal cannula was inserted into the lumen of the guide cannula to inject KA into the amygdala [0.3 μg in 0.2 μl vehicle; phosphate-buffered saline (PBS), pH adjusted to 7.4] at a flow rate of 0.02 μl per second over 10 s. Non-seizure control mice received an intra-amygdala injection of 0.2 μl of sterile PBS. Mice typically develop status epilepticus shortly following intra-amygdala KA injection undergoing typical behavioral changes scored according to a modified Racine Scale. This includes: Score 1, immobility and freezing; Score 2, forelimb and or tail extension, rigid posture; Score 3, repetitive movements, head bobbing; Score 4, rearing and falling; Score 5, continuous rearing and falling; Score 6, severe tonic–clonic seizures (Jimenez-Mateos et al., 2012). A single dose of the anticonvulsant lorazepam (8 mg/kg, intraperitoneal) was administered 40 min after KA to curtail status epilepticus and reduce mortality and morbidity. Mice were euthanized at different time-points (1 h, 4 h, 8 h, 24 h and 14 days) after anticonvulsant administration.

Microdissection of Hippocampal Subfields

To analyze the different hippocampal subfields separately, mouse brains were removed using sharp laboratory scissors and placed into a petri dish on top of a cold board. Following the separation of the cerebellum, the two brain hemispheres were separated. Then, using a dissecting microscope, the whole hippocampus was separated from the cortex. Following the identification of the boundaries between the dentate gyrus, cornus ammonis (CA)1 and CA3, the three hippocampal subfields were separated and immediately put on dry ice and stored at −80°C.

Drug Treatment

The GSK-3 inhibitor NP031112 [Tideglusib, NP12 (Domínguez et al., 2012); Sigma-Aldrich, Arklow, Ireland] was administered with a 2 μl infusion of intra-cerebro-ventricular (i.c.v.) Dimethyl sulfoxide (DMSO) 15 min after the administration of the anticonvulsant lorazepam into the ventricle (ventricle volume was calculated as 30 μl) to reach a final concentration of 100 μM (Engel et al., 2018). In the vehicle group, animals were injected with 2 μl of sterile DMSO.

Western Blotting

Western blotting was performed as described previously (Engel et al., 2017). Following quantification of protein concentration, 30 μg of protein samples were boiled in gel-loading buffer and separated by sodium dodecyl sulfate–polyacrylamide gel electrophoresis. Proteins were transferred to nitrocellulose membranes and probed with the following primary antibodies: Tau-1 (1:1,000, Merck Millipore, Arklow, Ireland), AT8 (1:100, Invitrogen, CA, USA), PHF-1 (1:1,000, Abcam, Cambridge, UK) and GAPDH (1:1,000, Cell Signalling, Dublin, Ireland). Next, membranes were incubated with horseradish peroxidase-conjugated goat anti-rabbit or anti-mouse secondary antibodies (Isis Limited, Bray, Ireland). Protein bands were visualized using Fujifilm LAS-4000 system (Fujifilm, Tokyo, Japan) with chemiluminescence.

RNA Extraction and Real-Time Quantitative Polymerase Chain Reaction

RNA extraction was undertaken as previously described using TRIzol® (QIAzol Lysis Reagent, Qiagen, Hilden, Germany; Jimenez-Mateos et al., 2015). Five-hundred microgram of total RNA was used to generate complementary DNA by reverse transcription using SuperScript® III reverse transcriptase enzyme (Thermo Fisher Scientific, Waltham, MA, USA). Quantitative real-time PCR was performed using a LightCycler 1.5 (Roche Diagnostics GmbH, Mannheim, Germany) in combination with QuantiTect® SYBR® Green PCR Kit (Qiagen, Hilden, Germany) as per the manufacturer's protocol, and 1.25 μM of primer pair was used. Data were analyzed by LightCycler 1.5 software and normalized to the expression of β-*actin* and represented as relative quantification values. Primers were designed using Primer3 software[1]. Primer sequences: *tau* F: aatcagtctccacaccccag, R: actacaacgtaacagggcga; *tau-3R* F: cccagc tctggtgaacctcca, R: tcacaaaccctgcttggccagand and β-*actin*, F: gggtgtgatggtgggaatgg, R: ggttggccttagggttcagg.

Fluoro-Jade B Staining

Fluoro-Jade B (FjB) staining was carried out as before (Engel et al., 2013). Twelve micrometer coronal sections at the medial level of the hippocampus (Bregma AP = −1.94 mm) were cut on a cryostat. Tissue was fixed in formalin, rehydrated in ethanol, and then transferred to a 0.006% potassium permanganate solution followed by incubation with 0.001% FjB (Chemicon Europe Limited, Chandlers Ford, UK). The sections were mounted in DPX mounting solution. Using an epifluorescence microscope, FjB-positive cells within the ipsilateral hippocampus including all subfields (dentate gyrus, CA1 and CA3 regions) were counted by a person unaware of treatment under a 40× lens in two adjacent sections and the average determined for each animal.

3,3′-Diaminobenzidine Immunohistochemistry

Mice were transcardially perfused with 4% paraformaldehyde (PFA) and postfixed for an additional 24 h. Brains were then transferred to PBS and immersed into 4% agarose before sectioning. 3,3′-Diaminobenzidine (DAB) staining was carried out as before (Engel et al., 2006). Slices were treated with 1% H_2O_2 for 45 min to inactivate endogenous peroxidases. This was followed by an incubation with blocking solution (10 ml: 8.3 ml 1× PBS, 1 ml 10% BSA, 0.5 ml 5% FBS, 0.2 ml Triton-X-100) for 1 h and primary antibody (AT8, 1:100, Invitrogen, CA, USA) overnight at 4°C. On the following day, tissue sections were washed 3× with PBS for 10 min each and incubated with Vectastain kit (Vector Laboratories, Burlingame, CA, USA; one drop of biotinylated antibody and three drops of horse/donkey serum were mixed in 10 ml of 1% BSA-PBS). This solution was added to the tissue and incubated for 90 min at room temperature. Three washes were performed with PBS for 10 min followed by a 90 min incubation with Avidin (ABC) peroxidase complex at room temperature (two drops of reagent A and reagent B in 10 ml of 1% BSA-PBS). Slices were washed with PBS for 20 min and immersed in DAB solution (Sigma-Aldrich, Arklow, Ireland) for approximately 10 min. Then, slices were mounted using FluorSave™. Staining was examined under a light microscope.

Immunofluorescence

As for DAB staining, mice were transcardially perfused with 4% PFA and postfixed for an additional 24 h. Following immersed into 4% agarose, brains were sectioned into 30 μm thick sagittal sections using the VT1000S vibratome (Leica Microsystems,

[1] http://frodo.wi.mit.edu

Wetzlar, Germany). Tissue sections were incubated with 0.1% Triton/PBS and 1 M glycine, followed by blocking with 1% BSA in PBS for 45 min. The sections were then incubated with the primary antibody AT8 (1:100, Invitrogen, CA, USA) overnight. This was followed by washing with PBS and a second incubation for 2 h at room temperature with a second primary antibody against NeuN (1:400, Millipore, Arklow, Ireland), GFAP (1:400, Sigma-Aldrich, Arklow, Ireland), Iba-1 (1:400, Wako, Fuggerstrasse, Germany) or Zinc Transporter 3 (ZnT3; 1:200, Synaptic Systems GmbH, Goettingen, Germany). After washing in PBS, tissue was incubated with fluorescent secondary antibodies [AlexaFluor-488 or AlexaFluor-568 (BioSciences, Dublin, Ireland)] followed by a short incubation with DAPI. FluorSave^{TM} (Millipore, Arklow, Ireland) was used to cover the tissue, and confocal images were taken with a TCR 6500 microscope (Leica Microsystems, Wetzlar, Germany) equipped with four laser lines (405, 488, 561, and 653 nm) using a 40× immersion oil objective (NA 1.3; Leica Microsystems).

Data Analysis

Data were analyzed for statistical significance using StatView. Parametric analysis was carried out using Student's t-test and one-way ANOVA with Fishers *post hoc* multiple comparisons analysis. Data are presented as mean ± standard error of the mean (SEM).

RESULTS

Increased Tau Phosphorylation in the Hippocampus Following Intra-Amygdala Kainic Acid-Induced Status Epilepticus

To study the effects of status epilepticus (prolonged, damaging seizure) on tau expression and phosphorylation in the hippocampus *in vivo*, status epilepticus was induced in C57Bl/6 wild-type mice by an intra-amygdala injection of KA (Engel et al., 2013). In this model, status epilepticus leads to a distinct cell death pattern in the brain which is mainly restricted to the ipsilateral cortex and hippocampus. Within the ipsilateral hippocampus, the CA3 subfield is the most affected while the dentate gyrus and CA1 are mainly spared from cell death (Mouri et al., 2008; **Figure 1A**). All mice treated with intra-amygdala KA develop epilepsy following a short latency period of 3–5 days experiencing 2–5 spontaneous seizures per day (Mouri et al., 2008).

As a first approach, we analyzed whether status epilepticus has an effect on the expression of tau in the ipsilateral hippocampus. RT-qPCR revealed hippocampal *tau* mRNA levels to be relatively unchanged compared to control at all time-points analyzed post-status epilepticus (1 h–24 h; **Figure 1B**). Moreover, no induction of the *3R tau* isoform was observed in the hippocampus following status epilepticus (**Supplementary Figure S1A**). In contrast to *tau* mRNA levels, hippocampal tau protein levels detected *via* the Tau-1 antibody were increased at 4 h post-status epilepticus and remained elevated for up to 24 h [Ctrl vs. 4 h, 1.65 ± 0.3373 (mean ± SEM), $p = 0.03$; ANOVA *post hoc* Fisher's test; **Figure 1C**]. Next, changes in the phosphorylation of tau in the hippocampus were analyzed using two antibodies recognizing different phosphorylation sites within the tau protein. This included AT8 (phosphorylation of Ser202/Thr205; Goedert et al., 1995) and PHF-1 (phosphorylation of Ser396/Ser404; Otvos et al., 1994). Western blotting of hippocampal samples revealed phosphorylation at the AT8 epitope was significantly increased at 4 h and 8 h post-status epilepticus when normalized to total tau levels [Ctrl vs. 4 h, 2.041 ± 0.384 (mean ± SEM), $p = 0.03$; Ctrl vs. 8 h, 2.413 ± 0.2357 (mean ± SEM), $p = 0.005$; ANOVA *post hoc* Fisher's test] with this increase tapering off at 24 h post-status epilepticus (**Figure 1D**). Increases in tau phosphorylation at the AT8 epitope were also present at 1 h, 4 h and 8 h when not corrected to total tau levels [Ctrl vs. 1 h post-status epilepticus: 2.954 ± 0.6304 (mean ± SEM), $p = 0.01$; Ctrl vs. 4 h post-status epilepticus: 3.111 ± 0.3991 (mean ± SEM), $p = 0.008$; Ctrl vs. 8 h: 3.401 ± 0.4129 (mean ± SEM), $p = 0.003$; ANOVA *post hoc* Fisher's test; **Supplementary Figure S1B**]. Western blots using the phospho-tau antibody PHF-1 revealed no significant increase when normalized to total tau levels (**Figure 1E**). PHF-1 was, however, increased at 4 h post-status epilepticus when not corrected to Tau-1 [Ctrl vs. 4 h: 2.261 ± 0.6531 (mean ± SEM), $p = 0.04$; ANOVA with Fisher's *post hoc* test; **Supplementary Figure S1B**].

Thus, intra-amygdala KA-induced status epilepticus leads to an increase in total tau levels and in tau phosphorylation in the hippocampus.

Subfield-Specific Tau Phosphorylation in the Hippocampus Post-Status Epilepticus

With AT8 showing the strongest increase in tau phosphorylation post-status epilepticus, we next sought to identify the localization of AT8 phospho-tau following status epilepticus using immunological staining of hippocampal tissue sections.

DAB immunostaining for AT8 4 h post-status epilepticus revealed a loss of phosphorylated tau within the stratum pyramidal and lucidum region of CA3 and an apparent increase in the mossy fibers (**Figure 2A**). Loss of AT8 immunoreactivity in the CA3 subfield was confirmed using co-immunostainings with the neuronal marker NeuN. Double immunofluorescence using antibodies recognizing AT8 phospho-tau and the synaptic and mossy fibers localized protein Zinc Transporter 3 (Znt3; Wenzel et al., 1997) confirmed co-localization of AT8 with mossy fibers (**Figures 2B,C**). Interestingly, AT8 immunoreactivity of hilar interneurons seemed to disappear post-status epilepticus (**Figure 2C**).

Next, we analyzed tau expression and phosphorylation post-status epilepticus within each hippocampal subfield (dentate gyrus, CA1 and CA3) separately *via* Western blotting. This revealed that total tau levels were increased at 8 h and 24 h in the dentate gyrus following status epilepticus [Ctrl vs. 8 h, 1.904 ± 0.4338 (mean ± SEM), $p = 0.045$; Ctrl vs. 24 h, 2.424 ± 0.3041 (mean ± SEM), $p = 0.005$; ANOVA *post hoc* Fischer's test; **Figure 3A**]. No changes occurred in CA1 (**Figure 3B**). In CA3, tau levels were found to be slightly decreased shortly following status epilepticus at 1 h [Ctrl vs. 1 h, 0.7211 ± 0.0731 (mean ± SEM), $p = 0.037$; ANOVA *post hoc*

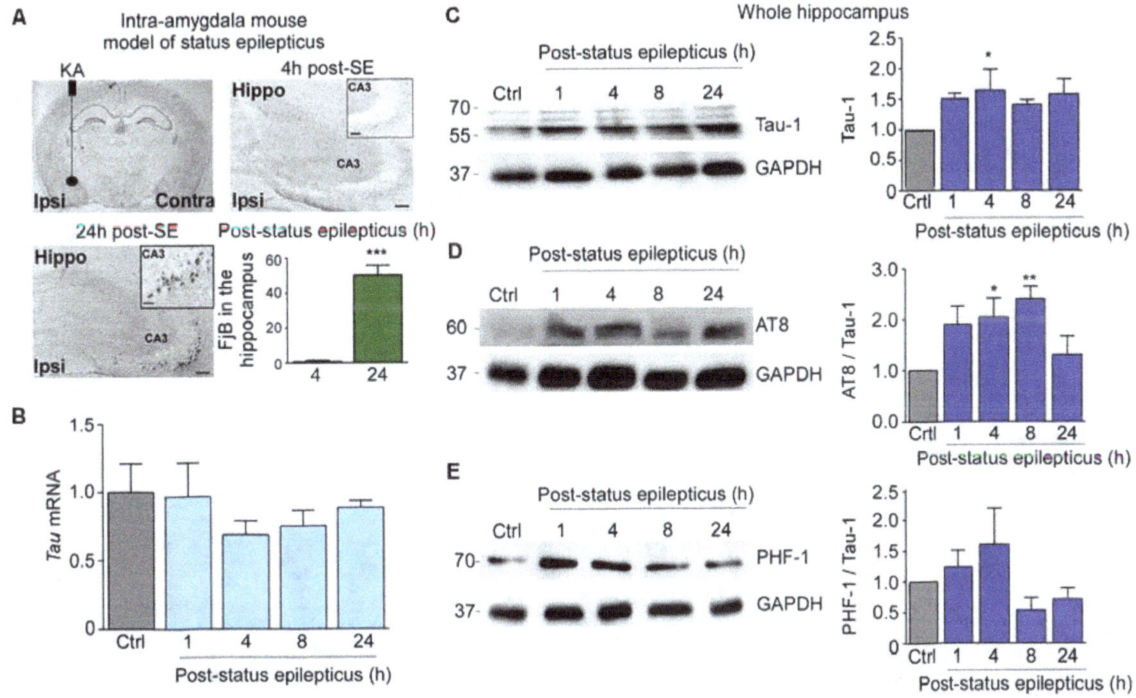

FIGURE 1 | Tau protein expression and tau phosphorylation in the hippocampus post-status epilepticus. **(A)** Illustration of intra-amygdala injection of Kainic acid (KA) in mice for the induction of status epilepticus and chronic epilepsy. Flouro-jade B (FjB) staining shows neurodegeneration in the ipsilateral hippocampus at 24 h post-KA injection. Note: absence of FjB-positive cells at 4 h post status epilepticus ($n = 4$ per group). FjB-positive cells are mainly localized to the ipsilateral CA3 subfield of the hippocampus. Scale bar = 200 μm. **(B)** *Tau* mRNA levels quantified by RT-qPCR showing no changes between control and post-status epilepticus ($n = 4$ per group). **(C–E)** Representative Western blot ($n = 1$/lane) and corresponding graphs showing an increase in total tau (Tau-1; Ctrl vs. 4 h, $p = 0.03$), AT8/Tau-1 (Ctrl vs. 4 h, $p = 0.03$; Ctrl vs. 8 h, $p = 0.005$) and PHF-1/Tau-1 protein levels in the ipsilateral hippocampus post-status epilepticus. GAPDH is shown as a loading control ($n = 4$ per group). One-way ANOVA with Fisher's *post hoc* test. Data are presented as mean ± standard error of the mean (SEM). $^*p < 0.05$, $^{**}p < 0.01$, $^{***}p < 0.001$.

Fisher's test; **Figure 3C**]. When normalized to total tau levels, the only statistically significant increase in tau phosphorylation on the AT8 epitope was at 1 h post-status epilepticus in the CA1 and CA3 hippocampal subfields, while no significant changes were present in the dentate gyrus [CA1 Ctrl vs. 1 h, 3.1 ± 0.79 (mean ± SEM), $p = 0.008$; CA3 Ctrl vs. 1 h, 1.756 ± 0.1471 (mean ± SEM), $p = 0.016$; ANOVA *post hoc* Fisher's test; **Figures 3A–C**]. AT8-dependent tau phosphorylation levels seemed then to progressively decreased in all subfields at each time point thereafter reaching significance at 4 h post-status epilepticus in the CA3 subfield [Ctrl vs. 4 h post-status epilepticus, 0.3496 ± 0.1625 (mean ± SEM), $p = 0.033$; ANOVA *post hoc* Fisher's test; **Figures 3A–C**]. A similar trend was observed when normalizing to the loading control GAPDH (**Supplementary Figure S1C**).

We have previously identified a functional involvement for GSK-3β, one of the main kinases targeting tau, during seizure generation and seizure-induced cell death in the intra-amygdala KA mouse model (Engel et al., 2018). To test whether GSK-3β contributes to tau phosphorylation during status epilepticus, mice were pre-treated with the GSK-3 inhibitor NP12 prior to the induction of status epilepticus. The inhibition of GSK-3 had no significant effect on the level of phosphorylation at the AT8 and PHF-1 epitope in the whole hippocampus indicating that GSK-3β alone may not be the primary driver of phosphorylation of tau during status epilepticus (**Supplementary Figure S2A**). In addition, the effect of the GSK-3 inhibitor NP12 was examined in the CA3 subfield of the hippocampus. Again, no changes in tau-phosphorylation could be observed (**Supplementary Figure S2B**).

In summary, tau expression and tau phosphorylation increases following intra-amygdala KA-induced status epilepticus in the hippocampus, with tau expression changes most evident in the dentate gyrus and CA3 and tau phosphorylation most evident in the CA1 and CA3 subfields.

Decreased Tau Levels and Increased Tau Phosphorylation in the Hippocampus of Mice During Epilepsy

To test whether tau phosphorylation is also increased during epilepsy, hippocampal tissue was analyzed using the same tau phosphorylation-recognizing antibodies as before in brain tissue of mice killed at 14 days post-intra-amygdala KA-induced status epilepticus, time-point when all mice have usually experienced at least 1 week of chronic epilepsy (Mouri et al., 2008;

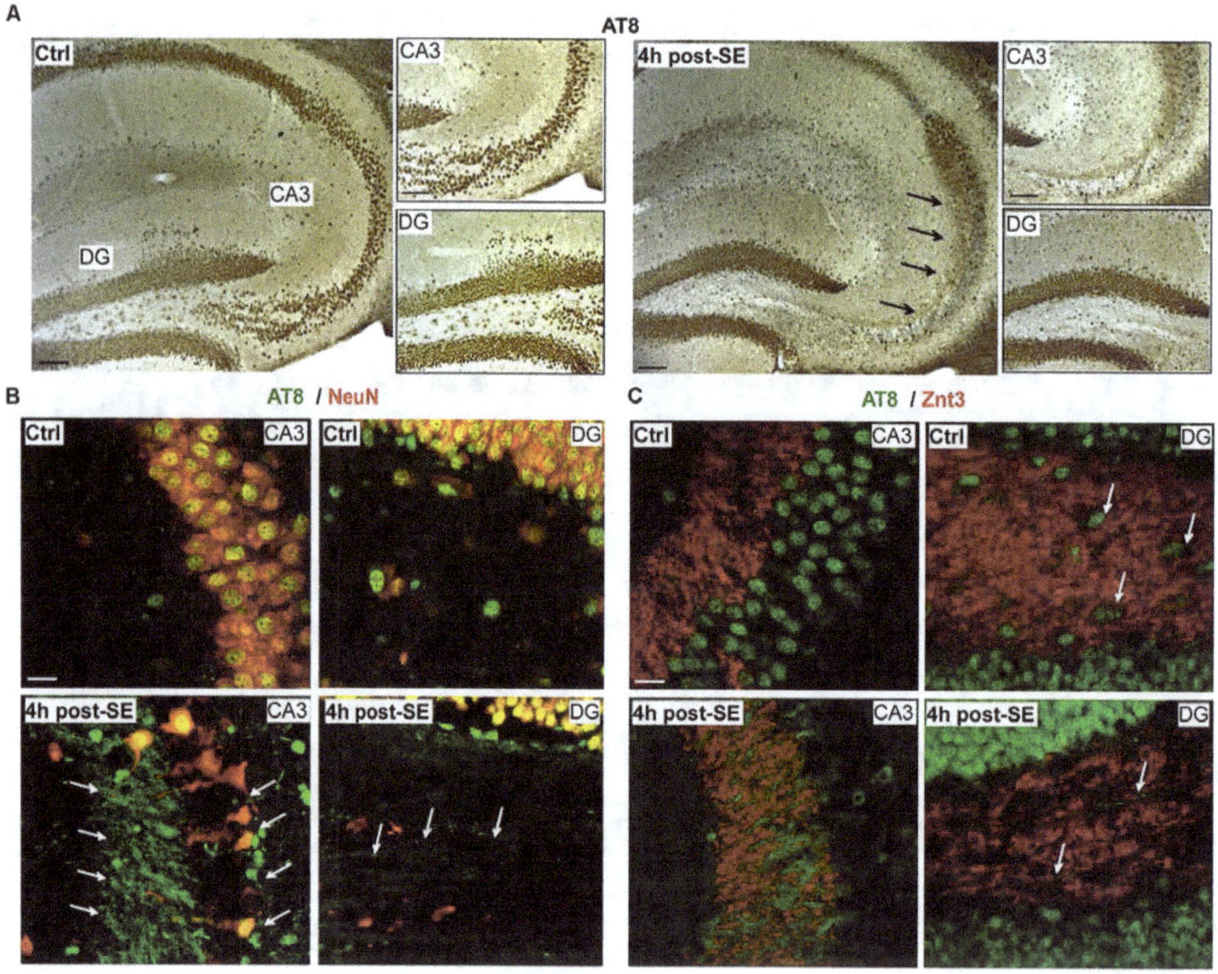

FIGURE 2 | Localization of tau phosphorylation in the hippocampus following status epilepticus. **(A)** Representative 3,3′-Diaminobenzidine (DAB) staining (from a total of three different mice) showing loss of AT8 phospho-tau in the stratum pyramidal and lucidum region (CA3). In contrast, AT8-positive tau was increased in mossy fibers 4 h post-status epilepticus. Arrows indicate AT8 phospho-tau localization to mossy fibers. Scale bar = 50 μm. **(B,C)** Representative photomicrographs (from a total of three different mice) showing AT8-positive phospho-tau co-localized with the neuronal marker NeuN under physiological conditions and 4 h post-status epilepticus. Co-localization of AT8 with the Zinc Transporter 3 (Znt-3) confirmed the presence of AT8-positive phospho-tau on mossy fibers in the CA3 subfield and the hilus. Of note, decreased AT8 immunoreactivity in hilar interneurons post-status epilepticus (green = AT8, red = NeuN or Znt-3). Scale bar = 25 μm.

Jimenez-Mateos et al., 2012; Engel et al., 2013; Jimenez-Pacheco et al., 2016). Western blotting using whole hippocampal extracts revealed, in contrast to our findings during status epilepticus, no changes in total tau expression compared to controls (**Figure 4A**). While AT8 phospho-tau was significantly increased in the hippocampus of epileptic mice [Ctrl vs. Epi, 3.315 ± 0.7054 (mean ± SEM), $p = 0.004$; *t*-test], PHF-1-positive phospho-tau showed no changes (**Figure 4A**). Tau phosphorylation at the AT8 epitope was also significantly higher in epileptic mice without correction for total tau [Ctrl vs. Epi, 2.860 ± 0.4957 (mean ± SEM), $p = 0.002$; *t*-test], while PHF-1 showed no significant changes (**Supplementary Figure S3A**).

As before for status epilepticus, we then analyzed tau expression and phosphorylation for each hippocampal subfield separately. While there was no obvious change in tau expression in the dentate gyrus, tau levels were significantly decreased in CA1 and CA3 [Ctrl vs. Epi: CA1, 0.5713 ± 0.06162 (mean ± SEM), $p = 0.0008$; CA3, 0.7537 ± 0.05271 (mean ± SEM), $p = 0.027$; *t*-test; **Figure 4B**]. In contrast, tau phosphorylation in AT8 was increased in CA1 and CA3, while no changes were observed in the dentate gyrus [Ctrl vs. Epi: CA1, 1.735 ± 0.1525 (mean ± SEM), $p = 0.014$; CA3: 2.452 ± 0.3394 (mean ± SEM), $p = 0.0073$; *t*-test; **Figure 4B**]. Without correction for total-tau levels, only the CA3 subfield showed significant differences in AT8 phosphorylation [*t*-test, 1.850 ± 0.3097 (mean ± SEM), $p = 0.038$)], while CA1 showed no changes (**Supplementary Figure S3B**).

In summary, while tau phosphorylation remained elevated during epilepsy at the AT8 epitope, total tau expression was reduced in the CA3 and CA1 subfield of the hippocampus.

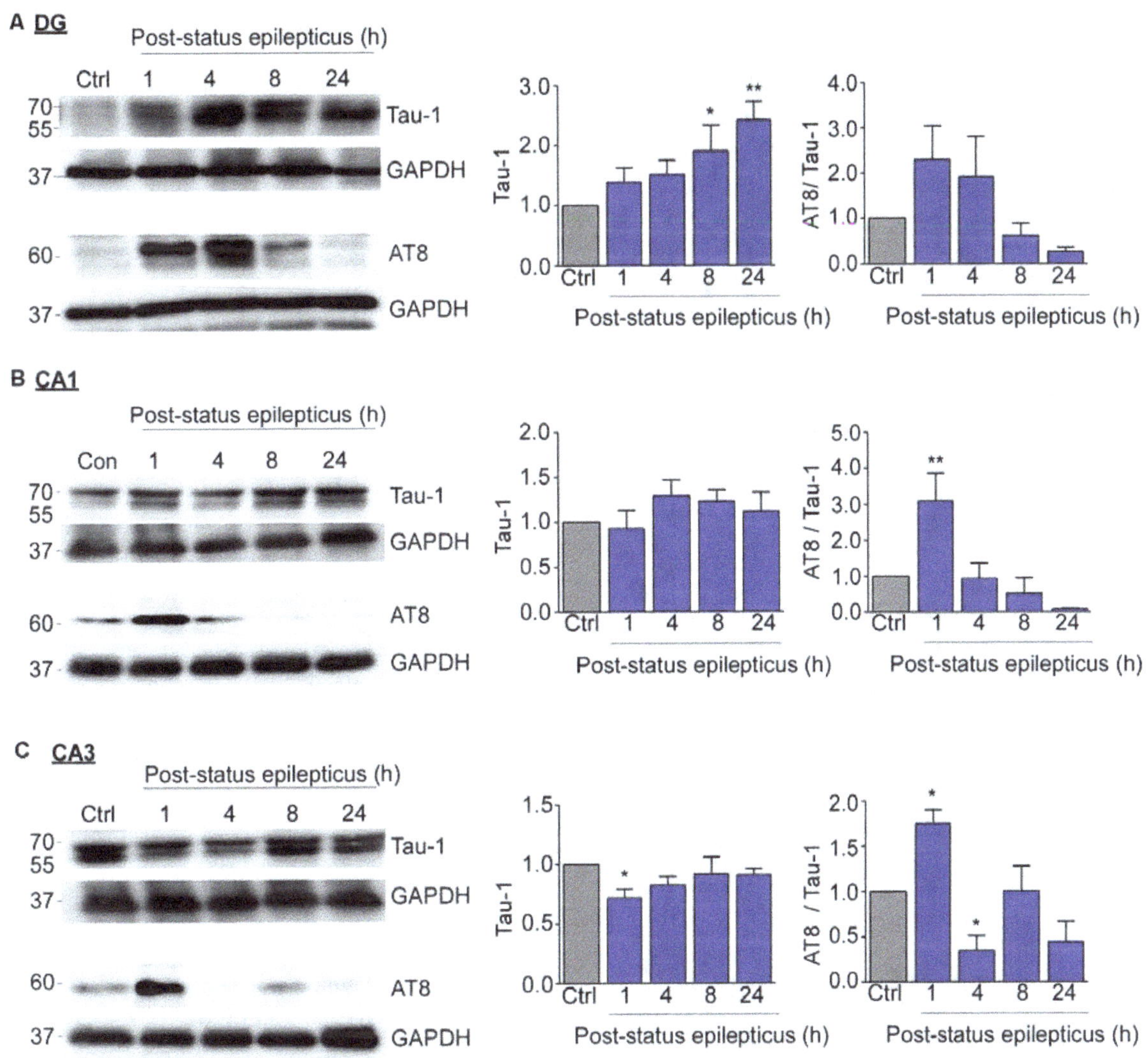

FIGURE 3 | Subfield-specific tau phosphorylation in the hippocampus following status epilepticus. **(A)** Representative Western blots (n = 1/lane) and corresponding graphs showing an increase in total tau levels at 8 h and 24 h post-status epilepticus in the dentate gyrus (Tau-1: Ctrl vs. 8 h, $p = 0.045$; Ctrl vs. 24 h, $p = 0.005$). No significant changes were found in AT8 phosphorylation in the dentate gyrus post-status epilepticus when normalized to Tau-1. **(B)** No changes in tau expression occurred in CA1 and, in CA3 **(C)**, tau levels were found to be slightly decreased 1 h following status epilepticus (Ctrl vs. 8 h, $p = 0.037$). When normalized to total tau levels, AT8 phosphorylated tau protein levels were increase at 1 h post-status epilepticus in the CA1 (AT8/Tau: Ctrl vs. 1 h, $p = 0.008$) and CA3 (AT8/Tau: Ctrl vs. 1 h, $p = 0.016$; Ctrl vs. 4 h, $p = 0.033$) hippocampal subfields. One-way ANOVA with Fisher's *post hoc* test. Data are presented as mean ± SEM. *$p < 0.05$, **$p < 0.01$.

Localization of AT8 Positive Phospho-Tau During Epilepsy

To determine in what cell types in the hippocampus phosphorylated tau was localized, immunostaining was carried out as before using the AT8 antibody, which showed the greatest change during epilepsy. In contrast to our results from post-status epilepticus tissue sections, AT8 phospho-tau localization to the mossy fibers was absent in the hippocampus of epileptic mice (**Figure 5A**). AT8-positive staining could, however, be observed throughout the entire hippocampus including all hippocampal subfields with an apparent glial-shaped appearance (**Figure 5A**). To establish which cell types express AT8-positive tau in the hippocampus, double immunofluorescence staining was carried out using the cell type-specific markers Iba-1 for microglia, GFAP for astrocytes and NeuN for neurons. This revealed that, AT8, as shown *via* DAB staining, was not detected in the mossy fibers (**Figure 5B**). While AT8-positive tau strongly co-localized with the microglia marker Iba-1 in all hippocampal subfields (**Figure 5C, Supplementary Figures S4A–C**), no co-localization was observed between AT8 and the astrocyte marker GFAP (**Figure 5D, Supplementary Figures S4A–C**).

Taken together, our results show that tau alterations persist within the epileptic state, however, suggest that the pattern of

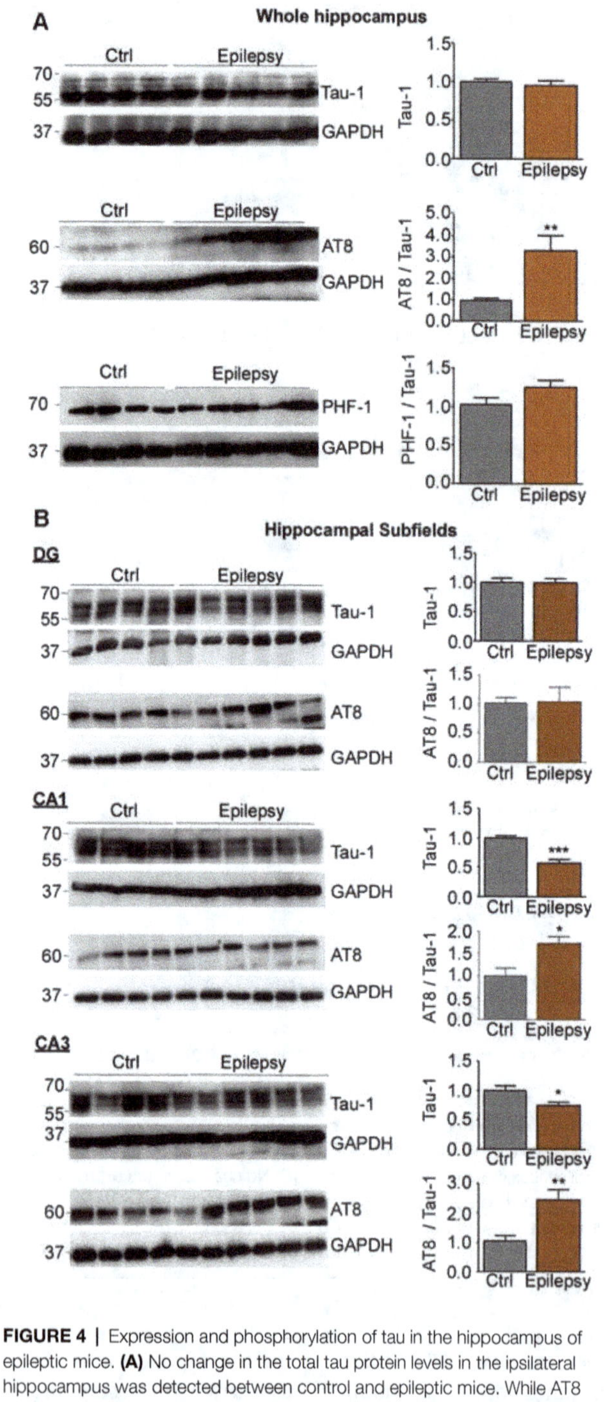

FIGURE 4 | Expression and phosphorylation of tau in the hippocampus of epileptic mice. **(A)** No change in the total tau protein levels in the ipsilateral hippocampus was detected between control and epileptic mice. While AT8 phospho-tau was significantly increased in the hippocampus of epileptic mice ($p = 0.004$), no change was observed for PHF-1-positive phospho-tau. **(B)** Representative Western blots and corresponding graphs showing no obvious change in tau expression in the dentate gyrus of epileptic mice. Tau levels were, however, significantly decreased in CA1 and CA3 in epileptic mice (CA1: Ctrl vs. Epilepsy, $p = 0.0008$; CA3: Ctrl vs. Epilepsy, $p = 0.027$). When normalized to total tau, tau phosphorylation in AT8 was increased in CA1 and CA3, while no changes were observed in the dentate gyrus (CA1: Ctrl vs. Epilepsy, $p = 0.014$; CA3: Ctrl vs. Epilepsy, $p = 0.0073$). GAPDH is shown as a loading control [CA1: $n = 4$ (Ctrl) and $n = 6$ (Epilepsy); CA3 and DG: $n = 5$ (Ctrl) and $n = 6$ (Epilepsy), unpaired Student's t-test. Data are presented as mean ± SEM]. $^{*}p < 0.05$, $^{**}p < 0.01$, $^{***}p < 0.001$.

abnormal tau phosphorylation during epilepsy is distinct from status epilepticus.

DISCUSSION

In the present study, we confirm and further elaborate on the effects of status epilepticus and epilepsy on the phosphorylation of tau in the hippocampus. We identify significant differences in the pattern of tau phosphorylation on specific epitopes between status epilepticus and chronic epilepsy with distinct localization of phosphorylated tau in epileptic mice compared to post-status epilepticus. The identification of a pattern of tau pathology in epilepsy distinct from status epilepticus could aid in elucidating the pathways by which seizure activity may drive neurodegeneration in epilepsies (Tai et al., 2016).

The phosphorylation of tau post-seizure activity has previously been described in models of intraperitoneal delivered KA-induced status epilepticus with the results of these studies being largely reproduced in our study in addition to the identification of a distinct tau phosphorylation pattern during epilepsy (Crespo-Biel et al., 2007; Liang et al., 2009). These mechanisms of tau phosphorylation have been given little attention as regards to epileptic disorders but could be central to explaining the high incidence of Alzheimer's disease in epilepsy patients (Téllez-Zenteno et al., 2005).

In our model, we detected an increase in protein levels of tau, which was not previously observed in other KA seizure models. Notably, the increase in tau protein levels did not correspond to any significant change in *tau* mRNA, indicating that the observed increase is not due to an increase in transcription and with no increase in total-tau present at 14 days it is likely a short-lived effect. Why tau was increased in the dentate gyrus and decreased in CA3 we do not know. A possible explanation is the inhibition of the ubiquitin-proteasome system (UPS) following status epilepticus. We have previously shown status epilepticus-induced inhibition of the UPS mainly to occur in the dentate gyrus, while proteasome activity has been shown to be slightly increased in the CA3 subfield of the hippocampus post-status epilepticus (Engel et al., 2017).

The subfield-specific changes in tau phosphorylation are possibly a result of the subfield-specific difference in kinase/phosphatase activity which may be dynamically altered in response to seizure activity which has similarly been described in other models (Liang et al., 2009). In line with this, we have previously shown that there are subfield-specific differences in GSK-3β activity following intraamygdala KA-induced status epilepticus (Engel et al., 2018). The reason for the observed early increase followed by a strong decrease in tau phosphorylation in CA3 post-status epilepticus remains elusive. The cell death-prone CA3 subfield seems to be, however, particularly susceptible to seizures in the intra-amygdala KA mouse model potentially leading to the activation of distinct intracellular signaling cascades during seizures when compared to the from cell death protected CA1 and dentate gyrus. Interestingly, previous studies have shown that the enhancement of tau phosphatase PP2A activity through the treatment with the PP2A activator sodium selenate to be an effective anti-epileptic treatment which further

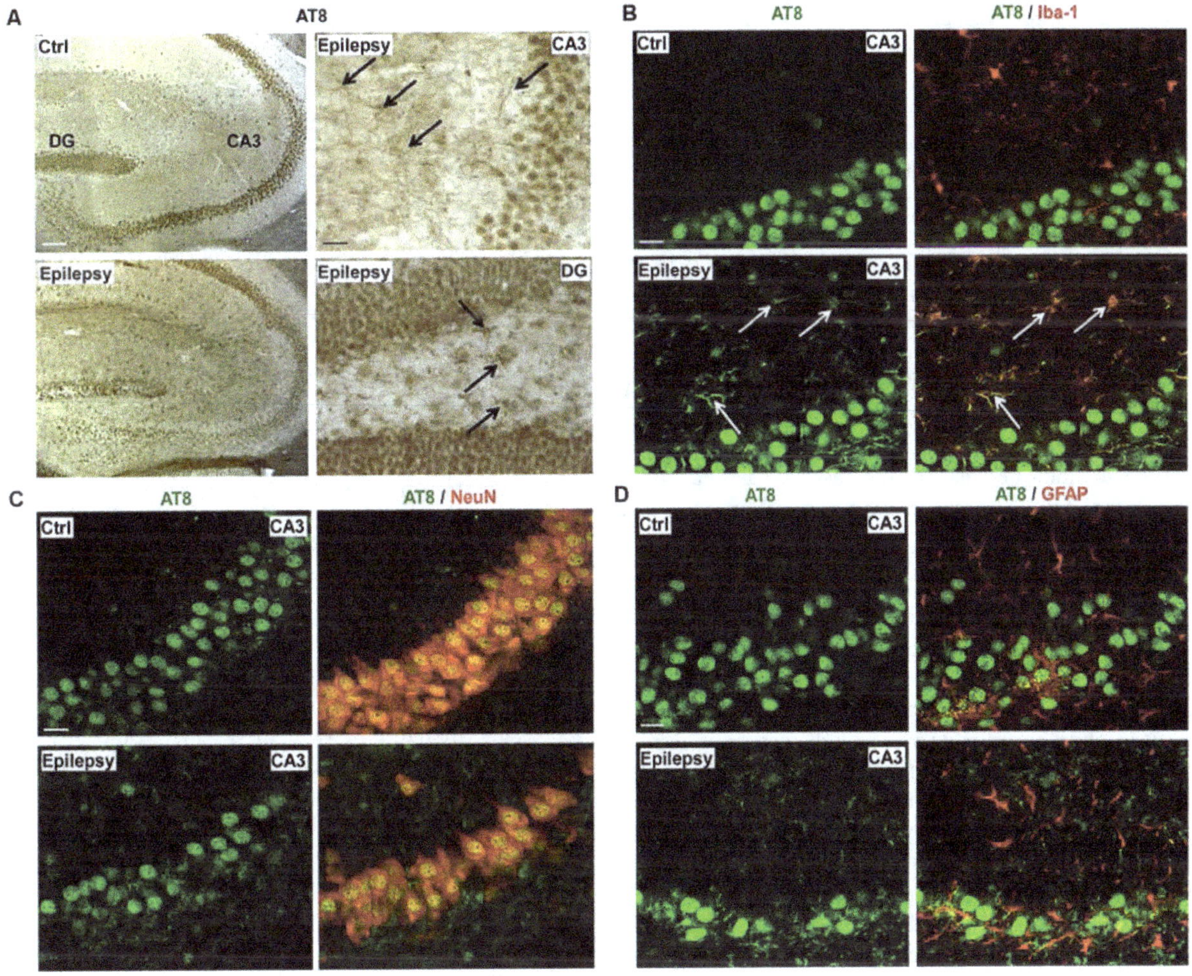

FIGURE 5 | Microglial localization of phospho-tau in the hippocampus of epileptic mice. **(A)** Representative photomicrographs of DAB staining (from a total of three different mice) for AT8 phospho-tau in control and epileptic mice showing the presence of AT8-phospho-tau throughout the entire hippocampus, with an apparent glial-shaped appearance. AT8-positive cells are indicated by black arrows. Scale bar = 200 μm. **(B)** Representative photomicrographs (from a total of three different mice) showing co-localization of AT8 phospho-tau with Iba1-positive microglia marker in the CA3 subfield (indicated by white arrows) during chronic epilepsy. Scale bar = 25 μm. **(C)** NeuN co-staining with AT8 phospho-tau in neurons from the CA3 subfield in epileptic mice. Scale bar = 25 μm. **(D)** Lack of co-localization between astrocyte marker GFAP and AT8 phospho-tau. Scale bar = 25 μm.

illustrates the dynamic relationship of tau and epileptiform activity and could present a novel therapeutic avenue for potentially protecting against seizures and the development of tau pathology (Jones et al., 2012). It must also be acknowledged that epilepsy and seizure activity have been repeatedly shown to have dramatic effects on post-transcriptional regulation *via* microRNAs, which could be implicated in the changes in tau expression observed in this study with various microRNAs altered in epilepsy models also known to target tau (Jimenez-Mateos and Henshall, 2013; Santa-Maria et al., 2015; Zheng et al., 2016). Cell death in the CA3 and hilus that occurs post-status epilepticus may also affect the levels of phospho-tau reducing the tau-containing cells and thus AT8-phosphorylated tau (Fuster-Matanzo et al., 2012). Status epilepticus stimulates sprouting of mossy fibers from the granule cell layer and interestingly, we observed AT8 phospho-tau co-localizing to the mossy fibers possibly contributing to sprouting observed during epileptogenesis (Parent et al., 1997).

Tau phosphorylation at 1–24 h time-points post-status epilepticus was most prominent on serine/threonine 202/205 (AT8) compared to serine 396/404 (PHF-1) with only AT8 phospho-tau increased in epileptic mice at 14 days. AT8 phosphorylation is the standard immunostaining utilized for the assessment of neurofibrillary tangle (NFT) formation and tau aggregation for Braak stage scoring and Alzheimer's Disease progressions, with a very strong correlation with cognitive decline in preclinical Alzheimer's Disease (Braak et al., 2006; Huber et al., 2018). The phosphorylation at Ser202/Thr205 (AT8) is associated with pre-tangle formation stage and among the earliest sites to be aberrantly phosphorylated in Alzheimer's Disease and is known to induce a toxic gain-of-function (Su et al., 1994; Luna-Muñoz et al., 2007;

Kanaan et al., 2011). AT8 phospho-tau aggregates were also identified in the hippocampus and cortex of TLE patients and correlated with cognitive decline (Tai et al., 2016). The lack of phosphorylation in PHF-1 (Ser-396/404) compared to AT8 (Ser202/Thr205) epitopes is interesting with regard to the activity of specific kinases on these sites as while GSK-3β and CDK5 both phosphorylate these epitopes, CDK5 acts on Ser-202 to a far greater extent with GSK-3β more prominently targeting Ser-396 (Cavallini et al., 2013). We had previously investigated the importance of GSK-3β during seizures through inhibition with NP12 and when investigated with regard to its effect on tau phosphorylation the lack of any significant effect in ameliorating the hyperphosphorylation of tau post-status suggests that the phosphorylation of tau occurs independently of GSK-3β. In addition, the lack of PHF-1 phosphorylation at 24 h and at 14 days, while AT8 phosphorylation remains elevated, could indicate that CDK5 activity has a more influential effect on the continued phosphorylation of tau in epileptic mice.

In contrast to status epilepticus, during epilepsy tau expression was not increased in the dentate gyrus, but reduced in the hippocampal subfields CA3 and CA1. Again, it is tempting to speculate that this is likely a protective response to potentially toxic levels of phosphorylated tau in the cells occurring during seizures. Another novel observation during the study was the presence of phosphorylated tau in microglia during chronic epilepsy. Tau is not natively expressed in microglia and its presence is most likely due to active microglia internalizing extracellular tau as has been previously described *in vitro* and *in vivo* using transgenic models of tauopathy (Luo et al., 2015; Bolós et al., 2016). Internalization of extracellular tau by microglia is thought to be protective, accelerating the clearance of toxic forms of tau in diseased brains although the activation of microglia is implicated in several pathways of epileptogenesis as well as driving the spread of tau pathology (Maphis et al., 2015). Extracellular tau is typically attributed to cell death but with no obvious cell death occurring during chronic epilepsy in our model, this is unlikely to be the primary contributor (Moran et al., 2013). One mechanism of extracellular tau release which could have a significant influence on tau present in epileptic mice is the neuronal excitation stimulated tau release described by Pooler et al. (2013) which could potentially result in a large release of tau through the aberrant excitation in the model. It must be noted that this mechanism has never been evaluated in response to seizures or experimental epilepsy and would require further investigation to confirm but could reveal an important mechanism in the development of tau pathology in epilepsies. These changes in tau phosphorylation in epileptic mice observed in this study have not been previously reported, which is possibly due to previous investigations being limited to status epilepticus without a confirmed epileptic state. To fully elucidate the impact of tau phosphorylation in epileptic mice further studies with longer periods of experimental epilepsy in mice would likely be required as even within tau overexpressing mouse models, tau pathology seeding takes over 1 month to onset (Holmes et al., 2014).

The aberrant tau hyperphosphorylation occurring in epileptic mice presents a convergence of numerous mechanisms that could have significant implications with epilepsies as well as Alzheimer's Disease. These findings point to experimental epilepsy models examined over a longer period of time to replicate the potential mechanisms of tau hyperphosphorylation and aggregation which have been observed in TLE patients. The intra-amygdala KA mouse model of status epilepticus represents, therefore, a valid model that could be utilized to further elucidate developing treatments against the propagation of hyperphosphorylated tau occurring in TLE patients.

ETHICS STATEMENT

The animal study was reviewed and approved by Research Ethics Committee of the Royal College of Surgeons in Ireland.

AUTHOR CONTRIBUTIONS

MA carried out Western blotting, PCRs, immunostainings and analyzed the data. AK analyzed the data and wrote parts of the manuscript. GL performed immunostainings. EB carried out experiments with GSK-3 inhibitors. TE wrote the manuscript.

REFERENCES

Angulo, S. L., Orman, R., Neymotin, S. A., Liu, L., Buitrago, L., Cepeda-Prado, E., et al. (2017). Tau and amyloid-related pathologies in the entorhinal cortex have divergent effects in the hippocampal circuit. *Neurobiol. Dis.* 108, 261–276. doi: 10.1016/j.nbd.2017.08.015

Bolós, M., Llorens-Martín, M., Jurado-Arjona, J., Hernández, F., Rábano, A., and Avila, J. (2016). Direct evidence of internalization of tau by microglia *in vitro* and *in vivo*. *J. Alzheimers Dis.* 50, 77–87. doi: 10.3233/jad-150704

Braak, H., Alafuzoff, I., Arzberger, T., Kretzschmar, H., and Del Tredici, K. (2006). Staging of Alzheimer disease-associated neurofibrillary pathology using paraffin sections and immunocytochemistry. *Acta Neuropathol.* 112, 389–404. doi: 10.1007/s00401-006-0127-z

Brennan, G. P., Jimenez-Mateos, E. M., Mckiernan, R. C., Engel, T., Tzivion, G., and Henshall, D. C. (2013). Transgenic overexpression of 14-3-3 zeta protects hippocampus against endoplasmic reticulum stress and status epilepticus *in vivo*. *PLoS One* 8:e54491. doi: 10.1371/journal.pone.0054491

Busche, M. A., Wegmann, S., Dujardin, S., Commins, C., Schiantarelli, J., Klickstein, N., et al. (2019). Tau impairs neural circuits, dominating amyloid-β effects, in Alzheimer models *in vivo*. *Nat. Neurosci.* 22, 57–64. doi: 10.1038/s41593-018-0289-8

Cavallini, A., Brewerton, S., Bell, A., Sargent, S., Glover, S., Hardy, C., et al. (2013). An unbiased approach to identifying tau kinases that phosphorylate tau at sites associated with Alzheimer disease. *J. Biol. Chem.* 288, 23331–23347. doi: 10.1074/jbc.m113.463984

Cisbani, G., Maxan, A., Kordower, J. H., Planel, E., Freeman, T. B., and Cicchetti, F. (2017). Presence of tau pathology within foetal neural allografts in patients with Huntington's and Parkinson's disease. *Brain* 140, 2982–2992. doi: 10.1093/brain/awx255

Crespo-Biel, N., Canudas, A. M., Camins, A., and Pallas, M. (2007). Kainate induces AKT, ERK and cdk5/GSK3β pathway deregulation, phosphorylates tau protein in mouse hippocampus. *Neurochem. Int.* 50, 435–442. doi: 10.1016/j.neuint.2006.10.002

Domínguez, J. M., Fuertes, A., Orozco, L., del Monte-Millán, M., Delgado, E., and Medina, M. (2012). Evidence for irreversible inhibition of glycogen synthase kinase-3β by tideglusib. *J. Biol. Chem.* 287, 893–904. doi: 10.1074/jbc.M111.306472

Engel, T., Gómez-Sintes, R., Alves, M., Jimenez-Mateos, E. M., Fernández-Nogales, M., Sanz-Rodriguez, A., et al. (2018). Bi-directional genetic modulation of GSK-3β exacerbates hippocampal neuropathology in experimental status epilepticus. *Cell Death Dis.* 9:969. doi: 10.1038/s41419-018-0963-5

Engel, T., Hernandez, F., Avila, J., and Lucas, J. J. (2006). Full reversal of Alzheimer's disease-like phenotype in a mouse model with conditional overexpression of glycogen synthase kinase-3. *J. Neurosci.* 26, 5083–5090. doi: 10.1523/JNEUROSCI.0604-06.2006

Engel, T., Martinez-Villarreal, J., Henke, C., Jimenez-Mateos, E. M., Sanz-Rodriguez, A., Alves, M., et al. (2017). Spatiotemporal progression of ubiquitin-proteasome system inhibition after status epilepticus suggests protective adaptation against hippocampal injury. *Mol. Neurodegener.* 12:21. doi: 10.1186/s13024-017-0163-2

Engel, T., Sanz-Rodgriguez, A., Jimenez-Mateos, E. M., Concannon, C. G., Jimenez-Pacheco, A., Moran, C., et al. (2013). CHOP regulates the p53-MDM2 axis and is required for neuronal survival after seizures. *Brain* 136, 577–592. doi: 10.1093/brain/aws337

Feinstein, S. C., and Wilson, L. (2005). Inability of tau to properly regulate neuronal microtubule dynamics: a loss-of-function mechanism by which tau might mediate neuronal cell death. *Biochim. Biophys. Acta* 1739, 268–279. doi: 10.1016/j.bbadis.2004.07.002

Fernández-Nogales, M., Cabrera, J. R., Santos-Galindo, M., Hoozemans, J. J., Ferrer, I., Rozemuller, A. J., et al. (2014). Huntington's disease is a four-repeat tauopathy with tau nuclear rods. *Nat. Med.* 20, 881–885. doi: 10.1038/nm.3617

Fuster-Matanzo, A., Llorens-Martín, M., Jurado-Arjona, J., Avila, J., and Hernández, F. (2012). Tau protein and adult hippocampal neurogenesis. *Front. Neurosci.* 6, 104–104. doi: 10.3389/fnins.2012.00104

Gangarossa, G., Sakkaki, S., Lory, P., and Valjent, E. (2015). Mouse hippocampal phosphorylation footprint induced by generalized seizures: focus on ERK, mTORC1 and Akt/GSK-3 pathways. *Neuroscience* 311, 474–483. doi: 10.1016/j.neuroscience.2015.10.051

García-Cabrero, A. M., Guerrero-López, R., Giráldez, B. G., Llorens-Martán, M., Avila, J., Serratosa, J. M., et al. (2013). Hyperexcitability and epileptic seizures in a model of frontotemporal dementia. *Neurobiol. Dis.* 58, 200–208. doi: 10.1016/j.nbd.2013.06.005

Goedert, M., Jakes, R., and Vanmechelen, E. (1995). Monoclonal antibody AT8 recognises tau protein phosphorylated at both serine 202 and threonine 205. *Neurosci. Lett.* 189, 167–169. doi: 10.1016/0304-3940(95)11484-e

Götz, J., Halliday, G., and Nisbet, R. M. (2019). Molecular pathogenesis of the tauopathies. *Annu. Rev. Pathol.* 14, 239–261. doi: 10.1146/annurev-pathmechdis-012418-012936

Henshall, D. C., Sinclair, J., and Simon, R. P. (2000). Spatio-temporal profile of DNA fragmentation and its relationship to patterns of epileptiform activity following focally evoked limbic seizures. *Brain Res.* 858, 290–302. doi: 10.1016/s0006-8993(99)02452-x

Holmes, B. B., Furman, J. L., Mahan, T. E., Yamasaki, T. R., Mirbaha, H., Eades, W. C., et al. (2014). Proteopathic tau seeding predicts tauopathy *in vivo*. *Proc. Natl. Acad. Sci. U S A* 111, E4376–E4385. doi: 10.1073/pnas.1411649111

Holth, J. K., Bomben, V. C., Reed, J. G., Inoue, T., Younkin, L., Younkin, S. G., et al. (2013). Tau loss attenuates neuronal network hyperexcitability in mouse and Drosophila genetic models of epilepsy. *J. Neurosci.* 33, 1651–1659. doi: 10.1523/JNEUROSCI.3191-12.2013

Hoover, B. R., Reed, M. N., Su, J., Penrod, R. D., Kotilinek, L. A., Grant, M. K., et al. (2010). Tau mislocalization to dendritic spines mediates synaptic dysfunction independently of neurodegeneration. *Neuron* 68, 1067–1081. doi: 10.1016/j.neuron.2010.11.030

Huber, C. M., Yee, C., May, T., Dhanala, A., and Mitchell, C. S. (2018). Cognitive decline in preclinical Alzheimer's disease: amyloid-β versus tauopathy. *J. Alzheimers Dis.* 61, 265–281. doi: 10.3233/jad-170490

Janning, D., Igaev, M., Sündermann, F., Brühmann, J., Beutel, O., Heinisch, J. J., et al. (2014). Single-molecule tracking of tau reveals fast kiss-and-hop interaction with microtubules in living neurons. *Mol. Biol. Cell* 25, 3541–3551. doi: 10.1091/mbc.e14-06-1099

Jimenez-Mateos, E. M., Arribas-Blazquez, M., Sanz-Rodriguez, A., Concannon, C., Olivos-Ore, L. A., Reschke, C. R., et al. (2015). microRNA targeting of the P2X7 purinoceptor opposes a contralateral epileptogenic focus in the hippocampus. *Sci. Rep.* 5:17486. doi: 10.1038/srep17486

Jimenez-Mateos, E. M., Engel, T., Merino-Serrais, P., Mckiernan, R. C., Tanaka, K., Mouri, G., et al. (2012). Silencing microRNA-134 produces neuroprotective and prolonged seizure-suppressive effects. *Nat. Med.* 18, 1087–1094. doi: 10.1038/nm.2834

Jimenez-Mateos, E. M., and Henshall, D. C. (2013). Epilepsy and microRNA. *Neuroscience* 238, 218–229. doi: 10.1016/j.neuroscience.2013.02.027

Jimenez-Pacheco, A., Diaz-Hernandez, M., Arribas-Blazquez, M., Sanz-Rodriguez, A., Olivos-Ore, L. A., Artalejo, A. R., et al. (2016). Transient P2X7 receptor antagonism produces lasting reductions in spontaneous seizures and gliosis in experimental temporal lobe epilepsy. *J. Neurosci.* 36, 5920–5932. doi: 10.1523/jneurosci.4009-15.2016

Jones, N. C., Nguyen, T., Corcoran, N. M., Velakoulis, D., Chen, T., Grundy, R., et al. (2012). Targeting hyperphosphorylated tau with sodium selenate suppresses seizures in rodent models. *Neurobiol. Dis.* 45, 897–901. doi: 10.1016/j.nbd.2011.12.005

Kanaan, N. M., Morfini, G. A., Lapointe, N. E., Pigino, G. F., Patterson, K. R., Song, Y., et al. (2011). Pathogenic forms of tau inhibit kinesin-dependent axonal transport through a mechanism involving activation of axonal phosphotransferases. *J. Neurosci.* 31, 9858–9868. doi: 10.1523/jneurosci.0560-11.2011

Lasagna-Reeves, C. A., Castillo-Carranza, D. L., Sengupta, U., Clos, A. L., Jackson, G. R., and Kayed, R. (2011). Tau oligomers impair memory and induce synaptic and mitochondrial dysfunction in wild-type mice. *Mol. Neurodegener.* 6:39. doi: 10.1186/1750-1326-6-39

Liang, Z., Liu, F., Iqbal, K., Grundke-Iqbal, I., and Gong, C.-X. (2009). Dysregulation of tau phosphorylation in mouse brain during excitotoxic damage. *J. Alzheimers Dis.* 17, 531–539. doi: 10.3233/jad-2009-1069

Luna-Muñoz, J., Chávez-Macías, L., García-Sierra, F., and Mena, R. (2007). Earliest stages of tau conformational changes are related to the appearance of a sequence of specific phospho-dependent tau epitopes in Alzheimer's disease. *J. Alzheimers Dis.* 12, 365–375. doi: 10.3233/JAD-2007-12410

Luo, W., Liu, W., Hu, X., Hanna, M., Caravaca, A., and Paul, S. M. (2015). Microglial internalization and degradation of pathological tau is enhanced by an anti-tau monoclonal antibody. *Sci. Rep.* 5:11161. doi: 10.1038/srep11161

Maphis, N., Xu, G., Kokiko-Cochran, O. N., Jiang, S., Cardona, A., Ransohoff, R. M., et al. (2015). Reactive microglia drive tau pathology and contribute to the spreading of pathological tau in the brain. *Brain* 138, 1738–1755. doi: 10.1093/brain/awv081

Martin, L., Latypova, X., Wilson, C. M., Magnaudeix, A., Perrin, M.-L., and Terro, F. (2013a). Tau protein phosphatases in Alzheimer's disease: The leading role of PP2A. *Ageing Res. Rev.* 12, 39–49. doi: 10.1016/j.arr.2012.06.008

Martin, L., Latypova, X., Wilson, C. M., Magnaudeix, A., Perrin, M.-L., Yardin, C., et al. (2013b). Tau protein kinases: involvement in Alzheimer's disease. *Ageing Res. Rev.* 12, 289–309. doi: 10.1016/j.arr.2012.06.003

Moran, C., Sanz-Rodriguez, A., Jimenez-Pacheco, A., Martinez-Villareal, J., Mckiernan, R. C., Jimenez-Mateos, E. M., et al. (2013). Bmf upregulation through the AMP-activated protein kinase pathway may protect the brain from seizure-induced cell death. *Cell Death Dis.* 4:e606. doi: 10.1038/cddis.2013.136

Mouri, G., Jimenez-Mateos, E., Engel, T., Dunleavy, M., Hatazaki, S., Paucard, A., et al. (2008). Unilateral hippocampal CA3-predominant damage and short latency epileptogenesis after intra-amygdala microinjection of kainic acid in mice. *Brain Res.* 1213, 140–151. doi: 10.1016/j.brainres.2008.03.061

Otvos, L. Jr., Feiner, L., Lang, E., Szendrei, G. I., Goedert, M., and Lee, V. M. (1994). Monoclonal antibody PHF-1 recognizes tau protein phosphorylated at serine residues 396 and 404. *J. Neurosci. Res.* 39, 669–673. doi: 10.1002/jnr.490390607

Parent, J. M., Yu, T. W., Leibowitz, R. T., Geschwind, D. H., Sloviter, R. S., and Lowenstein, D. H. (1997). Dentate granule cell neurogenesis is increased by seizures and contributes to aberrant network reorganization in the adult rat hippocampus. *J. Neurosci.* 17, 3727–3738. doi: 10.1523/JNEUROSCI.17-10-03727.1997

Pooler, A. M., Phillips, E. C., Lau, D. H., Noble, W., and Hanger, D. P. (2013). Physiological release of endogenous tau is stimulated by neuronal activity. *EMBO Rep.* 14, 389–394. doi: 10.1038/embor.2013.15

Santa-Maria, I., Alaniz, M. E., Renwick, N., Cela, C., Fulga, T. A., Van Vactor, D., et al. (2015). Dysregulation of microRNA-219 promotes neurodegeneration through post-transcriptional regulation of tau. *J. Clin. Invest.* 125, 681–686. doi: 10.1172/jci78421

Schmidt, D., and Löscher, W. (2005). Drug resistance in epilepsy: putative neurobiologic and clinical mechanisms. *Epilepsia* 46, 858–877. doi: 10.1111/j.1528-1167.2005.54904.x

Sloviter, R. S., Zappone, C. A., Bumanglag, A. V., Norwood, B. A., and Kudrimoti, H. (2007). On the relevance of prolonged convulsive status epilepticus in animals to the etiology and neurobiology of human temporal lobe epilepsy. *Epilepsia* 48, 6–10. doi: 10.1111/j.1528-1167.2007.01335.x

Su, J. H., Cummings, B. J., and Cotman, C. W. (1994). Early phosphorylation of tau in Alzheimer's disease occurs at Ser-202 and is preferentially located within neurites. *Neuroreport* 5, 2358–2362. doi: 10.1097/00001756-199411000-00037

Tai, X. Y., Koepp, M., Duncan, J. S., Fox, N., Thompson, P., Baxendale, S., et al. (2016). Hyperphosphorylated tau in patients with refractory epilepsy correlates with cognitive decline: a study of temporal lobe resections. *Brain* 139, 2441–2455. doi: 10.1093/brain/aww187

Téllez-Zenteno, J. F., Matijevic, S., and Wiebe, S. (2005). Somatic comorbidity of epilepsy in the general population in Canada. *Epilepsia* 46, 1955–1962. doi: 10.1111/j.1528-1167.2005.00344.x

Thom, M., Liu, J. Y. W., Thompson, P., Phadke, R., Narkiewicz, M., Martinian, L., et al. (2011). Neurofibrillary tangle pathology and Braak staging in chronic epilepsy in relation to traumatic brain injury and hippocampal sclerosis: a post-mortem study. *Brain* 134, 2969–2981. doi: 10.1093/brain/awr209

Wenzel, H. J., Cole, T. B., Born, D. E., Schwartzkroin, P. A., and Palmiter, R. D. (1997). Ultrastructural localization of zinc transporter-3 (ZnT-3) to synaptic vesicle membranes within mossy fiber boutons in the hippocampus of mouse and monkey. *Proc. Natl. Acad. Sci. U S A* 94, 12676–12681. doi: 10.1073/pnas.94.23.12676

Zheng, H., Tang, R., Yao, Y., Ji, Z., Cao, Y., Liu, Z., et al. (2016). MiR-219 protects against seizure in the kainic acid model of epilepsy. *Mol. Neurobiol.* 53, 1–7. doi: 10.1007/s12035-014-8981-5

2

The *MAPT* H1 Haplotype is a Risk Factor for Alzheimer's Disease in *APOE* ε4 Non-Carriers

Pascual Sánchez-Juan[1,2], Sonia Moreno[1,3], Itziar de Rojas[1,3], Isabel Hernández[1,3], Sergi Valero[1,3], Montse Alegret[1,3], Laura Montrreal[1], Pablo García González[1,3], Carmen Lage[1,2], Sara López-García[1,2], Eloy Rodríiguez-Rodríguez[1,2], Adelina Orellana[1], Lluís Tárraga[1,3], Mercè Boada[1,3] and Agustín Ruiz[1,3] on behalf of GR@ACE Study Group and DEGESCO Consortium*

[1] Center for Networked Biomedical Research on Neurodegenerative Diseases, National Institute of Health Carlos III, Ministry of Economy and Competitiveness, Madrid, Spain, [2] Service of Neurology, University Hospital Marqués de Valdecilla, IDIVAL, University of Cantabria, Santander, Spain, [3] Research Center and Memory Clinic, Fundació ACE, Institut Català de Neurociències Aplicades, Universitat Internacional de Catalunya, Barcelona, Spain

***Correspondence:**
Pascual Sánchez-Juan
pascualjesus.sanchez@scsalud.es;
psanjua@gmail.com

An ancestral inversion of 900 kb on chromosome 17q21, which includes the microtubule-associated protein tau (*MAPT*) gene, defines two haplotype clades in Caucasians (H1 and H2). The H1 haplotype has been linked inconsistently with AD. In a previous study, we showed that an SNP tagging this haplotype (rs1800547) was associated with AD risk in a large population from the Dementia Genetics Spanish Consortium (DEGESCO) including 4435 cases and 6147 controls. The association was mainly driven by individuals that were non-carriers of the *APOE* ε4 allele. Our aim was to replicate our previous findings in an independent sample of 4124 AD cases and 3290 controls from Spain (GR@ACE project) and to analyze the effect of the H1 sub-haplotype structure on the risk of AD. The H1 haplotype was associated with AD risk (OR = 1.12; p = 0.0025). Stratification analysis showed that this association was mainly driven by the *APOE* ε4 non-carriers (OR = 1.15; p = 0.0022). Pooled analysis of both Spanish datasets (n = 17,996) showed that the highest AD risk related to the *MAPT* H1/H2 haplotype was in those individuals that were the oldest [third tertile (>77 years)] and did not carry *APOE* ε4 allele (p = 0.001). We did not find a significant association between H1 sub-haplotypes and AD. H1c was nominally associated but lost statistical significance after adjusting by population sub-structure. Our results are consistent with the hypothesis that genetic variants linked to the *MAPT* H1/H2 are tracking a genuine risk allele for AD. The fact that this association is stronger in *APOE* ε4 non-carriers partially explains previous controversial results and might be related to a slower alternative causal pathway less dependent on brain amyloid load.

Keywords: Alzheimer's disease, *MAPT*, H1H2, *APOE*, genetic association

INTRODUCTION

Dementia is related to many underlying pathologies, with Alzheimer's disease (AD) being the most common. AD is pathologically defined by the deposits of two proteins: tau which accumulates intracellularly and β-amyloid that accumulates extracellularly and within the walls of the blood vessels of the central nervous system. Dementia of AD-type is a complex entity with a common clinical syndrome that is likely to be reached by different routes influenced by genetic and environmental factors. This complexity is likely to have contributed to the constant failures of AD clinical trials. In particular, therapies based on the amyloid cascade hypothesis have not demonstrated any disease-modifying effect, despite some of these attempts have been proved to be effective in permanently removing brain β-amyloid plaques (Nicoll et al., 2019). This has led the pharmaceutical industry to focus on other therapeutic targets such as the tau protein (Corvol and Buée, 2019).

Neurofibrillary tangles composed of truncated and hyperphosphorylated tau proteins are hallmarks of AD pathology (Goedert, 2004). Tau protein plays an essential role in the central nervous system by promoting microtubule assembly and stability in neuronal cells. Emerging evidence supports that tau function is essential for normal synaptic mechanisms and it may be dysregulated in AD potentially through interaction with genetic risk factors in an Aβ-dependent or Aβ-independent manner (Dourlen et al., 2019). Additionally, tau has been proposed to spread through the brain from neuron to neuron by a "prion-like" mechanism (Clavaguera et al., 2015).

Tau protein is encoded by the *MAPT* gene (*MAPT*: OMIM: *157140), located at chromosome 17q21-22. There are two common *MAPT* extended haplotypes in Caucasians resulting from an ancestral inversion: H1 and H2. The H1 haplotype has been linked with familial and sporadic neurodegenerative disorders like progressive supranuclear palsy (PSP) (Conrad et al., 1997; Baker et al., 1999; Higgins et al., 2000; Pastor et al., 2004, 2016), corticobasal degeneration (CBD) (Houlden et al., 2001), Frontotemporal Dementia (FTD) (Verpillat et al., 2002), and Parkinson's disease (PD) (Martin et al., 2001; Simón-Sánchez et al., 2009; Pastor et al., 2016). Genome-wide association studies (GWAS) have shown that the *MAPT* H1 haplotype is associated with CBD, PSP, and FTD (Yokoyama et al., 2017).

The H1 haplotype is further divided into sub-haplotypes, of those H1c has been associated with several neurodegenerative diseases (Myers et al., 2005; Heckman et al., 2019). H1c has been associated with higher levels of tau in plasma and CSF (Myers et al., 2007; Chen et al., 2017) and inconsistently with AD (Myers et al., 2005).

Although recent genetic studies show that several AD GWAS-associated genes, especially BIN1, are potentially involved in tau pathways (Dourlen et al., 2019), *MAPT* itself has not emerged until recently as a locus associated with AD. The IGAP consortium found a significant association between an SNP tagging *MAPT* H1 haplotype (rs2732703) and AD in subjects not carrying APOE ε4, however, the authors concluded that their conditional analysis pointed out that *MAPT* was probably not the causal gene (Jun et al., 2016).

Microtubule-associated protein tau H1/H2 haplotype frequency varies according to populations, with H2 frequency being maximum in the Mediterranean region and decreasing gradually as we move away from that area (Donnelly et al., 2010). These differences might contribute to explain controversial results among studies, as genetic stratification in genetically heterogeneous populations might constitute an important confounder. It is therefore essential to study these variants in large genetically homogeneous populations. In a previous study, we showed that H1 *MAPT* haplotype was strongly associated with risk of PSP, PD, and AD in 4435 cases and 6147 controls from Spain (Pastor et al., 2016). Therefore, it seems that *MAPT* H1/H2 haplotypes might play a relevant role within the genetic architecture of several neurodegenerative pathologies in our country. It is worth mention that the prevalence of the haplotype H2 in our control sample was one of the highest reported worldwide (29%) (Pastor et al., 2016).

In the present study, we aimed to replicate our previous findings in an independent sample. To do that, we assessed the association between the AD risk and the *MAPT* H1/H2 haplotype and H1 sub-haplotypes in 4,124 AD cases and 3,290 controls from Spain (GR@ACE/DEGESCO project).

MATERIALS AND METHODS

A detailed description of the methods and population of the GR@ACE study has been published elsewhere (Moreno-Grau et al., 2019)[1].

Population

The GR@ACE study comprises 4,120 AD cases and 3,289 control individuals. Cases were recruited from Fundació ACE, Institut Català de Neurociències Aplicades (Barcelona, Spain). Diagnoses were established by a neurology working-group according to the DSM-IV criteria for dementia and to the National Institute on Aging and Alzheimer's Association's (NIA-AA) 2011 guidelines for defining AD. In the present study, we considered AD cases, dementia individuals diagnosed with probable or possible AD at any moment of their clinical course.

Control individuals were recruited from three centers: Fundació ACE (Barcelona, Spain), Valme University Hospital (Seville, Spain) and the Spanish National DNA Bank Carlos III (University of Salamanca, Spain)[2]. Written informed consent was obtained from all participants. The Ethics and Scientific Committees have approved this research protocol (Acta 25/2016, Ethics Committee, Hospital Clinic I Provincial de Barcelona, Barcelona, Spain).

Genotyping, Quality Control, Imputation, and Statistical Analysis

Participants were genotyped using the Axiom 815K Spanish Biobank array (Thermo Fisher). Genotyping was performed in the Spanish National Center for Genotyping (CeGEN, Santiago de Compostela, Spain).

We removed samples with genotype call rates below 97%, excess heterozygosity, duplicates, samples genetically related to other individuals in the cohort or sample mix-up (PIHAT > 0.1875). If a sex discrepancy was detected, the sample was removed unless the discrepancy was safely resolved. To detect population outliers of non-European ancestry (>6 SD from European population mean), principal

[1] https://www.biorxiv.org/content/10.1101/528901v1
[2] www.bancoadn.org

component analysis (PCA) was conducted using SMARTPCA from EIGENSOFT 6.1.4.

We removed variants with a call rate < 95% or that grossly deviated from Hardy–Weinberg equilibrium in controls (P-value $\leq 1 \times 10^{-4}$), markers with a different missing rate between case and control (P-value $< 5 \times 10^{-4}$ for the difference) or minor allele frequency (MAF) below 0.01. Imputation was carried out using Haplotype reference consortium (HRC) panel in Michigan Imputation servers[3]. Only common markers (MAF > 0.01) with a high imputation quality ($R^2 > 0.30$) were selected to conduct downstream association analyses.

Statistical Analysis

Allelic and genotypic frequencies were compared using χ^2 statistics. Adjusted analyses were performed using multiple logistic regression. We used rs1800547 to tag *MAPT* H2 haplotype. Additionally, we used six tagging variants (rs1467967, rs242557, rs3785883, rs2471738, rs8070723, rs7521), to construct most common *MAPT* H1 sub-haplotypes as previously described (Pittman et al., 2005; Allen et al., 2014). To control for population sub-structure, results were co-variated by the main four principal components detected in this population (Moreno-Grau et al., 2019). All analyses were performed in PLINK 1.7.

RESULTS

We included 3290 controls with a mean age of 54.3 ± 14.4 years, and 48.9% of females, and 4124 AD cases with a mean age of 79.0 ± 7.5 years, 69.6% of females. No gross deviation from Hardy Weinberg equilibrium was found in controls for any of the *MAPT* studied variants (**Table 1**).

Table 2 shows the allelic and genotypic frequency distribution of the SNPrs1800547 tagging the H1/H2 haplotype. We found a statistically significant overrepresentation of the *MAPT* H1 haplotype, present in 73.3% of AD compared to 71.1% of controls (p = 0.00025). When we stratified the sample by *APOE* ε4 status, the association of the H1 haplotype was driven by non-carriers of *APOE* ε4 (p = 0.0022) (**Table 2**). The association followed exactly the same pattern as our previous study (Pastor et al., 2016). Pooling both Spanish population confirmed that *MAPT* H1 was significantly more common in AD compared to controls (73.5 versus 70.7% respectively; $p = 1.0 \times 10^{-5}$), and this association was predominantly due to the *APOE* ε4 non-carriers ($p = 8.0 \times 10^{-5}$) (**Table 2**).

Table 3 shows the sub-haplotypes of *MAPT* in cases and controls. In addition to the protective effect of H2, only H1c was statistically significantly associated with AD. However, when we adjusted by the four main genetic components H1c was not statistically significant. After stratifying by *APOE* ε4 these results did not change substantially, and in addition to H2, only two rare sub-haplotypes (H1u and H1v) were nominally associated with AD. After adjustment, none of the associations survived multiple comparisons correction (**Table 4**).

Figure 1 shows the genotypic distribution of the SNP rs1800547 (*MAPT* H1/H2) stratified by *APOE* ε4 across age tertiles for the pooled population. In the available entire sample of 15,522 individuals, we appreciated that within the APOE ε4 non-carriers the association between *MAPT* H1/H2 and AD increased with age, and it was stronger in the oldest individuals.

[3]https://imputationserver.sph.umich.edu

TABLE 1 | Hardy–Weinberg equilibrium test in controls.

SNP	Genotypes	Observed (HET)	Expected (HET)	*P*-value
rs1467967	264/1346/1679	0.41	0.41	0.83
rs242557	346/1426/1517	0.43	0.44	0.69
rs3785883	128/955/2206	0.29	0.30	0.06
rs2471738	89/991/2209	0.30	0.29	0.08
rs8070723	292/1328/1669	0.40	0.41	0.24
rs7521	614/1564/1111	0.48	0.49	0.13

DISCUSSION

Our data, from a large and homogeneous single country population, shows that individuals carrying the H1 *MAPT* haplotype are at higher risk to develop AD dementia. The association is predominantly present in the *APOE* ε4 non-carriers and it is stronger in the eldest. These results replicate our previous findings (Pastor et al., 2016) and are concordant with the IGAP study (Jun et al., 2016) showing an association of another SNP tagging H1 (rs2732703) with AD only in the *APOE* ε4 non-carriers.

Our pooled analysis, including 15522 individuals, strongly support an etiological role of the *MAPT* region in AD. This association has been difficult to replicate, and results of previous studies assessing *MAPT* H1/H2 haplotype as a risk factor for AD have been controversial, although some of them were considerably under-powered (Russ et al., 2001; Mukherjee et al., 2007; Babić Leko et al., 2018). A robust statistical association only emerged in large sample studies and meta-GWAS, after stratifying by *APOE* ε4 (Jun et al., 2016; Pastor et al., 2016). An alternative interpretation of our results would be that the causal variant could be in linkage disequilibrium with the *MAPT* H1 haplotype but outside the *MAPT* gene, as other authors have suggested (Jun et al., 2016). A less likely explanation might be contamination of non-AD tauopathies in *APOE* ε4 non-carriers.

There are several factors that might be related to our findings. Taken together, our two studies, comprise one of the largest single-country population assessing *MAPT* H1/H2 and AD risk to date. This is of special value, as the inversion haplotype frequency has been shown to differ significantly across populations, and it is estimated to be 20% in Europeans, 6% in Africans, and less than 1% in East Asians (Holzer et al., 2004). This ethnic variability might cause population sub-structure biasing the results in countries with a high degree of population admixture. This is likely to be less problematic in our study as our sample come from a single country, and we have tested population sub-structure in Spain which does not represent a substantial problem for common genetic variants analyses

TABLE 2 | Microtubule-associated protein tau H1/H2 haplotypes and AD risk.

	Control (%)	AD (%)	Genotype *P*-value	Allelic *P*-value	Allelic OR (95%CI)
ALL					
H2H2	290 (8.8)	328 (8.0)	$p = 0.008$	$p = 0.00025$	1.12 (1.04–1.20)
H1H2	1324 (40.2)	1546 (37.5)			
H1H1	1676 (50.9)	2250 (54.6)			
H1 frequency	0.711	0.733			
APOE4+					
H2H2	58 (8.3)	136 (8.3)	$p = 0.42$	$p = 0.32$	1.07 (0.93–1.23)
H1H2	286 (40.7)	625 (37.9)			
H1H1	358 (51.0)	887 (53.8)			
H1 frequency	0.714	0.728			
APOE4−					
H2H2	232 (9.0)	190 (7.7)	$p = 0.009$	$p = 0.0022$	1.15 (1.05–1.25)
H1H2	1033 (40.1)	913 (37.2)			
H1H1	1311 (50.9)	1353 (55.1)			
H1 frequency	0.709	0.737			
ALL (Pastor et al., 2016)					
H2H2	532 (9.15)	344 (8.34)	$p = 0.001$	$p = 0.00051$	1.12 (1.05–1.19)
H1H2	2444 (42.03)	1614 (39.11)			
H1H1	2839 (48.82)	2169 (52.56)			
H1 frequency	0.698	0.721			
APOE4+ (Pastor et al., 2016)					
H2H2	78 (9.07)	139 (8.50)	$p = 0.88$	$p = 0.65$	1.03 (0.91–1.18)
H1H2	345 (40.12)	655 (40.04)			
H1H1	437 (50.81)	842 (51.47)			
H1 frequency	0.709	0.715			
APOE4− (Pastor et al., 2016)					
H2H2	343 (8.46)	160 (8.16)	$p = 0.001$	$p = 0.0025$	1.14 (1.05–1.24)
H1H2	1701 (41.97)	730 (37.24)			
H1H1	2009 (49.57)	1070 (54.59)			
H1 frequency	0.706	0.732			
ALL pooled					
H2H2	822 (9.0)	672 (8.1)	$p = 1.03 \times 10^{-5}$	$p = 1.0 \times 10^{-5}$	1.126 (1.075–1.127)
H1H2	3769 (41.4)	3160 (38.3)			
H1H1	4515 (49.6)	4419 (53.6)			
H1 frequency	0.703	0.727			
APOE4+ pooled					
H2H2	136 (8.7)	275 (8.4)	$p = 0.52$	$p = 0.286$	1.053 (0.958–1.157)
H1H2	631 (40.4)	1280 (39.0)			
H1H1	795 (50.9)	1729 (52.6)			
H1 frequency	0.711	0.721			
APOE4− pooled					
H2H2	575 (8.7)	350 (7.9)	$p = 5.16 \times 10^{-5}$	$p = 8.0 \times 10^{-5}$	1.148 (1.08–1.22)
H1H2	2734 (41.2)	1643 (37.2)			
H1H1	3320 (50.1)	2423 (54.9)			
H1 frequency	0.707	0.735			

(Moreno-Grau et al., 2019). Additionally, in our sub-haplotype analysis, we controlled for population sub-structure by adjusting for genetic principal components. It is worth mentioning that, despite it is commonly reported that the inversion is found at a frequency of around 20% throughout Europe, it shows a great range of frequencies within Europe (from 5 to 37.5%). The H2 haplotype, which identifies the inversion, is most frequent around the Mediterranean decreasing outward in all directions (Donnelly et al., 2010). Our controls presented the inversion in nearly 30% of individuals, this high frequency of the H2 haplotype has increased our power to detect the association compared to other populations in which this variant is less prevalent.

A potential limitation of our study is the age difference between the cases and the controls, which are significantly

TABLE 3 | Microtubule-associated protein tau sub-haplotypes.

Haplotype ID	Haplotype*	Cases	Controls	*P*	Adjusted *P*-value**
H1o	AAACAA	0.022	0.021	0.63	0.47
H1y	AAATAG	0.013	0.011	0.31	0.22
H1d	AAGCAA	0.069	0.072	0.60	0.30
H1u	AAGCAG	0.025	0.022	0.19	0.14
H1q	AAGTAA	0.012	0.013	0.52	0.22
H1c	AAGTAG	0.114	0.104	0.05	0.14
H1h	AGACAA	0.050	0.047	0.51	0.25
H1l	AGACAG	0.046	0.044	0.65	0.44
H1t	AGATAG	0.011	0.010	0.64	0.30
H1e	AGGCAA	0.075	0.077	0.75	0.90
H1j	AGGCAG	0.016	0.016	0.78	0.95
H2	AGGCGG	0.283	0.309	0.0009	0.0008
H1z	GAATAG	0.014	0.011	0.12	0.07
H1i	GAGCAA	0.038	0.040	0.69	0.72
H1m	GAGCAG	0.026	0.023	0.32	0.36
H1f	GGACAA	0.014	0.014	0.95	0.75
H1v	GGATAG	0.014	0.012	0.27	0.08
H1b	GGGCAA	0.159	0.156	0.60	0.31

**rs1467967; rs242557; rs3785883; rs2471738; rs8070723; rs7521; **adjusted by the four genetic principal components.*

younger. However, this could only jeopardize the validity of our findings in the case of a survival bias. But to our knowledge, the MAPT H1/H2 haplotype has not been associated with mortality. The most likely consequence of our age unbalance is a decrease in our power to detect the association, as some of the controls carrying the H1 haplotype may still develop AD in the future. It is therefore likely that we are underestimating the true association between the H1/H2 haplotype and AD.

Microtubule-associated protein tau H1 has been associated with many neurodegenerative diseases: PSP, PD, CBD, FTD, and AD. It has been reported that the *MAPT* H1 is more efficient at driving gene expression than the H2 haplotype (Kwok et al., 2004). This has been shown to be particularly true with the H1c sub-haplotype (Myers et al., 2007). However, the H1 sub-haplotype association with AD is controversial, and H1c findings have been difficult to replicate (Myers et al., 2005; Abraham et al., 2009; Allen et al., 2014). It is likely that population stratification might have played a role. In our data H1c was nominally associated with AD, however, the statistical significance was lost after adjusting by the principal components supporting the notion that no H1sub-haplotype is specifically increasing AD-risk, and stratification by APOE ε4 did not change substantially these results.

Our results add further evidence for an etiological role of *MAPT* gene variants in clinical AD, supporting the role of the *APOE* ε4 allele as a modulator of this association. As seen in our previous study in population from Spain (Pastor et al., 2016) and by the international consortium IGAP (Jun et al., 2016), this association is significantly stronger in APOE ε4 non-carriers. Recent studies with tau and amyloid PET supports a view of AD as a tauopathy driven by amyloid, suggesting that tau pathology would appear in middle temporal lobe earlier than amyloid deposits, but the co-occurrence of both would be needed for tau pathology to expand beyond the temporal lobes (Schöll et al., 2016). This is also coherent with the new findings of AD meta-GWAS which shows the involvement of both amyloid and tau pathways (Dourlen et al., 2019; Kunkle et al., 2019). Therefore, it seems that tau and amyloid deposits might follow, at least initially, independent trajectories up to the point when they reach a threshold in which β-amyloid might accelerate tau pathology. A recent single case publication showing that a patient with a presenilin 1 mutation was resistant to cognitive impairment, likely due to a homozygous mutation in *APOE*, supports the hypothesis that *APOE* might play an important role in this tau pathology acceleration (Arboleda-Velasquez et al., 2019). On the other hand, *APOE* status is associated to prevalence of brain amyloid pathology, as shown by a large PET and CSF study in non-demented population that found that *APOE* ε4 carriers had two to three times higher prevalence than non-carriers (Jansen et al., 2015).

We hypothesize that the *MAPT* H1 variant might increase the risk of tau pathology which might be related to different amyloid thresholds to disparate tau pathology. We speculate that the association is only significant in the *APOE* ε4 non-carriers because in the carriers the amyloid would mask the H1 *MAPT* effect, while in the non-carriers the "tau etiologic pathway" would play a more relevant role and might be able to increase AD risk with a lower amyloid involvement. It is likely that this phenomenon might take longer to develop which might explain why this association is not significant in the youngest patients and stronger in the third tertile. This hypothesis could be tested studying the trajectory of individuals classified according to *APOE* ε4 status and *MAPT* H1/H2 haplotype in prospective cohorts with sequential amyloid and tau PET assessments.

Our study highlights the complexity of AD and suggests the existence of different pathogenic routes influenced by the genetic background. To look for successful therapeutic strategies it will be very important to take into account this mechanistic diversity and to combat specifically the pathology demonstrated on each afflicted individual.

MEMBERS OF THE GR@ACE STUDY GROUP

Research Center and Memory Clinic, Fundació ACE, Institut Català de Neurociències Aplicades, Universitat Internacional de Catalunya, Barcelona, Spain: C. Abdelnour, N. Aguilera, E. Alarcon, M. Alegret, M. Boada, M. Buendia, P. Cañabate, I. de Rojas, S. Diego, A. Espinosa, A. Gailhajenet, P. García González, S. Gil, M. Guitart, I. Hernández, M. Ibarria, A. Lafuente, E. Martín, A. Mauleón, G. Monté-Rubio, L. Montrreal, S. Moreno-Grau, M. Moreno, A. Orellana, G. Ortega, A. Pancho, E. Pelejà, A. Pérez-Cordon, S. Preckler, O. Rodríguez-Gómez, M. Rosende-Roca, A. Ruiz, S. Ruiz, A. Sanabria, M. A. Santos-Santos, O. Sotolongo-Grau, L. Tárraga, S. Valero, and L. Vargas. Center for Networked Biomedical Research on Neurodegenerative Diseases, National Institute of Health Carlos III, Ministry of Economy and Competitiveness, Madrid, Spain: C. Abdelnour, M. Alegret, M. Boada, P. Cañabate, A. Espinosa, I. Hernández, S. Moreno-Grau, G. Ortega, O. Rodríguez-Gómez, A. Ruiz, S. Ruiz, A. Sanabria, L. Tárraga, and S. Valero. Department of Surgery, Biochemistry and Molecular Biology, School of Medicine, University of Málaga, Málaga, Spain: E. Alarcon, I. Quintela, and L. M. Real. Grupo de Medicina Xenómica, Centro Nacional de Genotipado (CEGEN-PRB3-ISCIII), Universidade de Santiago de Compostela, Santiago, Spain: A. Carracedo and O. Maroñas. Fundación Pública Galega de Medicina Xenómica, CIBERER, IDIS, Santiago, Spain: A. Carracedo. Centro de Investigación Biomédica en Red de Diabetes y Enfermedades Metabólicas Asociadas, Hospital Clínico San Carlos, Madrid, Spain: A. Corbatón, M. T. Martínez, and M. Serrano-Rios. Centro Andaluz de Estudios Bioinformáticos, Seville, Spain: A. González Pérez and M. E. Sáez. Unidad Clínica de Enfermedades Infecciosas y Microbiología, Hospital Universitario de Valme, Seville, Spain: J. Macias, J. A. Pineda, and L. M. Real.

TABLE 4 | Microtubule-associated protein tau sub-haplotypes stratified by APOE ε4 status.

Haplotype ID	Haplotype*	OR	*P*-value	Adjusted *P*-value**
APOE4+				
H1o	AAACAA	1.17	0.61	0.63
H1f	GGACAA	1.55	0.31	0.20
H1h	AGACAA	0.96	0.81	0.93
H1i	GAGCAA	1.04	0.83	0.90
H1d	AAGCAA	0.85	0.26	0.18
H1b	GGGCAA	1.08	0.43	0.37
H1e	AGGCAA	1.02	0.88	0.93
H2	AGGCGG	0.93	0.28	0.23
H1z	GAATAG	1.77	0.14	0.10
H1v	GGATAG	0.95	0.86	0.92
H1t	AGATAG	1.46	0.37	0.28
H1c	AAGTAG	1.13	0.27	0.37
H1l	AGACAG	1.01	0.95	0.64
H1m	GAGCAG	1.07	0.78	0.89
H1u	AAGCAG	0.91	0.71	0.76
H1j	AGGCAG	0.66	0.18	0.21
APOE4−				
H1q	AAGTAA	1.12	0.56	0.86
H1g	GAACAA	0.94	0.81	0.92
H1o	AAACAA	1.12	0.46	0.40
H1f	GGACAA	0.93	0.74	0.93
H1h	AGACAA	1.11	0.34	0.19
H1i	GAGCAA	0.89	0.37	0.46
H1d	AAGCAA	1.02	0.83	0.83
H1b	GGGCAA	1.04	0.55	0.34
H1e	AGGCAA	0.94	0.46	0.90
H2	AGGCGG	0.88	0.00	0.00083
H1z	GAATAG	1.33	0.20	0.24
H1y	AAATAG	1.30	0.25	0.35
H1v	GGATAG	1.41	0.13	0.04
ND	AGATAG	1.03	0.91	0.65
H1c	AAGTAG	1.12	0.10	0.37
H1l	AGACAG	1.06	0.56	0.60
H1m	GAGCAG	1.21	0.20	0.33
H1u	AAGCAG	1.41	0.03	0.04
H1j	AGGCAG	1.15	0.46	0.30

**rs1467967; rs242557; rs3785883; rs2471738; rs8070723; rs7521; **adjusted by the four genetic principal components.*

MEMBERS OF THE DEGESCO CONSORTIUM

Unidad de Trastornos del Movimiento, Servicio de Neurología y Neurofisiología, Instituto de Biomedicina de Sevilla, Hospital Universitario Virgen del Rocío/CSIC/Universidad de Sevilla, Seville, Spain: A. D. Adarmes-Gómez, D. Buiza-Rueda, F. Carrillo, M. Carrión-Claro, P. Gómez-Garre, S. Jesús, M. A. Labrador Espinosa, D. Macias, P. Mir, and T. Periñán-Tocino. Network Center for Biomedical Research in Neurodegenerative Diseases, National Institute of Health Carlos III, Madrid, Spain: A. D. Adarmes-Gómez, R. Blesa, M. Boada, D. Buiza-Rueda, M. J. Bullido, M. Calero, F. Carrillo, M. Carrión-Claro, J. Clarimón, J. Fortea, A. Frank-García, P. Gómez-Garre, I. Hernández, S. Jesús, M. A. Labrador Espinosa, C. Lage, A. Lleó, S. López-García, D. Macias, A. Martín Montes, M. Medina, P. Mir, S. Moreno-Grau, J. Pérez Tur, T. Periñán-Tocino, G. Piñol Ripoll, A. Rábano, E. Rodríguez-Rodríguez, A. Ruiz, P. Sánchez-Juan, I. Sastre, L. Tárraga, and S. Valero. Research Center and Memory Clinic, Fundació ACE, Institut Català de Neurociències Aplicades, Universitat Internacional de Catalunya, Barcelona, Spain: E. Alarcón-Martín, M. Boada, I. de Rojas, I. Hernández, M. Marquié, G. Monté-Rubio, L. Montrreal, S. Moreno-Grau, A. Orellana, A. Ruiz, O. Sotolongo-Grau, L. Tárraga, and S. Valero. Department of Surgery, Biochemistry and Molecular Biology, School of Medicine, University of Málaga, Málaga, Spain: E. Alarcón-Martín, J. M. Cruz-Gamero, and J. L. Royo. Fundació per la Recerca Biomèdica i Social Mútua Terrassa, and

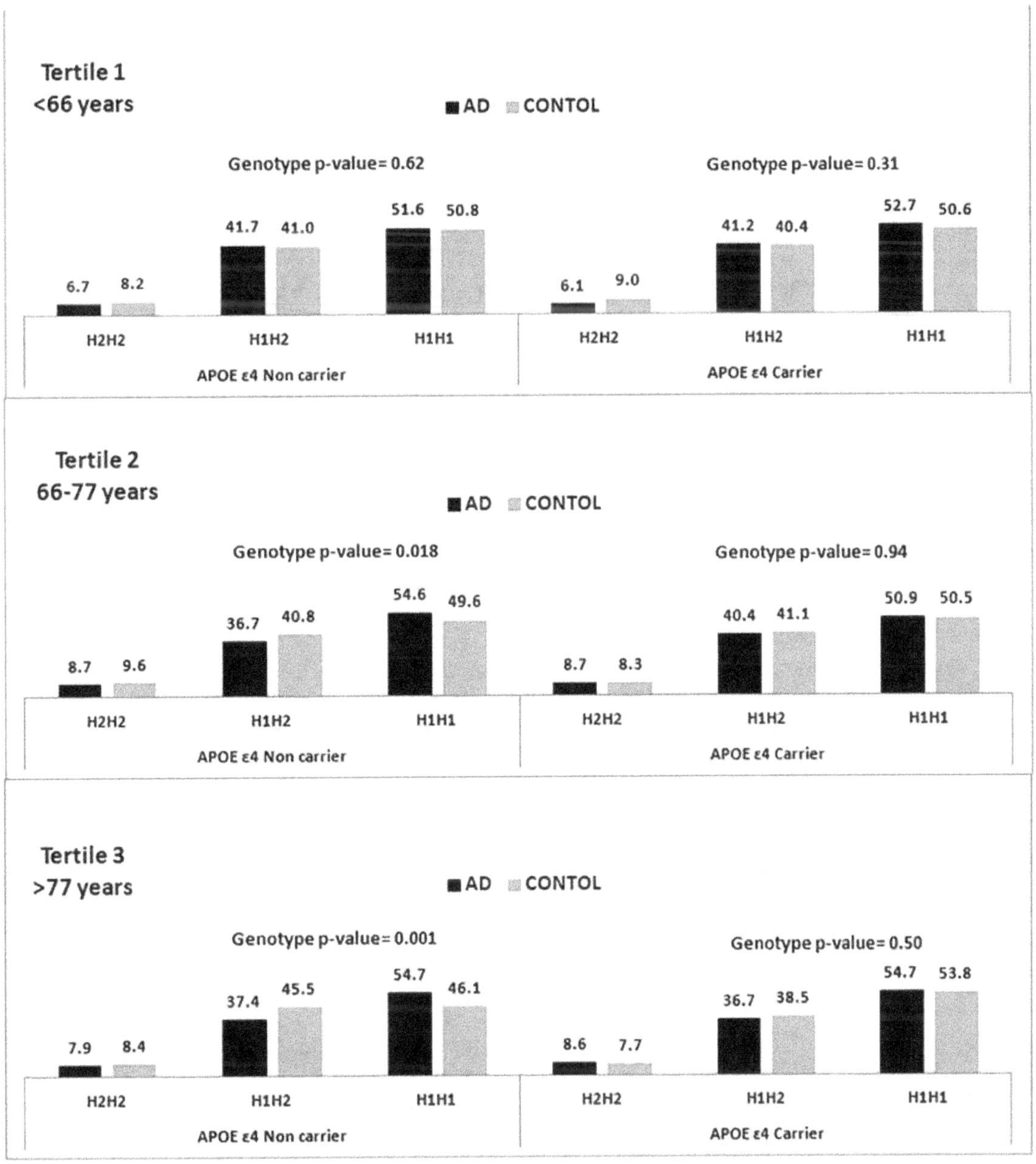

FIGURE 1 | Genotype frequency distribution of the rs1800547 SNP tagging *MAPT* H1/H2 haplotype stratified by *APOE* ε4 status and age tertiles.

Memory Disorders Unit, Department of Neurology, Hospital Universitari Mutua de Terrassa, School of Medicine, University of Barcelona, Barcelona, Spain: I. Álvarez, M. Diez-Fairen, and P. Pastor. Laboratorio de Genética, Hospital Universitario Central de Asturias, Oviedo, Spain: V. Álvarez. Instituto de Investigación Biosanitaria del Principado de Asturias, Oviedo, Spain: V. Álvarez, C. Martínez, and M. Menéndez-González. Department of Neurology, Hospital Universitario Son Espases, Palma, Spain: G. Amer-Ferrer. Unidad de Demencias, Hospital Clínico Universitario Virgen de la Arrixaca, Murcia, Spain: M. Antequera, C. Antúnez, A. Legaz, S. Manzanares, J. Marín-Muñoz, B. Martínez, V. Martínez, M. P. Vicente, and L. Vivancos. Servei de Neurologia, Hospital Universitari i Politècnic La Fe, Valencia, Spain: M. Baquero and J. A. Burguera. Unidad de Demencias, Servicio de Neurología y Neurofisiología, Instituto de Biomedicina de Sevilla, Hospital Universitario Virgen del Rocío/CSIC/Universidad de Sevilla, Seville, Spain: M. Bernal, E. Franco, M. Marín, and S. Rodrigo. Sant Pau Memory Unit, Neurology Department, Sant Pau Biomedical Research Institute, Hospital de la Santa Creu i Sant Pau, Universitat Autònoma de Barcelona, Barcelona, Spain: R. Blesa, J. Clarimón, J. Fortea, and A. Lleó. Centro de Biologia Molecular Severo Ochoa (CSIC), Universidad Autonoma de Madrid, Madrid, Spain: M. J. Bullido, A. Martín Montes, and I. Sastre. Instituto de Investigacion

Sanitaria "Hospital la Paz", Madrid, Spain: M. J. Bullido, T. del Ser, A. Frank-García, and M. Medina. CIEN Foundation, Queen Sofia Foundation Alzheimer Center, Madrid, Spain: M. Calero, A. B. Pastor, and A. Rábano. Instituto de Salud Carlos III, Madrid, Spain: M. Calero, S. Garcia Madrona, and G. Garcia-Ribas. Hospital Universitario Ramón y Cajal, Madrid, Spain: M. J. Casajeros. BIOMICs, Centro de Investigación Lascaray, Universidad del País Vasco UPV/EHU, Leioa, Spain: M. M. de Pancorbo. Neurology Service, Hospital Universitario La Paz (UAM), Madrid, Spain: A. Frank-García and A. Martín Montes. Alzheimer Research Center and Memory Clinic, Andalusian Institute for Neuroscience, Málaga, Spain: J. M. García-Alberca, S. Hevilla, and T. Marín. Neurology Service, Marqués de Valdecilla University Hospital, IDIVAL, University of Cantabria, Santander, Spain: C. Lage, S. López-García, E. Rodríguez-Rodríguez, and P. Sánchez-Juan. Hospital Donostia de San Sebastían, Donostia, Spain: A. López de Munáin. Fundación para la Formación e Investigación Sanitarias de la Región de Murcia, Murcia, Spain: S. Manzanares. Servicio de Neurología, Hospital de Cabueñes, Gijón, Spain: C. Martínez. Centro de Investigación y Terapias Avanzadas, Fundación CITA-Alzheimer, Donostia, Spain: P. Martínez-Lage Álvarez. Navarrabiomed, Pamplona, Spain: M. Mendioroz Iriarte. Servicio de Neurología, Hospital Universitario Central de Asturias, Oviedo, Spain: M. Menéndez-González. Barcelonaβeta Brain Research Center, Fundació Pasqual Maragall, Barcelona, Spain: J. L. Molinuevo. Unitat de Genètica Molecular, Institut de Biomedicina de València, CSIC, Valencia, Spain: J. Pérez Tur. Unidad Mixta de Neurologia y Genètica. Instituto de Investigación Sanitaria La Fe, Valencia, Spain: J. Pérez Tur. Unitat Trastorns Cognitius, Hospital Universitari Santa Maria de Lleida, Institut de Recerca Biomédica de Lleida, Lleida, Spain: G: Piñol Ripoll. BT-CIEN, Madrid, Spain: A. Rábano. Hospital Universitario La Princesa, Madrid, Spain: D. Real de Asúa. Hospital Clínic de Barcelona, Barcelona, Spain: R. Sanchez del Valle Díaz.

ETHICS STATEMENT

The studies involving human participants were reviewed and approved by Acta 25/2016, Ethics Committee, Hospital Clinic I Provincial de Barcelona, Barcelona, Spain. The patients/participants provided their written informed consent to participate in this study.

AUTHOR CONTRIBUTIONS

PS-J and AR: data collection, data analysis, study design, manuscript drafting, and manuscript critical review. SM, IR, IH, SV, MA, LM, PG, CL, SL-G, ER-R, and AO: data collection, data analysis, and manuscript critical review. LT and MB: data collection, data analysis, manuscript critical review, and study design.

ACKNOWLEDGMENTS

The Genome Research at Fundacio ACE/Dementia Genetics Spanish Consortium (GR@ACE/DEGESCO) would like to thank patients and controls who participated in this project. GR@ACE/DEGESCO GWAS program was funded by Grifols SA, Fundacion Bancaria "La Caixa," and Fundació ACE, Institut Català de Neurociències Aplicades. PS-J and AR have also received support by grant PI16/01861. Accion Estrategica en Salud integrated in the Spanish National I+D+i Plan and financed by Instituto de Salud Carlos III (ISCIII) - Subdireccion General de Evaluacion and the Fondo Europeo de Desarrollo Regional (FEDER - "Una Manera de Hacer Europa"). PS-J was supported by IDIVAL, Instituto de Salud Carlos III [Fondo de Investigacion Sanitario, PI08/0139, PI12/02288, PI16/01652, JPND (DEMTEST PI11/03028)], and the CIBERNED program. We thank Biobanco Valdecilla for their support. LM was supported by Consejería de Salud de la Junta de Andalucía (Grant PI-0001/2017). DEGESCO was also sponsored by the Centro de Investigación Biomédica en Red sobre Enfermedades Neurodegenerativas (CIBERNED, Spain). Control samples and data from patients included in this study were provided in part by the National DNA Bank Carlos III (www.bancoadn.org, University of Salamanca, Spain) and Hospital Universitario Virgen de Valme (Sevilla, Spain) and they were processed following standard operating procedures with the appropriate approval of the Ethical and Scientific Committee. The genotyping service to generate GR@ACE/DEGESCO GWAS data was carried out at CEGEN-PRB3-ISCIII; it was supported by grant PT17/0019, of the PE I+D+i 2013-2016, funded by ISCIII and ERDF. GR@ACE/DEGESCO consortia would also like to thank to all researchers contributing to this project. A complete list of collaborators involved in the GR@ACE/DEGESCO GWAS can be found at https://ciberned.es/proyectos/degesco.html.

REFERENCES

Abraham, R., Sims, R., Carroll, L., Hollingworth, P., O'Donovan, M. C., Williams, J., et al. (2009). An association study of common variation at the MAPT locus with late-onset Alzheimer's disease. *Am. J. Med. Genet.. Part B Neuropsychiatr. Genet.* 150B, 1152–1155. doi: 10.1002/ajmg.b.30951

Allen, M., Kachadoorian, M., Quicksall, Z., Zou, F., Chai, H. S., Younkin, C., et al. (2014). Association of MAPT haplotypes with Alzheimer's disease risk and MAPT brain gene expression levels. *Alzheimer's Res. Ther.* 6:39. doi: 10.1186/alzrt268

Arboleda-Velasquez, J. F., Lopera, F., O'Hare, M., Delgado-Tirado, S., Marino, C., Chmielewska, N., et al. (2019). Resistance to autosomal dominant Alzheimer's disease in an APOE3 Christchurch homozygote: a case report. *Nat. Med.* doi: 10.1038/s41591-019-0611-3 [Epub ahead of print].

Babić Leko, M., Willumsen, N., Nikolac Perković, M., Klepac, N., Borovečki, F., Hof, P. R., et al. (2018). Association of MAPT haplotype-tagging polymorphisms with cerebrospinal fluid biomarkers of Alzheimer's disease: a preliminary study in a croatian cohort. *Brain Behav.* 8:e01128. doi: 10.1002/brb3.1128

Baker, M., Litvan, I., Houlden, H., Adamson, J., Dickson, D., Perez-Tur, J., et al. (1999). Association of an extended haplotype in the tau gene with progressive supranuclear palsy. *Hum. Mol. Genet.* 8, 711–715. doi: 10.1093/hmg/8.4.711

Chen, J., Yu, J.-T., Wojta, K., Wang, H.-F., Zetterberg, H., Blennow, K., et al. (2017). Genome-wide association study identifies MAPT locus influencing human plasma tau levels. *Neurology* 88, 669–676. doi: 10.1212/WNL.0000000000003615

Clavaguera, F., Hench, J., Goedert, M., and Tolnay, M. (2015). Invited review: prion-like transmission and spreading of tau pathology. *Neuropathol. Appl. Neurobiol.* 41, 47–58. doi: 10.1111/nan.12197

Conrad, C., Andreadis, A., Trojanowski, J. Q., Dickson, D. W., Kang, D., Chen, X., et al. (1997). Genetic evidence for the involvement of tau in progressive supranuclear palsy. *Ann. Neurol.* 41, 277–281. doi: 10.1002/ana.410410222

Corvol, J.-C., and Buée, L. (2019). A new step towards targeting tau. *Lancet. Neurol.* 18, 517–518. doi: 10.1016/S1474-4422(19)30161-9

Donnelly, M. P., Paschou, P., Grigorenko, E., Gurwitz, D., Mehdi, S. Q., Kajuna, S. L. B., et al. (2010). The distribution and most recent common ancestor of the 17q21 inversion in humans. *Am. J. Hum. Genet.* 86, 161–171. doi: 10.1016/j.ajhg.2010.01.007

Dourlen, P., Kilinc, D., Malmanche, N., Chapuis, J., and Lambert, J.-C. (2019). The new genetic landscape of Alzheimer's disease: from amyloid cascade to genetically driven synaptic failure hypothesis? *Acta Neuropathol.* 138, 221–236. doi: 10.1007/s00401-019-02004-0

Goedert, M. (2004). Tau protein and neurodegeneration. *Sem. Cell Dev. Biol.* 15, 45–49. doi: 10.1016/j.semcdb.2003.12.015

Heckman, M. G., Brennan, R. R., Labbé, C., Soto, A. I., Koga, S., DeTure, M. A., et al. (2019). Association of MAPT Subhaplotypes with risk of progressive supranuclear palsy and severity of tau pathology. *JAMA Neurol.* 76, 710–717. doi: 10.1001/jamaneurol.2019.0250

Higgins, J. J., Golbe, L. I., De Biase, A., Jankovic, J., Factor, S. A., and Adler, R. L. (2000). An extended 5'-tau susceptibility haplotype in progressive supranuclear palsy. *Neurology* 55, 1364–1367. doi: 10.1212/wnl.55.9.1364

Holzer, M., Craxton, M., Jakes, R., Arendt, T., and Goedert, M. (2004). Tau gene (MAPT) sequence variation among primates. *Gene* 341, 313–322. doi: 10.1016/j.gene.2004.07.013

Houlden, H., Baker, M., Morris, H. R., MacDonald, N., Pickering-Brown, S., Adamson, J., et al. (2001). Corticobasal degeneration and progressive supranuclear palsy share a common tau haplotype. *Neurology* 56, 1702–1706. doi: 10.1212/wnl.56.12.1702

Jansen, W. J., Ossenkoppele, R., Knol, D. L., Tijms, B. M., Scheltens, P., Verhey, F. R. J., et al. (2015). Prevalence of cerebral amyloid pathology in persons without dementia: a meta-analysis. *JAMA* 313, 1924–1938. doi: 10.1001/jama.2015.4668

Jun, G., Ibrahim-Verbaas, C. A., Vronskaya, M., Lambert, J.-C., Chung, J., Naj, A. C., et al. (2016). A novel Alzheimer disease locus located near the gene encoding tau protein. *Mol. Psychiatry* 21, 108–117. doi: 10.1038/mp.2015.23

Kunkle, B. W., Grenier-Boley, B., Sims, R., Bis, J. C., Damotte, V., Naj, A. C., et al. (2019). Genetic meta-analysis of diagnosed Alzheimer's disease identifies new risk loci and implicates Aβ, tau, immunity and lipid processing. *Nat. Genet.* 51, 414–430. doi: 10.1038/s41588-019-0358-2

Kwok, J. B. J., Teber, E. T., Loy, C., Hallupp, M., Nicholson, G., Mellick, G. D., et al. (2004). Tau haplotypes regulate transcription and are associated with Parkinson's disease. *Ann. Neurol.* 55, 329–334. doi: 10.1002/ana.10826

Martin, E. R., Scott, W. K., Nance, M. A., Watts, R. L., Hubble, J. P., Koller, W. C., et al. (2001). Association of single-nucleotide polymorphisms of the tau gene with late-onset Parkinson disease. *JAMA* 286, 2245–2250.

Moreno-Grau, S., Rojas, I., de, Hernandez, I., Quintela, I., Montrreal, L., Alegret, M., et al. (2019). Genome-wide association analysis of dementia and its clinical endophenotypes reveal novel loci associated with Alzheimer disease and three causality networks of AD: the GR@ACE project. *bioRxiv.* [preprint]. doi: 10.1101/528901

Mukherjee, O., Kauwe, J. S. K., Mayo, K., Morris, J. C., and Goate, A. M. (2007). Haplotype-based association analysis of the MAPT locus in late onset Alzheimer's disease. *BMC Genet.* 8:3. doi: 10.1186/1471-2156-8-3

Myers, A. J., Kaleem, M., Marlowe, L., Pittman, A. M., Lees, A. J., Fung, H. C., et al. (2005). The H1c haplotype at the MAPT locus is associated with Alzheimer's disease. *Hum. Mol. Genet.* 14, 2399–2404. doi: 10.1093/hmg/ddi241

Myers, A. J., Pittman, A. M., Zhao, A. S., Rohrer, K., Kaleem, M., Marlowe, L., et al. (2007). The MAPT H1c risk haplotype is associated with increased expression of tau and especially of 4 repeat containing transcripts. *Neurobiol. Dis.* 25, 561–570. doi: 10.1016/j.nbd.2006.10.018

Nicoll, J. A. R., Buckland, G. R., Harrison, C. H., Page, A., Harris, S., Love, S., et al. (2019). Persistent neuropathological effects 14 years following amyloid-β immunization in Alzheimer's disease. *Brain* 142, 2113–2126. doi: 10.1093/brain/awz142

Pastor, P., Ezquerra, M., Perez, J. C., Chakraverty, S., Norton, J., Racette, B. A., et al. (2004). Novel haplotypes in 17q21 are associated with progressive supranuclear palsy. *Ann. Neurol.* 56, 249–258. doi: 10.1002/ana.20178

Pastor, P., Moreno, F., Clarimón, J., Ruiz, A., Combarros, O., Calero, M., et al. (2016). (MAPT)H1 haplotype is associated with late-onset Alzheimer's Disease risk in APOE ε4 noncarriers: results from the dementia genetics spanish consortium. *J. Alzheimer's Dis.* 49, 343–352. doi: 10.3233/JAD-150555

Pittman, A. M., Myers, A. J., Abou-Sleiman, P., Fung, H. C., Kaleem, M., Marlowe, L., et al. (2005). Linkage disequilibrium fine mapping and haplotype association analysis of the tau gene in progressive supranuclear palsy and corticobasal degeneration. *J. Med. Genet.* 42, 837–846. doi: 10.1136/jmg.2005.031377

Russ, C., Powell, J. F., Zhao, J., Baker, M., Hutton, M., Crawford, F., et al. (2001). The microtubule associated protein Tau gene and Alzheimer's disease–an association study and meta-analysis. *Neurosci. Lett.* 314, 92–96. doi: 10.1016/s0304-3940(01)02289-3

Schöll, M., Lockhart, S. N., Schonhaut, D. R., O'Neil, J. P., Janabi, M., Ossenkoppele, R., et al. (2016). PET imaging of tau deposition in the aging human brain. *Neuron* 89, 971–982. doi: 10.1016/j.neuron.2016.01.028

Simón-Sánchez, J., Schulte, C., Bras, J. M., Sharma, M., Gibbs, J. R., Berg, D., et al. (2009). Genome-wide association study reveals genetic risk underlying Parkinson's disease. *Nat. Genet.* 41, 1308–1312. doi: 10.1038/ng.487

Verpillat, P., Camuzat, A., Hannequin, D., Thomas-Anterion, C., Puel, M., Belliard, S., et al. (2002). Association between the extended tau haplotype and frontotemporal dementia. *Arch. Neurol.* 59, 935–939.

Yokoyama, J. S., Karch, C. M., Fan, C. C., Bonham, L. W., Kouri, N., Ross, O. A., et al. (2017). Shared genetic risk between corticobasal degeneration, progressive supranuclear palsy, and frontotemporal dementia. *Acta Neuropathol.* 133, 825–837. doi: 10.1007/s00401-017-1693-y

3

EFhd2 Affects Tau Liquid–Liquid Phase Separation

Irving E. Vega[1,2,3]*, *Andrew Umstead*[1] *and Nicholas M. Kanaan*[1,2,4]

[1] *Department of Translational Science and Molecular Medicine, College of Human Medicine, Grand Rapids, MI, United States,* [2] *Neuroscience Program, Michigan State University, Grand Rapids, MI, United States,* [3] *Department of Neurology, University of Michigan, Ann Arbor, MI, United States,* [4] *Hauenstein Neuroscience Center, Mercy Health Saint Mary's, Grand Rapids, MI, United States*

Correspondence:
Irving E. Vega
vegaie@msu.edu;
irvingvega@gmail.com

The transition of tau proteins from its soluble physiological conformation to the pathological aggregate forms found in Alzheimer's disease and related dementias, is poorly understood. Therefore, understanding the process that modulates the formation of toxic tau oligomers and their conversion to putative neuroprotective neurofibrillary tangles will lead to better therapeutic strategies. We previously identified that EFhd2 is associated with aggregated tau species in AD brains and the coiled-coil domain in EFhd2 mediates the interaction with tau. To further characterize the association between EFhd2 and tau, we examined whether EFhd2 could affect the liquid–liquid phase separation properties of tau under molecular crowding conditions. We demonstrate that EFhd2 alters tau liquid phase behavior in a calcium and coiled-coil domain dependent manner. Co-incubation of EFhd2 and tau in the absence of calcium leads to the formation of solid-like structures containing both proteins, while in the presence of calcium these two proteins phase separate together into liquid droplets. EFhd2's coiled-coil domain is necessary to alter tau's liquid phase separation, indicating that protein–protein interaction is required. The results demonstrate that EFhd2 affects the liquid–liquid phase separation of tau proteins *in vitro*, suggesting that EFhd2 modulates the structural dynamics of tau proteins.

Keywords: EFhd2, tau, liquid–liquid phase separation, neurodegeneration, tauopathy, Alzheimer's disease

INTRODUCTION

Proteinopathies are a group of diseases whose pathological hallmark is aberrant accumulation of protein aggregates (Dugger and Dickson, 2017; Sweeney et al., 2017). The molecular processes leading to the transition from physiological to pathological protein conformations is a research area of significant interest. The microtubule-associated protein tau undergoes transitions from soluble monomer to oligomer and subsequently into paired helical filaments that comprise the neurofibrillary tangles (NFTs), a pathological hallmark in Alzheimer's disease (AD) and other neurodegenerative disorders (Lee et al., 2001; Guo et al., 2017; Polanco et al., 2017). The molecular mechanisms involved in the formation and accumulation of tau aggregates is poorly understood. Several studies indicate that tau oligomers are a toxic form, while NFTs may represent a neuroprotective form due to sequestration of the more toxic tau species (Alonso et al., 2006; Vega et al., 2008; Kuchibhotla et al., 2014; Goedert and Spillantini, 2017). Understanding how these two thermodynamically different tau structures are formed and coexist is crucial to deciphering the molecular mechanisms involved in tau-mediated neurodegeneration.

We previously identified EFhd2 as a tau-associated protein in a tauopathy mouse model (JNPL3) and AD brains (Vega et al., 2008; Ferrer-Acosta et al., 2013a). EFhd2 is highly expressed in the central nervous system in comparison to other tissues but the function of neuronal EFhd2 is poorly understood (Vega et al., 2008). EFhd2 mouse and human protein sequences are 93% identical (Ferrer-Acosta et al., 2013b). EFhd2 is a 240 amino acid protein with two structural units mediating protein–protein interactions, a polyalanine motif at the N-terminus and a coiled-coil domain at the C-terminus (**Figure 1**). EFhd2 has two functional EF-hand motifs, demonstrating that EFhd2 is a calcium binding protein (Vega et al., 2008; Ferrer-Acosta et al., 2013b). Cdk5, a kinase associated with the pathophysiology of AD, phosphorylates EFhd2 at serine 74, significantly reducing its calcium binding activity (Vázquez-Rosa et al., 2014). Further characterization of the EFhd2-tau association demonstrated that EFhd2 colocalized with pathological tau in the somatodendric compartment in AD and this association is increasingly detected as neurodegeneration progresses in JNPL3 mice (Vega et al., 2008; Ferrer-Acosta et al., 2013a). EFhd2 co-purified with sarkosyl insoluble tau (Vega et al., 2008; Ferrer-Acosta et al., 2013a). Immuno-gold labeling of the sarkosyl insoluble tau fraction from AD temporal lobe demonstrated that EFhd2 and tau coexist in filamentous structures and electron microscopy analysis confirmed that EFhd2 self-associates forming filamentous structures *in vitro* (Ferrer-Acosta et al., 2013a). The presence of calcium reduces the formation of these structures and the coiled-coil domain is required for EFhd2 self-association (Ferrer-Acosta et al., 2013a). Deletion of EFhd2's coiled-coil domain also affected its associations with tau proteins, while deletion of the N-terminus had no effect (Ferrer-Acosta et al., 2013a). Recently, we demonstrated that incubation of EFhd2 with tau's three repeat domain promote the formation of amyloid structures as detected by increased Thioflavin S signal (Vega et al., 2018). However, it is unclear whether EFhd2 can modulate the formation of tau aggregates.

The physiological and pathological role of intracellular phase separation is starting to be appreciated as the formation of functional and dynamic entities within the cellular milieu (Aguzzi and Altmeyer, 2016; Banani et al., 2017). The ability of intrinsically disordered proteins to demix into liquid droplets or form solid-like structures suggests that mechanisms that regulate these transitions could demark the boundaries between health and diseased states (Aguzzi and Altmeyer, 2016; Banani et al., 2017). Recent studies showed that tau proteins can undergo liquid phase condensation *in vitro*, forming distinct and dynamic liquid droplets under molecular crowding conditions (Ambadipudi et al., 2017; Hernández-Vega et al., 2017; Shin and Brangwynne, 2017). Tau can facilitate tubulin polymerization, driving the nucleation of microtubules, within these liquid droplets (Ambadipudi et al., 2017). Thus, tau proteins preserve biological function within liquid droplets, suggesting that tau physiological and pathological functions could be mediated within distinct intracellular protein condensate states. Here, we demonstrate that EFhd2 forms solid-like and liquid droplets structures, which are mediated by its coiled-coil domain. We also show that EFhd2 modulates liquid–liquid phase separation behavior of tau, demonstrating, for the first time, that EFhd2 directly converts tau liquid phase behavior to solid-like structures *in vitro* and this phenomenon is controlled by calcium.

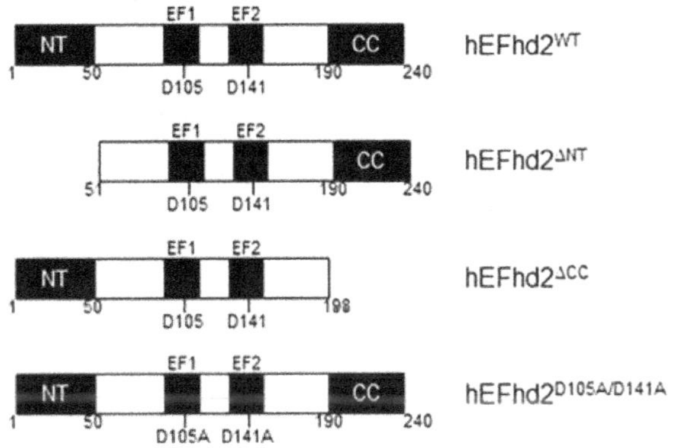

FIGURE 1 | Human EFhd2 protein. Illustrated representation of recombinant human proteins used in this study. EFhd2 is a 240 amino acids protein that has two EF-hand motifs that expand from amino acids 96–114 (EF1) and 132–160 (EF2). As part ate residues at the EF-loops mediate calcium binding. At the N-terminus (NT) has a poly-Alanine motif and a coiled-coil domain (CC) at the C-terminus. The illustration is not at scale.

MATERIALS AND METHODS

EFHD2 Gene Cloning

Human EFHD2 (Accession # Q96C19) wild type gene, N-terminal and C-terminal truncated and D105A/D141A mutants were produced by custom gene synthesis (Integrated DNA Technologies). The synthesized genes were subcloned into a bacterial expression vector pp-80L (5Prime Cat No. 2400850) in frame with an N-terminal 6x-Histidine tag, between *Bam*HI (5′ site) and *Hin*dIII (3′ site) restriction sites. After ligation, the plasmids were transformed into One Shot^{TM} BL21 (DE3) *E. coli* chemically competent cells (Thermo Fisher Scientific, Cat No. # C600003). Colonies were checked for protein expression. Plasmid DNA was extracted from colonies with positive expression of the expected protein molecular weight and subjected to DNA sequencing (GENEWIZ). Protein bands were also excised and subjected to trypsin in-gel digestion and tandem mass spectrometry analysis to confirm protein sequence (**Supplementary Figure 1**).

Recombinant Protein

For recombinant EFhd2 protein purification, a 50 mL LB/Ampicillin (50μ g/mL) pre-culture was incubated overnight at 37°C with constant shaking. 300 mL LB/Ampicillin was inoculated to 0.2 $OD_{600\ rmnm}$ using the saturated pre-culture and incubated at 37°C with constant shaking for 1 h or until the culture reach 0.5–0.7 $OD_{600\ nm}$. Then, IPTG was added to the culture to a final concentration of 0.5 mM. The culture was incubated for 3 h at 37°C. The culture was centrifuge at 10,000 rpm for 10 min at 4°C. The bacteria pellet was resuspended in 10 mL of Lysate Buffer [1x PBS with 5 mM Imidazole (pH 8.0)] and lysed by sonication on ice. The resulting lysate was centrifuged at 14,000 rpm for 10 min at 4°C. The supernatant was incubated with 500µ L of HIS-SELECT (Sigma, Cat No. # H0537-25 mL) beads (pre-calibrated in Lysate Buffer) and incubated overnight at 4°C with constant rotation. The beads were allowed to settle by gravity and the supernatant was removed. The beads were resuspended in 10 mL of Lysate buffer and transferred to an empty 10 mL column. The Lysate buffer was allowed to flow through until reaching the top of the beads bed and the recombinant protein was eluted with 500µ L of 1x PBS containing 250 mM Imidazole (pH 8.0). Four 500µ L fractions were collected and checked on SDS-PAGE. Those fractions containing recombinant protein were pooled and buffer exchanged to 1x PBS pH 8.0, using centricon spin filters 3 kDa cutoff. The final volume was 250µ L and concentration was kept below 3µ g/µL to prevent EFhd2 spontaneous self-aggregation. GFP tagged (Tau-GFP) and untagged (Tau) recombinant tau (Accession # P10636-8) proteins with C-terminal 6x poly-histidine tags were produced and purified as previously described (Combs et al., 2017). Briefly, T7 express *E. coli* cells were induced to express proteins with IPTG, followed by collection of cells and lysis of the cell pellet. Proteins were extracted through a three-step chromatography process with a GE Akta Pure system. First, proteins were purified on a Talon metal affinity resin column, the resulting proteins were further cleaned using size exclusion chromatography with an S500 column, and finally the samples were further polished over an anion exchange column. DTT (1 mM) was added to the proteins stocks, which were aliquoted and stored at −80°C until used for experiments.

Recombinant Protein Labeling and Quantification

The recombinant proteins were labeled using Alexa Fluor®594 Protein Labeling Kit (Molecular Probe Cat No. # A10238) or FluoReporter™ FITC Protein Labeling Kit (Molecular Probe Cat No. # F6436) following the manufacture instructions. Briefly, purified recombinant protein was buffer exchanged into 1x PBS. Sodium Bicarbonate was added to final concentration of 100 mM (1M stock solution). Then, 100 µL of purified recombinant protein was added to a vial of reactive dye. The labeling reaction was stirred for 1 h at room temperature. The labeled protein was purified using the provided resin bed and centrifugation at 1100 × *g* for 3 min. A protein series dilution and BSA as concentration standard (1, 2, 4, 8, 16 µg/µL) were resolved on SDS-PAGE and stained with Coomassie (R250). The distained gel was imaged in a GelDoc (BioRad) and the intensity of the stained protein bands was determined using the quantity tools of Image Lab software (Version 5.2.1 build 11).

Liquid–Liquid Phase Separation

A pre-determined concentration of labeled recombinant protein was diluted in 40µ L of reaction buffer containing 10% Polyethylene glycol (PEG) 3000 monodisperse solution, 10 mM HEPES (pH7.6), 150 mM NaCl, 5 mM DTT, and 0.1 mM EGTA. EGTA was not added when $CaCl_2$ was used in the reaction. The proteins were visualized using a confocal microscope at 60x with oil immersion (Nikon Confocal Microscope A1). All images were collected within 1 h after the samples were prepared. After each experiment, the samples were collected and 10 µL of the protein solution was resolved in SDS-PAGE and visualized by Coomassie staining. The presence of PEG induces a noticeable mobility shift on the migration of EFhd2 proteins in SDS-PAGE (**Figure 2B**). A mixture of recombinant Tau-GFP (2µ M) and Tau (2µ M) was used to avoid signal saturation. The experiments were repeated, at least, three times and independently validated in a different lab from recombinant protein purification to liquid phase separation.

Fluorescence Recovery After Photobleaching (FRAP) Analysis

EFhd2 samples were prepared as described in the Liquid–liquid phase separation section. Only samples with crowding agent (PEG 3000) plus or minus 10 mM $CaCl_2$ were subject to FRAP analysis. Briefly, at 60x magnification and 6x optical zooming, EFhd2 solid-like and liquid droplets were outlined with a circular overlay object and assigned as "stimulation" (bleaching) or "reference" (unbleached) (~8 per field of view). Similar number of circular objects were placed on areas without either of the structures and assigned as "background." This process was repeated in, at least, three different view fields, per sample. The FRAP parameters were as follows: a single pre-bleaching image (T0), bleaching at laser power set at 100 and 1 frame/2 s rate, an immediate post-bleach image, and several images over a total of 7 min. The FRAP curves were calculated by normalizing fluorescence signal to the background and reference signals was determined using these functions in the Nikon Elements Software. The extracted data was normalized to the intensity of the first image before photobleaching and analyzed in GraphPad Prism 6. The values were graph as mean and standard error of the mean. All imaging was done with the same acquisition settings (i.e., scan speed, resolution, magnification, optical zoom, gain, offset, and laser intensity).

RESULTS

EFhd2 Proteins Condense Into Distinct High-Order Structures

Previous studies showed that EFhd2 self-associates and forms amyloid structures in a concentration dependent manner and independent of nucleation factors such as heparin (Ferrer-Acosta et al., 2013a). Recently it was shown that tau, FUS, TDP3, and other amyloid proteins form liquid droplets under molecular crowding conditions, suggesting that these proteins may maintain different intracellular liquid phase states (Ambadipudi et al., 2017; Banani et al., 2017; Hernández-Vega et al., 2017; Shin and Brangwynne, 2017; Zhang et al., 2017). To determine if EFhd2 also undergoes liquid–liquid phase separation, both recombinant mouse and human EFhd2 protein orthologs were purified and labeled with fluorescent dyes. Labeled proteins were subjected to different conditions to induce liquid–liquid phase separation similar to that reported for tau and other proteins. In our experiments, PEG 3000 was used as a molecular crowding agent and the reaction buffer contained 150 mM NaCl. Recombinant EFhd2 protein was used at much lower concentrations (4–16 μM) than previously used to report its self-association (30–40 μM) (Ferrer-Acosta et al., 2013a).

The results demonstrate that EFhd2 condenses into different high order structures in response to specific chemical environments (**Figure 2**). In the absence of molecular crowding, EFhd2 did not undergo liquid–liquid phase separation (**Figure 2A**; −PEG/-$CaCl_2$ and −PEG/ + $CaCl_2$). In contrast, both mouse and human EFhd2 orthologs formed amorphous structures under molecular crowding (**Figure 2A**; +PEG/-$CaCl_2$) that resemble solid-like structures observed with other intrinsically disordered proteins (Patel et al., 2015; Zhang et al., 2017; Wegmann et al., 2018). In the presence of 10 mM calcium chloride ($CaCl_2$), EFhd2 formed liquid droplets like those formed by tau and other intrinsically disordered proteins. EFhd2 condensation is not due to the presence of the fluorescent tag, since EFhd2 labeled with two different fluorescent tags show the same protein dynamic in presence and absence of calcium (**Figure 2A**) and unlabeled EFhd2 proteins formed these same structures as observed using differential interference contrast in the transmitted light channel of the confocal microscope system (**Supplementary Figure 2**). Both mouse and human EFhd2 protein orthologs showed the same condensation behavior, indicating that EFhd2 condensation capacity is conserved. After confocal imaging, the protein samples were resolved in SDS-PAGE and visualized by Coomassie staining (**Figure 2B**). As previously reported, PEG affected the mobility of recombinant proteins in SDS-PAGE (Odom et al., 1997). This effect is due to changes in SDS-PAGE that affects the electrophoretic mobility of proteins that run behind the PEG front (Odom et al., 1997). Human EFhd2 protein was used in all subsequent experiments.

Previous studies, using fluorescence recovery after photobleaching (FRAP), showed that proteins within liquid droplets are highly dynamic, whereas proteins within solid-like structures are arrested in glassy solid or amyloid fiber states (Patel et al., 2015; Ambadipudi et al., 2017; Banani et al., 2017; Hernández-Vega et al., 2017; Riback et al., 2017; Shin and Brangwynne, 2017; Zhang et al., 2017; Wegmann et al., 2018). FRAP analyses were performed to determine the dynamic behavior of EFhd2 within the two condensate states (**Figure 2C**). EFhd2 liquid-droplets' fluorescence signal recovered ~50% after photobleaching (**Figure 2C**). However, EFhd2's solid-like structures, formed in the absence of calcium, did not show FRAP. These results confirmed the dynamic nature of EFhd2's droplets formed in the presence of calcium and the static structure of the solid-like state in absence of calcium. Additionally, the results suggest that calcium enhances EFhd2 protein dynamics.

Mutation of EFhd2's Calcium Binding Sites Prevents Liquid-Droplet Formation

We conducted several controls experiments to study the effect that calcium has on EFhd2 protein dynamics. To determine if NaCl contributes, in combination with $CaCl_2$, to EFhd2 condensation, experiments were performed in the absence of 150 mM NaCl and under molecular crowding conditions (**Supplementary Figure 3**). Even with the absence of 150 mM NaCl, EFhd2 formed solid-like and liquid droplet structures in absence or presence of $CaCl_2$, respectively, under crowding conditions (**Supplementary Figure 3**). The same results were obtained in experiments containing 2 mM NaCl in the presence and absence of $CaCl_2$ (data not shown). These results demonstrate that NaCl does not play a role in EFhd2 condensation. We also assessed whether other divalent ions, such as Mg^{2+}, could contribute to EFhd2 changes in protein dynamic (**Supplementary Figure 4**). Recombinant EFhd2 incubated in different concentrations of $MgCl_2$ did not form liquid droplets under molecular crowding conditions (**Supplementary Figure 4**). These results indicate that calcium ions, and neither chloride nor other divalent ions, play an important role in EFhd2 protein dynamics. Additionally, electrostatic interaction in aqueous salt solutions does not drive the observed structures.

To determine if the integrity of EFhd2's calcium binding sites are required for the formation of liquid-droplets, we used human EFhd2 protein bearing a missense mutation of conserved aspartate residues (D105A and D141A) within each EF-hand motif (**Figure 1**). We and others previously demonstrated that mutating these aspartate residues to alanine render EFhd2 unable to bind calcium (Ferrer-Acosta et al., 2013a; Park et al., 2016). hEFhd2$^{D105A/D141A}$ formed solid-like structures in the absence and presence of crowding agent (**Figure 3**). The addition of calcium did not promote the formation of liquid droplets (**Figure 3**). These results indicate that mutation of EFhd2's calcium binding sites affects the formation of EFhd2 liquid droplet but not solid-like structures. Importantly, since all EFhd2 recombinant proteins used are 6x His-tagged, this experiment also helps rule out the effect that 6x His-tagging could exert on the formation of EFhd2 liquid droplets. The result indicates that calcium and not the 6x His-tagged is what promotes the formation of EFhd2 liquid droplets.

EFhd2's Coiled-Coil Domain Is Required for Liquid–Liquid Phase Separation

Previously, we demonstrated that deletion of EFhd2's coiled-coil domain affected its dimerization and association with tau proteins, while deletion of the N-terminus did not affect these protein–protein interactions (Ferrer-Acosta et al., 2013a). To demonstrate that EFhd2 condensation behavior is due to intermolecular interaction and not solely to the presence of the crowding agent, we investigated the role that the N-terminus and coiled-coil domain play in liquid–liquid phase separation (**Figure 4**). The EFhd2 N-terminal truncation mutant (hEFhd2$^{\Delta NT}$) formed solid-like structures when calcium was absent and liquid droplets when calcium was present under molecular crowding conditions, similar to the structures observed with wild type EFhd2 (hEFhd2^{WT}; **Figure 4**). The results indicate that the N-terminus is not required for the formation of EFhd2's solid-like structures

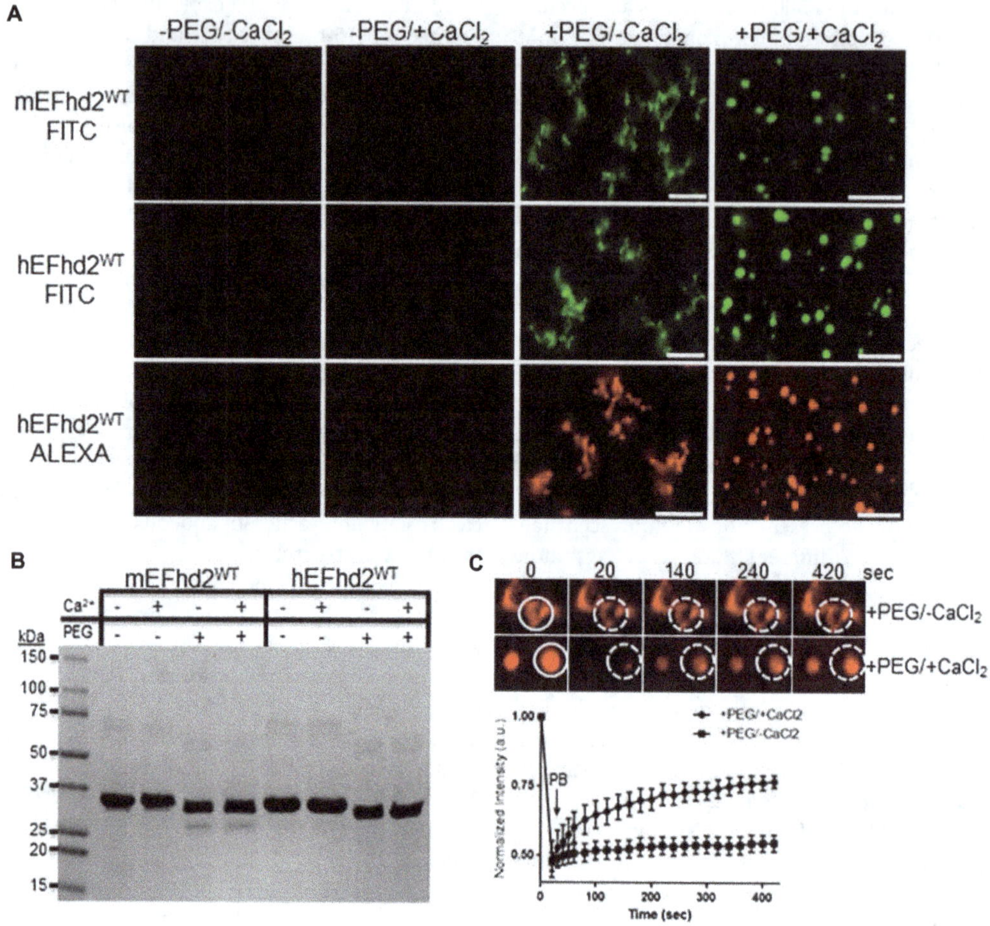

FIGURE 2 | EFhd2 condense into distinct high-order structures. **(A)** Mouse (mEFhd2) and human (hEFhd2) EFhd2 orthologous were labeled with fluorescence dyes (FITC or ALEXA). The labeled proteins (16 gμM) were subjected to liquid–liquid phase separation in absence (–PEG) or presence (+PEG) of 10% Polyethylene glycol (PEG) as crowding agent plus or minus 10 mM $CaCl_2$ and visualized by confocal microscopy. **(B)** Representative Coomassie stained protein gel of mEFhd2 and hEFhd2 proteins used. **(C)** Human EFhd2 wild type protein (16 μM) in the presence or absence of 10 mM $CaCl_2$ was subjected to fluorescence recovery after photobleaching (FRAP). The graph shows fluorescence recovery with time in seconds (sec) after photo-bleaching (PB). The intensity was normalized to the first time point before photo-bleaching and shown as the mean and standard error of the mean (SEM), $n = 8$. The white circles illustrate the photobleached (PB) area in the sample without $CaCl_2$- The images are representative of, at least, three independent experiments. Scale bar = 10 μm.

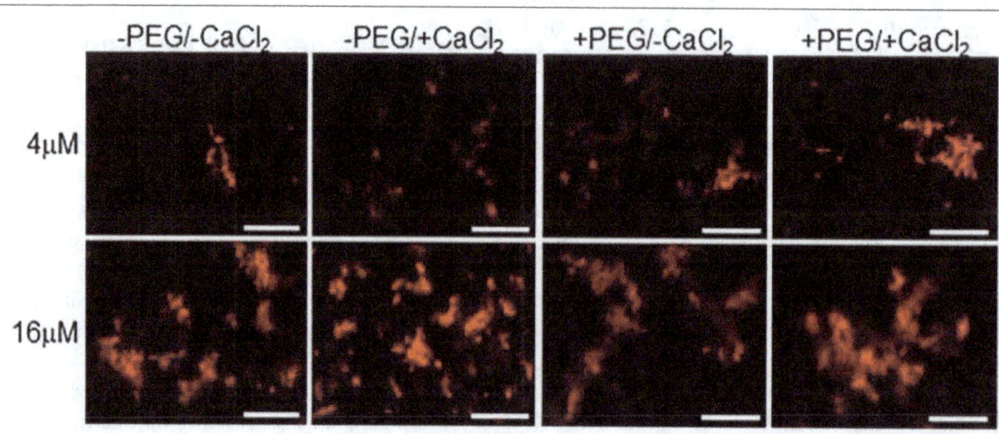

FIGURE 3 | Calcium binding drives EFhd2 liquid-droplet formation. Human EFhd2 D105A/DH41A mutant was subjected to liquid–liquid phase separation in absence [–PEG) or presence [+PEG) of 10% Polyethylene glycol (PEG) as crowding agent plus or minus 10 mM $CaCl_2$- The proteins were visualized by confocal microscopy. The images are representative of, at least, three independent experiments. Scale bar = 10 μm.

or liquid droplets (**Figure 4**). In contrast, deletion of the C-terminus coiled-coil domain (hEFhd2$^{\Delta CC}$) prevented EFhd2 condensation (**Figure 4**). hEFhd2$^{\Delta CC}$ protein did not undergo liquid–liquid phase separation in the absence or presence of crowding agent and calcium, indicating that while calcium changes structural dynamics, the coiled-coil domain is required for EFhd2 phase condensation. These results indicate that EFhd2 liquid condensation is mediated by protein–protein interaction. Under the same conditions and protein concentration used for EFhd2, recombinant tau formed liquid droplets similar to those previously reported in the presence or absence of $CaCl_2$ (**Figure 4**) (Patel et al., 2015; Ambadipudi et al., 2017; Hernández-Vega et al., 2017; Riback et al., 2017; Zhang et al., 2017; Wegmann et al., 2018). Thus, calcium does not affect tau liquid phase condensation as it does for EFhd2 (**Figure 4**).

EFhd2 Protein Affects Tau Liquid–Liquid Phase Separation

The effect that EFhd2 has on tau proteins and its role in tauopathy is still unknown. Since both EFhd2 and tau undergo liquid–liquid phase separation, we assessed whether EFhd2 could influence tau liquid phase separation. Recombinant EFhd2 (red) and tau (green) proteins were combined at equimolar concentration in conditions that induced liquid–liquid phase

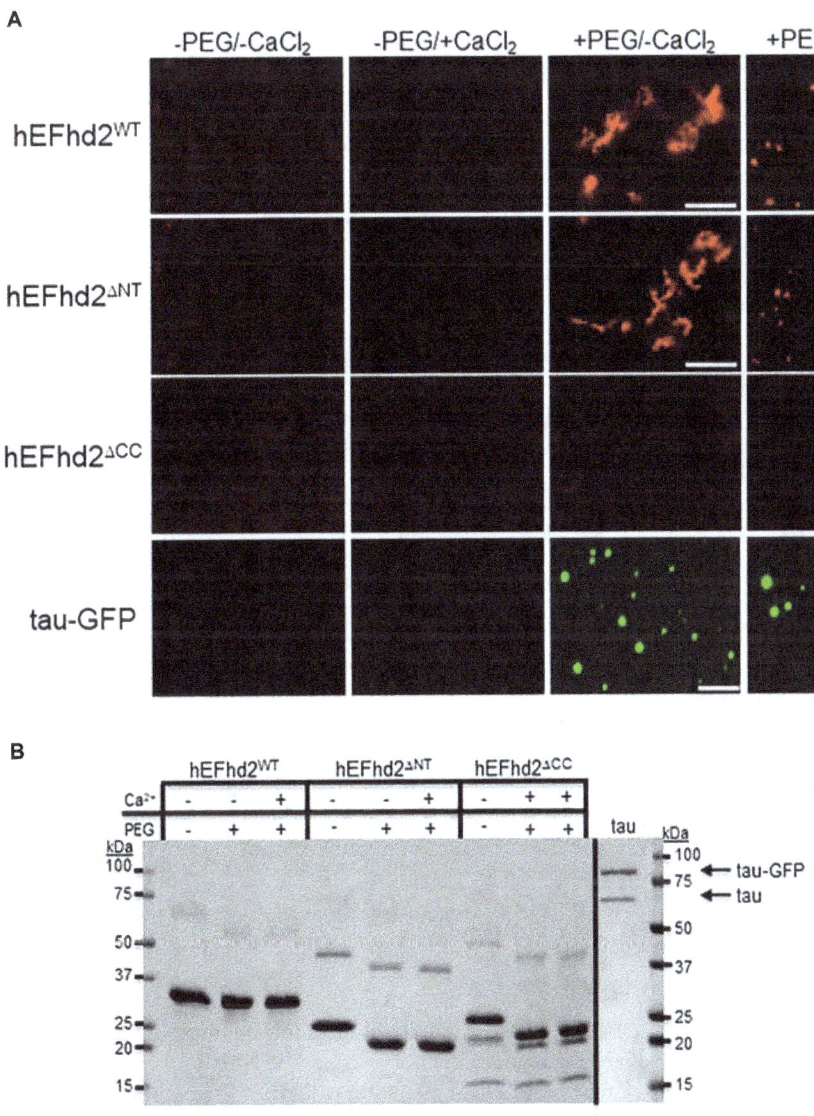

FIGURE 4 | Coiled-coil domain is required for EFhd2 liquid–liquid phase separation. **(A)** Wild type human EFhd2 (hEFhd2^{WT}), N-terminal (hEFhd2$^{\Delta NT}$), and coiled-coil (hEFhd2$^{\Delta CC}$) truncated mutants ALEXA-labeled recombinant proteins (4 μM) were subjected to liquid–liquid phase separation in absence (–PEG) or presence (+PEG) of 10% Polyethylene glycol (PEG) as crowding agent plus or minus 10 mM $CaCl_2$-Recombinant tau (4 μM) was subjected to the same conditions as EFhd2. **(B)** EFhd2 wild type (WT), N-terminal (ΔNT), and coiled-coil (ΔCC) truncation mutant proteins and Tau proteins were resolved in SDS-PAGED and visualized by Coomassie blue staining. The images are representative of, at least, three independent experiments. Scale bar = 10 μm.

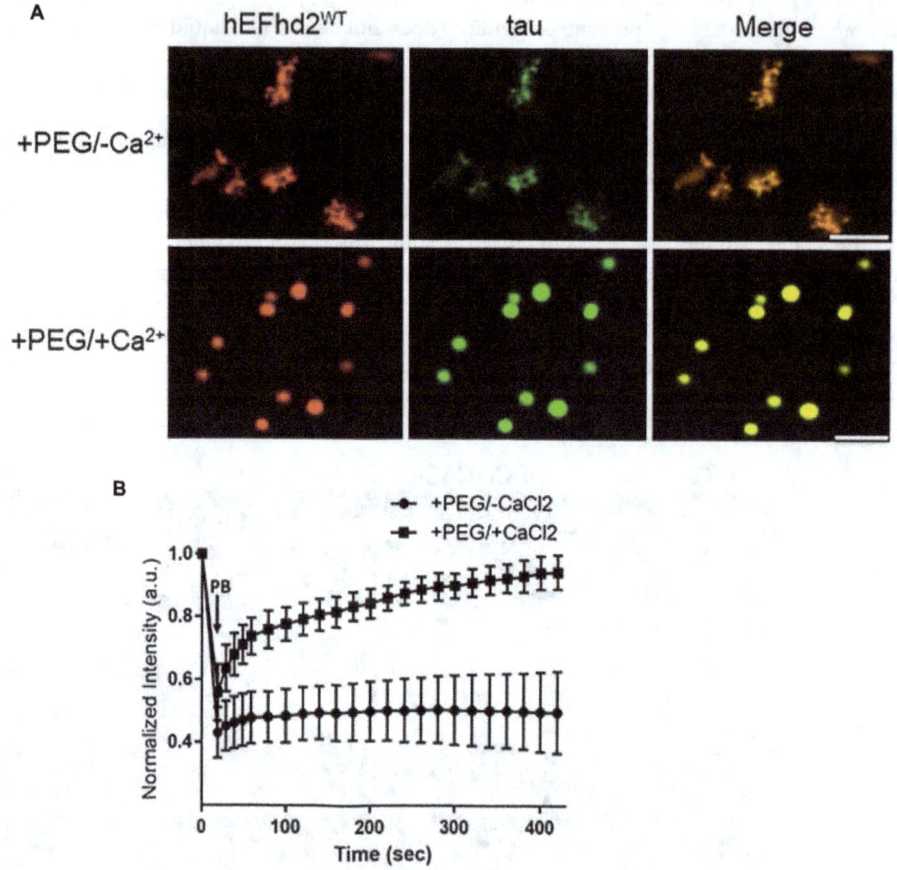

FIGURE 5 | EFhd2 affects tau liquid–liquid phase separation. **(A)** Wild type human EFhd2 (hEFhd2^{WT}) recombinant protein (4 μM) and equimolar concentration of recombinant tau (4 μM) were subjected to liquid–liquid phase separation in absence (–PEG; not shown) or presence (+PEG) of 10% Polyethylene glycol (PEG) as crowding agent plus or minus 10 mM $CaCl_2$- The images are representative of, at least, three independent experiments. Scale bar = 10 μm. **(B)** Co-incubated EFhd2 wild type protein (4 μM) and tau (4 μM) in the presence or absence of 10 mM $CaCl_2$ was subjected to FRAP. The graph shows fluorescence recovery with time in seconds (sec) after photo-bleaching (PB). The intensity was normalized to the first time point before photo-bleaching and shown as the mean and standard error of the mean (SEM) through time, *n* = 11.

separation (**Figure 5**). As expected, EFhd2 and tau did not demix in the absence of the crowding agent (**Supplementary Figure 5**). In contrast, EFhd2 and tau co-localized in solid-like structures in the presence of the crowding agent and absence of calcium (**Figure 5A**; +PEG/-Ca^{2+}). As shown on **Figure 3**, tau alone forms liquid droplets while EFhd2 forms solid-like structures under this condition. Thus, this result indicates that EFhd2 changes tau proteins liquid phase separation to solid-like structures. Conversely, EFhd2 and tau come together into liquid droplets in the presence of calcium and crowding agent (**Figure 5A**; +PEG/ + Ca^{2+}). To further assess the effect that EFhd2 has on tau liquid–liquid phase separation, we conducted FRAP analyses of co-incubated EFhd2 and tau in presence and absence of calcium under molecular crowding conditions (**Figure 5B**). The results showed that solid-like structures did not recover after photobleaching, confirming that these structures formed by EFhd2 and tau are not dynamic (**Figure 5B**). In contrast, EFhd2-tau droplets formed in the presence of calcium showed recovery after photobleaching, indicating that calcium influences the molecular dynamics of EFhd2-tau structures formed under molecular crowding conditions.

To determine if EFhd2 concentration plays a role in its effect on tau liquid–liquid phase separation, submolar concentrations of recombinant EFhd2 were incubated with 4 μM of recombinant tau in absence of $CaCl_2$ under molecular crowding conditions (**Figure 6**). In the absence of calcium, EFhd2 at 1 and 2 μM promoted the formation of solid-like structures containing both EFhd2 and tau proteins (**Figure 6**). No tau droplets were observed despite the lower concentration of EFhd2, indicating that submolar EFhd2 concentrations can affect tau dynamics. These results indicate that EFhd2 modulates tau condensate phase behavior *in vitro*.

Deletion of EFhd2 N-terminus does not affect its association with tau proteins (Ferrer-Acosta et al., 2013a). Thus, we investigated whether EFhd2 N-terminal truncation mutant (EFhd2$^{\Delta NT}$) could affect tau liquid phase behavior as shown with wild type EFhd2 (**Figure 7**). EFhd2$^{\Delta NT}$ and tau co-localized in amyloid structures in the presence of crowding agent without calcium (**Figure 6**; +PEG/-Ca^{2+}) and in liquid

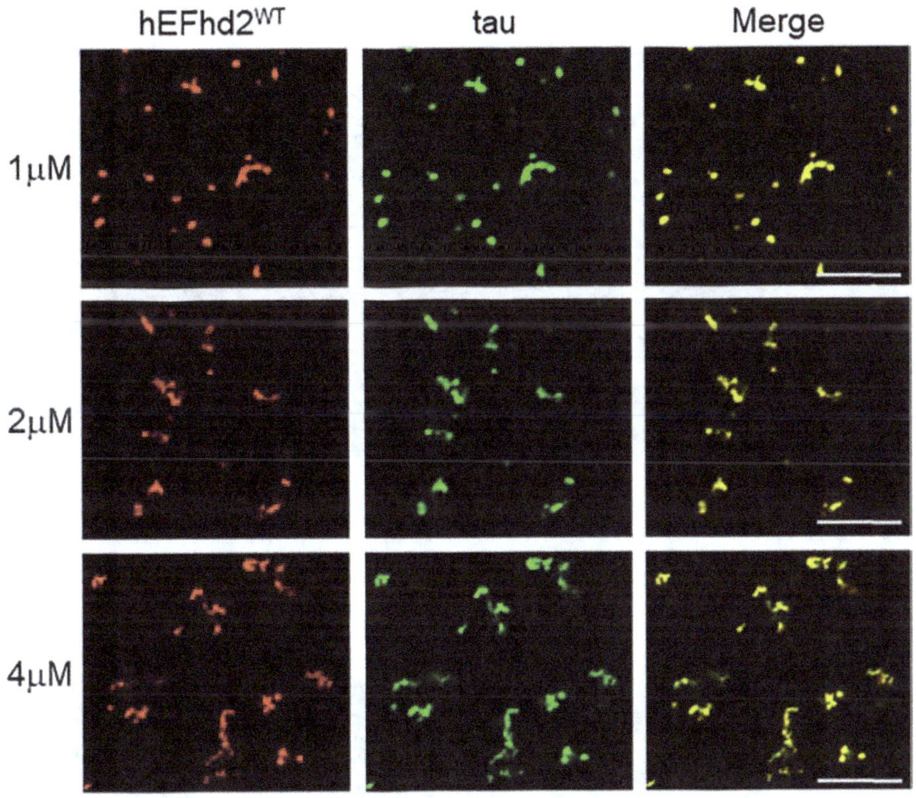

FIGURE 6 | EFhd2 submolar concentrations promotes the formation of tau solid-like structures in absence of calcium. Wild type human EFhd2 (hEFhd2^{WT}) recombinant protein at 1, 2, and 4 μM concentrations with recombinant tau (4 μM) were subjected to liquid–liquid phase separation in presence of 10% Polyethylene glycol (PEG) as crowding agent without $CaCl_2$. The images are representative of, at least, three independent experiments. Scale bar = 10 μm.

droplets when incubated with crowding agent and calcium (**Figure 6**; +PEG/ + Ca^{2+}). These results indicate that EFhd2's N-terminus is not required to affect tau liquid phase behavior *in vitro*.

Previously, we showed that EFhd2's coiled-coil domain is required for its association with tau proteins (Ferrer-Acosta et al., 2013a). Therefore, we investigated the role of EFhd2's coiled-coil domain in affecting tau liquid phase behavior (**Figure 8**). As shown in **Figure 3**, EFhd2 coiled-coil domain deletion mutant (EFhd2$^{\Delta CC}$) did not form detectable liquid-droplets or solid-like structures. Moreover, EFhd2$^{\Delta CC}$ did not affect tau liquid phase separation in the presence of crowding agent and calcium (**Figure 8**). This result indicates that EFhd2's coiled-coil domain is required to affect tau's liquid phase behavior, suggesting that protein–protein interactions drive EFhd2 modulation of tau condensate state.

DISCUSSION

EFhd2 condensate phase behavior ranges from solid-like to liquid droplets structures under crowding conditions. In the absence of calcium, EFhd2 is arrested in solid-like structures that are not dynamic, while calcium induces the formation of dynamic EFhd2 liquid droplets. These results indicate that the concentration of calcium and/or regulatory signals that modulate EFhd2's calcium binding capacity can have an impact on EFhd2 protein dynamics. The coiled-coil domain is required to form solid-like and liquid droplet structures, indicating that EFhd2 protein–protein interaction drives the formation of these structures while calcium promotes enhanced EFhd2 protein dynamics. These changes in protein dynamics may have consequences on EFhd2 physiology. For example, EFhd2 serves as a scaffold for the function of Syk, SLP-65, and PLCγ2 downstream of the activation of the B-cell receptor, inducing calcium influx (Kroczek et al., 2010). EFhd2 has also facilitates F-actin remodeling necessary for migration and invasion of cancer cells (Huh et al., 2013, 2015; Park et al., 2016). Although the role of calcium signaling dysregulation in cancer cells is still poorly understood, increases in calcium levels could be the driving force to facilitate the effect of EFhd2 on nucleation and polymerization of actin filaments.

We also show that EFhd2 affects tau's condensate phase behavior. EFhd2, in the absence of calcium, promotes tau to co-localize in solid-like structures. In the presence of calcium, however, EFhd2 and tau phase separate together into liquid droplets. The effect that EFhd2 has on tau condensate phase behaviors requires EFhd2's coiled-coil domain, indicating that EFhd2 interaction with tau proteins affects tau condensate phase behavior.

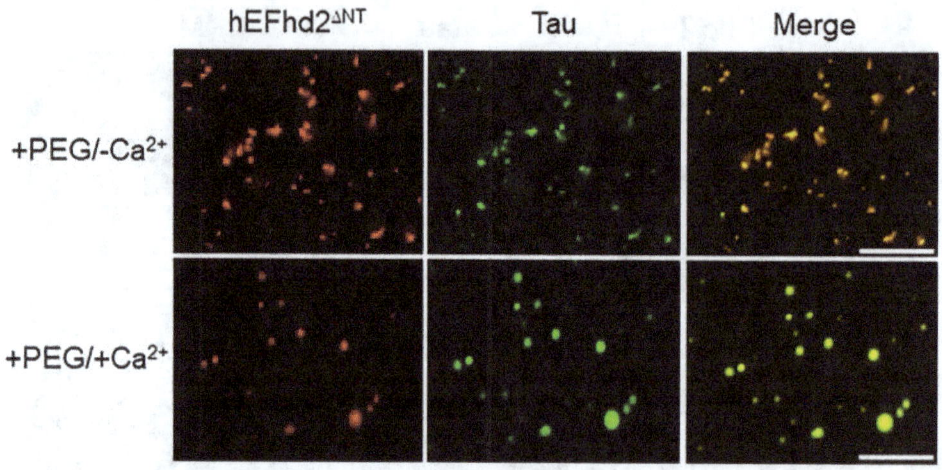

FIGURE 7 | EFhd2 N-terminus is not required for affecting Tau liquid phase condensation, human EFhd2 NT-terminal truncation mutant (hEFhd2$^{\Delta NT}$) protein (4 μM) and equimolar concentration of recombinant Tau (4 μM) were subjected to liquid–liquid phase separation in presence (+PEG) of 10% Polyethylene glycol (PEG) as crowding agent plus or minus 10 mM $CaCl_2$- The images are representative of, at least, three independent experiments.

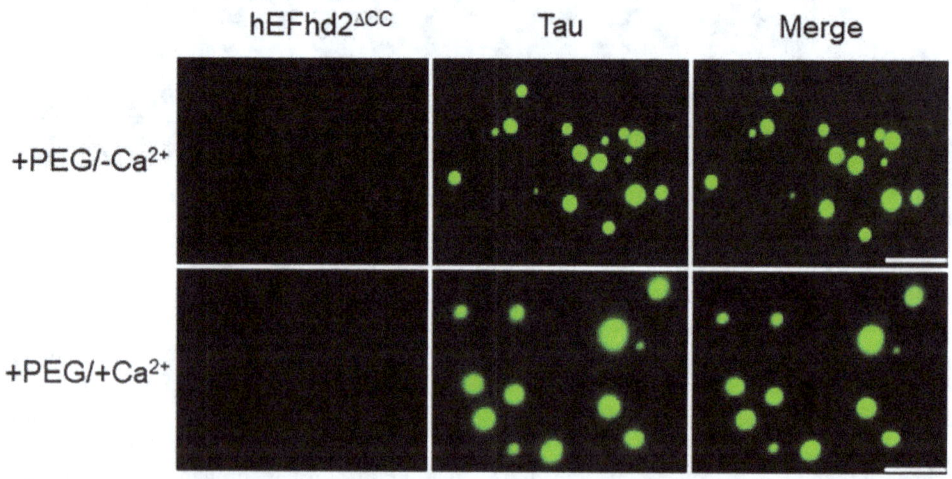

FIGURE 8 | EFhd2 coiled-coil domain is required for affecting Tau liquid phase condensation, human EFhd2 coiled-coil deletion mutant (hEFhd2$^{\Delta CC}$) protein (4 μM) and equimolar concentration of recombinant Tau (4 μM) were subjected to liquid–liquid phase separation in presence (+PEG) of 10% Polyethylene glycol (PEG) as crowding agent plus or minus 10 mM $CaCl_2$- The images are representative of, at least, three independent experiments. Scale bar = 10 μm.

The role that EFhd2 plays in neurodegeneration is still unclear (Vega, 2016). The association of EFhd2 and tau in AD, identification of EFhd2 and tau in filamentous structures, their colocalization in the somatodendritic compartment and copurification in the sarkosyl-insoluble fraction indicates that EFhd2 is associated with pathological tau in AD (Vega et al., 2008; Ferrer-Acosta et al., 2013a). We previously showed that Cdk5 phosphorylation of EFhd2 affects its calcium binding capacity (Vázquez-Rosa et al., 2014). Hyperactivation of Cdk5 in AD brain is associated with phosphorylation of tau proteins, leading to its dissociation from microtubules and formation of oligomers (Wilkaniec et al., 2016). Taken together, hyperactivated Cdk5 could phosphorylate EFhd2, affecting its calcium binding activity and, consequently, its protein dynamics. The accumulation of EFhd2 in solid-like state could then drive tau aggregation into oligomers and/or NFTs. Further studies are required to test this working hypothesis.

CONCLUSION

The data provide further evidence that EFhd2 shares molecular and biochemical characteristics with known intrinsically disordered proteins associated with neurodegenerative diseases. This suggests that EFhd2 may play an important role in the pathophysiology of neurodegenerative diseases. In this regard, EFhd2 expression is increased in substantia nigra and was found associated with Lrrk2 in Parkinson's disease (Meixner et al., 2011; Liscovitch and French, 2014). EFhd2 was also identified as associated with poly-GA C9Orf72 aggregates in amyotrophic lateral sclerosis and frontotemporal lobar degeneration, suggesting that EFhd2 may modulate the formation of pathological protein aggregates other than tau (May et al., 2014). Further characterization of EFhd2's role in AD and other neurological disorders could lead to better understanding of the transition from physiological to pathological protein conformations that could serve as the basis for the identification of therapeutic strategies.

AUTHOR CONTRIBUTIONS

IV did the experimental design, conducted the experiments, analyzed the data, and prepared the manuscript. AU performed the experiments, contributed to the data analysis, and proofread the manuscript. NK provided the purified recombinant tau protein, contributed to the data analysis, and proofread the manuscript.

ACKNOWLEDGMENTS

Thanks to Dr. Roger Albin for the critical reading of the manuscript.

REFERENCES

Aguzzi, A., and Altmeyer, M. (2016). Phase separation: linking cellular compartmentalization to disease. *Trends Cell Biol.* 26, 547–558. doi: 10.1016/j.tcb.2016.03.004

Alonso, A. C., Li, B., Grundke-Iqbal, I., and Iqbal, K. (2006). Polymerization of hyperphosphorylated tau into filaments eliminates its inhibitory activity. *Proc. Natl. Acad. Sci. U.S.A.* 103, 8864–8869. doi: 10.1073/pnas.0603214103

Ambadipudi, S., Biernat, J., Riedel, D., Mandelkow, E., and Zweckstetter, M. (2017). Liquid-liquid phase separation of the microtubule-binding repeats of the Alzheimer-related protein Tau. *Nat. Commun.* 8:275. doi: 10.1038/s41467-017-00480-0

Banani, S. F., Lee, H. O., Hyman, A. A., and Rosen, M. K. (2017). Biomolecular condensates: organizers of cellular biochemistry. *Nat. Rev. Mol. Cell Biol.* 18, 285–298. doi: 10.1038/nrm.2017.7

Combs, B., Tiernan, C. T., Hamel, C., and Kanaan, N. M. (2017). Production of recombinant tau oligomers in vitro. *Methods Cell Biol.* 141, 45–64. doi: 10.1016/bs.mcb.2017.06.005

Dugger, B. N., and Dickson, D. W. (2017). Pathology of neurodegenerative diseases. *Cold Spring Harb. Perspect. Biol.* 9:a028035. doi: 10.1101/cshperspect.a028035

Ferrer-Acosta, Y., Rodríguez-Cruz, E. N., Orange, F., De Jesús-Cortés, H., Madera, B., Vaquer-Alicea, J., et al. (2013a). EFhd2 is a novel amyloid protein associated with pathological tau in Alzheimer's disease. *J. Neurochem.* 125, 921–931. doi: 10.1111/jnc.12155

Ferrer-Acosta, Y., Rodríguez Cruz, E. N., Vaquer, A., del, C., and Vega, I. E. (2013b). Functional and structural analysis of the conserved EFhd2 protein. *Protein Pept. Lett.* 20, 573–583. doi: 10.2174/0929866511320050011

Goedert, M., and Spillantini, M. G. (2017). Propagation of Tau aggregates. *Mol. Brain.* 10:18. doi: 10.1186/s13041-017-0298-7

Guo, T., Noble, W., and Hanger, D. P. (2017). Roles of tau protein in health and disease. *Acta Neuropathol.* 133, 665–704. doi: 10.1007/s00401-017-1707-9

Hernández-Vega, A., Braun, M., Scharrel, L., Jahnel, M., Wegmann, S., Hyman, B. T., et al. (2017). Local nucleation of microtubule bundles through tubulin concentration into a condensed tau phase. *Cell Rep.* 20, 2304–2312. doi: 10.1016/j.celrep.2017.08.042

Huh, Y. H., Kim, S. H., Chung, K. H., Oh, S., Kwon, M. S., Choi, H. W., et al. (2013). Swiprosin-1 modulates actin dynamics by regulating the F-actin accessibility to cofilin. *Cell. Mol. Life Sci.* 70, 4841–4854. doi: 10.1007/s00018-013-1447-5

Huh, Y. H., Oh, S., Yeo, Y. R., Chae, I. H., Kim, S. H., Lee, J. S., et al. (2015). Swiprosin-1 stimulates cancer invasion and metastasis by increasing the Rho family of GTPase signaling. *Oncotarget* 6, 13060–13071. doi: 10.18632/oncotarget.3637

Kroczek, C., Lang, C., Brachs, S., Grohmann, M., Dütting, S., Schweizer, A., et al. (2010). Swiprosin-1/EFhd2 controls B cell receptor signaling through the assembly of the B cell receptor, Syk, and phospholipase C gamma2 in membrane rafts. *J. Immunol.* 184, 3665–3676. doi: 10.4049/jimmunol.0903642

Kuchibhotla, K. V., Wegmann, S., Kopeikina, K. J., Hawkes, J., Rudinskiy, N., Andermann, M. L., et al. (2014). Neurofibrillary tangle-bearing neurons are functionally integrated in cortical circuits in vivo. *Proc. Natl. Acad. Sci. U.S.A.* 111, 510–514. doi: 10.1073/pnas.1318807111

Lee, V. M.-Y., Goedert, M., and Trojanowski, J. Q. (2001). Neurodegenerative tauopathies. *Annu. Rev. Neurosci.* 24, 1121–1159. doi: 10.1006/exnr.1993.1074

Liscovitch, N., and French, L. (2014). Differential co-expression between α-Synuclein and IFN-γ signaling genes across development and in Parkinson's disease. *PLoS One.* 9:e115029. doi: 10.1371/journal.pone.0115029

May, S., Hornburg, D., Schludi, M. H., Arzberger, T., Rentzsch, K., Schwenk, B. M., et al. (2014). C9orf72 FTLD/ALS-associated Gly-Ala dipeptide repeat proteins cause neuronal toxicity and Unc119 sequestration. *Acta Neuropathol.* 128, 485–503. doi: 10.1007/s00401-014-1329-4

Meixner, A., Boldt, K., Van Troys, M., Askenazi, M., Gloeckner, C. J., Bauer, M., et al. (2011). A QUICK screen for Lrrk2 interaction partners–leucine-rich repeat kinase 2 is involved in actin cytoskeleton dynamics. *Mol. Cell. Proteomics* 10, M110.001172. doi: 10.1074/mcp.M110.001172

Odom, O. W., Kudlicki, W., Kramer, G., and Hardesty, B. (1997). An effect of polyethylene glycol 8000 on protein mobility in sodium dodecyl sulfate-polyacrylamide gel electrophoresis and a method for eliminating this effect. *Anal. Biochem.* 245, 249–252. doi: 10.1006/abio.1996.9993

Park, K. R., Kwon, M. S., An, J. Y., Lee, J. G., Youn, H. S., Lee, Y., et al. (2016). Structural implications of Ca2+-dependent actin-bundling function of human EFhd2/Swiprosin-1. *Sci. Rep.* 6:39095. doi: 10.1038/srep39095

Patel, A., Lee, H. O., Jawerth, L., Maharana, S., Jahnel, M., Hein, M. Y., et al. (2015). A Liquid-to-solid phase transition of the ALS protein FUS accelerated by disease mutation. *Cell* 162, 1066–1077. doi: 10.1016/j.cell.2015.07.047

Polanco, J. C., Li, C., Bodea, L. G., Martinez-Marmol, R., Meunier, F. A., and Götz, J. (2017). Amyloid-β and tau complexity - towards improved biomarkers and targeted therapies. *Nat. Rev. Neurol.* 14, 22–39. doi: 10.1038/nrneurol.2017.162

Riback, J. A., Katanski, C. D., Kear-Scott, J. L., Pilipenko, E. V., Rojek, A. E., Sosnick, T. R., et al. (2017). Stress-Triggered phase separation is an adaptive, evolutionarily tuned response. *Cell* 168, 1028–1040. doi: 10.1016/j.cell.2017.02.027

Shin, Y., and Brangwynne, C. P. (2017). Liquid phase condensation in cell physiology and disease. *Science* 357:eaaf4382. doi: 10.1126/science.aaf4382

Sweeney, P., Park, H., Baumann, M., Dunlop, J., Frydman, J., Kopito, R., et al. (2017). Protein misfolding in neurodegenerative diseases: implications and strategies. *Transl. Neurodegener.* 6:6. doi: 10.1186/s40035-017-0077-5

Vázquez-Rosa, E., Rodríguez-Cruz, E. N., Serrano, S., Rodríguez-Laureano, L., and Vega, I. E. (2014). Cdk5 phosphorylation of EFhd2 at S74 affects its calcium binding activity. *Protein Sci.* 23, 1197–1207. doi: 10.1002/pro.2499

Vega, I. E. (2016). EFhd2, a protein linked to Alzheimer's disease and other neurological disorders. *Front. Neurosci.* 10:150. doi: 10.3389/fnins.2016.00150

Vega, I. E., Sutter, A., Parks, L., Umstead, A., and Ivanova, M. I. (2018). Tau's three-repeat domain and EFhd2 co-incubation leads to increased thioflavin signal. *Front. Neurosci.* 12:879. doi: 10.3389/fnins.2018.00879

Vega, I. E., Traverso, E. E., Ferrer-Acosta, Y., Matos, E., Colon, M., Gonzalez, J., et al. (2008). A novel calcium-binding protein is associated with tau proteins in tauopathy. *J. Neurochem.* 106, 96–106. doi: 10.1111/j.1471-4159.2008.05339.x

Wegmann, S., Eftekharzadeh, B., Tepper, K., Zoltowska, K. M., Bennett, R. E., Dujardin, S., et al. (2018). Tau protein liquid-liquid phase separation can initiate tau aggregation. *EMBO J.* 37:e98049. doi: 10.15252/embj.20179804

Wilkaniec, A., Czapski, G. A., and Adamczyk, A. (2016). Cdk5 at crossroads of protein oligomerization in neurodegenerative diseases: facts and hypotheses. *J. Neurochem.* 136, 222–233. doi: 10.15252/embj.201798049

Zhang, X., Lin, Y., Eschmann, N. A., Zhou, H., Rauch, J. N., Hernandez, I., et al. (2017). RNA stores tau reversibly in complex coacervates. *PLoS Biol.* 15:e2002183. doi: 10.1371/journal.pbio.2002183

4

Genetic Background Influences the Propagation of Tau Pathology in Transgenic Rodent Models of Tauopathy

Tomas Smolek[1,2], Veronika Cubinkova[1,2], Veronika Brezovakova[1], Bernadeta Valachova[2], Peter Szalay[1,2], Norbert Zilka[1,2] and Santosh Jadhav[1,2]*

[1] *Institute of Neuroimmunology, Slovak Academy of Sciences, Bratislava, Slovakia,* [2] *Axon Neuroscience R&D Services SE, Bratislava, Slovakia*

***Correspondence:**
Santosh Jadhav
santosh.jadhav@savba.sk*

Alzheimer's disease (AD), the most common tauopathy, is an age-dependent, progressive neurodegenerative disease. Epidemiological studies implicate the role of genetic background in the onset and progression of AD. Despite mutations in familial AD, several risk factors have been implicated in sporadic AD, of which the onset is unknown. In AD, there is a sequential and hierarchical spread of tau pathology to other brain areas. Studies have strived to understand the factors that influence this characteristic spread. Using transgenic rat models with different genetic backgrounds, we reported that the genetic background may influence the manifestation of neurofibrillary pathology. In this study we investigated whether genetic background has an influence in the spread of tau pathology, using hippocampal inoculations of insoluble tau from AD brains in rodent models of tauopathy with either a spontaneously hypertensive (SHR72) or Wistar-Kyoto (WKY72) genetic background. We observed that insoluble tau from human AD induced AT8-positive neurofibrillary structures in the hippocampus of both lines. However, there was no significant difference in the amount of neurofibrillary structures, but the extent of spread was prominent in the W72 line. On the other hand, we observed significantly higher levels of AT8-positive structures in the parietal and frontal cortical areas in W72 when compared to SHR72. Interestingly, we also observed that the microglia in these brain areas in W72 were predominantly phagocytic in morphology (62.4% in parietal and 47.3% in frontal), while in SHR72 the microglia were either reactive or ramified (67.2% in parietal and 84.7% in frontal). The microglia in the hippocampus and occipital cortex in both lines were reactive or ramified structures. Factors such as gender or age are not responsible for the differences observed in these animals. Put together, our results, for the first time, show that the immune response modulating genetic variability is one of the factors that influences the propagation of tau neurofibrillary pathology.

Keywords: tauopathy, neurofibrillary tangles, microglia, genetic background, ramified

INTRODUCTION

Alzheimer's disease (AD), a primary tauopathy, is the most prevalent neurodegenerative disorder characterized by neurodegeneration and dementia. The risk factors for AD include lower mental and physical activity during old age, trauma to the head, cardiovascular diseases, diabetes, smoking, and obesity. Although the role of genetic factors, such as mutation, in early-onset familial AD has been extensively characterized (Campion et al., 1999; Bekris et al., 2010), the exact modality of the onset and progression of the disease pathogenesis in sporadic forms of AD is unknown.

Besides factors such as environmental exposure or psychological factors, epidemiological studies also implicate the role of genetic susceptibility in the onset and progression of sporadic AD (Miech et al., 2002; Cacabelos et al., 2005; Stozicka et al., 2007; Qiu et al., 2009). Genome-wide association studies and their meta-analyses implicate more than 20 genetic loci, mainly involved in the immune system (directly or indirectly related to microglia), lipid metabolism, and endocytosis, as potential risk factors in sporadic late-onset Alzheimer's disease (Ridge et al., 2016; Jansen et al., 2019; Kunkle et al., 2019). However, clinic-pathological heterogeneity between AD cases complicate the understanding of the role these genetic components play in the manifestation of the disease (Moreno-Grau et al., 2019). It is suggested that genetic susceptibility may influence the effect of environmental and psychological factors on cognitive phenotypes during aging (Wang et al., 2019). Several studies have investigated the influence of genetic susceptibility and environment modifiers on transgenic models of Alzheimer's disease (Ryman and Lamb, 2006; Stozicka et al., 2010; Zilka et al., 2012b; Pardossi-Piquard et al., 2016). Moreover, we have also demonstrated the influence of genetic background on the manifestation of neurofibrillary pathology and associated neuroinflammation (Stozicka et al., 2010; Zilka et al., 2012b). Despite retaining similar levels of transgene expression, the W72 line showed higher levels of activated microglia than the SHR72 line (Stozicka et al., 2010), suggesting that there exists a strain-dependent difference in response to neurofibrillary pathology.

One of the characteristic features of AD and a few other tauopathies is the propagation of tau pathology in a hierarchical manner to anatomically connected regions (Braak and Braak, 1991; Delacourte et al., 1999). Although studies have, in recent years, strived to recapitulate and understand the modality of the characteristic spread, it is still unknown if genetic background also influences the seeding propensity and propagation of tau pathology. Therefore in this study, we investigated the potency of insoluble tau from human AD to induce tau pathology in well-characterized transgenic rat models of tauopathy expressing human truncated tau aa151–391 in two different genetic backgrounds (Zilka et al., 2006; Koson et al., 2008). Our results show that, regardless of the genetic background, the misfolded tau seeds from AD were able to induce tau pathology; however, genetic background had an influence on the spread of tau pathology in the rodents. To the best of our knowledge, the current study is the first to investigate the role of genetic background in the seeding and propagation of tau pathology.

MATERIALS AND METHODS

Human Brain

Alzheimer's disease brains (Braak stage 5) were procured from the brain collection of the University of Geneva, Geneva, Switzerland, in compliance with the material transfer agreement. The parietal cortex was used for the isolation of sarkosyl insoluble tau fraction.

Animals

The study was performed on 3-month-old transgenic female rats expressing human truncated tau aa151–391 with four repeat domains in a spontaneously hypertensive (line SHR72) or Wistar-Kyoto (line W72) genetic background. The SHR72 line was back-crossed to the Wistar-Kyoto genetic background to generate the W72 line, and the normotensive and hypertensive properties of the W72 and SHR72 lines, respectively, have been characterized (Stozicka et al., 2010). The neurofibrillary pathology is localized mainly in the brainstem and spinal cord of these transgenic rats (Zilka et al., 2006; Koson et al., 2008). All animals were housed under standard laboratory conditions with free access to water and food and were kept under diurnal lighting conditions. A total of 12 transgenic animals (n = 6/group) were used in the study. Age-matched non-transgenic Wistar-Kyoto (WKY) and spontaneous hypertensive rats (SHR), transgenic W72, and SHR72 lines were used as controls for the morphological examination of Iba-1 positive microglia (n = 3/group).

Ethics Statement

All experiments were performed in accordance with the Slovak and European Community Guidelines, with the approval of the Institute's Ethical Committee, and the study was approved by the State Veterinary and Food Administration of the Slovak Republic.

Isolation of Sarkosyl-Insoluble Tau and Western Blotting

Sarkosyl-insoluble tau was extracted as previously described (Jadhav et al., 2015). Briefly, tissues were homogenized in a buffer containing 20 mM *Tris*, 0.8 M NaCl, 1 mM EGTA, 1 mM EDTA, and 10% sucrose that was supplemented with protease inhibitors (Complete, EDTA free, Roche Diagnostics, United States) and phosphatase inhibitors (1 mM sodium orthovanadate and 20 mM sodium fluoride). After centrifugation at 20,000 × g for 20 min, the supernatant (S1) was collected and a small fraction was saved as the total protein extract; 40% w/v of N-lauroylsarcosine (sarkosyl) in water was added to a final concentration of 1% and mixed by stirring it for 1 h at room temperature. The sample was then centrifuged at 100,000 × g for 1 h at 25°C using Beckmann TLA-100 (Beckmann instrument Inc., CA, United States). Pellets (P2) were washed and re-suspended in PBS to 1/50 volume of the S1 fraction and sonicated briefly; 10 μg w/v of the P2 fraction corresponding to the S1 fraction was used for the SDS-PAGE analysis.

Western blotting was performed as previously described (Jadhav et al., 2015). Briefly, known amounts of recombinant human tau 2N4R (tau 40) and insoluble tau extract were resolved using 12% SDS-PAGE gels and transferred to nitrocellulose membranes. After blocking, the membranes were incubated using a pan-tau antibody DC25 (1:1 with 5% fat free milk; Axon Neuroscience, Bratislava, Slovakia). Following washing, membranes were incubated with anti-mouse secondary antibody (Dako, Glostrup, Denmark). Blots were developed using a SuperSignal West Pico chemiluminescent Substrate (Thermo Scientific, IL, United States) on an Image Reader LAS-3000 (FUJI Photo Film Co., Ltd., Tokyo, Japan). The semi-quantitative estimation of sarkosyl-insoluble tau was performed as previously described (Smolek et al., 2019). The intensities of the samples and tau 40 were quantified by densitometry using an AIDA Biopackage (Advanced Image Data Analyzer software; Raytest, Germany). The concentration of insoluble tau protein was estimated using a standard curve with reference intensities of known concentrations of recombinant tau 2N4R (Tau 40).

Stereotaxic Surgery

Rats were anesthetized through intraperitoneal injection of a cocktail containing Zoletil (30 mg/kg) and Xylariem (10 mg/kg). Animals were fixed to a stereotaxic apparatus (Kopf Instruments, CA, United States) and an UltraMicroPump III Micro-syringe injector and Micro4 Controller (World Precision Instruments, FL, United States) were used for applying substances. Animals received 900 ng (concentration 300 ng/ul) of sarkosyl-insoluble tau at a rate of 1.25 μl/minute, and the needle was kept in position for 5 min before slow withdrawal to prevent leakage of the liquid infused. Stereotaxic coordinates for the injection were W72: A/P: −3.6 mm, L: ± 2.0 mm, D/V: 3.1 mm from bregma and SHR72: A/P: −3.6 mm, L: ± 2.0 mm, D/V: 3.3 from bragma (Paxinos and Watson, 1997).

Immunohistochemistry

Rats were deeply anesthetized before being sacrificed and perfused transcardially with 1× phosphate-buffered saline. Brains were removed and fixed in 4% PFA overnight, followed by permeabilization in sucrose solutions (15, 25, and 30% for 24 h each), freezing in 2-methyl butane, and stored at a temperature of −80°C. Frozen brains were cut serially into sagittal 40 μm-thick sections using a cryomicrotome (Leica CM1850, Leica Biosystems). The sections were blocked with Aptum Section block (Aptum, United Kingdom), and this was followed by incubation with primary antibodies AT8 (epitope anti-tau pS202/pT205, 1:1000; Thermo Scientific, IL, United States), anti-phospho tau pT212 (1:1000; Invitrogen, CA, United States), or Iba1 (1:500; Wako, Japan) overnight at 4°C. Sections were stained with biotin-conjugated secondary antibodies and developed using a Vectastain ABC Kit (Vector Laboratories, CA, United States). After mounting, sections were evaluated using an Olympus BX51 microscope (Olympus microscope solutions). For immunohistological staining, every eighth sagittal section was used; 10 sections were used for quantification and the total distance in range (lateral from the medial line 0.40–3.9 mm). Quantification was performed manually, with every tangle or Iba 1 positive macrophages in the respective regions of interest being counted by a blind observer. Iba 1 positive microglia with two or less processes were considered as phagocytic in morphology.

Statistical Analysis

Data were analyzed using Prism (Graph Pad Software version 6, CA, United States). An unpaired *t*-test (Mann–Whitney) was used for comparison of histological analysis between two groups. Data are presented as mean ± standard deviation. Differences were considered to be statistically significant if $p < 0.05$. $^{*}p < 0.05$, $^{**}p < 0.01$, and $^{***}p < 0.001$ were used to denote statistical significance.

RESULTS

Insoluble Tau From Alzheimer's Disease Brains Induces Neurofibrillary Pathology in Transgenic Rat Model in a Wistar-Kyoto Background

We demonstrated earlier that insoluble tau from the human AD brain induces tau pathology in a transgenic rat model of tauopathy that had an SHR background (Smolek et al., 2019). Therefore, we were intrigued to see whether a similar phenomenon could also be observed in a transgenic rat model with a different genetic background. Similar to SHR72 line, the W72 transgenic rat model also does not develop hippocampal tau pathology despite expressing human truncated tau aa151-391. We performed bilateral injections of insoluble tau from AD brains (900 ng, AD-PHF in **Figure 1A**) in a transgenic rat model of tauopathy expressing human truncated tau aa151–391 with a Wistar-Kyoto and SHR background at the age of 3 months. After 3 months, we performed histological analyses using phospho-tau specific AT8 and pT212 antibodies. We observed the presence of AT8- and pT212-positive neurofibrillary structures in the hippocampus of transgenic Wistar-Kyoto rats (**Figures 1B,E**).

We then compared the degree of neurofibrillary pathology in the hippocampus of two transgenic lines after inoculation of insoluble tau from AD brains. Using AT8 (**Figures 1B,C,H–Q**) and pT212 (**Figures 1E,F**) antibodies, we did not observe any difference in the levels of neurofibrillary pathology in the hippocampus of both transgenic rats (**Figures 1B–G**; AT8 $p = 0.818$ and pT212 $p = 0.999$). However, there was a mild difference in the pattern of distribution of neurofibrillary pathology (**Figures 1H–K,M–P**). In W72, the neurofibrillary pathology displayed more rostral distribution, mainly in CA3 (yet insignificant, $p > 0.05$), from the site of injection when compared to SHR72 (**Figures 1J,O**). The CA2 (**Figures 1I,N**) and dentate gyrus (**Figures 1K,P**) showed identical patterns of distribution. The brainstem, the region where the two transgenic lines innately develop neurofibrillary pathology, was used as a positive control

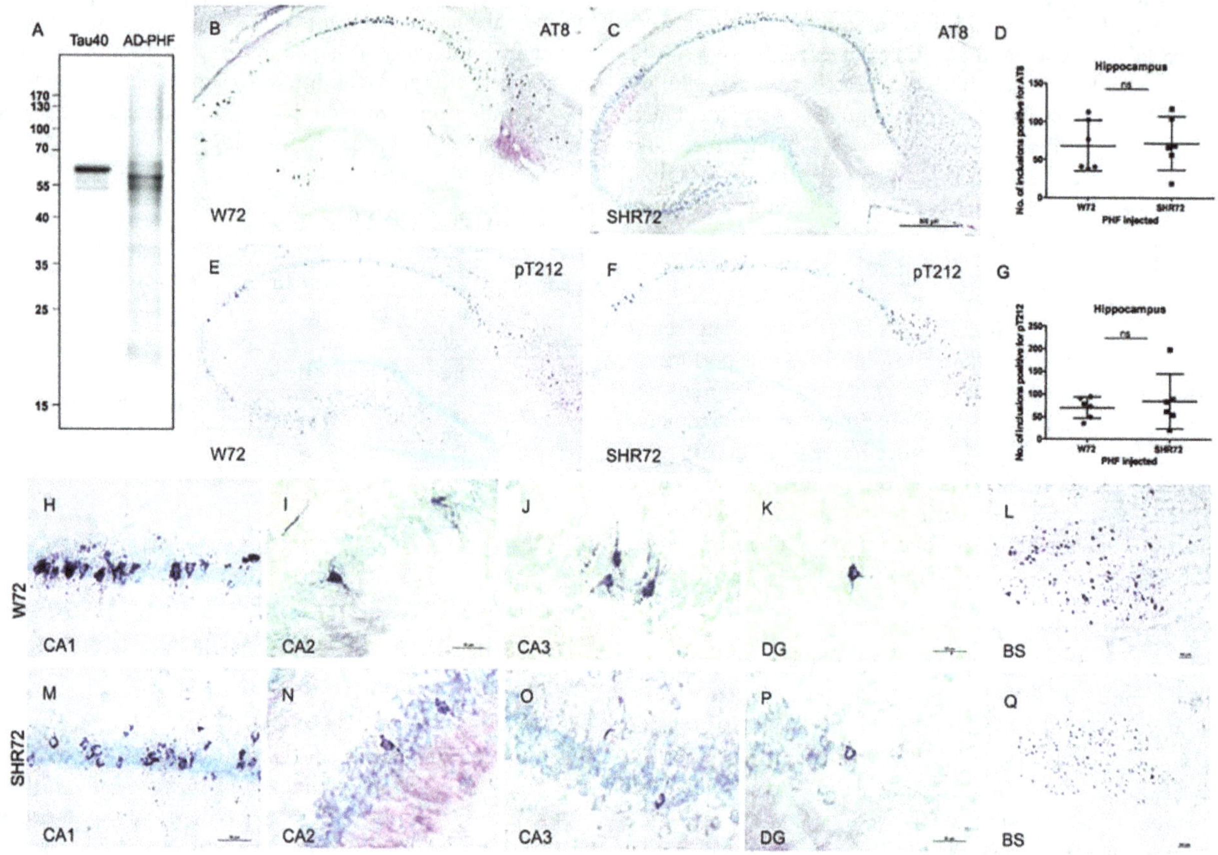

FIGURE 1 | Histological analysis for neurofibrillary pathology in the hippocampus of SHR72 and W72 rats after inoculation of insoluble tau. **(A)** Immuno-blot using pan-tau antibody DC25 showing insoluble tau isolated from human AD brain (AD-PHF). Recombinant human 2N4R (Tau 40) was used as positive control. Histological images showing AT8-positive structures in the hippocampus of W72 **(B, H–L)** and SHR72 transgenic line **(C, M–Q)**. **(E, F)** The presence of neurofibrillary pathology was confirmed using a pT212 phospho-tau specific antibody in the hippocampus of the transgenic lines. A statistical analysis did not reveal any difference in the levels of AT8-positive **(D)** or pT212 positive **(G)** structures in the hippocampus of the two transgenic lines (unpaired *t*-test: AT8 $p = 0.818$; pT212 $p = 0.999$). However, AT8-positive structures were prominent in the CA3 region of the W72 line **(J)** when compared to the SHR72 line **(O)**. There was not difference in the levels of AT8-positive structures in CA1 **(H,M)**, CA2 **(I,N)**, or dentate gyrus **(K,P)**. The brainstem of the transgenic lines was used as a positive control for the presence of genuine AT8-positive structures **(L,Q)**. Scale bar **B,C,E,F:** 500 μm and **H–Q:** 50 μm.

to confirm the presence of genuine AT8-positive staining in our tissue sections (**Figures 1L,Q**).

Cortical Distribution of Neurofibrillary Structures Was Markedly Different Between the Two Transgenic Lines

We proceeded to observe if the inoculation of insoluble tau induced neurofibrillary pathology in adjacent cortical areas. We observed neurofibrillary pathology in cortices of both transgenic lines; however, the extent of neurofibrillary pathology was different between the two lines. We observed that the number of AT8-positive structures were higher in the cortex of W72 transgenic rats (**Figures 2A,C**; $p = 0.004$), than in the SHR72 line (**Figures 2B,C**). The frontal cortex also showed higher levels of neurofibrillary structures in W72 when compared to the SHR72 line (**Figure 2D**; $p = 0.0043$). The parietal cortex also demonstrated higher levels of AT8-positive structures then the SHR72 ($p = 0.0152$) (**Figure 2E**). The occipital cortex displayed a tendency to develop higher neurofibrillary pathology in the W72 line but was not statistically significant (**Figure 2F**; $p = 0.2251$).

Microglia Displayed Morphological Differences in Regions With Neurofibrillary Pathology Between the Two Transgenic Lines

We previously reported that genetic background-mediated immunomodulation, dependent on microglia, plays a role in the development of neurofibrillary pathology in these transgenic lines (Stozicka et al., 2010; Zilka et al., 2012b). We therefore used anti-Iba 1 antibody to investigate the microglial status between the two transgenic lines after the induction of tau pathology. Upon response to stimuli, microglia undergoes morphological changes (**Figure 3A**; Streit et al., 1999). Initially, there was an increase in the ramification of microglial processes (ramified state), followed by hypertrophy (reactive phase). In the end, the microglia became

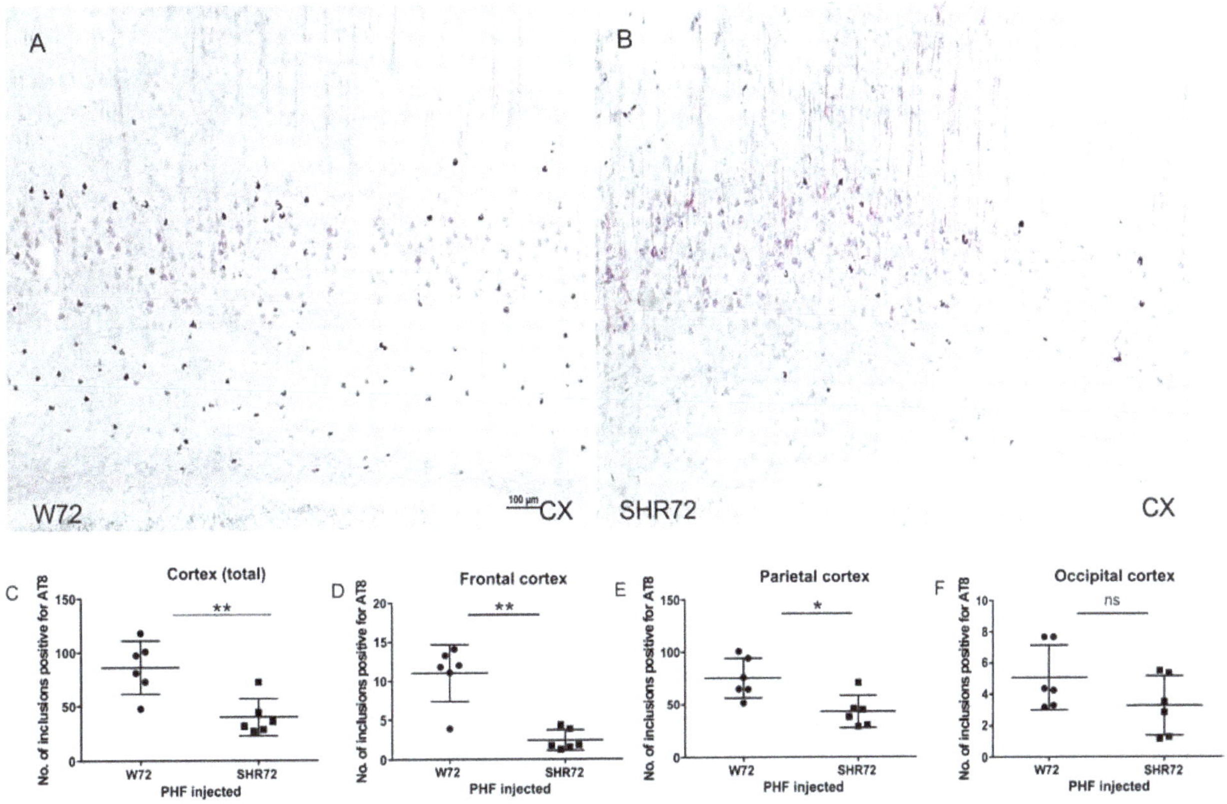

FIGURE 2 | Representative histological images showing AT8-positive neurofibrillary structures in the cortices of the transgenic lines **(A,B)**. **(C,D)** A statistical analysis revealed that the number of AT8-positive structures was higher in the W72 line when compared to SHR72 line (Cortex: $p = 0.004$). **(E)** Higher levels of AT8-positive neurofibrillary tangles were also observed in the frontal cortex ($p = 0.0043$). In the parietal cortex, the levels of AT8-positive structures were higher than the SHR72 line ($p = 0.0152$). **(F)** The occipital cortex showed moderately higher levels of AT8-positive structures; this was, however, insignificant ($p = 0.2251$). $^{*}p < 0.05$ and $^{**}p < 0.01$ is used to denote statistical significance. An unpaired t-test was used for statistical analysis. Scale bar: 100 μm.

phagocytic, characterized by de-ramification, with few or no processes (**Figure 3A**).

In the hippocampus of both transgenic lines, the anti-Iba1 antibody revealed microglia with ramified or phagocytic morphology (**Figures 3B–E**). However, we did not observe any differences in microglial morphology in the hippocampus between the two lines (percentage of phagocytic microglia: W72: 17.8% vs. SHR72: 16.6%). On the other hand, the anti-Iba1 antibody revealed a marked difference in the microglial morphology of the cortex between the two transgenic lines. In the parietal cortex (**Figures 3F,G**) and frontal cortex (**Figures 3N,O**) of the W72 line, regions that develop significantly higher levels of neurofibrillary pathology, the majority of microglia either displayed phagocytic morphology with few degenerating processes or were completely devoid of them. In comparison, the microglia in those regions in the SHR72 line prominently displayed ramified to reactive morphology with numerous digitating processes (**Figures 3H,I,P,Q**). The levels of phagocytic microglia in the parietal cortex in the W72 and SHR72 lines were 62.4 and 32.7%, respectively. In the frontal cortex, the levels were 47.3% in W72 and 15.2% in SHR72 (W72 vs. SHR72). Interestingly, we did not observe any differences in the microglial morphology in the occipital cortex, which displayed either reactive or ramified microglia in both lines (**Figures 3J–M**) (phagocytic microglia: W72: 53.6% and SHR72: 52.11%). We did not observe any difference in the microglial morphology of non-transgenic Wistar-Kyoto, SHR, and transgenic non-injected W72 and SHR72 in any of the examined regions (**Supplementary Figures S1, S2**). This suggested that there was a genuine difference in morphology in Iba 1 positive microglia after inoculation of exogenous tau seeds between the two transgenic lines in the study.

DISCUSSION

In this study, using two transgenic rat models of tauopathy, we demonstrated the influence of genetic background on the induction and propagation of tau pathology. In our earlier study (Stozicka et al., 2010), we observed cardinal differences in Iba1-positive microglia between the two transgenic lines. Therefore, we only used the transgenic lines in the study. In order to avoid bias, we utilized our well-established transgenic rodent models (Zilka et al., 2006; Koson et al., 2008; Stozicka et al., 2010) expressing the same human truncated tau aa151–391 under the same type of promoter in the study. The two

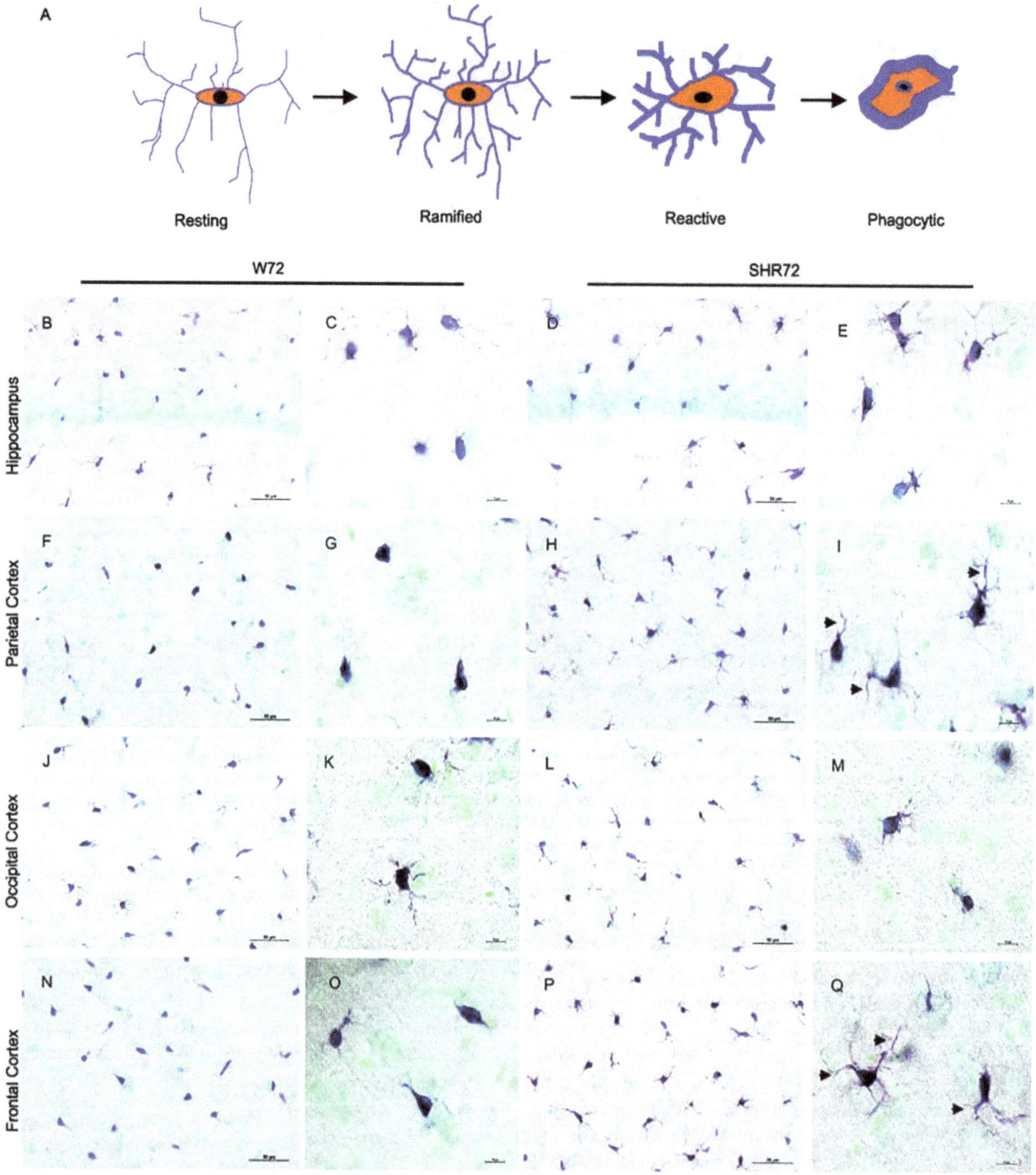

FIGURE 3 | Histological images showing Iba1 positive microglia in the hippocampus and cortical regions. **(A)** Schematic illustration showing changes in microglial morphology in response to stimuli. Upon activation, microglia become hyper-ramified, developing numerous processes, and subsequently become reactive and phagocytic. Iba1-positive structures in the hippocampus of the W72 line **(B,C)** and SHR72 **(D,E)** revealed microglia with both reactive and ramified morphology in both lines (W72: 17.8% and SHR72: 16.6%). However, as evidenced by the size and form of the soma, the microglia showed phagocytic morphology in the parietal cortex **(F,G)** and frontal cortex **(N,O)** of the W72 line (62.4 and 47.3%, respectively). The microglia from the SHR72 were predominantly displaying reactive or ramified morphology, with numerous processes (arrowheads) in the cortex **(H,I)**–the frontal cortex in particular **(P,Q**; 84.7%). The microglia in occipital cortex from both lines were ramified or phagocytic in morphology **(J–M**; W72: 53.6% and SHR72: 52.1% of phagocytic microglia). Scale bar **B**,**D**,**F**,**H**,**J**,**L**,**N**,**P**; 50 μm, rest 10 μm.

animal models had the same copy number of transgenes in their genome and had similar expression levels of truncated tau. The transgenic rat models of tauopathy replicated crucial features of Alzheimer's disease, such as tau hyperphosphorylation, insoluble tau formation, neurofibrillary pathology, and reduction in life span (Zilka et al., 2006; Koson et al., 2008). The animal models did not develop neurofibrillary pathology in the hippocampus. In order to induce tau pathology, we injected insoluble tau from a human AD brain into the hippocampus. We recently demonstrated that inoculation of insoluble tau from an AD brain induced neurofibrillary pathology in the hippocampus of SHR72 transgenic rats (Smolek et al., 2019). Moreover, the neurofibrillary pathology spread to other regions from the site of injection and induced misfolding of endogenous rat tau, culminating in inclusions containing both exogenous and endogenous tau species (Smolek et al., 2019). We therefore used a similar approach to investigate the influence of genetic background on the propagation of tau pathology.

We first showed that the inoculation of tau seeds from a human AD brain induced neurofibrillary pathology in the hippocampus of the W72 line, similar to SHR72. However, we observed that the lines demonstrated significant differences in the propagation of tau neurofibrillary pathology. We observed that the W72 line developed more pathology in the rostral cortical areas from the hippocampus, even in the frontal cortex, when compared to SHR72 line. We previously reported that W72, the animal model with higher levels of activated microglia, were more susceptible to neurofibrillary degeneration (Stozicka et al., 2010). Our results further extended these observations and showed that the W72 line is also more susceptible to propagation of tau pathology than the SHR72 line.

Studies have observed that the presence of neurofibrillary inclusions corresponded to the distribution of active microglia in AD (Sheng et al., 1997; Sheffield et al., 2000), and activated microglia were frequently present in close proximity to neurofibrillary tangles (Cras et al., 1991; DiPatre and Gelman, 1997; Zilka et al., 2012b). Studies show that region-specific microglial morphology has been observed in models of neuroinflammation (Fernandez-Arjona et al., 2017) and stress (Avignone et al., 2015). Interestingly, we also observed major differences in the morphology of microglia in both transgenic lines in response to induced neurofibrillary pathology. In the W72 line, the cortical areas with higher levels of neurofibrillary pathology than SHR72 showed higher levels of microglia demonstrating phagocytic morphology. On the other hand, most microglia showed ramified or reactive morphology in the SHR72 line. Factors such as age or gender were not responsible for the difference in microglial morphology in our study since the experiments were performed on animals of the same age and gender and for the same period. Therefore, the distinct responses of microglia between the two transgenic lines may be due to their unique genetic background, as we previously described (Stozicka et al., 2010).

Despite the presence of active phagocytic microglia in the W72, we observed significantly higher levels of neurofibrillary pathology in this line, mainly in the cortical areas. We have previously reported that the levels of neurofibrillary tangles correlated well with the levels of activated microglia in transgenic model of tauopathy (Stozicka et al., 2010). Studies have also shown that microglia-mediated inflammatory responses may contribute to the development of tau pathology and thus accelerate the course of disease (Zilka et al., 2012b; Maphis et al., 2015). Furthermore, amelioration of AD pathology using immunomodulatory agents in transgenic models of AD has been shown to inhibit the inflammatory consequences of tau aggregation (Martinez and Peplow, 2019). Numerous studies have also implicated the direct role of microglia in tau propagation (Asai et al., 2015; Maphis et al., 2015). A recent study evidenced the presence of competent microglia capable of the uptake and release of tau in an AD brain and transgenic model of tauopathy (Hopp et al., 2018); however, the microglia were only partially able to neutralize the seed-competent tau. Since we observed higher levels of phagocytic microglia in the W72 line, in areas accompanied by higher levels of tau pathology, we speculate that strain-dependent role of microglia may be responsible for the manifestation of higher levels of neurofibrillary pathology in the cortices of W72 line.

In the end, the rat lines were developed based on an SHR or Wistar-Kyoto background, and the two lines are genetically different (H'Doubler et al., 1991). Interestingly, chronic inflammation in SHR probably causes an altered reaction to acute immune challenges (Bernard et al., 1998; Bauhofer et al., 2003). The SHR rats demonstrated resistance to LPS stimuli and had better survival rates than the Wistar-Kyoto counterparts. This attenuated response was independent of hypertension in these rats but was due to an altered inflammatory response (Bernard et al., 1998). In our previous study, we demonstrated that the WKY tg rats developed a more robust immunologic response in comparison to SHR tg rats (Stozicka et al., 2010). Therefore, the overall response to exogenous tau in SHR tg or WKY tg to tau spreading in our study was independent of the hypertension and was dependent on the difference in immunological susceptibility between the two lines. Although hypertension is considered a risk factor, inflammation may have a more prominent role in the progression of pathology in neurodegenerative tauopathies.

Several studies have discussed the interrelationship between the immune response and tau neurofibrillary pathology (Zilka et al., 2012a; Perea et al., 2018; Spanic et al., 2019). Reactive microglia are associated with neurofibrillary tangles, suggesting that the tau can trigger neuroinflammation. However, the exact relationship between tau propagation and the immune response is less known. Interestingly, higher levels of microglia were observed in hippocampus CA1, the entorhinal cortex, and the parasubiculum in humans (Sheffield et al., 2000)—the regions that demonstrate propagation of tau pathology in AD brains during disease progression. Similar distributions of microglia were also observed in the mouse model of tauopathy, where microglial activation preceded tangle formation (Yoshiyama et al., 2007). Based on this evidence, one can speculate that the regional distribution of microglia and its activation may contribute to propagation of tau pathology. Our study demonstrates that, irrespective of the presence of microglia, the genetic background had an influence on the microglial activation status and, subsequently, the propagation of tau pathology.

Several factors are responsible for the propagation of tau pathology *in vivo*, including genetic factors (Ryman and Lamb, 2006; McQuade and Blurton-Jones, 2019), the presence of a proper seeding partner in the host (Levarska et al., 2013), and the stability and inter-individual variability of the tau strains (Smolek et al., 2019). Our results further extended these observations and showed, for the first time, that the immune response modifying the genetic background is one of the factors that also has an influence on the susceptibility to, and propagation of, tau neurofibrillary pathology in AD and other tauopathies. Our study also demonstrated, for first time, the strain-dependent response of microglia to neurofibrillary pathology in a rodent model of tauopathies. The study opens new vistas in our understanding of the pathogenesis of neurodegenerative disorders, such as Alzheimer's disease and other tauopathies.

ETHICS STATEMENT

The animal study was reviewed and approved by Ethical Committee of Institute of Neuroimmunology, Slovak Academy of Sciences and State Veterinary and Food Administration of the Slovak Republic.

AUTHOR CONTRIBUTIONS

TS performed the histological analysis and imaging. VC performed the stereological injections. VB and SJ performed the isolation and characterization of insoluble tau. BV was involved in the handling of animals and stereological analysis. PS was involved in the histological analysis. SJ supervised the project. NZ and SJ wrote the manuscript. All authors approved the final manuscript.

ACKNOWLEDGMENTS

We thank the brain bank of the University of Geneva (Geneva, Switzerland) for providing the brain tissue.

REFERENCES

Asai, H., Ikezu, S., Tsunoda, S., Medalla, M., Luebke, J., Haydar, T., et al. (2015). Depletion of microglia and inhibition of exosome synthesis halt tau propagation. *Nat. Neurosci.* 18, 1584–1593. doi: 10.1038/nn.4132

Avignone, E., Lepleux, M., Angibaud, J., and Nagerl, U. V. (2015). Altered morphological dynamics of activated microglia after induction of status epilepticus. *J. Neuroinflamm.* 12:202. doi: 10.1186/s12974-015-0421-6

Bauhofer, A., Tischer, B., Middeke, M., Plaul, U., Lorenz, W., and Torossian, A. (2003). The genetic background of hypertensive, septic rats determines outcome improvement with antibiotic and G-CSF prophylaxis. *Shock* 20, 326–331. doi: 10.1097/01.shk.0000084342.58020.1e

Bekris, L. M., Yu, C. E., Bird, T. D., and Tsuang, D. W. (2010). Genetics of Alzheimer disease. *J. Geriatr. Psychiatry Neurol.* 23, 213–227. doi: 10.1177/0891988710383571

Bernard, C., Merval, R., Esposito, B., and Tedgui, A. (1998). Resistance to endotoxin shock in spontaneously hypertensive rats. *Hypertension* 31, 1350–1356. doi: 10.1161/01.hyp.31.6.1350

Braak, H., and Braak, E. (1991). Neuropathological stageing of Alzheimer-related changes. *Acta Neuropathol.* 82, 239–259. doi: 10.1007/bf00308809

Cacabelos, R., Fernandez-Novoa, L., Lombardi, V., Kubota, Y., and Takeda, M. (2005). Molecular genetics of Alzheimer's disease and aging. *Methods Find. Exp. Clin. Pharmacol.* 27(Suppl. A), 1–573.

Campion, D., Dumanchin, C., Hannequin, D., Dubois, B., Belliard, S., Puel, M., et al. (1999). Early-onset autosomal dominant Alzheimer disease: prevalence, genetic heterogeneity, and mutation spectrum. *Am. J. Hum. Genet.* 65, 664–670. doi: 10.1086/302553

Cras, P., Kawai, M., Siedlak, S., and Perry, G. (1991). Microglia are associated with the extracellular neurofibrillary tangles of Alzheimer disease. *Brain Res.* 558, 312–314. doi: 10.1016/0006-8993(91)90783-r

Delacourte, A., David, J. P., Sergeant, N., Buee, L., Wattez, A., Vermersch, P., et al. (1999). The biochemical pathway of neurofibrillary degeneration in aging and Alzheimer's disease. *Neurology* 52, 1158–1165.

DiPatre, P. L., and Gelman, B. B. (1997). Microglial cell activation in aging and Alzheimer disease: partial linkage with neurofibrillary tangle burden in the hippocampus. *J. Neuropathol. Exp. Neurol.* 56, 143–149. doi: 10.1097/00005072-199702000-00004

Fernandez-Arjona, M. D. M., Grondona, J. M., Granados-Duran, P., Fernandez-Llebrez, P., and Lopez-Avalos, M. D. (2017). Microglia morphological categorization in a rat model of neuroinflammation by hierarchical cluster and principal components analysis. *Front. Cell Neurosci.* 11:235. doi: 10.3389/fncel.2017.00235

H'Doubler, P. B. Jr., Peterson, M., Shek, W., Auchincloss, H., Abbott, W. M., and Orkin, R. W. (1991). Spontaneously hypertensive and Wistar Kyoto rats are genetically disparate. *Lab Anim. Sci.* 41, 471–473.

Hopp, S. C., Lin, Y., Oakley, D., Roe, A. D., Devos, S. L., Hanlon, D., et al. (2018). The role of microglia in processing and spreading of bioactive tau seeds in Alzheimer's disease. *J. Neuroinflamm.* 15:269. doi: 10.1186/s12974-018-1309-z

Jadhav, S., Katina, S., Kovac, A., Kazmerova, Z., Novak, M., and Zilka, N. (2015). Truncated tau deregulates synaptic markers in rat model for human tauopathy. *Front. Cell Neurosci.* 9:24. doi: 10.3389/fncel.2015.00024

Jansen, I. E., Savage, J. E., Watanabe, K., Bryois, J., Williams, D. M., Steinberg, S., et al. (2019). Genome-wide meta-analysis identifies new loci and functional pathways influencing Alzheimer's disease risk. *Nat. Genet.* 51, 404–413. doi: 10.1038/s41588-018-0311-9

Koson, P., Zilka, N., Kovac, A., Kovacech, B., Korenova, M., Filipcik, P., et al. (2008). Truncated tau expression levels determine life span of a rat model of tauopathy without causing neuronal loss or correlating with terminal neurofibrillary tangle load. *Eur. J. Neurosci.* 28, 239–246. doi: 10.1111/j.1460-9568.2008.06329.x

Kunkle, B. W., Grenier-Boley, B., Sims, R., Bis, J. C., Damotte, V., Naj, A. C., et al. (2019). Genetic meta-analysis of diagnosed Alzheimer's disease identifies new risk loci and implicates Abeta, tau, immunity and lipid processing. *Nat. Genet.* 51, 414–430. doi: 10.1038/s41588-019-0358-2

Levarska, L., Zilka, N., Jadhav, S., Neradil, P., and Novak, M. (2013). Of rodents and men: the mysterious interneuronal pilgrimage of misfolded protein tau in Alzheimer's disease. *J. Alzheimers. Dis.* 37, 569–577. doi: 10.3233/JAD-131106

Maphis, N., Xu, G., Kokiko-Cochran, O. N., Jiang, S., Cardona, A., Ransohoff, R. M., et al. (2015). Reactive microglia drive tau pathology and contribute to the spreading of pathological tau in the brain. *Brain* 138, 1738–1755. doi: 10.1093/brain/awv081

Martinez, B., and Peplow, P. V. (2019). Amelioration of Alzheimer's disease pathology and cognitive deficits by immunomodulatory agents in animal models of Alzheimer's disease. *Neural. Regen. Res.* 14, 1158–1176. doi: 10.4103/1673-5374.251192

McQuade, A., and Blurton-Jones, M. (2019). Microglia in Alzheimer's Disease: exploring how genetics and phenotype influence risk. *J. Mol. Biol.* 431, 1805–1817. doi: 10.1016/j.jmb.2019.01.045

Miech, R. A., Breitner, J. C., Zandi, P. P., Khachaturian, A. S., Anthony, J. C., and Mayer, L. (2002). Incidence of AD may decline in the early 90s for men, later for women: the cache county study. *Neurology* 58, 209–218. doi: 10.1212/wnl.58.2.209

Moreno-Grau, S., De Rojas, I., Hernandez, I., Quintela, I., Montrreal, L., Alegret, M., et al. (2019). Genome-wide association analysis of dementia and its clinical endophenotypes reveal novel loci associated with Alzheimer's disease and three causality networks: the GR@ACE project. *Alzheimers Dement.* 15, 1333–1347. doi: 10.1016/j.jalz.2019.06.4950

Pardossi-Piquard, R., Lauritzen, I., Bauer, C., Sacco, G., Robert, P., and Checler, F. (2016). Influence of genetic background on apathy-like behavior in triple transgenic AD mice. *Curr. Alzheimer Res.* 13, 942–949. doi: 10.2174/1567205013666160404120106

Paxinos, G., and Watson, C. (1997). The rat brain in stereotaxic coordinates, 3rd Edn, *J. Anat.* 191, 315–317.

Perea, J. R., Llorens-Martin, M., Avila, J., and Bolos, M. (2018). The role of microglia in the spread of tau: relevance for tauopathies. *Front. Cell Neurosci.* 12:172. doi: 10.3389/fncel.2018.00172

Qiu, C., Kivipelto, M., and Von Strauss, E. (2009). Epidemiology of Alzheimer's disease: occurrence, determinants, and strategies toward intervention. *Dial. Clin. Neurosci.* 11, 111–128.

Ridge, P. G., Hoyt, K. B., Boehme, K., Mukherjee, S., Crane, P. K., Haines, J. L., et al. (2016). Assessment of the genetic variance of late-onset Alzheimer's disease. *Neurobiol. Aging* 41, 200.e13–200.e20. doi: 10.1016/j.neurobiolaging.2016.02.024

Ryman, D., and Lamb, B. T. (2006). Genetic and environmental modifiers of Alzheimer's disease phenotypes in the mouse. *Curr. Alzheimer Res.* 3, 465–473. doi: 10.2174/156720506779025198

Sheffield, L. G., Marquis, J. G., and Berman, N. E. (2000). Regional distribution of cortical microglia parallels that of neurofibrillary tangles in Alzheimer's disease. *Neurosci. Lett.* 285, 165–168. doi: 10.1016/s0304-3940(00)01037-5

Sheng, J. G., Mrak, R. E., and Griffin, W. S. (1997). Glial-neuronal interactions in Alzheimer disease: progressive association of IL-1alpha+ microglia and S100beta+ astrocytes with neurofibrillary tangle stages. *J. Neuropathol. Exp. Neurol.* 56, 285–290. doi: 10.1097/00005072-199703000-00007

Smolek, T., Jadhav, S., Brezovakova, V., Cubinkova, V., Valachova, B., Novak, P., et al. (2019). First-in-rat study of human Alzheimer's disease tau propagation. *Mol. Neurobiol.* 56, 621–631. doi: 10.1007/s12035-018-1102-0

Spanic, E., Langer Horvat, L., Hof, P. R., and Simic, G. (2019). Role of microglial cells in Alzheimer's disease tau propagation. *Front. Aging Neurosci.* 11:271. doi: 10.3389/fnagi.2019.00271

Stozicka, Z., Zilka, N., and Novak, M. (2007). Risk and protective factors for sporadic Alzheimer's disease. *Acta Virol.* 51, 205–222.

Stozicka, Z., Zilka, N., Novak, P., Kovacech, B., Bugos, O., and Novak, M. (2010). Genetic background modifies neurodegeneration and neuroinflammation driven by misfolded human tau protein in rat model of tauopathy: implication for immunomodulatory approach to Alzheimer's disease. *J. Neuroinflamm.* 7:64. doi: 10.1186/1742-2094-7-64

Streit, W. J., Walter, S. A., and Pennell, N. A. (1999). Reactive microgliosis. *Prog. Neurobiol.* 57, 563–581. doi: 10.1016/s0301-0082(98)00069-0

Wang, Y., Du, Y., Li, J., and Qiu, C. (2019). Lifespan intellectual factors, genetic susceptibility, and cognitive phenotypes in aging: implications for interventions. *Front. Aging Neurosci.* 11:129. doi: 10.3389/fnagi.2019.00129

Yoshiyama, Y., Higuchi, M., Zhang, B., Huang, S. M., Iwata, N., Saido, T. C., et al. (2007). Synapse loss and microglial activation precede tangles in a P301S tauopathy mouse model. *Neuron* 53, 337–351. doi: 10.1016/j.neuron.2007.01.010

Zilka, N., Filipcik, P., Koson, P., Fialova, L., Skrabana, R., Zilkova, M., et al. (2006). Truncated tau from sporadic Alzheimer's disease suffices to drive neurofibrillary degeneration *in vivo*. *FEBS Lett.* 580, 3582–3588. doi: 10.1016/j.febslet.2006.05.029

Zilka, N., Kazmerova, Z., Jadhav, S., Neradil, P., Madari, A., Obetkova, D., et al. (2012a). Who fans the flames of Alzheimer's disease brains? Misfolded tau on the crossroad of neurodegenerative and inflammatory pathways. *J. Neuroinflamm.* 9:47. doi: 10.1186/1742-2094-9-47

Zilka, N., Stozicka, Z., Cente, M., Kazmerova, Z., Kovacech, B., and Novak, M. (2012b). Immunomodulation of memory-impairing protein tau in Alzheimer's disease. *Neurodegener. Dis.* 10, 242–245. doi: 10.1159/000333125

5

Restoration of Olfactory Memory in *Drosophila* Overexpressing Human Alzheimer's Disease Associated Tau by Manipulation of L-Type Ca^{2+} Channels

James P. Higham†, Sergio Hidalgo†, Edgar Buhl and James J. L. Hodge*

School of Physiology, Pharmacology and Neuroscience, University of Bristol, Bristol, United Kingdom

***Correspondence:**
James J. L. Hodge
james.hodge@bristol.ac.uk

† These authors have contributed equally to this work

The cellular underpinnings of memory deficits in Alzheimer's disease (AD) are poorly understood. We utilized the tractable neural circuits sub-serving memory in *Drosophila* to investigate the role of impaired Ca^{2+} handling in memory deficits caused by expression of human 0N4R isoform of tau which is associated with AD. Expression of tau in mushroom body neuropils, or a subset of mushroom body output neurons, led to impaired memory. By using the Ca^{2+} reporter GCaMP6f, we observed changes in Ca^{2+} signaling when tau was expressed in these neurons, an effect that could be blocked by the L-type Ca^{2+} channel antagonist nimodipine or reversed by *RNAi* knock-down of the L-type channel gene. The L-type Ca^{2+} channel itself is required for memory formation, however, *RNAi* knock-down of the L-type Ca^{2+} channel in neurons overexpressing human tau resulted in flies whose memory is restored to levels equivalent to wild-type. Expression data suggest that *Drosophila* L-type Ca^{2+} channel mRNA levels are increased upon tau expression in neurons, thus contributing to the effects observed on memory and intracellular Ca^{2+} homeostasis. Together, our Ca^{2+} imaging and memory experiments suggest that expression of the 0N4R isoform of human tau increases the number of L-type Ca^{2+} channels in the membrane resulting in changes in neuronal excitability that can be ameliorated by *RNAi* knockdown or pharmacological blockade of L-type Ca^{2+} channels. This highlights a role for L-type Ca^{2+} channels in tauopathy and their potential as a therapeutic target for AD.

Keywords: tau, tauopathy, Alzheimer's disease, memory, L-type Ca2+ channels, *Drosophila*, GCaMP Ca2+ imaging

INTRODUCTION

The accumulation of the microtubule-associated protein tau (MAPT) within central neurons is a key histopathological feature of Alzheimer's disease (AD) (Kaufman et al., 2018; Nisbet and Gotz, 2018). Post-mortem AD brain samples contain the hallmark accumulation of extracellular amyloid beta (Aβ) plaques and intracellular neurofibrillary tangles (NFTs) of hyperphosphorylated tau, resulting in neurodegeneration and brain atrophy. The accumulation of tau is more correlated with the progression of AD pathology and symptoms than the magnitude of Aβ plaques

(Arendt et al., 2016). However, the mechanisms by which tau disrupts neuronal function, and consequently behavior, are not clear. Tau exists in six major isoforms formed by alternative splicing of exons 2 and/or 3 (0N, 1N or 2N) and 10 (3R or 4R) of the MAPT-17 gene (Buee et al., 2000). There is some evidence that 4R isoforms are upregulated in post-mortem brains, particularly within the hippocampus of AD patients (Boutajangout et al., 2004; Espinoza et al., 2008; Hasegawa et al., 2014), and show stronger affinity binding to tubulin and aggregation than 3R forms (Arendt et al., 2016). However, both 3R and 4R isoforms are present in NFTs, suggesting both play a role in pathology. The expression of 0N4R tau in model organisms can yield neuronal and behavioral dysfunction prior to the onset of neurodegeneration (Wittmann et al., 2001; Mershin et al., 2004). This suggests that tau's detrimental effect on neurons is sufficient to drive behavioral changes before neuronal death.

Patients with AD display memory impairment, and once the onset of neurodegeneration has occurred, treating the symptoms of AD becomes exceedingly difficult, so targeting the earlier signs of neuronal dysfunction is likely to be more efficacious. To this end, an understanding of how tau influences neuronal function is required. Disrupted calcium (Ca^{2+}) homeostasis including increased Ca^{2+} levels causing excitotoxicity has been posited as a key pathophysiology in AD, which may underpin the early stages of disease and precipitate neurodegeneration (Mattson and Chan, 2001; Brzyska and Elbaum, 2003; Canzoniero and Snider, 2005). Recent work suggests that these changes in neuronal excitability and Ca^{2+} signaling provide an important link between Aβ and tau pathology and disease progression (Spires-Jones and Hyman, 2014; Wu et al., 2016), but exactly how remains unknown. Different rodent models of tauopathy recapitulate some features of AD pathology including changes in excitability (Booth et al., 2016a,b), increased Ca^{2+} signaling (Wang and Mattson, 2014), neurodegeneration (Spillantini and Goedert, 2013), and impaired synaptic plasticity and memory (Arendt et al., 2016; Biundo et al., 2018). It is not clear what the source of increased Ca^{2+} is, however, increased levels of Ca^{2+} channels, such as the L-type voltage-gated Ca^{2+} channel (Ca_V1), have been shown to be upregulated in rodent models of AD, with blockers, such as nifedipine, being effective in trails to prevent the cognitive decline that occurs in AD (Coon et al., 1999; Anekonda et al., 2011; Goodison et al., 2012; Nimmrich and Eckert, 2013; Daschil et al., 2015). The role of voltage-gated Ca^{2+} channels in memory or AD has not been studied in *Drosophila*. *Drosophila* contains three different voltage-gated Ca^{2+} channel genes including the *DmCa1D* or *Ca-α1D* gene that encodes a high voltage-activated current and is equivalent to the vertebrate $Ca_V1.1$-1.4 genes that encode L-type Ca^{2+} channels (Worrell and Levine, 2008).

Alzheimer's disease and tauopathies have been modeled in *Drosophila* (Iijima-Ando and Iijima, 2010; Wentzell and Kretzschmar, 2010; Papanikolopoulou and Skoulakis, 2011), with targeted neuronal expression of human 0N4R tau causing neurodegeneration, shortened lifespan, circadian, sleep and motor deficits (Wittmann et al., 2001; Kerr et al., 2011; Sealey et al., 2017; Buhl et al., 2019; Higham et al., 2019). Furthermore, during development at the larval neuromuscular junction, motor neurons overexpressing human 0N3R or 0N4R caused a reduction in size and irregular and abnormally shaped synaptic terminals, a reduction in endocytosis and exocytosis and a reduction in high frequency synaptic transmission (Chee et al., 2005; Zhou et al., 2017). Also, while expression of tau 0N3R in the adult giant fiber system caused increased failure rate at high frequency stimulation, expression of 0N4R caused defects in stimulus conduction, response speed and conduction velocity (Kadas et al., 2019).

Learning and memory deficits can also be assessed in *Drosophila* using aversive olfactory classical conditioning (Malik et al., 2013; Malik and Hodge, 2014). Different mushroom body (MB) neuropils underpin specific phases of memory and are redundant during others (Pascual and Preat, 2001; Krashes et al., 2007; Davis, 2011). MB neurons send axons that terminate in lobed structures, with memory acquisition being mediated by the α′β′ lobe neurons and memory-storage by the αβγ neurons. In addition, a number of additional pairs of neurons innervate or are innervated by the MB and mediate different aspects of memory. For instance, the amnesiac expressing dorsal paired medial (DPM) and anterior paired lateral (APL) neurons are thought to consolidate and stabilize labile memory (Pitman et al., 2011). Finally, the MB innervate a pair of M4/6 MB output neurons via a cholinergic synapse, with optogenetic manipulation of the M4/6 neurons switching between appetitive and aversive memory (Barnstedt et al., 2016). Previous work has demonstrated that expression of tau in γ neurons caused a reduction in learning and 1.5 h memory in 3–5 days old young flies which were shown to still have their γ neurons intact, prior to their degeneration around day 45 (Mershin et al., 2004). Moreover, pan-neuronal 0N4R expression caused learning and long-term memory loss while 0N3R tau expression failed to do so (Sealey et al., 2017).

Therefore, *Drosophila* expressing human tau can be used to study AD relevant behaviors and their underlying neuronal mechanism, with loss of memory being possible prior to neurodegeneration. Although tau-mediated changes in neuronal properties are likely underpinning the memory impairment observed in *Drosophila* AD models, these changes have not been extensively studied in *Drosophila* MB neurons.

In this study, we determined the effect of human 0N4R tau expression in different neuropils of the *Drosophila* memory circuit on one-hour memory. We measured the effect of 0N4R tau on MB output neuron mediated memory and Ca^{2+} signaling and described a potential interaction between 0N4R tau with L-type voltage-gated Ca^{2+} channels which may underpin memory impairment.

RESULTS

To determine the effect of human tau 0N4R on memory, we targeted expression of the transgene to different neuronal populations of the *Drosophila* memory circuit and performed one-hour olfactory aversive conditioning. Driving expression of a human tau 0N4R transgene (Wittmann et al., 2001; Kerr et al., 2011; Higham et al., 2019) in the entire MB (*OK107-Gal4*

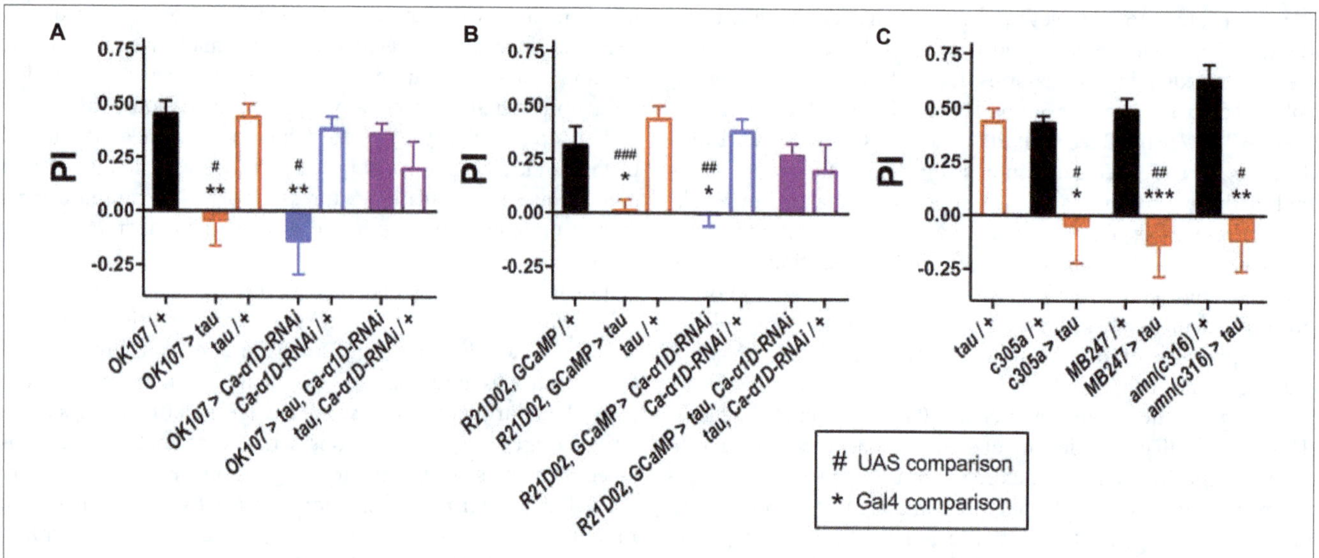

FIGURE 1 | Knock-down of L-type Ca^{2+} channels rescued tau-induced memory defects. **(A)** Tau expression in the MB (*OK107-Gal4*) ablated one-hour memory ($n = 7$ experiments with 50–100 flies each, red bar), as did the expression of an *RNAi* to the gene encoding the L-type Ca^{2+} channel alpha subunit (*Ca-α1D-RNAi*, $n = 8$, blue bar) compared to both Gal4 ($n = 12$, black bar) and UAS controls (tau, $n = 11$, open red bars; *Ca-α1D-RNAi*, $n = 9$, open blue bars). Co-expression of both transgenes ($n = 12$, purple bar) resulted in flies with a memory performance equivalent to that of control animals, as did the UAS controls ($n = 4$, open purple bar). **(B)** Likewise, expression of tau ($n = 9$) or *Ca-α1D-RNAi* ($n = 6$) in the MB efferent M4/6 neurons (*R21D02-Gal4*, $n = 10$) abolished memory. Memory was restored to wild-type levels by co-expression of both transgenes ($n = 15$). **(C)** Expression of tau in neuronal subpopulations of the MB impaired memory. Expression was driven in the α′β′ neurons (*c305a-Gal4*, $n = 6$ control, $n = 4$ tau), αβγ neurons (*MB247-Gal4*, $n = 10$ control, $n = 7$ tau) and dorsal paired medial neurons (*amn(c316)-Gal4*, $n = 5$ control, $n = 4$ tau). Data analyzed with Kruskal–Wallis test with Dunn's *post hoc* tests **(A,C)** or with one-way ANOVA with Dunnett's *post hoc* tests **(B)**. $^{*/\#}p < 0.05$, $^{**/\#\#}p < 0.01$, and $^{***/\#\#\#}p < 0.001$. Note that *UAS / +* controls are the same for each panel.

(Malik et al., 2013), $p_{Gal4} = 0.004$, $p_{UAS} = 0.01$, **Figure 1A**) yielded memory deficient flies. Similarly, when expressed in the memory-relevant M4/6 MB output neurons (Barnstedt et al., 2016), *R21D02-Gal4, GCaMP6f > tau* flies displayed greatly reduced memory performance compared to control counterparts ($p_{Gal4} = 0.02$, $p_{UAS} < 0.001$, **Figure 1B**). We also found that tau caused a significant reduction in one-hour memory when expressed in the α′β′ MB neurons (*c305a-Gal4* (Krashes et al., 2007), $p_{Gal4} = 0.02$, $p_{UAS} = 0.01$, **Figure 1C**), which mediate memory acquisition and in the memory-storing αβγ neurons (*MB247-Gal4* (Krashes et al., 2007), $p_{Gal4} < 0.001$, $p_{UAS} = 0.003$) and dorsal paired medial (DPM) neurons (*amn(c316)-Gal4*, $p_{Gal4} = 0.002$, $p_{UAS} = 0.03$), which consolidate and stabilize labile memory (Pitman et al., 2011). All animals used for aversive conditioning were aged 2–5 days and displayed naïve avoidance of shock (**Supplementary Table S1**). Likewise, all genotypes showed similar naïve avoidance of the odors used for olfactory conditioning (**Supplementary Table S1**). Thus, all genotypes were able to detect both odors and shock, verifying that memory defects were *bone fide* and not attributable to a sensorimotor defect.

To assess changes in Ca^{2+} handling which may underpin behavioral dysfunction, we imaged the M4/6 neurons in whole *ex vivo* brains using GCaMP6f as these neurons are pertinent to memory and single neurons can be visualized (Barnstedt et al., 2016). There did not appear to be a difference in baseline fluorescence of these neurons between control and tau-expressing animals ($p = 0.5$, **Figure 2A**), suggesting no effect on basal Ca^{2+} handling, assuming comparable GCaMP6f expression between genotypes. Bath application of high potassium chloride (KCl) concentration resulted in a robust and transient elevation in fluorescence which could be ameliorated by removing Ca^{2+} from the external solution ($12.8 \pm 1.0\%$ of control, $p = 0.003$) or by adding cadmium (200 μM, $11.75 \pm 11.75\%$ of control, $p = 0.009$), a general blocker of *Drosophila* voltage-gated Ca^{2+} channels (Ryglewski et al., 2012), to the external solution (**Supplementary Figure S2A**). This indicated that the transient relies upon Ca^{2+} influx through voltage-gated Ca^{2+} channels, or that cadmium blocked presynaptic Ca^{2+} channels and, consequently, neurotransmitter release and activation of M4/6 neurons.

KCl-evoked Ca^{2+} transients in tau-expressing M4/6 neurons were almost three-fold greater than in control neurons ($268.9 \pm 45.2\%$ of control, $p = 0.005$, **Figure 2B**). Since previous reports have documented the potential involvement of L-type Ca^{2+} channels in AD (Wang and Mattson, 2014; Coon et al., 1999), we tested whether the change in magnitude of Ca^{2+} transients in M4/6 neurons was dependent on these channels by applying the clinically-used L-type channel-selective blocker nimodipine (Nimmrich and Eckert, 2013; Terada et al., 2016). The addition of 5 μM nimodipine to the external solution had no effect on the magnitude of Ca^{2+} transients in control brains ($p > 0.9$, **Figure 2C**). However, the peak of the transient in tau-expressing neurons was sensitive to nimodipine and was reduced to a magnitude indistinguishable from control ($98.9 \pm 21.1\%$ of control, $p > 0.9$). The elevated Ca^{2+} influx seen in these neurons may, therefore, be due to augmented L-type Ca^{2+} channels. To further investigate which type of voltage-gated Ca^{2+} channel

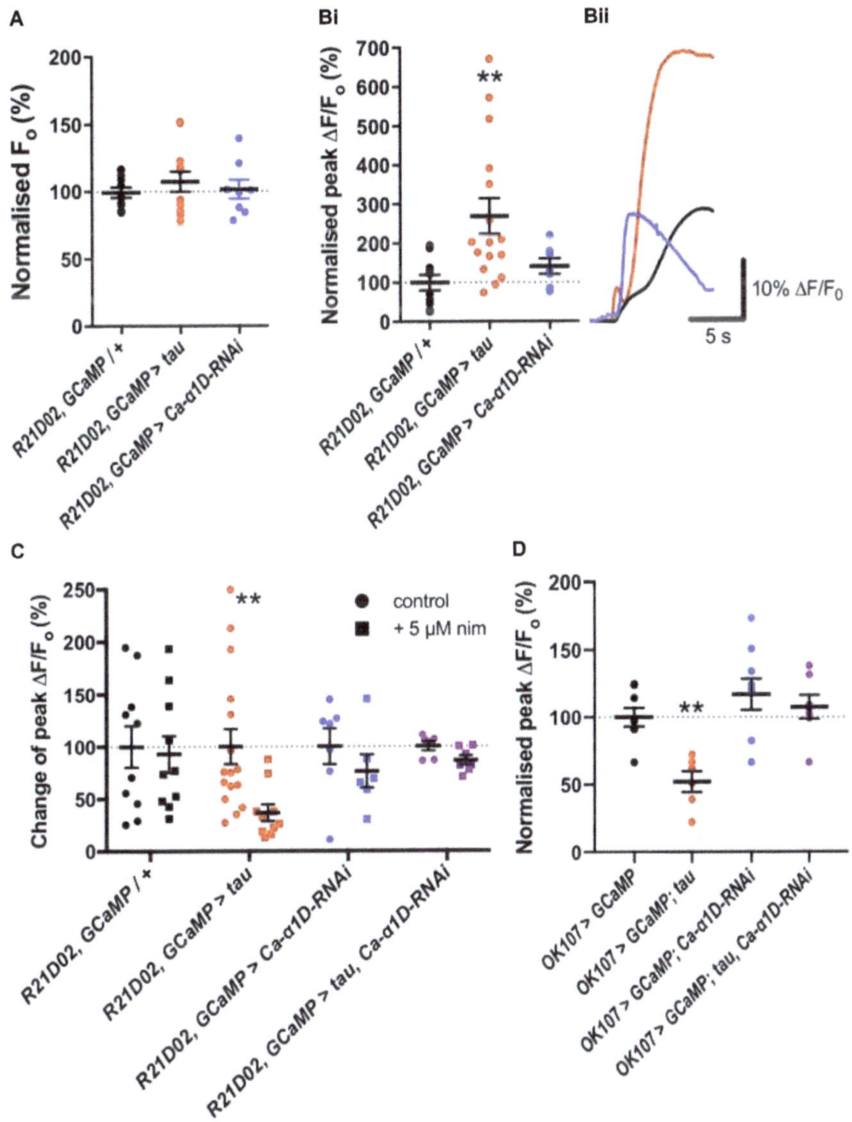

FIGURE 2 | Tau expression elevated nimodipine-sensitive Ca^{2+} channels in mushroom body (MB) and M4/6 neurons. **(A)** Basal Ca^{2+} levels were no different between control neurons and those expressing tau or *Ca-α1D-RNAi*. **(Bi)** However, the peak magnitude of Ca^{2+} transients were greater in the tau-expressing neurons than in control or *Ca-α1D-RNAi*-expressing neurons. **(Bii)** GCaMP6f relative fluorescence changes over time traces of M4/6 neurons in response to 100 mM KCl for control (black trace), tau (red trace) and *Ca-α1D-RNAi* (blue trace). **(C)** Ca^{2+} transients in control and *Ca-α1D-RNAi*-expressing neurons were not sensitive to the L-type Ca^{2+} channel blocker nimodipine (black and blue symbols, respectively). Driving tau expression in M4/6 neurons conferred sensitivity of Ca^{2+} transients to nimodipine (red symbols). The effect of tau on Ca^{2+} transient nimodipine sensitivity was ablated by co-expression of tau and *Ca-α1D-RNAi* in these neurons (purple symbols). Control for each genotype normalized to 100%. **(D)** Tau expression in the MB reduced peak fluorescence following a high KCl challenge; an effect reversed by co-expression of *Ca α1D-RNAi*. Data analyzed with one-way ANOVA with Dunnett's *post hoc* tests panels **(A,D)**, with Kruskal–Wallis test with Dunn's *post hoc* tests panel **(B)** or with two-way ANOVA with Sidak's *post hoc* tests panel **(C)**. $^{*/\#}p < 0.05$, $^{**/\#\#}p < 0.01$, and $^{***/\#\#\#}p < 0.001$. Note that data for *OK107 > GCaMP* and *OK107 > GCaMP, tau* are reproduced from Higham et al. (2019).

mediated the Ca^{2+} influx, we also tested the effect of addition of the L-type and T-type Ca^{2+} channel blocker, amiloride (1 mM), to nimodipine on the KCl-induced Ca^{2+} transient, as this compound greatly reduced Ca^{2+} currents in cultured embryonic *Drosophila* giant neurons (Peng and Wu, 2007). Amiloride did not significantly reduce the peak of the Ca^{2+} transient in M4/6 neurons ($p = 0.2$, **Supplementary Figure S2B**). The lack of effect of amiloride likely indicates developmental or cell-specific differences in Ca^{2+} channel expression or that the voltage-gated Ca^{2+} channels blocked by amiloride largely overlap with nimodipine which do not contribute significantly to the Ca^{2+} transient in wild-type M4/6 neurons.

To corroborate our pharmacological data, we tested the nimodipine sensitivity of Ca^{2+} transients in M4/6 neurons co-expressing tau and an *RNAi* to the L-type Ca^{2+} channel gene (*UAS-Ca-α1D-RNAi*), that has been shown to reduce

L-type Ca^{2+} channel currents and protein levels by over 75% in *Drosophila* neurons (Kadas et al., 2017). Ca^{2+} transients in these neurons displayed a much reduced, and statistically insignificant ($p > 0.05$, **Figure 2C**), block by nimodipine compared to transients in neurons expressing tau alone (13.2% vs. 62.3% reduction in peak). This data shows that the elevated Ca^{2+} transients in tau-expressing M4/6 neurons rely on L-type Ca^{2+} channels. As L-type channels negatively regulate neuronal excitability (Worrell and Levine, 2008), *RNAi* mediated reduction of L-type Ca^{2+} channels increases neuronal activity (Kadas et al., 2017).

We went on to test the involvement of the L-type Ca^{2+} channel itself in memory by knocking down its expression with *RNAi*. Knock-down of *Ca-α1D* in the M4/6 neurons abolished one-hour memory ($p_{Gal4} = 0.03$, $p_{UAS} = 0.007$, **Figure 1B**). These animals exhibited no sensorimotor defects (**Supplementary Table S1**), verifying the observed phenotype as a genuine memory defect. In alignment with the lack of effect of nimodipine on the Ca^{2+} transient in control neurons, knock-down of the L-type channel had no effect on KCl-evoked Ca^{2+} influx in M4/6 cells ($p = 0.6$, **Figure 2B**).

We sought to resolve whether there was a behavioral interaction between 0N4R tau and the L-type Ca^{2+} channel by testing whether knocking down *Ca-α1D* could ameliorate the effect of tau on memory as it did on Ca^{2+} signaling. Strikingly, even though expression of human tau or *Ca-α1D-RNAi* removed memory alone, co-expression in M4/6 neurons yielded flies with memory performance indistinguishable from wild-type animals ($p_{Gal4} > 0.9$, $p_{UAS} > 0.9$, **Figure 1B**). We tested whether this restoration of memory could have been a consequence of *Gal4* dilution due to the presence of multiple transgenes. Expression of an innocuous gene, *UAS-GFP*, with either *UAS-tau* or *UAS-Ca-α1D-RNAi* yielded animals with impaired memory ($p = 0.02$ and 0.005, respectively, **Supplementary Figure S1**). This demonstrates that dilution of transgene expression is not responsible for the observed change in memory performance. Lastly, the expression of transgenes in the M4/6 output neurons had no effect on the animals' naïve sensorimotor behavior indicating that the effects seen in memory are not due to defective sensory responses (**Supplementary Table S1**).

To test if the apparent interaction between tau and L-type Ca^{2+} channels occurred in other neurons, we performed Ca^{2+} imaging of the entire MB (*OK107-Gal4*). The KCl-evoked Ca^{2+} response in this large population of neurons was reduced by the expression of tau (48.1% reduction, $p = 0.006$, **Figure 2D**; Higham et al., 2019), likely reflecting a reduction in excitability. MB neuronal architecture appeared grossly intact in tau-expressing animals (data not shown), and neurodegeneration has been shown not to play a significant role in memory defects at this age (Higham et al., 2019). In alignment with observations in M4/6 neurons, the expression of *Ca-α1D-RNAi* in the MB abolished one-hour memory ($p_{Gal4} = 0.001$, $p_{UAS} = 0.04$, **Figure 1A**) but did not affect the magnitude of the Ca^{2+} transient in these neurons ($p = 0.4$, **Figure 2D**). The co-expression of these two transgenes in the MB resulted in a Ca^{2+} transient which was no different in magnitude compared to control animals ($p > 0.9$, **Figure 2D**). The ablation of one-hour memory caused by tau or *Ca-α1D-RNAi* expression in MB neurons was also reversed by co-expression of both transgenes as these animals exhibited a memory performance equivalent to control animals ($p_{Gal4} > 0.9$, $p_{UAS} > 0.9$, **Figure 1A**).

The mechanism underlying tau-mediated augmentation of Ca^{2+} influx through L-type channels is not clear. It could be due to elevated expression of the *Ca-α1D* gene, increased trafficking to, or reduced recycling from, the plasma membrane or changes in single channel properties such as conductance or open probability. To investigate this further, we measured *Ca-α1D* expression in whole brain extracts by RT-qPCR. All transgenes were expressed in all neurons (*elav-Gal4*) to ensure changes in gene expression were detectable (**Figure 3**). *Ca-α1D-RNAi* knock-down reduced expression of the channel by 58% ($p < 0.05$), while expression of tau lead to a 68% ($p = 0.04$) increase in *Ca-α1D*. Interestingly, co-expression of tau and *Ca-α1D-RNAi* restored *Ca-α1D* to 72% ($p = 0.3$) of control fly levels. This strongly suggests that the effects observed in behavior and Ca^{2+} imaging are due to a change in *Ca-α1D* expression in the brain.

DISCUSSION

Selectively expressing tau in MB neuronal subsets revealed a non-specific adverse effect on memory processing (**Figure 1**). MB neurons sub-serving specific memory phases rely on different signaling molecules. For example, CaMKII is required in α′β′ neurons, but not αβγ, and vice versa for KCNQ channels (Cavaliere et al., 2013; Malik et al., 2013). This suggests that

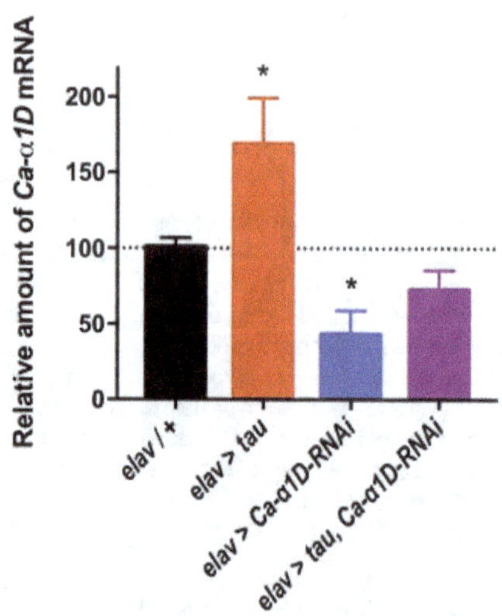

FIGURE 3 | Tau expression increased Ca^{2+} *channelα1D mRNA* levels. Pan-neuronal Tau expression led to a 68% increase in *Ca-α1D mRNA* levels compared to controls, while expressing a *RNAi* against *Ca-α1D* reduced its expression by 58%. Co-expression of the *RNAi* in tau expressing flies partially restored levels of *Ca-α1D* compared to controls. $n = 6$ biological replicates of 23 or more heads each for all groups. Data analyzed with one-way ANOVA with Holm-Sidak's *post hoc* tests. $^*p < 0.05$.

tau either promiscuously interacts with and disrupts numerous intracellular components or disrupts a pathway common to all MB neurons. *In vivo* Ca^{2+} imaging of different MB neuronal subsets has revealed the importance of Ca^{2+} transient plasticity in olfactory associative memory (Yu et al., 2006; Sejourne et al., 2011). Following conditioning, MB neurons exhibit differential Ca^{2+} responses to the CS+ and CS- odors (Yu et al., 2006; Sejourne et al., 2011). In the β′ lobe dendrites of M4/6 neurons, exposure to an aversively conditioned CS+ odour results in a greater Ca^{2+} influx compared with CS-, with the reverse being true for appetitively conditioned odors (Owald et al., 2015). Other MB neurons display a similar distinction between CS+ and CS-, with these differences believed to coordinate avoidance or approach behavior. Given that tau expression aberrantly elevated stimulus-evoked Ca^{2+} influx, it is plausible that this interferes with conditioning-induced Ca^{2+} transient plasticity. Augmented Ca^{2+} entry via L-type channels in tau-expressing neurons may ablate the difference in Ca^{2+} influx between CS+ and CS-, rendering them indistinguishable at the cellular level.

The knock-down of the *Drosophila* L-type Ca^{2+} channel demonstrated its importance in both the MB and the M4/6 neurons for memory. This aligns with data from $Ca_V1.2$ knock-out mice, which are deficient in spatial memory tasks (Moosmang et al., 2005; White et al., 2008). Despite *R21D02, GCaMP6f* > *Ca-α1D-RNAi* and *OK107* > *Ca-α1D-RNAi* flies being memory deficient, the M4/6 and MB neurons of these animals displayed no reduction in evoked Ca^{2+} entry, nor did nimodipine have any effect on the Ca^{2+} transient in control M4/6 neurons (**Figure 2**). This suggests that perhaps only a small population of L-type channels is present in these neurons. A previous electrophysiological study of Ca^{2+} currents in cultured *Drosophila* giant embryonic neurons revealed only a very small block by nifedipine, likely reflecting a low number of L-type channels (Peng and Wu, 2007). Likewise an electrophysiological and pharmacological study of the adult *OK107-Gal4* MB neurons again showed only a small contribution of L-type channels to their Ca^{2+} transients (Jiang et al., 2005). Fluorescence imaging using GCaMP may not be sufficiently sensitive to resolve such a small contribution to global Ca^{2+} influx – a contribution that is nonetheless important for cellular function and, hence, memory.

It is not known whether the L-type channel plays any role in the plasticity of Ca^{2+} transients in *Drosophila per se*. However, these channels are vital for the function of memory-associated neurons. The generation of medium and slow afterhyperpolarizations (AHPs), which are a period of prolonged hyperpolarized membrane potential following action potential firing, in hippocampal neurons is dependent on Ca^{2+} entry through L-type channels (Lancaster and Adams, 1986; Marrion and Tavalin, 1998; Bowden et al., 2001). Elevated Ca^{2+} entry would augment AHPs and suppress neuronal firing, thereby disrupting neural circuit function and the behavior subserved by that circuit. This is apparent in mice and rabbits, which exhibit an age-related memory decline with concomitant elevation of L-type Ca^{2+} channel expression and AHP magnitude in the hippocampus (Moyer et al., 1992; Nunez-Santana et al., 2014). This impairs stimulus-evoked changes in neuronal activity which underpin learning (Moyer et al., 2000). Blocking augmented AHPs in aged rabbits with nimodipine facilitated enhanced performance in associative learning tasks (Straube et al., 1990). L-type Ca^{2+} channels also negatively regulate neuronal excitability in *Drosophila* neurons (Worrell and Levine, 2008), and so their augmentation by tau may exert a similar effect on *Drosophila* neurons to that observed in aging mammals, with their knock-down resulting in increased firing of neurons (Kadas et al., 2017).

In M4/6 neurons, we observed raised evoked Ca^{2+} influx due to tau expression, while Ca^{2+} influx was suppressed in MB neurons (**Figures 2B,D**). Augmentation of the Ca^{2+} transient in single tau-expressing M4/6 neurons reflects the elevated Ca^{2+} influx through L-type channels, as the transients were reduced by nimodipine and L-type channel knock-down. However, in a large population of MB neurons (~2500 neurons) the elevated Ca^{2+} influx through L-type channels is likely small relative to the reduced Ca^{2+} levels due to suppressed neuronal activity, therefore a reduction in the Ca^{2+} transient was observed. The reduced excitability of MB neurons was rescued by co-expression of *Ca-α1D-RNAi* as this manipulation opposes the suppression of excitability caused by tau (Kadas et al., 2017). Not only were the tau-induced Ca^{2+} signaling defects rescued by manipulation of L-type Ca^{2+} channels, but so was olfactory memory (**Figures 1A,B**). This lends further credence to the suggestion that tau interacts with the L-type Ca^{2+} channel and also shows that this interaction solely mediates memory dysfunction, at least in young animals.

Raised L-type Ca^{2+} channel expression has also been documented in other AD models, as well as in aging. In agreement with our data, L-type Ca^{2+} current density was elevated in CA1 neurons of 3 × Tg mice (Wang and Mattson, 2014), as were AHPs in the dorsomedial entorhinal cortex of rTg4510 mice (Booth et al., 2016a). Our data shows that wild-type 0N4R tau, as well as the frontotemporal dementia-associated P301L mutant expressed in 3 × Tg and rTg4510 mice, is capable of augmenting Ca^{2+} influx in neurons. What is more, elevated expression of a mammalian L-type Ca^{2+} channel ($Ca_V1.2$) was observed in a neuroblastoma cell line following transgenic $A\beta_{42}$ expression; this resulted in reduced cell viability and six-fold increase in Ca^{2+} influx, that could be ameliorated by the L-type Ca^{2+} channel dihydropyridine blockers, nimodipine and isradipine (Copenhaver et al., 2011). This study went on to show that the L-type channel blocker, isradipine could increase survival of *Drosophila* overexpressing human amyloid precursor protein (APP_{695}), as well as decreasing the accumulation of Aβ and phosphorylated tau in the triple transgenic AD mice (3 × TgAD) which express human Presenilin 1_{M146V}, $APP_{Swedish}$ and tau_{P30L}. This indicates that correcting defective Ca^{2+} handling in AD may be of therapeutic benefit, particularly as L-type Ca^{2+} channels appear to be relevant in the human AD brain, too.

Raised L-type Ca^{2+} channel expression has been documented in the brains of AD patients (Coon et al., 1999), with increased L-type channels thought to underlie the memory loss and neurodegeneration that occurs in dementia (Missiaen et al., 2000; Mattson and Chan, 2001; Canzoniero and Snider, 2005; Thibault et al., 2007). Our data shows that there is increased expression of the *Drosophila* L-type Ca^{2+} channel, *Ca-α1D,* in tau expressing neurons, therefore suggesting conserved mechanisms of Aβ and tau-related calcium deficits across species (**Figure 3**). Importantly, clinical trials of L-type blockers show a slowing of cognitive decline in AD patients (Anekonda et al., 2011; Goodison et al., 2012; Nimmrich and Eckert, 2013).

In summary, using behavioral, physiological, pharmacological and molecular methods, we show that knock-down of the *Drosophila* L-type Ca^{2+} channel *Ca-α1D* can rescue tau mediated olfactory learning deficits by restoring Ca^{2+} handling in MB neurons.

MATERIALS AND METHODS

Drosophila Genetics

Flies were raised at a standard density with a 12 h:12 h light dark (LD) cycle on standard *Drosophila* medium (0.7% agar, 1.0% soya flour, 8.0% polenta/maize, 1.8% yeast, 8.0% malt extract, 4.0% molasses, 0.8% propionic acid, and 2.3% nipagen) at 25°C. Wild-type control was *Canton S w- (CSw-)* and *R21D02-GAL4, UAS-GCaMP6f* were kind gifts from Prof. Scott Waddell (University of Oxford). *UAS-human MAPT (TAU 0N4R) wild-type* (Wittmann et al., 2001; Kerr et al., 2011) was a kind gift from Prof. Linda Partridge (University College London), *UAS-GFP* was a gift from Prof. Mark Wu (John Hopkins University). The following flies were obtained from the Bloomington and Vienna fly stock centers: *OK107-Gal4* (Bloomington *Drosophila* stock center number BDSC:854), *c305a-Gal4* (BDSC:30829), *amn(c316)-Gal4* (BDSC:30830), *MB247-Gal4* (BDSC:50742), *elav-Gal4* (BDSC:8760), *UAS-GCaMP6f* (BDSC:42747) and *UAS-Ca-α1D-RNAi* flies [Vienna *Drosophila* resource center GD51491 (Kadas et al., 2017)].

Aversive Olfactory Conditioning

All memory experiments were carried out at 25°C and 70% relative humidity under dim red light. Flies were used for experiments after 2–5 days of aging at 25°C and 70% relative humidity in a 12-hour light: 12-hour dark environment. Using a previously published protocol (Mershin et al., 2004; Krashes et al., 2007; Kosmidis et al., 2010; Malik et al., 2013; Malik and Hodge, 2014; Barnstedt et al., 2016), groups of 25–50 flies were first transferred from food tubes into the training tube lined with an electrifiable grid. After acclimatization to the electrified tube for 90 s, flies were exposed to either 3-octanol (OCT, Sigma) or 4-methylcyclohexanol (MCH, Sigma) (conditioned stimulus, CS+) paired with twelve 70 V DC electric shocks (unconditioned stimulus, United States) over 60 s (shocks of duration 1.25 s with inter-shock latency of 3.75 s). This was followed by a 30 s rest period with no stimulus. Flies were then exposed to the reciprocal odour (CS−) for 60 s with no electric shock. Memory retention was tested one-hour post-conditioning (intermediate-term memory). To account for any innate bias the flies may have towards an odour, the CS + odour was reversed in alternate groups of flies and the performances from these two groups averaged to give $n = 1$. Moreover, the order of delivery of CS+ and CS− was alternately reversed.

To test memory, flies were placed at the choice point of a T-maze with one pathway exposed to CS+ and the other to CS−. After 120 s, the number of flies choosing each pathway was counted. Memory was quantified using the performance index (PI):

$$PI = \frac{N_{CS-} - N_{CS+}}{N_{CS-} + N_{CS+}}$$

where N_{CS-} and N_{CS+} is the number of flies choosing CS− and CS+, respectively. A $PI = 1$ indicates perfect learning where all flies chose CS−, and $PI = 0$ indicates a 50:50 split between CS− and CS+ and, therefore, no learning.

Calcium Imaging

GCaMP imaging was performed using previously published protocols (Cavaliere et al., 2012; Gillespie and Hodge, 2013; Malik et al., 2013; Schlichting et al., 2016; Shaw et al., 2018) with flies being anaesthetized on CO_2, decapitated and their brains dissected out of the head in extracellular saline containing (in mM): 101 NaCl, 1 $CaCl_2$, 4 $MgCl_2$, 3 KCl, 5 D-glucose, 1.25 NaH_2PO_4, and 20.7 $NaHCO_3$ adjusted to a final pH of pH 7.2 with an osmolality of 247–253 mmol/kg. Brains were held ventral side up in a recording chamber using a custom-made anchor and visualized with a 40× water-immersion lens on an upright microscope (Zeiss Examiner Z1).

Brains were superfused with extracellular saline (5 mL/min) as above and cells were depolarized by bath application of 100 mM KCl in extracellular solution (362 mmol/kg) for 15 s at 5 mL/min. Drug-containing or Ca^{2+}-lacking solutions were superfused over the brain for 60 s prior to imaging. The Ca^{2+}-lacking external solution contained 8 mM $MgCl_2$.

Images were acquired at 8 Hz with 50 ms exposure using a CCD camera (ZEISS Axiocam) and a 470 nm LED light source (Colibri, ZEISS) and recorded with ZEN (Zeiss, 4 frames/sec). Baseline fluorescence (F_0) was taken as the mean fluorescence during the 10 s (80 images) prior to the start of KCl perfusion. The change in fluorescence relative to baseline [$(F-F_0)/F_0$, where F is fluorescence at a given time] following KCl addition was recorded, and the peak change [$(F_{max}-F_0)/F_0$] was used as a metric of transient [Ca^{2+}] increase. Example traces were plotted using Origin 9 (Origin Lab).

All chemicals were purchased from Sigma-Aldrich (Gillingham, United Kingdom), except for nimodipine which was purchased from Tocris (Bristol, United Kingdom) and amiloride which was donated by Prof. David Sheppard (University of Bristol).

RT-qPCR

Relative measure of Ca-α1D expression levels was assessed by two-step qPCR. 2–5 days old male flies were anesthetized with CO_2 and decapitated, obtaining six biological replicates with 23 heads each. Total *RNA* was extracted from head lysates by organic phenol/chloroform method using TRIzol reagent (Invitrogen). *RNA* quantification was carried out in Nanodrop spectrophotometer (Thermo Scientific) and *RNA* integrity was checked by electrophoresis in 1% agarose gel. Samples were treated with TURBO DNA-free kit (Invitrogen) in order to remove genomic DNA contamination. Reverse transcription was carried out using RevertAid First Strand cDNA Synthesis Kit (Thermo Scientific) following manufacturer's instructions, with 500 ng of *RNA* as template and Oligo (dT) as primer to amplify total *mRNA*. cDNA samples were stored at −20°C or used immediately for qPCR reactions.

Quantitative PCR reactions were carried out in QuantStudio 3 Real-Time PCR system (Applied Biosystems) using HOT FIREPol EvaGreen qPCR Mix Plus (Solis BioDyne). The primers used to amplify Ca-α1D *mRNA* were as follows: Ca1DF 5′-CCTTGAGGGCTGGACTGATG-3′ and Ca1DR 5′-ATCACGAAGAAGGCACCCAG-3′ with a PCR product expected size of 108 bp and 104% primer efficiency (**Supplementary Figure S3**). As a housekeeping gene, the following primers for GAPDH2 *mRNA* were used: GAPDH2F 5′-CGTTCATGCCACCACCGCTA-3′ and GAPDH2R 5′-CCACGTCCATCACGCCACAA-3′. The expected PCR product size was 72 bp and the primer efficiency was 100%. To activate DNA polymerase, a first step of 15 min at 95°C was used, followed by 50 cycles of 30 s at 95°C, 30 s at 60°C, followed by a 1 min 72°C elongation step. At the end of the experiment, a temperature ramp from 60°C to 95°C was used for melting curve analysis and the product fit to the predicted melting curve obtained by uMelt software (Dwight et al., 2011). Quantification for each genotype and each gene was carried out using the $2^{(-\Delta\Delta Ct)}$ method and data was expressed as a percentage of change.

Analysis

All data were analyzed using Prism 7 (GraphPad Inc.). Data were scrutinized to check they met the assumptions of parametric statistical tests, and non-parametric, rank-based alternatives were used where appropriate. Details of statistical tests used are in figure legends. Data are presented as mean ± standard error of mean.

AUTHOR CONTRIBUTIONS

All authors devised and performed the experiments, and wrote and edited the manuscript. JH secured the funding.

ACKNOWLEDGMENTS

The authors are grateful to Drs. Linda Partridge, Scott Waddell, and Mark Wu for providing the fly stocks, and Drs. Kofan Chen, Bilal Malik, and Neil Marrion for helpful advice and comments on the manuscript.

REFERENCES

Anekonda, T. S., Quinn, J. F., Harris, C., Frahler, K., Wadsworth, T. L., and Woltjer, R. L. (2011). L-type voltage-gated calcium channel blockade with isradipine as a therapeutic strategy for Alzheimer's disease. *Neurobiol. Dis.* 41, 62–70. doi: 10.1016/j.nbd.2010.08.020

Arendt, T., Stieler, J. T., and Holzer, M. (2016). Tau and tauopathies. *Brain Res. Bull.* 126, 238–292. doi: 10.1016/j.brainresbull.2016.08.018

Barnstedt, O., Owald, D., Felsenberg, J., Brain, R., Moszynski, J. P., Talbot, C. B., et al. (2016). Memory-Relevant mushroom body output synapses are cholinergic. *Neuron* 89, 1237–1247. doi: 10.1016/j.neuron.2016.02.015

Biundo, F., Del Prete, D., Zhang, H., Arancio, O., and D'Adamio, L. (2018). A role for tau in learning, memory and synaptic plasticity. *Sci. Rep.* 8:3184. doi: 10.1038/s41598-018-21596-3

Booth, C. A., Ridler, T., Murray, T. K., Ward, M. A., de Groot, E., Goodfellow, M., et al. (2016a). Electrical and network neuronal properties are preferentially disrupted in dorsal, but not ventral, medial entorhinal cortex in a mouse model of tauopathy. *J. Neurosci.* 36, 312–324. doi: 10.1523/JNEUROSCI.2845-14.2016

Booth, C. A., Witton, J., Nowacki, J., Tsaneva-Atanasova, K., Jones, M. W., Randall, A. D., et al. (2016b). Altered intrinsic pyramidal neuron properties and pathway-specific synaptic dysfunction underlie aberrant hippocampal network function in a mouse model of tauopathy. *J. Neurosci.* 36, 350–363. doi: 10.1523/JNEUROSCI.2151-15.2016

Boutajangout, A., Boom, A., Leroy, K., and Brion, J. P. (2004). Expression of tau mRNA and soluble tau isoforms in affected and non-affected brain areas in Alzheimer's disease. *FEBS Lett.* 576, 183–189. doi: 10.1016/j.febslet.2004.09.011

Bowden, S. E., Fletcher, S., Loane, D. J., and Marrion, N. V. (2001). Somatic colocalization of rat SK1 and D class ($Ca_V1.2$) L-type calcium channels in rat CA1 hippocampal pyramidal neurons. 21:RC175. doi: 10.1523/JNEUROSCI.21-20-j0006.2001

Brzyska, M., and Elbaum, D. (2003). Dysregulation of calcium in Alzheimer's disease. *Acta Neurobiol. Exp.* 63, 171–183.

Buee, L., Bussiere, T., Buee-Scherrer, V., Delacourte, A., and Hof, P. R. (2000). Tau protein isoforms, phosphorylation and role in neurodegenerative disorders. *Brain Res. Brain Res. Rev.* 33, 95–130. doi: 10.1016/s0165-0173(00)00019-9

Buhl, E., Higham, J. P., and Hodge, J. J. L. (2019). Alzheimer's disease-associated tau alters *Drosophila* circadian activity, sleep and clock neuron electrophysiology. *Neurobiol. Dis.* 130:104507. doi: 10.1016/j.nbd.2019.104507

Canzoniero, L. M., and Snider, B. J. (2005). Calcium in Alzheimer's disease pathogenesis: too much, too little or in the wrong place? *J. Alzheimers Dis.* 8, 147–154; discussion 209–115.

Cavaliere, S., Gillespie, J. M., and Hodge, J. J. (2012). KCNQ channels show conserved ethanol block and function in ethanol behaviour. *PLoS One* 7:e50279. doi: 10.1371/journal.pone.0050279

Cavaliere, S., Malik, B. R., and Hodge, J. J. (2013). KCNQ channels regulate age-related memory impairment. *PLoS One* 8:e62445. doi: 10.1371/journal.pone.0062445

Chee, F. C., Mudher, A., Cuttle, M. F., Newman, T. A., MacKay, D., Lovestone, S., et al. (2005). Over-expression of tau results in defective synaptic transmission in *Drosophila* neuromuscular junctions. *Neurobiol. Dis.* 20, 918–928. doi: 10.1016/j.nbd.2005.05.029

Coon, A. L., Wallace, D. R., Mactutus, C. F., and Booze, R. M. (1999). L-type calcium channels in the hippocampus and cerebellum of Alzheimer's disease brain tissue. *Neurobiol. Aging* 20, 597–603. doi: 10.1016/s0197-4580(99)00068-8

Copenhaver, P. F., Anekonda, T. S., Musashe, D., Robinson, K. M., Ramaker, J. M., Swanson, T. L., et al. (2011). A translational continuum of model systems for evaluating treatment strategies in Alzheimer's disease: isradipine as a candidate drug. *Dis. Models Mech.* 4, 634–648. doi: 10.1242/dmm.006841

Daschil, N., Kniewallner, K. M., Obermair, G. J., Hutter-Paier, B., Windisch, M., Marksteiner, J., et al. (2015). L-type calcium channel blockers and substance P induce angiogenesis of cortical vessels associated with beta-amyloid plaques in an Alzheimer mouse model. *Neurobiol. Aging* 36, 1333–1341. doi: 10.1016/j.neurobiolaging.2014.12.027

Davis, R. L. (2011). Traces of *Drosophila* memory. *Neuron* 70, 8–19. doi: 10.1016/j.neuron.2011.03.012

Dwight, Z., Palais, R., and Wittwer, C. T. (2011). uMELT: prediction of high-resolution melting curves and dynamic melting profiles of PCR products in a rich web application. *Bioinformatics* 27, 1019–1020. doi: 10.1093/bioinformatics/btr065

Espinoza, M., de Silva, R., Dickson, D. W., and Davies, P. (2008). Differential incorporation of tau isoforms in Alzheimer's disease. *J. Alzheimers Dis.* 14, 1–16. doi: 10.3233/jad-2008-14101

Gillespie, J. M., and Hodge, J. J. (2013). CASK regulates CaMKII autophosphorylation in neuronal growth, calcium signaling, and learning. *Front. Mol. Neurosci.* 6:27. doi: 10.3389/fnmol.2013.00027

Goodison, W. V., Frisardi, V., and Kehoe, P. G. (2012). Calcium channel blockers and Alzheimer's disease: potential relevance in treatment strategies of metabolic syndrome. *J. Alzheimes Dis.* 30(Suppl. 2), S269–S282. doi: 10.3233/JAD-2012-111664

Hasegawa, M., Watanabe, S., Kondo, H., Akiyama, H., Mann, D. M., Saito, Y., et al. (2014). 3R and 4R tau isoforms in paired helical filaments in Alzheimer's disease. *Acta Neuropathol.* 127, 303–305. doi: 10.1007/s00401-013-1191-9

Higham, J. P., Malik, B. R., Buhl, E., Dawson, J. M., Ogier, A. S., Lunnon, K., et al. (2019). Alzheimer's disease associated genes ankyrin and tau cause shortened lifespan and memory loss in *Drosophila*. *Front. Cell. Neurosci.* 13:260. doi: 10.3389/fncel.2019.00260

Iijima-Ando, K., and Iijima, K. (2010). Transgenic *Drosophila* models of Alzheimer's disease and tauopathies. *Brain Struct. Funct.* 214, 245–262. doi: 10.1007/s00429-009-0234-4

Jiang, S. A., Campusano, J. M., Su, H., and O'Dowd, D. K. (2005). *Drosophila* mushroom body Kenyon cells generate spontaneous calcium transients mediated by PLTX-sensitive calcium channels. *J. Neurophysiol.* 94, 491–500. doi: 10.1152/jn.00096.2005

Kadas, D., Klein, A., Krick, N., Worrell, J. W., Ryglewski, S., and Duch, C. (2017). Dendritic and Axonal L-Type calcium channels cooperate to enhance motoneuron firing output during *Drosophila* larval locomotion. *J. Neurosci.* 37, 10971–10982. doi: 10.1523/JNEUROSCI.1064-17.2017

Kadas, D., Papanikolopoulou, K., Xirou, S., Consoulas, C., and Skoulakis, E. M. C. (2019). Human Tau isoform-specific presynaptic deficits in a *Drosophila* central nervous system circuit. *Neurobiol. Dis.* 124, 311–321. doi: 10.1016/j.nbd.2018.12.004

Kaufman, S. K., Del Tredici, K., Thomas, T. L., Braak, H., and Diamond, M. I. (2018). Tau seeding activity begins in the transentorhinal/entorhinal regions and anticipates phospho-tau pathology in Alzheimer's disease and PART. *Acta Neuropathol.* 136, 57–67. doi: 10.1007/s00401-018-1855-6

Kerr, F., Augustin, H., Piper, M. D., Gandy, C., Allen, M. J., Lovestone, S., et al. (2011). Dietary restriction delays aging, but not neuronal dysfunction, in *Drosophila* models of Alzheimer's disease. *Neurobiol. Aging* 32, 1977–1989. doi: 10.1016/j.neurobiolaging.2009.10.015

Kosmidis, S., Grammenoudi, S., Papanikolopoulou, K., and Skoulakis, E. M. (2010). Differential effects of Tau on the integrity and function of neurons essential for learning in *Drosophila*. *J. Neurosci.* 30, 464–477. doi: 10.1523/JNEUROSCI.1490-09.2010

Krashes, M. J., Keene, A. C., Leung, B., Armstrong, J. D., and Waddell, S. (2007). Sequential use of mushroom body neuron subsets during *Drosophila* odor memory processing. *Neuron* 53, 103–115. doi: 10.1016/j.neuron.2006.11.021

Lancaster, B., and Adams, P. R. (1986). Calcium-dependent current generating the afterhyperpolarization of hippocampal neurons. *J. Neurophysiol.* 55, 1268–1282. doi: 10.1152/jn.1986.55.6.1268

Malik, B. R., Gillespie, J. M., and Hodge, J. J. (2013). CASK and CaMKII function in the mushroom body alpha'/beta' neurons during *Drosophila* memory formation. *Front. Neural Circ.* 7:52. doi: 10.3389/fncir.2013.00052

Malik, B. R., and Hodge, J. J. (2014). *Drosophila* adult olfactory shock learning. *J. Vis. Exp.* 90:e50107.

Marrion, N. V., and Tavalin, S. J. (1998). Selective activation of Ca^{2+}-activated K^+ channels by co-localized Ca^{2+} channels in hippocampal neurons. *Nature* 395, 900–905. doi: 10.1038/27674

Mattson, M. P., and Chan, S. L. (2001). Dysregulation of cellular calcium homeostasis in Alzheimer's disease: bad genes and bad habits. *J. Mol. Neurosci.* 17, 205–224. doi: 10.1385/jmn:17:2:205

Mershin, A., Pavlopoulos, E., Fitch, O., Braden, B. C., Nanopoulos, D. V., and Skoulakis, E. M. (2004). Learning and memory deficits upon TAU accumulation in *Drosophila* mushroom body neurons. *Learn Mem.* 11, 277–287. doi: 10.1101/lm.70804

Missiaen, L., Robberecht, W., van den Bosch, L., Callewaert, G., Parys, J. B., Wuytack, F., et al. (2000). Abnormal intracellular Ca^{2+}homeostasis and disease. *Cell Calcium* 28, 1–21. doi: 10.1054/ceca.2000.0131

Moosmang, S., Haider, N., Klugbauer, N., Adelsberger, H., Langwieser, N., Muller, J., et al. (2005). Role of hippocampal $Ca_V1.2$ Ca^{2+} channels in NMDA receptor-independent synaptic plasticity and spatial memory. *J. Neurosci.* 25, 9883–9892. doi: 10.1523/jneurosci.1531-05.2005

Moyer, J. R. Jr., Power, J. M., Thompson, L. T., and Disterhoft, J. F. (2000). Increased excitability of aged rabbit CA1 neurons after trace eyeblink conditioning. *J. Neurosci.* 20, 5476–5482. doi: 10.1523/jneurosci.20-14-05476.2000

Moyer, J. R. Jr., Thompson, L. T., Black, J. P., and Disterhoft, J. F. (1992). Nimodipine increases excitability of rabbit CA1 pyramidal neurons in an age- and concentration-dependent manner. *J. Neurophysiol.* 68, 2100–2109. doi: 10.1152/jn.1992.68.6.2100

Nimmrich, V., and Eckert, A. (2013). Calcium channel blockers and dementia. *Br. J. Pharmacol.* 169, 1203–1210.

Nisbet, R. M., and Gotz, J. (2018). Amyloid-beta and Tau in Alzheimer's Disease: novel pathomechanisms and non-pharmacological treatment strategies. *J. Alzheimers Dis.* 64, S517–S527. doi: 10.3233/JAD-179907

Nunez-Santana, F. L., Oh, M. M., Antion, M. D., Lee, A., Hell, J. W., and Disterhoft, J. F. (2014). Surface L-type Ca^{2+} channel expression levels are increased in aged hippocampus. *Aging Cell* 13, 111–120. doi: 10.1111/acel.12157

Owald, D., Felsenberg, J., Talbot, C. B., Das, G., Perisse, E., Huetteroth, W., et al. (2015). Activity of defined mushroom body output neurons underlies learned olfactory behavior in *Drosophila*. *Neuron* 86, 417–427. doi: 10.1016/j.neuron.2015.03.025

Papanikolopoulou, K., and Skoulakis, E. M. (2011). The power and richness of modelling tauopathies in *Drosophila*. *Mol. Neurobiol.* 44, 122–133. doi: 10.1007/s12035-011-8193-1

Pascual, A., and Preat, T. (2001). Localization of long-term memory within the *Drosophila* mushroom body. *Science* 294, 1115–1117. doi: 10.1126/science.1064200

Peng, I. F., and Wu, C. F. (2007). *Drosophila cacophony* channels: a major mediator of neuronal Ca^{2+} currents and a trigger for K^+ channel homeostatic regulation. *J. Neurosci.* 27, 1072–1081. doi: 10.1523/jneurosci.4746-06.2007

Pitman, J. L., Huetteroth, W., Burke, C. J., Krashes, M. J., Lai, S. L., Lee, T., et al. (2011). A pair of inhibitory neurons are required to sustain labile memory in the *Drosophila* mushroom body. *Curr. Biol.* 21, 855–861. doi: 10.1016/j.cub.2011.03.069

Ryglewski, S., Lance, K., Levine, R. B., and Duch, C. (2012). Ca_V2 channels mediate low and high voltage-activated calcium currents in *Drosophila* motoneurons. *J. Physiol.* 590, 809–825. doi: 10.1113/jphysiol.2011.222836

Schlichting, M., Menegazzi, P., Lelito, K. R., Yao, Z., Buhl, E., Dalla Benetta, E., et al. (2016). A neural network underlying circadian entrainment and photoperiodic adjustment of sleep and activity in *Drosophila*. *J. Neurosci.* 36, 9084–9096. doi: 10.1523/JNEUROSCI.0992-16.2016

Sealey, M. A., Vourkou, E., Cowan, C. M., Bossing, T., Quraishe, S., Grammenoudi, S., et al. (2017). Distinct phenotypes of three-repeat and four-repeat human tau in a transgenic model of tauopathy. *Neurobiol. Dis.* 105, 74–83. doi: 10.1016/j.nbd.2017.05.003

Sejourne, J., Placais, P. Y., Aso, Y., Siwanowicz, I., Trannoy, S., Thoma, V., et al. (2011). Mushroom body efferent neurons responsible for aversive olfactory memory retrieval in *Drosophila*. *Nat. Neurosci.* 14, 903–910. doi: 10.1038/nn.2846

Shaw, R. E., Kottler, B., Ludlow, Z. N., Buhl, E., Kim, D., Morais da Silva, S., et al. (2018). In vivo expansion of functionally integrated GABAergic interneurons by targeted increase in neural progenitors. *EMBO J.* 37:e98163. doi: 10.15252/embj.201798163

Spillantini, M. G., and Goedert, M. (2013). Tau pathology and neurodegeneration. *Lancet Neurol.* 12, 609–622. doi: 10.1016/s1474-4422(13)70090-5

Spires-Jones, T. L., and Hyman, B. T. (2014). The intersection of amyloid beta and tau at synapses in Alzheimer's disease. *Neuron* 82, 756–771. doi: 10.1016/j.neuron.2014.05.004

Straube, K. T., Deyo, R. A., Moyer, J. R. Jr., and Disterhoft, J. F. (1990). Dietary nimodipine improves associative learning in aging rabbits. *Neurobiol. Aging* 11, 659–661. doi: 10.1016/0197-4580(90)90033-v

Terada, S., Matsubara, D., Onodera, K., Matsuzaki, M., Uemura, T., and Usui, T. (2016). Neuronal processing of noxious thermal stimuli mediated by dendritic Ca^{2+} influx in *Drosophila* somatosensory neurons. *eLife* 5:e12959. doi: 10.7554/eLife.12959

Thibault, O., Gant, J. C., and Landfield, P. W. (2007). Expansion of the calcium hypothesis of brain aging and Alzheimer's disease: minding the store. *Aging Cell* 6, 307–317. doi: 10.1111/j.1474-9726.2007.00295.x

Wang, Y., and Mattson, M. P. (2014). L-type Ca^{2+} currents at CA1 synapses, but not CA3 or dentate granule neuron synapses, are increased in 3xTgAD mice in an age-dependent manner. *Neurobiol. Aging* 35, 88–95. doi: 10.1016/j.neurobiolaging.2013.07.007

Wentzell, J., and Kretzschmar, D. (2010). Alzheimer's disease and tauopathy studies in flies and worms. *Neurobiol. Dis.* 40, 21–28. doi: 10.1016/j.nbd.2010.03.007

White, J. A., McKinney, B. C., John, M. C., Powers, P. A., Kamp, T. J., and Murphy, G. G. (2008). Conditional forebrain deletion of the L-type calcium channel $Ca_V1.2$ disrupts remote spatial memories in mice. *Learn. Mem.* 15, 1–5. doi: 10.1101/lm.773208

Wittmann, C. W., Wszolek, M. F., Shulman, J. M., Salvaterra, P. M., Lewis, J., Hutton, M., et al. (2001). Tauopathy in *Drosophila*: neurodegeneration without neurofibrillary tangles. *Science* 293, 711–714. doi: 10.1126/science.1062382

Worrell, J. W., and Levine, R. B. (2008). Characterization of voltage-dependent Ca2+ currents in identified *Drosophila* motoneurons in situ. *J. Neurophysiol.* 100, 868–878. doi: 10.1152/jn.90464.2008

Wu, J. W., Hussaini, S. A., Bastille, I. M., Rodriguez, G. A., Mrejeru, A., Rilett, K., et al. (2016). Neuronal activity enhances tau propagation and tau pathology in vivo. *Nat. Neurosci.* 19, 1085–1092. doi: 10.1038/nn.4328

Yu, D., Akalal, D. B., and Davis, R. L. (2006). *Drosophila* alpha/beta mushroom body neurons form a branch-specific, long-term cellular memory trace after spaced olfactory conditioning. *Neuron* 52, 845–855. doi: 10.1016/j.neuron.2006.10.030

Zhou, L., McInnes, J., Wierda, K., Holt, M., Herrmann, A. G., Jackson, R. J., et al. (2017). Tau association with synaptic vesicles causes presynaptic dysfunction. *Nat. Commun.* 8:15295. doi: 10.1038/ncomms15295

6

Chronic PD-1 Checkpoint Blockade does not Affect Cognition or Promote Tau Clearance in a Tauopathy Mouse Model

*Yan Lin[1], Hameetha B. Rajamohamedsait[1], Leslie A. Sandusky-Beltran[1], Begona Gamallo-Lana[1], Adam Mar[1] and Einar M. Sigurdsson[1,2]**

[1]*Department of Neuroscience and Physiology, Neuroscience Institute, New York University School of Medicine, New York, NY, United States,* [2]*Department of Psychiatry, New York University School of Medicine, New York, NY, United States*

Correspondence:
Einar M. Sigurdsson
einar.sigurdsson@nyumc.org

Programmed cell death protein 1 (PD-1) checkpoint blockade with an antibody has been shown to reduce amyloid-β plaques, associated pathologies and cognitive impairment in mouse models. More recently, this approach has shown effectiveness in a tauopathy mouse model to improve cognition and reduce tau lesions. Follow-up studies by other laboratories did not see similar benefits of this type of therapy in other amyloid-β plaque models. Here, we report a modest increase in locomotor activity but no effect on cognition or tau pathology, in a different more commonly used tauopathy model following a weekly treatment for 12 weeks with the same PD-1 antibody and isotype control as in the original Aβ- and tau-targeting studies. These findings indicate that further research is needed before clinical trials based on PD-1 checkpoint immune blockage are devised for tauopathies.

Keywords: tau, Alzheimer's disease, tauopathy, PD-1 blockade, antibody, therapy, mouse models, behavior

INTRODUCTION

Programmed death ligand 1 (PD-L1) binds to its receptor, programmed cell death protein 1 (PD-1), resulting in complex effects on the immune system (Chamoto et al., 2017; Wei et al., 2018). PD-1 and PD-L1 inhibitors block this association and are primarily used today to treat cancer, in which interaction of PD-L1 on tumor cells with PD-1 on T-cells reduces T-cell function and thereby prevents the immune system from attacking the tumor cells (Chamoto et al., 2017; Wei et al., 2018).

In 2016, it was reported that PD-1 immune checkpoint blockage cleared amyloid-β (Aβ) in two mouse models following a few antibody injections at ages when Aβ plaques are abundant (Baruch et al., 2016). Cognition was assessed in one of the models and was improved as well. The putative mechanism put forward was that PD-1 blockage led to the recruitment of monocyte-derived macrophages to the brain, which then cleared Aβ resulting in improved cognition. Following these interesting findings, several pharmaceutical companies that were developing PD-1 antibody blockers for other conditions pursued this approach with their own compounds and in different Aβ plaque mouse models. In their hands, PD-1 immunotherapy stimulated systemic activation of the peripheral immune system as expected, but monocyte-derived macrophage infiltration into the brain was not detected, and brain Aβ pathology was not altered (Latta-Mahieu et al., 2018).

Recently, the same group that showed beneficial effects of PD-1 blockade on Aβ clearance and cognition followed up on their pioneering findings demonstrating that similar benefits could be obtained in a tauopathy model using the same PD-1 antibody and isotype control as in their original study (Rosenzweig et al., 2019). Comparable results were observed with a PD-L1 antibody. We have examined this approach in a different more commonly used tauopathy model, intervening also at a stage when tau pathology is clearly evident. Twelve weekly injections of the same PD-1 antibody as used in both of the effective Aβ and tau-targeting studies, slightly increased locomotor activity but failed to significantly reduce tau pathology or affect cognitive performance in five different tasks.

MATERIALS AND METHODS

Mice

Homozygous female JNPL3 tauopathy mice of a mixed background were used for this study (Taconic, Germantown, NY, USA, Stock # 2508), starting at 10–11 months of age (n = 22: 11 treated and 11 controls) and concluding at 14–15 months following extensive behavioral testing (n = 18 brains analyzed: 10 treated and eight controls). Six mice died during the study, four controls and two treated. Two controls died after the first and eighth injection, respectively. One mouse in each group was euthanized before the Barnes maze. Those two brains were saved and included in the analyses. In addition, one mouse in each group died before the fear conditioning test. This mouse model expresses ubiquitously the human P301L tau mutation within the 0N4R isoform under the direction of a prion promoter and is one of the most widely used tauopathy mouse models. The homozygous animals have an early onset of tau pathology, which is most severe in the brainstem and spinal cord but is evident throughout the brain. In the original description of this model, the motor phenotype was severe with progressive hindleg paralysis leading the animals to not being able to ambulate or feed themselves properly (Lewis et al., 2000). This was more severe in females and in homozygous animals, with functional deficits starting at about 5 months and not many females survived past 1 year of age. Because of the motor phenotype, cognitive tests were not commonly employed in this model in the first years after it was developed because those typically require intact motor functions. Currently, the tau pathology and related motor deficits have shifted to an older age in this model, with motor deficits starting at 8–12 months and most animals survive well into their second year of age, in particular the males, with females showing more severe pathology (EM Sigurdsson, personal observation). Because of sex differences in pathology, only females were used in the present study and all appeared healthy at the onset of the study. The mice were housed in Association for Assessment and Accreditation of Laboratory Animal Care (AAALAC) approved facilities. All mouse care and experimental procedures were compliant with guidelines of animal experimentation and were approved by the Institutional Animal Care and Use Committee at New York University School of Medicine.

Antibody Administration

PD-1 checkpoint inhibitor (anti m PD-1; Rat IgG2a isotype, clone RPM1-14, Bioxcell Catalog# BE0146) or its isotype control (rat IgG2a, clone 2A3 Bioxcell Catalog# BE0089) were administered intraperitoneally at a dose of 10 mg/kg every week for 12 weeks. The PD-1 antibody blocks PD-1 and PD-L1 binding and boosts the immune response. The mice went through sensorimotor tests following the 12th injection at 13–14 months of age, followed by cognitive testing. The brains were subsequently harvested at 14–15 months of age.

Behavior

Each instrument was wiped down with 30% ethanol and allowed to completely dry between each mouse tested. Before each testing session, the mice were acclimated to the testing room conditions for a minimum of 30 min.

Sensorimotor Tests

Locomotor Activity

A circular open field activity chamber (56 cm in diameter, 31 cm in height) was used to measure exploratory locomotor activity over 15 min as we have routinely assessed previously in this model (Asuni et al., 2007; Boutajangout et al., 2011). A camera placed above the field recorded animal movements (Ethovision XT, Noldus, Leesburg, VA, USA). Measured parameters were distance traveled (cm) and mean velocity (cm/s).

Rotarod

This test was conducted to measure limb motor coordination and balance (San Diego Instruments, San Diego, CA, USA). Initially, the mice were habituated to the instrument and the task by a four trial training session to obtain a baseline level of performance. Each training trial consisted of 5 min, with 15 min break between sessions, and the speed of the rotating rod increased linearly from 0 to 50 revolutions per min (rpm) during the 5 min period. The next day, the mice went through four trials with 15 min break between sessions. Each testing trial consisted of 10 min, with the speed of the rod increasing linearly from 0 to 40 rpm during that period until the mouse fell off or inverted (by clinging) from the rotating rod. The distance traveled and latency at that point were recorded. To prevent injury, a soft foam cushion was placed beneath the rod.

Cognitive Tests

Object Recognition Test

The spontaneous object recognition test (ORT) that was used measures deficits in short-term memory, and was conducted in the circular open field activity arena mentioned above (56 cm in diameter). A video camera mounted above the arena automatically recorded mouse movement and time spent by the objects and in different zones. At the training session, two identical novel objects were placed in opposite quadrants of the arena, and the mouse was allowed to explore for 15 min. For any given trial, the objects in a pair were 10 cm high and composed of the same material so that they could not readily be distinguished by olfactory cues. The time spent exploring each object was recorded by a tracking system (Ethovision XT, Noldus), and at the end of the training phase, the mouse was removed from the arena for the duration of the retention delay (3 h). Normal mice remember a specific object after a delay of 3 h and spend the majority of their time investigating the novel object during the retention trial. During the retention test, the animals were placed back into the same arena, in which one of the previous familiar objects used during training was replaced by a novel object, and allowed to explore freely for 6 min. The time spent exploring the novel and familiar objects was recorded for the 6 min period. The percentage short-term memory score is the time spent exploring the novel object compared to the old object during the retention session. Typically, an animal with intact memory spends about 70% of the time with the novel object. For the long-term memory test, the mice were replaced back into the same arena 24 h after the short-term test, with a different novel object used, whereas the familiar object was the same as before. For both tests, each mouse was exposed to the same familiar and novel objects but their location was counterbalanced across animals within each treatment condition.

Spontaneous Alternation Test

The spontaneous alternation test was conducted in a Y-maze apparatus. The Y-maze apparatus (Med Associates) was comprised of a central hub (working area: 8.3 cm L × 8.3 cm W × 12.7 cm H) attached to three arms (working area: 36 cm L × 7.3 cm W × 12.7 cm H) equally spaced 120° apart. Clear polycarbonate walls and removable ventilated lids ensured that mice were confined to the maze but had access to all surrounding visual cues in the testing room.

The test consisted of a single 5 min trial in which the mouse was allowed to freely explore all three arms of the Y-maze. Mice were started in the central hub facing a wall to help avoid placement or initial arm bias. Mice were tracked by an overhead camera and video acquired and analyzed using Noldus Ethovision software (v11.5). Locomotor activity was assessed using metrics of the total number of arm entries (from the central hub) and the total distance traveled. Spontaneous Alternation [%] was defined as consecutive entries in three different arms (ABC), divided by the number of possible alternations [total arm entries minus 2; (Sarter et al., 1988)]. Re-entries into the same arm were rated as separate entries, which resulted in a 22.2% chance level for continuous alternation.

Novel Location Test

The Novel Location test was conducted in the same Y-maze apparatus described above. To maximize novelty, a different set of arms was used and the maze configuration was rotated by 45° relative to the position for the Spontaneous Alternation test so that the vantage of distal cues would differ between tests. Mice were tracked by an overhead camera and video acquired and analyzed using Noldus Ethovision software (v11.5).

The novel location test consisted of two 3 min trials. In trial 1, each mouse was started in the central hub facing a wall. The mouse was permitted to explore two arms of the Y-maze, while entry into the third arm was blocked by an opaque acrylic door. The location of the blocked arm was randomized across mice. After trial 1, the mouse was briefly returned to its home cage and the maze was cleaned with 30% ethanol and left to dry completely. The inter-trial interval (ITI) was 1 h. In trial 2, the door in front of the blocked arm was removed and the mouse was again placed into the central hub facing a wall and then allowed to access all three arms of the maze. Locomotor activity was assessed using metrics of the total number of arm entries (from the central hub) and the total distance traveled. Time in Novel Arm [%] was defined as the time spent in the novel arm divided by the time spent in all arms during the 3 min trial. The chance performance on this measure is 33.3%.

Barnes Maze

The Barnes Maze procedure was designed to provide an index of visuospatial learning and memory. The test comprises a series of trials in which rodents learn to navigate to a hole box location providing shelter from a noisy, brightly-lit platform (Barnes, 1979). The protocol we implemented was adapted based on a hybrid of prior studies suggesting optimal parameters for platform characteristics (O'Leary and Brown, 2013), as well as for the number and spacing of training and probe trials (Sunyer et al., 2007; Illouz et al., 2016). Our previous experience using these parameters has produced reliable spatial learning in wild type mice, based primarily on the use of extra-maze cues.

The maze apparatus consists of a beige, textured plastic platform surface, 36" in diameter, elevated 36" from the floor on a black-painted wooden stand (San Diego Instruments, San Diego, CA, USA). The platform has 20 2" holes equally spaced around the periphery of the platform (~1" from the edge). For a given subject, a gray plastic escape box (~10 cm × 8.5 cm × 4 cm) was located under one of the holes that were kept consistent across trials. Visible distal cues were placed around the room and remained constant throughout the testing period. The maze was illuminated by an overhead lamp (100W) placed 30" above the center of the platform. Behavior was recorded using an overhead camera for later tracking and analysis using Noldus Ethovision software (v11.5).

On the first day, mice were given two trials: a guided, habituation trial and a standard escape trial. For the habituation trial, each mouse was gently removed from their home cage by the base of their tail and placed in the center of the platform under an inverted, transparent 500 ml beaker for 1 min. A white noise generator (~90–100 dB at platform level) was turned on when the mouse was placed onto the maze. After the 1 min period, the beaker was slowly moved with the mouse inside to guide them to the target hole. The mouse was then allowed or was gently guided by the experimenter using the beaker, to enter the escape box. Once inside, the mouse was permitted 2 min to explore the escape box before being transported back to its home cage within the box. On both the habituation and standard escape trials, the white noise was turned off as soon as the mouse entered the escape box. Between each training trial, the maze was rotated such that the hole positions were maintained relative to the room and distal cues. This was done to ensure that only distal spatial cues (not local or non-spatial landmark cues) could be used to guide successful escape navigation. The target hole was counterbalanced across animals within each treatment condition.

After the initial beaker trial (2 h ITI), each mouse was given a standard escape trial in which the mouse was gently placed onto the center of the maze within a plastic 6" (L) × 6" (W) × 8" (H) start box. The white noise was turned on and, after 10–15 s, the start box was lifted. The mouse was given a maximum of 3 min to find the designated hole and escape box. When a mouse entered the escape box, the white noise was turned off and the animal was given 1 min inside the box before being transferred back to the home cage. If the mouse did not find the escape hole within the 3 min limit, it was slowly guided to the target hole under the inverted beaker (as described above), and given 1 min inside the box (with white noise turned off) before being transferred back to the home cage.

After the first two trials on day 1, each mouse was given three standard escape trials per day—with the maze rotated after each trial—over the next three consecutive days.

The day following the 10th standard escape trial, a probe trial was conducted in which the escape box was removed to help control for possible strategies that used local cues from the box, This trial was started similar to training but was only 120 s in duration. Latency, distance and the number of mistakes (non-target holes visited) until finding the target hole as well as average proximity to the target hole on the probe trial were recorded as indices of spatial memory.

Fear Conditioning

Fear conditioning is an associative learning task in which mice are presented with a behaviorally neutral conditioning stimulus (CS), such as an auditory stimulus, that is presented in temporal proximity with a mild foot shock that acts as an aversive unconditioned stimulus (US; Maren, 2001). In the task, the mice learn that the CS predicts the US and will subsequently elicit specific behavioral responses such as freezing when the CS is presented on its own. Mice additionally learn to associate the environment or context of the chamber in which the CS-US pairings take place with the US, and will elicit specific behavioral responses when in the environment/context in the absence of the CS.

The fear conditioning apparatus consists of four identical square-shaped chambers (Coulbourn Instruments). The floor of the chamber has a metal grid through which the shock US is delivered, and the walls of the testing chamber are made of aluminum and clear acrylic. All chambers are mounted within specially designed light and sound attenuating outer boxes ventilated by a small fan. To aid in establishing a context, chambers were scented with three drops of mild natural extract (vanilla or lilac) added to a gauze inside a small plastic dish placed within the waste pan below the grid floor and out of reach of the subject. Each chamber was illuminated by small white, blue and/or infrared LEDs to provide low-ambient light, with speakers mounted on one wall and a camera mounted overhead to record video of behaviors during the training and testing sessions. Chamber, scent and lighting conditions were counterbalanced across the drug testing groups.

The fear conditioning protocol comprised four phases: (1) a conditioning phase in which mice receive CS-US context/tone-shock pairings; (2) a short term (1 h post-conditioning); (3) a long term (24 h postconditioning) testing phase in which the extent of associative fear memory for the context is assessed by examining behavior during re-exposure to the same testing chambers (without tone CS or US shocks); and (4) a testing phase for associative fear memory for the auditory white noise cue in different chamber context (with tone CS but no shocks 48 h post-conditioning). The conditioning phase comprised one 6 min session, in which each mouse was placed alone into a specified chamber and given a 2 min acclimation period in which no stimuli or shocks were delivered. Then animals were given two noise-shock pairings, each of which comprised a 30 s auditory white noise CS (78 dB) presented prior to delivery of 2 s 0.2 mA shock current US *via* a scrambled signal across the stainless steel grid floor overlapping with the last 2 s of the noise stimulus. Spacing between the noise-shock CS-US pairing was 2 min (each pairing initiated at 3 min and 5 min within the trial). After the second shock, animals were left in the chamber another 30 s prior to being gently removed from the chamber and placed back into their home cage.

Associative learning and memory were evaluated in the subsequent three sessions. To assess short-term and long-term associative fear memory for the context, mice were gently placed into the same chamber used to assess the extent of contextual learning for 5 min at 1 h and 24 h time points after the conditioning session, respectively. To assess associative fear conditioning for the white noise cue, a 20 min session was given in a novel chamber context 48 h after the conditioning session. The white noise stimulus was presented alone for 3 min after 3 min within the chamber and then a 30 s white noise was played and an additional six times at 3 min intervals. After each session, mice were gently removed from the chamber and placed back into their home cage.

Associative learning was determined by the amount of time the mice spend freezing or immobile during these sessions, in the presence or absence of the white noise. Percent freezing was extracted using the automated Freeze Frame 3 software (threshold = 10, duration criterion = 2 s).

Western Blotting

The left hemisphere brain tissue was homogenized in (5× vol/w) modified radioimmunoprecipitation assay (RIPA) buffer (50 mM Tris-HCl, 150 mM NaCl, 1 mM ethylene diamine tetra-acetic acid (EDTA), 1% Nonidet P-40, pH 7.4) containing protease and phosphatase inhibitors (4 nM phenylmethylsulfonyl fluoride (PMSF), 1 mM NaF, 1 mM Na_3VO_4, 1× Complete protease inhibitor cocktail (Roche, Indianapolis, IN, USA), and 0.25% sodium deoxycholate). The homogenate was then centrifuged (20,000× *g*) for 20 min at 4°C and the supernatant collected as soluble tau fraction [low-speed supernatant (LSS)]. To obtain the sarkosyl insoluble tau fraction, equal amounts of protein from the LSS were mixed with 10% sarkosyl solution to a final 1% sarkosyl concentration and incubated on a rotator for 30 min at room temperature. The samples were then centrifuged at 100,000× *g* in a Beckman TL-100 ultracentrifuge at 20°C for 1 h. The pellet was resuspended in 100 μl 1% sarkosyl solution and spun again at 100,000× g at 20°C for 1 h. The supernatant was then discarded and the pellet air-dried for

30 min. Then, 50 μl of modified O+ buffer (62.5 mM Tris-HCl, 10% glycerol, 5% β-mercaptoethanol, 2.3% SDS, 1 mM EDTA, 1 mM ethylene glycol-bis(β-aminoethyl ether)-tetraacetic acid (EGTA), 1 mM NaF, 1 mM Na_3VO_4, 1 nM PMSF and 1× Complete protease inhibitor cocktail, including about 1 μg/ml of bromophenol blue) was added and the sample vortexed for 1 min, and then boiled for 5 min [Sarkosyl Pellet (SP) fraction] and kept frozen at −80°C until used for Westerns. The LSS fraction (500 μg—about 30 μl) was diluted with the modified RIPA buffer (about 220 μl) and modified O+ buffer (50 μl), resulting in a final protein concentration of 25 μg/15 μl, and processed in the same way (boiled for 5 min and frozen). For Western blots, the soluble and insoluble tau fractions were thawed, reboiled for 5 min and electrophoresed (15 μl per lane) on a 12% (w/v) polyacrylamide gel. The proteins were then transferred to a nitrocellulose membrane that was subsequently blocked in 5% nonfat milk with 0.1% Tween-20 in TBS for 1 h, and incubated with different antibodies at 4°C overnight (Tau-5 (SantaCruz, sc-58860, 1:1,000, tau epitope 210–241), PHF1 (1:1,000, tau epitope around aa P-Ser396) and CP27 (1:500, human tau specific epitope aa 130–150) generously provided as cell culture supernatants by Peter Davies). Following washes, the membranes were then incubated for 2 h with 1:2,000 horseradish-peroxidase (HRP) conjugated goat anti-mouse antibody (ThermoFisher Scientific), developed in ECL (ThermoFisher Scientific), imaged with Fuji LAS-4000, and the signal quantified with by ImageQuant software. All the samples within each figure panel were run on the same gel, and each set of blots was repeated at least twice with one set used for quantitation.

Tau Sandwich Enzyme-Linked Immunosorbent Assay (ELISA)

For assessing human tau levels, a Corning Costar® Assay Plate, 96 well Clear Flat Bottom Half Area High Binding Polystyrene (Ref 3690), was coated (50 μl/well) with the anti-human tau monoclonal antibody BT2 (1 μg/ml, ThermoFisher Scientific, MN1010, epitope aa 194–198) for 72 h at 4°C on a shaker. The plate was washed four times with wash buffer and then blocked with SuperBlock Blocking Buffer in TBS (ThermoFisher Scientific) for 90 min at room temperature on a shaker. Low-speed supernatant (LSS) samples (soluble tau) were first normalized to 2 mg/ml total protein concentration and then diluted 1:100 using RIPA base buffer. SP samples (insoluble tau) were diluted 1:100 using an O+ base buffer. Human recombinant tau standards [Tau-441 (2N4R), rPeptide], LSS, and SP samples were loaded in duplicate (20 μl/well) and then diluted 1:5 with 20% Super Block in 1× TBS in the plate and incubated overnight at 4°C on a shaker. The following day, the plate was washed four times with wash buffer and 0.2 μg/ml anti-human tau monoclonal antibody, biotin-labeled (HT7B; ThermoFisher Scientific, MN1000B, epitope aa 159–163) in 20% Super Block in 1× TBS was added to the plate (50 μl/well) and incubated at 37°C for 90 min. The plate was then washed four times with wash buffer and then Streptavidin Poly-HRP50 Conjugate (1:6,000 in 20% Super Block in 1× TBS, Fitzgerald Industries International, 65R-S10PHRP) was added (50 μl/well) and incubated in the dark at room temperature for 40 min on a shaker. The plate was then washed four times with wash buffer and then developed with 3,3′,5,5′-Tetramethylbenzidine Liquid Substrate, Super Slow, for enzyme-linked immunosorbent assay (ELISA; 50 μl/well) and the absorbance was read at 650 nm using a BioTek Synergy 2 plate reader.

Data Analysis

All the data were plotted and analyzed using GraphPad 8.0. Normality was assessed with the D'Agostino-Pearson test. Data that passed the test, were analyzed with an unpaired *t*-test, and data that failed the test were analyzed with the Mann–Whitney test. Both tests were two-tailed. A *P*-value of less than 0.05 was considered significant.

RESULTS

Following weekly treatment with PD-1 antibody or isotype control IgG for 12 weeks, starting at 10–11 months of age, the homozygous JNPL3 mice underwent a battery of behavioral tests as outlined below, and in that particular order. Subsequently, their brains were analyzed for tau and phospho-tau levels in soluble and sarkosyl insoluble fractions by Western blots and ELISA to determine if the PD-1 treatment led to clearance of pathological tau protein.

Behavior

Sensorimotor Tests

Locomotor Activity

The PD-1 treatment group was more active in the open field compared to the IgG control group, traveling 23% further ($p < 0.05$; **Figure 1A**) and at a 23% greater speed {IgG: 3.59 ± 0.18 cm/s, PD-1: 4.43 ± 0.30 cm/s [average ± standard error of the mean (SEM)], $p < 0.05$}.

Rotarod

The PD-1 treatment group and the IgG control group did not differ in their performance on the rotarod as measured by the distance traveled (**Figure 1B**, $p = 0.35$) and the time to fall off the rotating rod (IgG: 107.50 ± 15.70 s, PD-1: 125.10 ± 14.34 s, $p = 0.42$).

Cognitive Tests

Object Recognition

The PD-1 treatment group did not differ from the IgG control group in the time spent with the novel object in the short-term test (3 h, $p = 0.33$) or the long-term test (24 h, $p = 0.17$; **Figure 1C**).

Spontaneous Alternation

The PD-1 treatment group did not differ from the IgG control group in the spontaneous alternation index ($p = 0.96$; **Figure 1D**), total arm visits (IgG: 24.13 ± 1.86, PD-1: 29.00 ± 3.32, $p = 0.25$), total distance traveled (IgG: 1576.02 ± 120.98 cm, PD-1: 1870.79 ± 181.09 cm, $p = 0.22$) and total time spent in the arms (IgG: 210.41 ± 8.66 s, PD-1: 211.52 ± 7.73 s, $p = 0.93$).

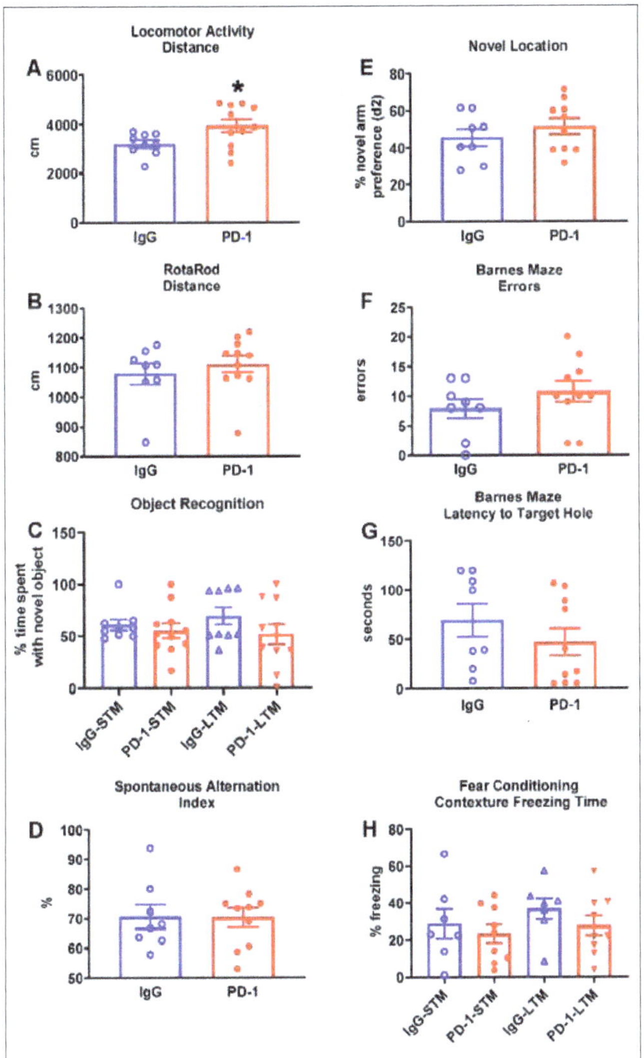

FIGURE 1 | Programmed cell death protein 1 (PD-1) treatment slightly increased locomotor activity but did not improve rotarod performance or affect cognition. **(A)** PD-1 antibody treatment increased distance traveled in a locomotor test compared to the control group. **(B)** PD-1 treatment did not improve rotarod performance compared to the control group. **(C)** PD-1 treatment did not affect memory in an object recognition task. **(D)** PD-1 treatment did not alter spontaneous alternation in the Y-maze or **(E)** preference for the novel arm location in the 2-trial **(F,G)** PD-1 treatment did not alter the number of errors or the latency to find the target hole in the Barnes Maze. **(H)** PD-1 treatment did not affect short- or long-term contextual memory in a fear-conditioning task. Each bar represents the group average +/− standard error of the mean (SEM). $^*p < 0.05$. As shown in individual scatterplots, 9–11 PD-1 treated- and 7–9 IgG control mice went through each test. The rotarod results failed normality test and were, therefore, analyzed by the Mann–Whitney test. All the other results passed the normality test and were, therefore, analyzed by unpaired *t*-test.

Novel Location

The PD-1 treatment group did not differ from the IgG control group in the preference (d2) for the novel object (p = 0.36; **Figure 1E**), total arm visits (IgG: 9.75 ± 1.74, PD-1: 10.90 ± 2.16, p = 0.81), total distance traveled (IgG: 630.83 ± 90.39 cm, PD-1: 779.49 ± 162.41 cm, p = 0.70) and the total time spent in the arms (IgG: 130.23 ± 11.12 s, PD-1: 110.55 ± 12.35 s, p = 0.27). In trial 1, there was no difference between treatment groups in terms of arm preference (IgG: 58.85 ± 3.61%, PD-1: 57.43 ± 6.25%, p = 0.44), total arm visits (IgG: 9.13 ± 0.83, PD-1: 9.50 ± 1.20, p = 0.81), total distance traveled (IgG: 560.21 ± 60.49 cm, PD-1: 608.02 ± 69.90 cm, p = 0.62) and total time spent in the arms (IgG: 101.95 ± 8.03, PD-1: 90.96 ± 9.88, p = 0.42).

Barnes Maze

In the probe trial, the PD-1 treatment group did not differ from the IgG control group in the number of errors committed (p = 0.41; **Figure 1F**) or in the latency to reach the target hole (p = 0.31; **Figure 1G**). There were also no differences between groups in the distance traveled to find the platform (IgG: 238.71 ± 51.36 cm, PD-1: 308.82 ± 62.20 cm, p = 0.41) or in the average proximity to the target hole during the probe trial (IgG: 68.71 ± 6.11 cm, PD-1: 70.98 ± 7.77 cm, p = 0.83).

Fear Conditioning

The PD-1 treatment group and the IgG control group did not differ in freezing time when examined under the short-term (p = 0.55) and long-term (p = 0.27) contextual memory assessment (**Figure 1H**). There was also no effect of PD-1 treatment on percent freezing time when the white noise cue was on (IgG: 46.10 ± 7.67%, PD-1: 50.59 ± 10.95%, p = 0.76) or off (IgG: 15.69 ± 4.61%, PD-1: 22.88 ± 8.30%, p = 0.50) in the novel context for the cue conditioning test. In addition, there was no difference between treatment groups in freezing during the initial conditioning session (IgG: 11.45 ± 3.85%, PD-1: 9.98 ± 1.32%, p = 0.70).

Measurements of Tau Clearance

Western blot analysis of soluble and sarkosyl insoluble tau fractions did not reveal any significant differences between the PD-1 treatment group and the IgG control group (**Figure 2**). Specifically, analysis of the low speed brain homogenate supernatant fraction showed no significant differences in phospho-tau (PHF-1, p = 0.74), total tau (Tau-5, p = 0.24) total human tau (CP27, p = 0.71) or ratios thereof (PHF-1/CP27, p = 0.46 and Tau-5/CP27, p = 0.78), between the two groups (**Figures 2A–F**). Likewise, levels of sarkosyl insoluble tau did not differ significantly between the groups (**Figures 2A,G**, p = 0.16).

The lack of effect of PD-1 treatment on tau clearance was confirmed by ELISA measurements of total tau in the soluble (p = 0.67) and an insoluble fraction (p = 0.23), revealing comparable levels in treatment and control groups (**Figures 2H,I**).

DISCUSSION

Several different groups were not able to replicate the original beneficial effects of PD-1 antibody therapy in Aβ plaque models (Baruch et al., 2016; Latta-Mahieu et al., 2018). Although the antibodies and the experimental design, including animal models, were not identical to the pioneering study, a reasonable counter-argument can be made that robust findings under various related experimental conditions are necessary

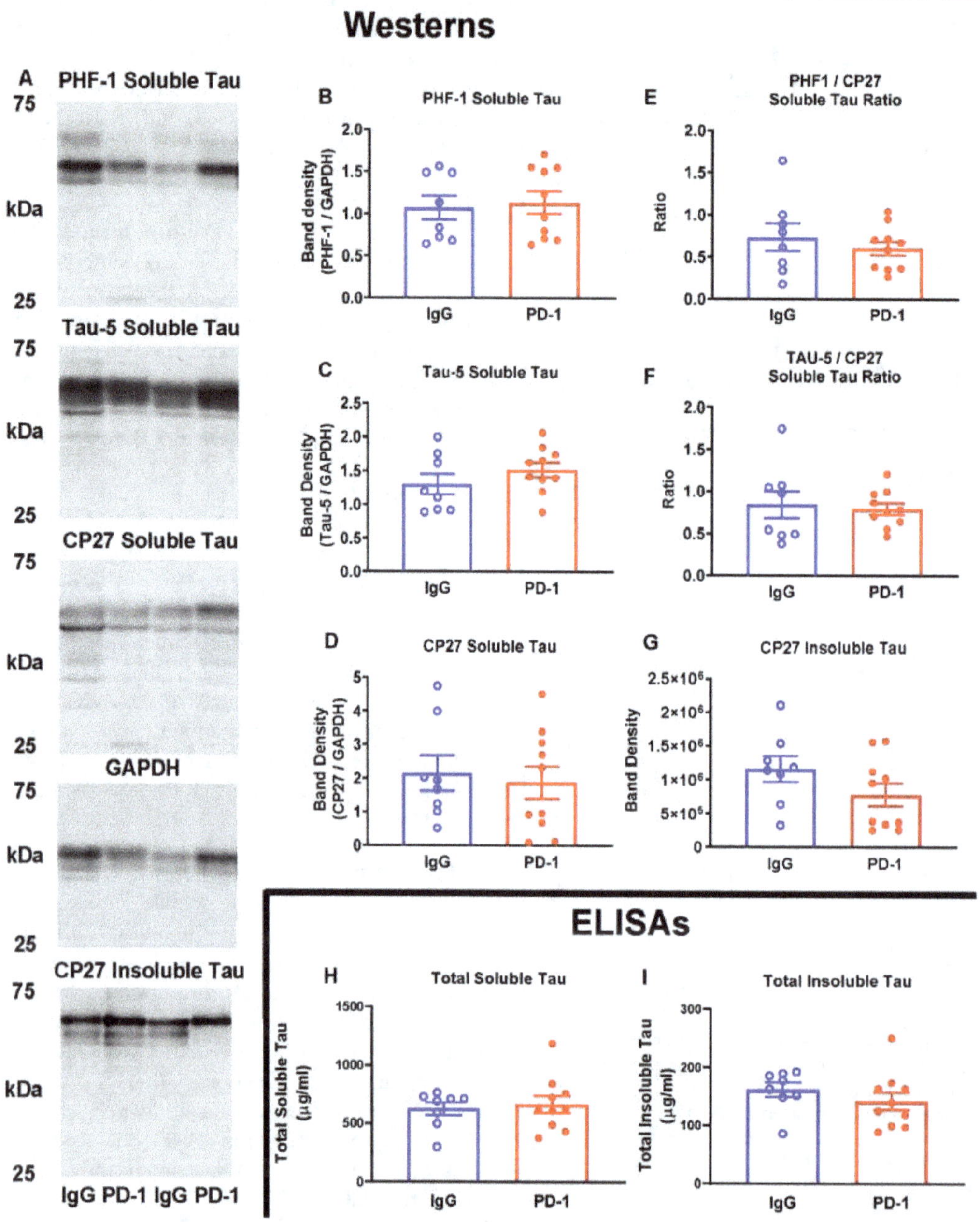

FIGURE 2 | PD-1 treatment did not enhance tau clearance. **(A–F)** PD-1 antibody treatment had no effect on soluble phospho-tau (PHF-1), total tau (Tau-5), total human tau (CP27) or ratios thereof on Western blots of tauopathy mouse brain homogenates, compared to control group. **(A,G)** PD-1 treatment had no effect on insoluble Western blot tau levels in the brain. **(H,I)** Enzyme-linked immunosorbent assay (ELISA) analyses of the same brain homogenates analyzed by Western blots confirmed lack of efficacy of the PD-1 therapy in clearing tau from the brain. Each bar represents the group average +/− SEM. As shown in individual scatterplots, 10 PD-1 treated- and eight control IgG mice were analyzed in each blot or ELISA assay. The total insoluble tau ELISA data failed normality test (IgG group) and was, therefore, analyzed by the Mann–Whitney test. All the other data passed the normality test and were, therefore, analyzed by unpaired *t*-test.

to consider examining this therapeutic approach further in clinical trials.

With regard to the tauopathy study, Swartz and colleagues administered the same PD-1 antibody as in their Aβ model study to tauopathy mice at 8 months of age (a single intraperitoneal injection of 0.5 mg; Rosenzweig et al., 2019). The DM-hTAU mouse model has two tau mutations (K257T and P301S) and has impaired cognition and extensive tau pathology at this age (Rosenzweig et al., 2019). The single antibody injection improved cognition in a T-maze when examined 1 month later in a mixed-sex group. Follow-up analysis of the males revealed similarly improved performance in a Y-maze. Subsequent brain analyses showed a reduction in inflammatory cytokines and diminished tau pathology.

Comparable findings were observed with two different PD-L1 antibodies.

To examine the potential of this therapeutic approach, we used the JNPL3 tauopathy mouse model, in which we have previously shown beneficial effects of active and passive tau immunotherapies (Asuni et al., 2007; Boutajangout et al., 2011). The mice received weekly intraperitoneal injections (10 mg/kg or 0.35 mg for a 35 g mouse) for 12 weeks of the same PD-1 antibody and isotype control as used by the Swartz group in their Aβ and tau pathology mice. We used this dosing paradigm in our original passive tau immunotherapy study (Boutajangout et al., 2011), and it was modeled after similar approaches by others in Aβ plaque models, and subsequently by numerous laboratories targeting Aβ, tau or other protein aggregates. This dose is also a typical dose in human trials of Aβ and tau antibodies. Treatment started at 10–11 months of age when this model has already moderate to severe tau pathology, presumably comparable to their DM-hTAU model. If a single injection is effective as per the original study, one would expect 12 weekly injections of a slightly lower dose to be effective as well. Only a minor increase in locomotor activity was observed in the tauopathy mice and no effect in five different cognitive tasks (Object recognition task, Spontaneous alternation task, Novel location task, Barnes maze, and Fear-conditioning task). Furthermore, soluble phosphorylated or non-phosphorylated tau levels or sarkosyl insoluble tau levels were not altered with the prolonged PD-1 antibody therapy as per Western blot analyses, although there was a trend for reduction in soluble PHF1/CP27 tau ratio, and in insoluble CP27 tau. ELISA analyses confirmed a lack of efficacy of the PD-1 antibody therapy on tau clearance.

In addition to the differences in models, the extent of the treatment period, and the number and types of behavioral tests as detailed above, the tau pathology was analyzed differently. Rosensweig primarily analyzed phospho-tau immunoreactivity in the hippocampus (P-Thr212, P-Ser214 and P-Thr231) and aggregated tau in protein extracts, whereas we focused on Western blot analyses of whole-brain homogenate for soluble and insoluble tau and phospho-tau (P-Ser396), followed by ELISA analyses of soluble and insoluble tau. While our approach is more easily quantifiable than histological assessment, it may not detect increased tau clearance within certain brain regions, and there may also be differences in which epitopes are being cleared. However, the efficacy of candidate treatments for clinical development should ideally be sufficiently robust and measurable by any of the standard approaches used to examine the clearance of pathological tau. Considering these negative key findings, it was not warranted to determine if this approach altered cytokine levels and/or led to brain infiltration of monocyte-derived macrophages. Notably, Latta-Mahieu et al. (2018) did not detect macrophage infiltration into the brain in Aβ plaque models following PD-1 treatment.

Cognition has not been extensively examined in the JNPL3 model, presumably because of its motor phenotype, which now is substantially delayed compared to the early days of this model. A prior report indicated that young (5–8.5 months of age) hemizygous JNPL3 mice ($n = 10$) were not impaired as a group in various cognitive tests, compared to non-transgenic littermates ($n = 11$; Arendash et al., 2004). A subsequent study showed normal cognition of hemizygous JNPL3 mice ($n = 6$) in the radial arm water maze and Y-maze at 7–8 months of age, compared to non-transgenic littermates ($n = 9$; Morgan et al., 2008). Similar to these two studies, our JNPL3 mice were of a mixed genetic background, however they were not derived from breeding with the Tg2576 Aβ deposition model. In addition, our mice were homozygous and older at testing (13–15 months of age). In this study, we were not able to compare our JNPL3 mice to non-transgenic mice of the same strain background but based on prior historical data from the Sigurdsson lab and the literature, the JNPL3 mice appear to be impaired in novel object recognition and in the fear conditioning task. In the former test, wild-type mice, younger JNPL3 tauopathy mice, and tauopathy mice in which treatment has been effective, typically spend about 70% of their time with the novel object (Asuni et al., 2007; Boutajangout et al., 2010; Gulinello et al., 2019). In the current study, object preference in both IgG- and PD-1-treated JNPL3 mice did not significantly differ from chance performance (50%). In the latter test, we have previously reported impairments in short- and long-term memory in 12–13 months old JNPL3 mice compared to wild-type mice (Levenga et al., 2013). Similar to our previous work, aged JNPL3 mice exhibited around 35% freezing, which is markedly lower than 50–60% levels of freezing observed in wild-type mice under similar conditions (Levenga et al., 2013; O'Leary et al., 2018).

Various amyloid diseases have over the years been associated with inflammation and an inflammatory stimulus can promote or resolve amyloidosis depending on its strength and various factors in experimental design (Sigurdsson et al., 2002; Lee et al., 2013). It is interesting to note as well that activation of microglia/macrophages is typically associated with increased tau phosphorylation, presumably because of cytokine-mediated activation of cellular kinases (Lee et al., 2013). Accumulation of microglia/macrophages is closely associated with Aβ deposits and these cells are likely involved in plaque clearance. Their link to tau pathology is less clear. With most of the tau lesions being intracellular, the accumulation of phagocytic microglia/macrophages and associated inflammatory signals are much less prominent in pure tauopathies than for Aβ pathology, which is mainly found extracellularly. Hence, linking PD-1 inhibition to Aβ clearance is in many ways feasible, whereas such a mechanistic association with tau clearance is not as apparent. Only a small fraction of tau is found extracellularly (Sigurdsson, 2019). Therefore, it is rather unlikely that acute clearance of extracellular tau within a 1 month period following a single antibody injection could have an extensive effect on intracellular tau aggregates. In addition, any indirect effect of PD-1 blockade on intracellular tau is more likely to promote tau hyperphosphorylation based on prior studies as mentioned above (Lee et al., 2013). If the effect is mainly extracellular, a prolonged treatment such as ours, with weekly antibody injections for 12 weeks, would be more likely to eventually lead to removal of intraneuronal tau aggregates. However, that was not the case in our study.

Finally, it can be argued that the effects of PD-1 blockade on tau pathology and associated behavioral impairments may differ between acute vs. chronic treatment. Although possible, prolonged treatment will be necessary to effectively treat chronic slowly progressing diseases like Alzheimer's disease and other tauopathies. Unfortunately, chronic treatment with a PD-1 blocking antibody, as could be envisioned to be applied clinically, did not clear tau pathology or substantially improve behavior under our experimental conditions. Therefore, further research is needed before clinical trials based on PD-1 checkpoint immune blockage are devised for tauopathies.

ETHICS STATEMENT

The animal study was reviewed and approved by New York University School of Medicine, IACUC committee.

AUTHOR CONTRIBUTIONS

HR took care of the mouse colony and immunized the mice. YL performed the behavioral studies with help from BG-L and AM who designed some of the tests. YL performed the western blots and related analyses. LS-B designed and performed the ELISAs. All the authors contributed to the method section. ES designed the experiment and wrote the article. YL and AM edited the article.

ACKNOWLEDGMENTS

We thank Peter Davies at the Feinstein Institute for generously providing the PHF1 and CP27 antibodies for the western blots.

REFERENCES

Arendash, G. W., Lewis, J., Leighty, R. E., McGowan, E., Cracchiolo, J. R., Hutton, M., et al. (2004). Multi-metric behavioral comparison of APPsw and P30IL models for Alzheimer's disease: linkage of poorer cognitive performance to tau pathology in forebrain. *Brain Res.* 1012, 29–41. doi: 10.1016/s0006-8993(04)00468-8

Asuni, A. A., Boutajangout, A., Quartermain, D., and Sigurdsson, E. M. (2007). Immunotherapy targeting pathological tau conformers in a tangle mouse model reduces brain pathology with associated functional improvements. *J. Neurosci.* 27, 9115–9129. doi: 10.1523/JNEUROSCI.2361-07.2007

Barnes, C. A. (1979). Memory deficits associated with senescence: a neurophysiological and behavioral study in the rat. *J. Comp. Physiol. Psychol.* 93, 74–104. doi: 10.1037/h0077579

Baruch, K., Deczkowska, A., Rosenzweig, N., Tsitsou-Kampeli, A., Sharif, A. M., Matcovitch-Natan, O., et al. (2016). PD-1 immune checkpoint blockade reduces pathology and improves memory in mouse models of Alzheimer's disease. *Nat. Med.* 22, 135–137. doi: 10.1038/nm.4022

Boutajangout, A., Ingadottir, J., Davies, P., and Sigurdsson, E. M. (2011). Passive immunization targeting pathological phospho-tau protein in a mouse model reduces functional decline and clears tau aggregates from the brain. *J. Neurochem.* 118, 658–667. doi: 10.1111/j.1471-4159.2011.07337.x

Boutajangout, A., Quartermain, D., and Sigurdsson, E. M. (2010). Immunotherapy targeting pathological tau prevents cognitive decline in a new tangle mouse model. *J. Neurosci.* 30, 16559–16566. doi: 10.1523/JNEUROSCI.4363-10.2010

Chamoto, K., Al-Habsi, M., and Honjo, T. (2017). Role of PD-1 in immunity and diseases. *Curr. Top. Microbiol. Immunol.* 410, 75–97. doi: 10.1007/82_2017_67

Gulinello, M., Mitchell, H. A., Chang, Q., Timothy O'Brien, W., Zhou, Z., Abel, T., et al. (2019). Rigor and reproducibility in rodent behavioral research. *Neurobiol. Learn. Mem.* 165:106780. doi: 10.1016/j.nlm.2018.01.001

Illouz, T., Madar, R., Clague, C., Griffioen, K. J., Louzoun, Y., and Okun, E. (2016). Unbiased classification of spatial strategies in the Barnes maze. *Bioinformatics* 32, 3314–3320. doi: 10.1093/bioinformatics/btw376

Latta-Mahieu, M., Elmer, B., Bretteville, A., Wang, Y., Lopez-Grancha, M., Goniot, P., et al. (2018). Systemic immune-checkpoint blockade with anti-PD1 antibodies does not alter cerebral amyloid-β burden in several amyloid transgenic mouse models. *Glia* 66, 492–504. doi: 10.1002/glia.23260

Lee, D. C., Rizer, J., Hunt, J. B., Selenica, M. L., Gordon, M. N., and Morgan, D. (2013). Review: experimental manipulations of microglia in mouse models of Alzheimer's pathology: activation reduces amyloid but hastens tau pathology. *Neuropathol. Appl. Neurobiol.* 39, 69–85. doi: 10.1111/nan.12002

Levenga, J., Krishnamurthy, P., Rajamohamedsait, H., Wong, H., Franke, T. F., Cain, P., et al. (2013). Tau pathology induces loss of GABAergic interneurons leading to altered synaptic plasticity and behavioral impairments. *Acta Neuropathol. Commun.* 1, 34–47. doi: 10.1186/2051-5960-1-34

Lewis, J., McGowan, E., Rockwood, J., Melrose, H., Nacharaju, P., Van Slegtenhorst, M., et al. (2000). Neurofibrillary tangles, amyotrophy and progressive motor disturbance in mice expressing mutant (P301L) tau protein. *Nat. Genet.* 25, 402–405. doi: 10.1038/78078

Maren, S. (2001). Neurobiology of Pavlovian fear conditioning. *Annu. Rev. Neurosci.* 24, 897–931. doi: 10.1146/annurev.neuro.24.1.897

Morgan, D., Munireddy, S., Alamed, J., DeLeon, J., Diamond, D. M., Bickford, P., et al. (2008). Apparent behavioral benefits of tau overexpression in P301L tau transgenic mice. *J. Alzheimers Dis.* 15, 605–614. doi: 10.3233/jad-2008-15407

O'Leary, T. P., and Brown, R. E. (2013). Optimization of apparatus design and behavioral measures for the assessment of visuo-spatial learning and memory of mice on the Barnes maze. *Learn. Mem.* 20, 85–96. doi: 10.1101/lm.028076.112

O'Leary, T. P., Hussin, A. T., Gunn, R. K., and Brown, R. E. (2018). Locomotor activity, emotionality, sensori-motor gating, learning and memory in the APPswe/PS1dE9 mouse model of Alzheimer's disease. *Brain Res. Bull.* 140, 347–354. doi: 10.1016/j.brainresbull.2018.05.021

Rosenzweig, N., Dvir-Szternfeld, R., Tsitsou-Kampeli, A., Keren-Shaul, H., Ben-Yehuda, H., Weill-Raynal, P., et al. (2019). PD-1/PD-L1 checkpoint blockade harnesses monocyte-derived macrophages to combat cognitive impairment in a tauopathy mouse model. *Nat. Commun.* 10:465. doi: 10.1038/s41467-019-08352-5

Sarter, M., Bodewitz, G., and Stephens, D. N. (1988). Attenuation of scopolamine-induced impairment of spontaneous alteration behaviour by antagonist but not inverse agonist and agonist β-carbolines. *Psychopharmacology* 94, 491–495. doi: 10.1007/bf00212843

Sigurdsson, E. M. (2019). Alzheimer's therapy development: a few points to consider. *Prog. Mol. Biol. Transl. Sci.* 168, 205–217. doi: 10.1016/bs.pmbts.2019.06.001

Sigurdsson, E. M., Wisniewski, T., and Frangione, B. (2002). Infectivity of amyloid diseases. *Trends Mol. Med.* 8, 411–413. doi: 10.1016/s1471-4914(02)02403-6

Sunyer, B., Patil, S., Frischer, C., Höger, H., Selcher, J., Brannath, W., et al. (2007). Strain-dependent effects of SGS742 in the mouse. *Behav. Brain Res.* 181, 64–75. doi: 10.1016/j.bbr.2007.03.025

Wei, S. C., Duffy, C. R., and Allison, J. P. (2018). Fundamental mechanisms of immune checkpoint blockade therapy. *Cancer Discov.* 8, 1069–1086. doi: 10.1158/2159-8290.cd-18-0367

7

Role of Tau Protein in Remodeling of Circadian Neuronal Circuits and Sleep

*Mercedes Arnes[1,2], Maria E. Alaniz[1,2], Caline S. Karam[3], Joshua D. Cho[1,2], Gonzalo Lopez[4], Jonathan A. Javitch[3,5,6] and Ismael Santa-Maria[1,2]**

[1] Taub Institute for Research on Alzheimer's Disease and the Aging Brain, Columbia University, New York, NY, United States, [2] Department of Pathology and Cell Biology, Columbia University, New York, NY, United States, [3] Department of Psychiatry, Vagelos College of Physicians and Surgeons, Columbia University, New York, NY, United States, [4] Department of Genetics and Genomic Sciences, Icahn School of Medicine at Mount Sinai, New York, NY, United States, [5] Division of Molecular Therapeutics, New York State Psychiatric Institute, New York, NY, United States, [6] Department of Pharmacology, Vagelos College of Physicians and Surgeons, Columbia University, New York, NY, United States

***Correspondence:**
Ismael Santa-Maria
is2395@cumc.columbia.edu

Multiple neurological, physiological, and behavioral functions are synchronized by circadian clocks into daily rhythms. Neurodegenerative diseases such as Alzheimer's disease and related tauopathies are associated with a decay of circadian rhythms, disruption of sleep patterns, and impaired cognitive function but the mechanisms underlying these alterations are still unclear. Traditional approaches in neurodegeneration research have focused on understanding how pathology impinges on circadian function. Since in Alzheimer's disease and related tauopathies tau proteostasis is compromised, here we sought to understand the role of tau protein in neuronal circadian biology and related behavior. Considering molecular mechanisms underlying circadian rhythms are conserved from *Drosophila* to humans, here we took advantage of a recently developed tau-deficient *Drosophila* line to show that loss of tau promotes dysregulation of daily circadian rhythms and sleep patterns. Strikingly, tau deficiency dysregulates the structural plasticity of the small ventral lateral circadian pacemaker neurons by disrupting the temporal cytoskeletal remodeling of its dorsal axonal projections and by inducing a slight increase in the cytoplasmic accumulation of core clock proteins. Taken together, these results suggest that loss of tau function participates in the regulation of circadian rhythms by modulating the correct operation and connectivity of core circadian networks and related behavior.

Keywords: tau, circadian rhythm, sleep, PDF, structural plasticity

INTRODUCTION

Circadian rhythms impose daily cycles to many behaviors and physiological processes in a wide variety of organisms. In mammals, the master biological clock is a group of about 20000 neurons that form a structure called the suprachiasmatic nucleus (SCN). In *Drosophila melanogaster* (fruit fly) the small ventral Lateral Neurons (sLNvs) are the master circadian pacemaker cells that set the pace of locomotor activity rhythms (Stoleru et al., 2005). At the molecular level, the molecules that regulate daily circadian behavioral rhythms are well known and conserved between mammals and insects like *Drosophila*. These molecular clocks consist of interlocked transcriptional-translational feedback loops that drive circadian rhythms in gene expression (Hardin, 2011).

The dysregulation of circadian clocks contributes to the decline in optimal functioning of the nervous system, ultimately leading to a reduction in the quality of life due to cognitive impairments and emotional stress (Touitou and Haus, 2000; Hastings et al., 2003; Hafycz and Naidoo, 2019). Therefore, since damaged circadian rhythms and sleep/wake cycles have been associated with an increase in disease susceptibility (Hastings et al., 2003; Gibson et al., 2009) it is important to determine the rather complex source of age-related circadian or sleep/wake dysfunction. Some of the observed sources of circadian dysfunction are low-functioning neuronal connections or loss of neurotransmitter or neuropeptide production, transport, or secretion (Kolker et al., 2003).

Maintenance of circadian rhythms requires exquisite synaptic coordination at multiple molecular and cellular levels of brain organization. The emergence of this complex circadian clock network requires both stable and dynamic properties of the neuronal cytoskeleton (Shweiki, 1999). Microtubules are key components of the cytoskeleton and their localization, mass, and dynamics are very important in many intracellular processes in neuronal health and disease (Brandt and Bakota, 2017; Dent, 2017). In addition, it has been demonstrated that microtubules have an influence on circadian activity patterns (Jarzynka et al., 2006, 2009). Microtubule stability is regulated by various microtubule-associated proteins (MAPs), like tau, MAP1B and MAP2 (Matus, 1988). Among them, tau protein adds stability and dynamic properties to the neuronal cytoskeleton, facilitating the maturation and establishment of synaptic networks involved in a large number of complex behaviors (Voelzmann et al., 2016; Tracy and Gan, 2018).

The multiple functions and different locations of tau in neurons have revealed novel insights into its importance in a diverse range of molecular pathways including cell signaling, synaptic plasticity, and regulation of genomic stability (Guo et al., 2017). However, little is currently known about the role tau protein plays in circadian regulation and sleep and the possible mechanisms involved (Cantero et al., 2010). Conversely, only few reports have shown how sleep regulates tau (Holth et al., 2019).

Drosophila has been used as a powerful model system to investigate *in vivo* the role of proteins linked to human diseases, including AD (Gistelinck et al., 2012; Rincon-Limas et al., 2012). Interestingly, the human tau protein has a fly homolog called *Drosophila* tau (dTau) which also displays microtubule-binding properties (Heidary and Fortini, 2001). Moreover, to further dissect the functions of the endogenous dTau protein, a new tau knock-out (Tau$^{-/-}$) fly line has been generated by homologous recombination (Burnouf et al., 2016).

The work presented here is focused on addressing the current gap in our knowledge on the role tau protein plays in regulating circadian rhythms and sleep patterns in *Drosophila*. Using this new *Drosophila* tau KO (dTau$^{-/-}$) line, we found alterations in daily circadian activities and dysregulation of sleep accompanied with molecular and structural changes in circadian pacemaker neurons, suggesting a new role for tau protein in circadian regulation and sleep. Taken together, our results demonstrate that tau in *Drosophila* has an impact on behavioral rhythms and sleep patterns, likely due to its role in modulating the structural plasticity of the terminal projections of circadian pacemaker neurons, demonstrated by the temporal dynamics of dTau levels in sLNv neurons.

MATERIALS AND METHODS

Drosophila Stocks

All *Drosophila* stocks were maintained on standard food (Bloomington recipe, Archon Scientific) in incubators at constant 70% relative humidity and 25°C on a 12-h/12-h light/dark cycle (unless otherwise specified). *Drosophila* dTau knockout line (dTau$^{-/-}$) was generated and kindly provided to us by Prof. Dr. Linda Partridge (Burnouf et al., 2016). dTau$^{-/-}$ line was isogenized and backcrossed for more than 10 generations with control line w^{1118} (Stock #5905) obtained from the Bloomington Drosophila Stock Center (Indiana University, United States). dTau-GFP line (Stock #60199) was also obtained from Bloomington Drosophila Stock Center.

Measurement of *Drosophila* Circadian Activity

Circadian activity of flies was measured as previously described (Chiu et al., 2010). Briefly, single 7 days-old male flies were placed in 5 × 65 mm glass tubes that fit a custom-built Multibeam Activity Monitors (DAM5M, Trikinetics Inc.) with four sets of infrared beams for activity detection. All tubes contained 2% agarose with 5% sucrose food. The monitors were connected to a computer to record beam breaks every minute for each animal using standard data acquisition software (DAMSystem 3, Trikinetics Inc.). Beam breaks occur due to locomotor activity of the single flies through the tubes. At the conclusion of the experiment, raw binary data collected was processed using DAM FileScan 111X (Trikinetics Inc.) and summed in 30 min bins when analyzing circadian parameters. DAM5M monitors were housed in a 25°C and 70% relative humidity incubator. Day/night activity was measured by maintaining the flies in a 12 h Light/Dark (LD) cycle for 5 days. Circadian activity rhythms was measured under constant darkness (DD) for 6–9 days after an entraining period of 5 days in LD cycles. Data analysis of Drosophila activity shown in actograms and eduction graphs (**Figure 1**) were performed using FaasX software. Further analyses of circadian activity in DD conditions (**Table 1**) were done in Matlab using the SCAMP scripts developed by Vecsey lab from Skidmore College (Donelson et al., 2012).

Sleep Analysis

For sleep analysis, 7 day-old male Drosophila locomotor activity data was collected and summed in 1 min bins. Sleep was quantified in Matlab using SCAMP scripts (Donelson et al., 2012). Wakefulness was defined as any period of at least 1 min characterized by activity (≥1 count/min) and sleep was defined as any period of inactivity (0 counts/min) lasting ≥5 min (Hendricks et al., 2000; Shaw et al., 2000; Van Swinderen et al., 2004). Sleep parameters analyzed were total sleep, number of sleep episodes, mean sleep episode duration (is a measure of

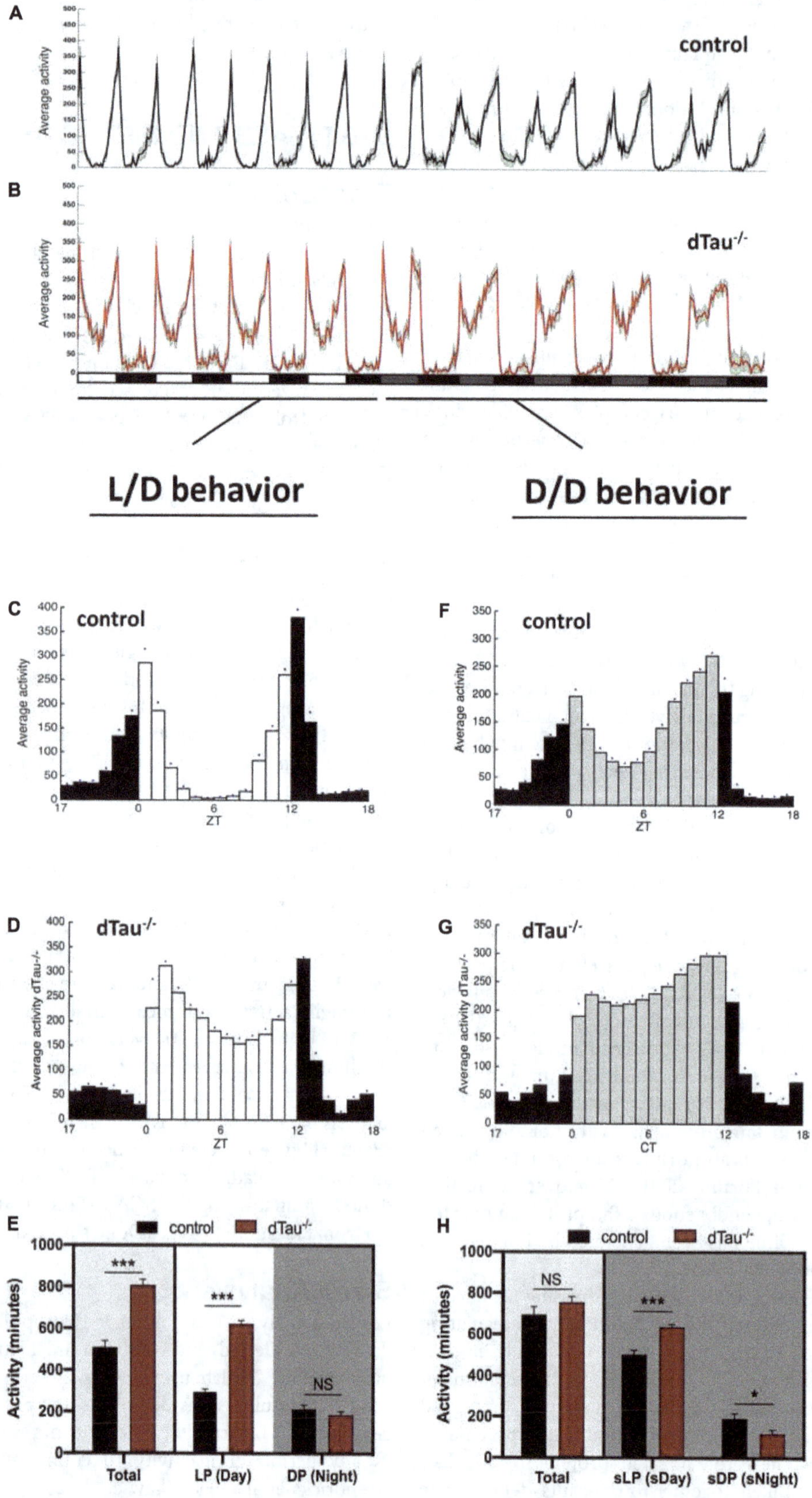

FIGURE 1 | Continued

FIGURE 1 | Effect of tau deficiency on circadian activity in *Drosophila*. **(A,B)** Averaged activity profiles across four 12 h LD cycles followed by another four DD cycles, of 7 day-old male flies from the denoted genotypes (w1118 in black and dTau$^{-/-}$ in red). White rectangles represent light period (LP), or day, and black rectangles represent dark period (DP) or night. During DD cycles, subjective light period (sLP) is represented in gray, and subjective dark period (sDP) in black. Activity peaks in dTau$^{-/-}$ flies show a different pattern when compared to controls, with noticeably more activity values during the "siesta" period in the light period during LD cycles, and the subjective day during the DD cycles. **(C–H)** Averaged activity profiles across five LD and DD cycles of the corresponding genotypes. White bars represent the light period (day), and black bars represent the dark period (night) in LD cycles **(C,D)**. During DD cycles **(F,G)** subjective daytime is represented in gray. Blue dots represent SEM for each Zeitgeber time. Both in LD and DD cycles, dTau$^{-/-}$ flies **(D,G)** were more active than controls **(C,F)** during the day and subjective daytime, with higher activity values and shows affection of the normal "siesta" pattern that control flies elicit during this particular period. **(E,H)** Total averaged locomotion activity quantification demonstrates that dTau mutant flies were significantly more active than controls, specifically during the LP in LD cycles. In DD cycles, dTau mutant flies were also significantly more active than controls during both the sLP and the sDP. However, no changes were found in total locomotor activity during DD cycles. Data represent mean and SEM analyzed with non-parametric Mann–Whitney statistical test, with $^{*}p < 0.05$ and $^{***}p < 0.001$ or NS if no statistical significance ($n = 21$–27 flies).

how consolidated the sleep is and can illustrate the quality of sleep), total time awake and sleep latency (time in minutes from lights out transition that marks the starting of total recoding time to the first sleep episode) for day- and night-time, averaged over five LD cycles.

Immunohistochemistry

Adult heads were fixed and dissected in 4% formaldehyde in 1X PBS and then washed three times in PBS containing 0.2% Triton X-100 (PBST). Heads were then blocked in blocking solution (5% goat serum in 0.2% PBST). Primary antibodies were mouse-anti-PDF (Developmental Studies Hybridoma Bank), guinea pig-anti-Clockwork Orange (CWO) (gift from Dr. Paul Hardin laboratory), goat-anti-PER (gift from Dr. Michael Rosbash laboratory), rat-anti-TIM (gift from Dr. Amita Seghal laboratory); and secondary antibodies were Alexa Fluor 488, 568, and 647 (Invitrogen). Finally, wholemount dissected brains were washed again and mounted with Vectashield mounting media containing DAPI (Vector Laboratories). GFP-tagged dTau was directly visualized without anti-GFP antibody incubation.

Confocal Microscopy

Visualization of *Drosophila* brain optical sections was performed on a Zeiss LSM800 confocal microscope. Image acquisition was made with 40X objective (oil-immersion) with optical zoom. For intensity quantification studies, laser parameters were maintained invariable.

Sholl Analysis

Quantification of the PDF (Pigment Dispersing Factor) positive signal across LNv neuron projections was analyzed with Sholl analysis (Sholl, 1953), in which six concentric and evenly spaced (10 μm) rings are drawn. The centers of the rings are localized at the point where the first dorsal ramification starts in each hemisphere. The number of intersections per ring as well as the total number of intersections were compared using a one-way ANOVA statistical test. Scoring was performed blindly. FIJI software was used for axonal crosses, and quantification was according to software instructions.

TABLE 1 | Circadian behavior analysis of flies in D/D conditions.

Genotype	Period (h)	RI	RS	% rhythmic	n
control	23.99 ± 0.03	0.5593 ± 0.03	5.264 ± 0.37	100%	22
dTau$^{-/-}$	24.04 ± 0.09	0.5816 ± 0.03	5.437 ± 0.42	94.4%	25

Data are mean ± SEM. Table representing period length, the rhythmic index (RI), the rhythmic strength (RS), the percentage of rhythmic flies, and the number of total flies used for the study.

Statistics

Statistical analysis was performed using GraphPad Prism 8 (GraphPad Inc.). A Normality test was performed for every data set from the different experimental results and statistical tests were used accordingly. Details of statistical tests used in described in the figure legends. Statistical significance is indicated as $^{*}p < 0.05$, $^{**}p < 0.01$, $^{***}p < 0.001$, and $^{****}p < 0.0001$ or NS if no statistical significance is obtained.

RESULTS

Loss of Tau Alters Daily Rhythms and Sleep in *Drosophila melanogaster*

Drosophila melanogaster is a valuable model organism in investigating novel regulators (direct or indirect) of circadian rhythms and sleep. Locomotor activity in *Drosophila* is organized such that, in a 12:12 h light:dark (LD) cycle, flies exhibit peaks of activity during dawn and dusk (morning and evening peaks), with increases in activity typically occurring slightly before (anticipating) the lights-on and lights-off transitions (**Figure 1**). We found that tau deficient animals (dTau$^{-/-}$) (Burnouf et al., 2016) display a different activity pattern than isogenic controls (w^{1118}). Control animals showed expected day/night locomotor activities under a 12:12 h light:dark (LD) cycles (**Figures 1A,C**) with higher activity observed during the day than at night. Control flies also display a typical drop in activity (siesta) around mid-day between the two activity peaks, one at dawn and one at dusk (lights on: zeitgeber time (ZT) = 0, lights off: ZT = 12). Tau deficient flies were found to display higher total activity during the day (**Figures 1B,D,E**). We observed tau deficient flies to have significantly higher activity at mid-day, where control flies displayed a drop in their locomotor activity. In addition, tau deficient flies show a significantly higher peak of activity in the morning, compared to control flies (**Figures 1A–E**). However, we did not observe any change in activity patterns at night for the tau deficient flies (**Figures 1A–E**). In order to assess the robustness and integrity of the circadian clock, we monitored locomotor activity in the absence of any external stimulus (i.e., constant darkness, DD). Typically, in constant dark conditions, the morning activity peak in Drosophila shrinks and only the evening peak persists, reoccurring with a period of ~23.8 h. Control and tau deficient flies were entrained for at least 3 days. Upon transition into DD, control and tau deficient flies maintained sustained differences in activity between subjective day and night (**Figures 1A,B,F–H**). As we previously observed in Light/Dark conditions, tau deficient flies showed significantly higher activity during the subjective day (sDay, **Figure 1H**). No changes in rhythmicity or in free-running period were observed in tau deficient flies (**Table 1**).

In addition to eclosion and locomotor activity, circadian rhythms also drive other aspects of physiology and behavior, including sleep and metabolism. Circadian control of all of these processes relies not only on the intracellular clock, but also on networks of cells that interact to influence circadian outputs. In light of the results obtained, we went on to examine the sleep behaviors of these flies. Tau deficient flies showed sleep alterations when compared to controls (**Figures 2A–E,G**). Tau deficient flies sleep significantly less during the day, including the afternoon, with no significant changes observed during the night (**Figure 2C**). The number of sleep episodes are also significantly different at daytime and night time between controls and tau deficient flies (**Figure 2D**). When we measured the mean sleep episode duration of the dTau$^{-/-}$ flies analysis demonstrated a significantly low- consolidated sleep during the daytime indicating a poor quality of sleep for the dTau$^{-/-}$ flies (**Figure 2E**). Poor quality of sleep resulted in longer periods of time awake (**Figure 2F**). Importantly, the daytime sleep latency of tau deficient flies was surprisingly longer than that of control flies (**Figure 2G**). The increased time that it takes for the tau deficient flies to get to sleep is observed only during the day. These observed alterations in sleep are in accordance with similar alterations previously reported in mice (Cantero et al., 2010), supporting tau's role in circadian modulation and sleep as a mechanism that is conserved among different species.

Role of *Drosophila* Tau in the Core Circadian Neuronal Operation

Next, we attempted to narrow down the cause of the locomotor and sleep defects in tau deficient flies. First, we tested whether rhythmic phenotypes observed in tau deficient flies might involve defective core clock operation. Two groups of central brain circadian neurons are particularly important for behavioral rhythms, including both morning (M) and evening (E) cells (Grima et al., 2004; Stoleru et al., 2004). The PDF-expressing small ventrolateral neurons (sLNvs or M cells) dictate morning activity as well as the rhythmicity in constant darkness (Renn et al., 1999; Blanchardon et al., 2001; Stoleru et al., 2004). Because of this latter feature, free running locomotor activity rhythms, the sLNvs are considered the major fly pacemaker neurons. The normal period of tau deficient flies implied that these clock cells functioned appropriately (**Figure 1** and **Table 1**). To assess this more directly, we stained for periodic nuclear accumulation of PER and TIM in tau deficient flies and controls. **Figure 3** shows a slightly significant difference in the magnitude of oscillatory dynamics between tau deficient flies and controls in sLNvs (**Figure 3C**). However, as the molecular clock is functional in tau deficient flies, this implies that tau protein regulates clock output function.

Drosophila Tau Modulates Rhythmic Axonal Structural Remodeling

Given the effect of tau observed on daily activity and sleep behavior, we analyzed expression of PDF and CWO, which respectively label LNvs, including the sLNvs (or M cells), and all major circadian groups (including both M and E cells). These markers display normally in tau deficient brains and controls, and LNvs extended normal axonal and dendritic projections (**Figure 4A**). It has previously been shown that the dorsal projections of the sLNv neurons show rhythmic remodeling and that an operational clock is required for this circadian structural plasticity (Fernandez et al., 2008). In light of our previous results, we decided to assess if this process was affected in tau deficient flies. Day-night (ZT2 and ZT14) changes in PDF terminal morphology were measured in tau deficient flies and control flies (**Figures 4C,D**). The degree of axonal arborization was quantified by using an adaptation of Sholl's method to study the dendritic branching pattern (Sholl, 1953; Fernandez et al., 2008). As illustrated in **Figure 4B**, the number of intersections between the concentric rings and the projections were determined. In controls, we observed, as expected, a significant difference in the axonal morphology between early morning (ZT2) and early night (ZT14). The decrease in the complexity of the axonal arbor of the PDF circuit at ZT14 is represented by fewer intersections. When we analyzed the effect of tau deficiency, we found a significantly reduced number of axonal crosses at ZT2, representing a reduction in the structural morphology of the sLNv (**Figure 4D**) that correlated with an increased circadian activity and decreased sleep at this given zeitgeber time (ZT2).

Daily Expression of *Drosophila* Tau in PDF Neurons

To further investigate the role of tau in the structural plasticity of the PDF-positive sLNv neurons, we decided to analyze the expression pattern of dTAu in the sLNv neurons. To this aim, we took advantage of a *Drosophila* line expressing the endogenous dTau tagged with GFP. Interestingly, we found that dTau expression in PDF-positive neurons changes depending on the time of day (**Figure 5**). Quantification of dTau protein immunostaining levels revealed that dTau expression was significantly higher in early morning than in early night (**Figure 5B**). It is important to mention that dTau and PDF expression is increased in the morning, paralleling this peak of activity. In addition, we analyzed dTau gene expression using available RNA-seq data sets from LNv (PDF positive) neurons (Abruzzi et al., 2017). Strikingly, a 6-fold increase in dTau gene expression was found in the early morning (ZT2) (**Figure 5C**),

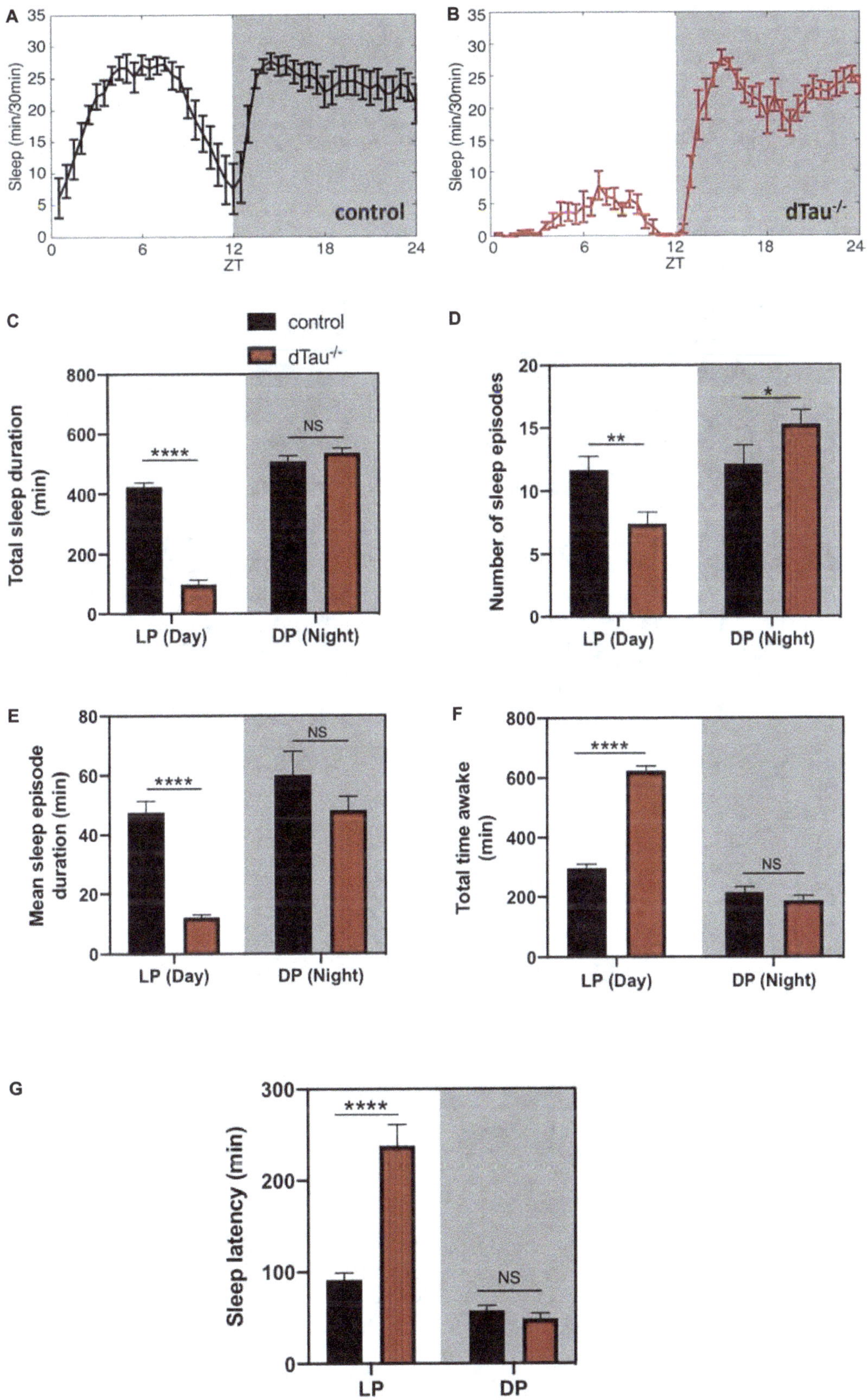

FIGURE 2 | Continued

FIGURE 2 | Loss of tau induces alterations in sleep in *Drosophila*. **(A,B)** Sleep plot representing the minutes of sleep per 30 min for control (in black) **(A)** and dTau mutant (in red) **(B)** of 7 day-old male flies in five averaged LD cycles. Gray shaded area represents the dark period (DP) or night. Results show a reduction in sleep in tau mutant flies in the day (LP) (white left side of the plots) but not in the night. **(C)** Total sleep duration quantification demonstrated significant differences between control and dTau$^{-/-}$ flies. Total sleep quantification in LP and DP showed that the differences only occur during the day, and not during the night (DP). **(D)** Graph representing the number of sleep episodes in the LP and DP for dTau$^{-/-}$ and control flies. Data show that the absence of tau significantly alters the number of sleep episodes, both in LP and DP. **(E)** Graph indicating differences in mean sleep episode duration, which shows a significant decrease in the case of dTau mutants specifically in LP and not in DP. **(F)** Total wake duration for light and dark periods. **(G)** Plot representing latency quantification. Data shows that latency to sleep was significantly increased during the day in Tau mutants, although there was no effect at night. Data represent mean and SEM, analyzed by non-parametric Mann–Whitney statistical test, with $^{*}p < 0.05$, $^{**}p < 0.01$, and $^{****}p < 0.0001$ or NS if no statistical significance (n = 20–25 flies).

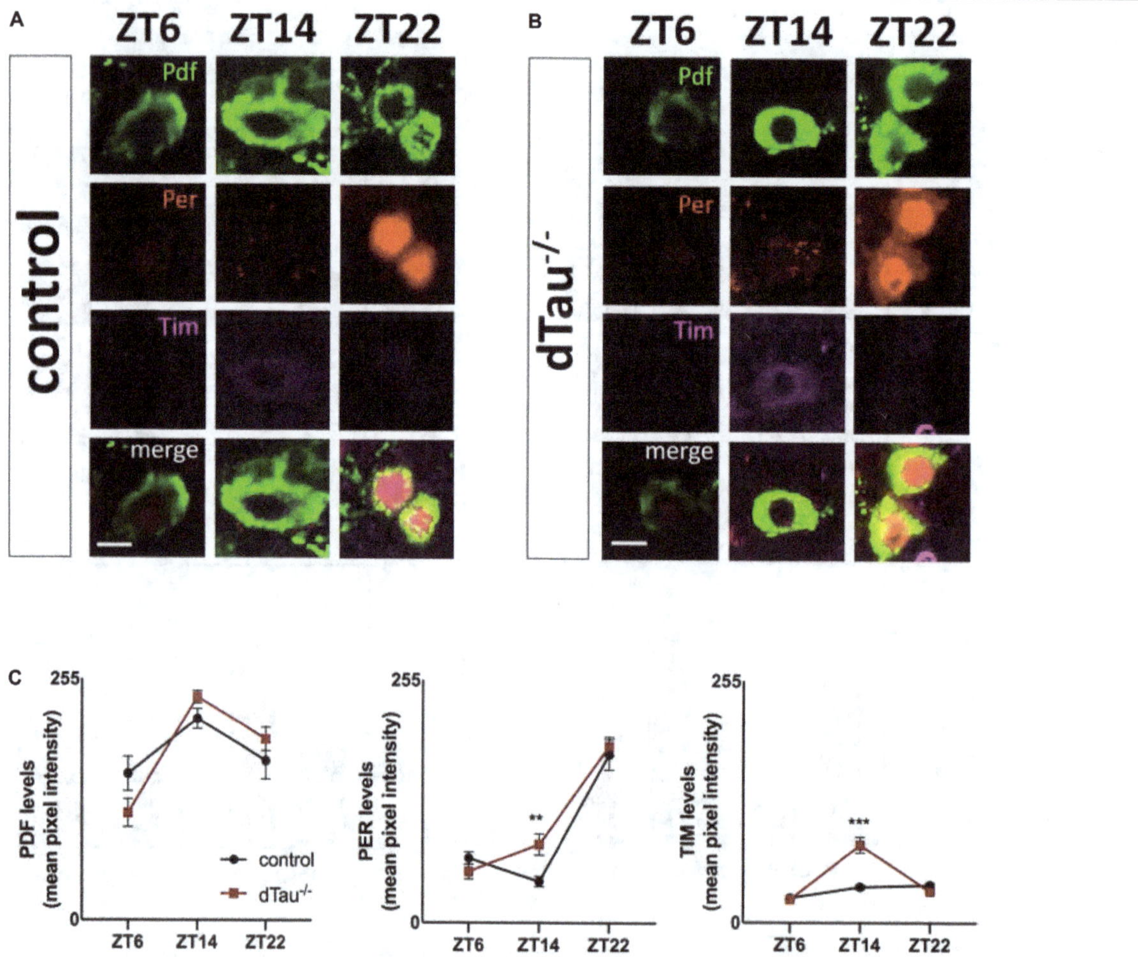

FIGURE 3 | Minimal alteration of core clock operation in tau deficient flies. **(A,B)** Confocal images of LNv neurons immunostained for PDF, PER, and TIM, at different Zeitgeber times (ZT). Wholemount dissections of adult brains were done in control and dTau mutant of 7 day-old. **(C)** Quantification of PER, TIM, and PDF intensity levels across the indicated circadian time points (ZT-6, ZT-14, and ZT-22) shows significant increase in TIM and PER signals at ZT-14 when compared with controls. No changes were found at ZT-6 or ZT-22. Data represent mean and SEM analyzed by non-parametric Mann–Whitney statistical test ($^{**}p < 0.01$ and $^{***}p < 0.001$; n = 12–14 hemispheres). Scale bar is 5 μm.

suggesting tau expression is necessary for the observed structural plasticity of the sLNv terminals.

DISCUSSION

Our results show major abnormalities in circadian activity and sleep in dTau$^{-/-}$ flies, including higher morning activity and reduced sleep during the day-light period of the bimodal circadian rhythm (**Figures 1–2**). These results are also in agreement with previous results obtained in tau KO mice (Cantero et al., 2010). Sleep alterations are observed as a function of normal aging, yet in AD, an exacerbated dysregulation of circadian sleep patterns increases in severity as the disease progresses, contributing to impairment in cognitive function (Musiek et al., 2015; Homolak et al., 2018).

Here, similar patterns of sleep to those observed in human patients with AD and related tauopathies (Aldrich et al., 1989;

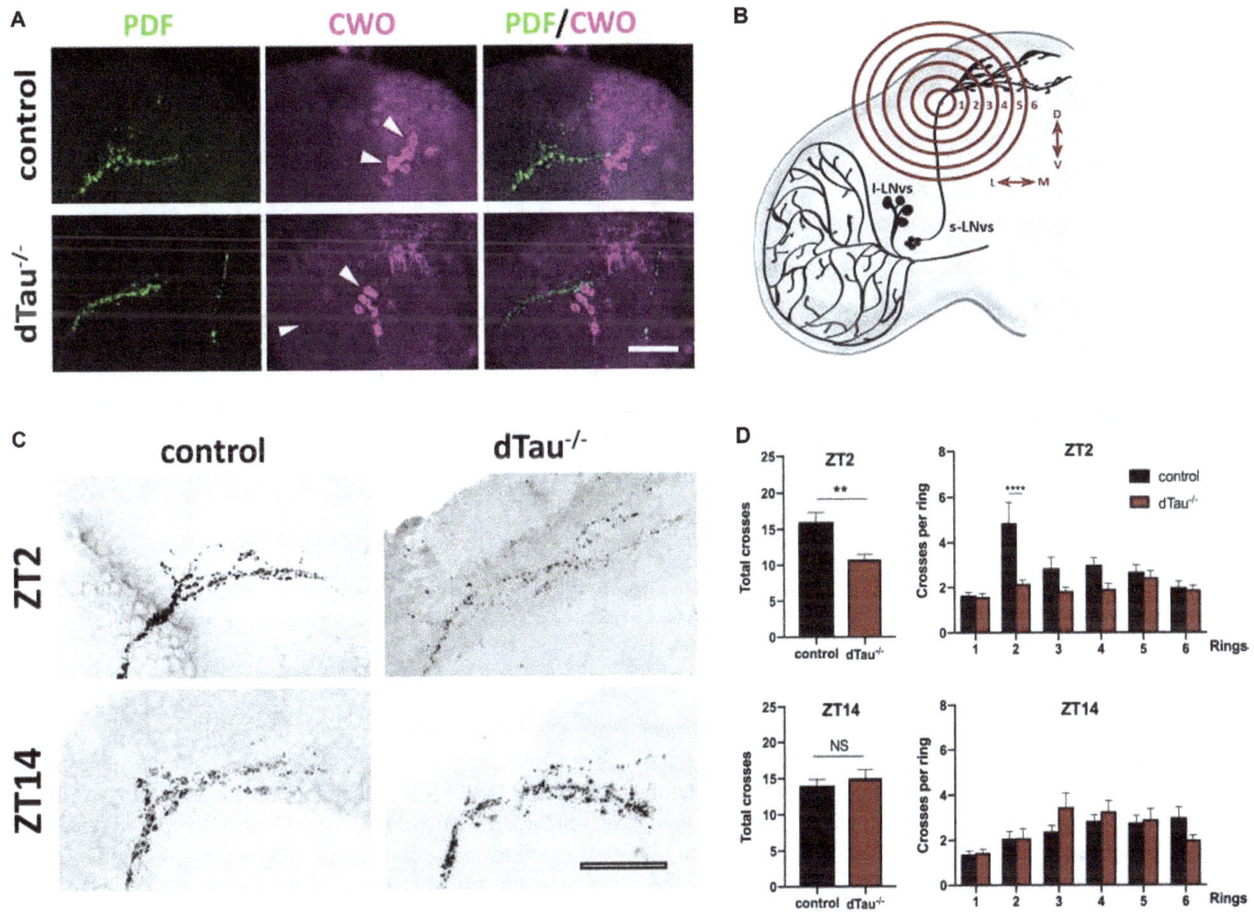

FIGURE 4 | Effect of tau deficiency on daily rhythms of axonal structural remodeling. **(A)** Immunolabeling with anti-PDF and anti-CWO antibodies in LNv and DN neurons of adult brains from 7 day-old male flies. CWO immunostaining denotes the proper localization and morphology of DN neurons (arrow heads). Scale bar is 20 μm. **(B)** Scheme representing Sholl analysis in PDF-positive (black) LNv projections. Six concentric and evenly spaced (10 μm) rings (in red) are drawn. The centers of the rings are localized at the point where the first dorsal ramification starts in each hemisphere. **(C)** Representative confocal images of LNv neurons immunolabeled with anti-PDF antibody at ZT-2 and ZT-14, early morning and early evening, respectively. Panels show PDF-positive signal in LNv projections. Scale bar is 25 μm. **(D)** Plots representing Sholl analysis quantification at ZT2 and ZT14 for the corresponding genotypes. dTau$^{-/-}$ flies showed a significant reduction in the spreading across the concentric rings specifically at ZT-2, when compared to controls. No changes were found at ZT-14. Data represent mean and SEM analyzed by one-way ANOVA test, with $^{**}p < 0.01$ and $^{****}p < 0.0001$ or NS if no statistical significance (n = 12–14 hemispheres).

Logsdon et al., 1998; Vitiello and Borson, 2001) were observed in dTau$^{-/-}$ flies (**Figure 2**). The prolonged sleep latency observed in the dTau$^{-/-}$ flies following lights-off seems to mimic the sundowning syndrome observed in human tauopathic patients (Aldrich et al., 1989) to some extent, supporting tau loss-of-function as a possible pathogenic mechanism of the disease.

Experimental evidence suggests that slow and fast neural oscillations are strongly involved in motor behavior and sleep (Saleh et al., 2010; Posluszny, 2014; Niethard et al., 2018). In this regard, previous results in tau KO mice have indicated slowing of theta rhythms (5–11 Hz) in the hippocampus, and loss of functional connectivity between the hippocampus and the frontal cortex in the gamma range (30–80 Hz) (Cantero et al., 2011). Our results in dTau$^{-/-}$ flies agree with previous observations in tau KO mice on motor behavior and sleep, however, future studies showing neural activity recordings of clock neurons of dTau$^{-/-}$ flies may uncover alterations on electrophysiological properties and will further confirm the role tau protein appears to play in the regulation of these neuronal responses and behaviors. In addition, a recent study has shown that abnormal hyperphosphorylated tau alters circadian clock operation supporting tau loss-of-function (Stevanovic et al., 2017) similar to our obtained results in dTau$^{-/-}$ flies.

The circadian alterations observed in tau deficient flies may involve aberrant environmental perception, defective core clock operation, or perhaps altered clock output. We first considered whether tau deficiency affected visual phototransduction. This was conceivable given the altered light-on responses (**Figure 1**). However, electrophysiological recordings performed in the dTau$^{-/-}$ line did not show any abnormalities (Burnouf et al., 2016). In addition, electroretinogram recordings in young tau KO mice are normal (Rodriguez et al., 2018), suggesting loss of tau does not induce developmental defects on retinal neurons.

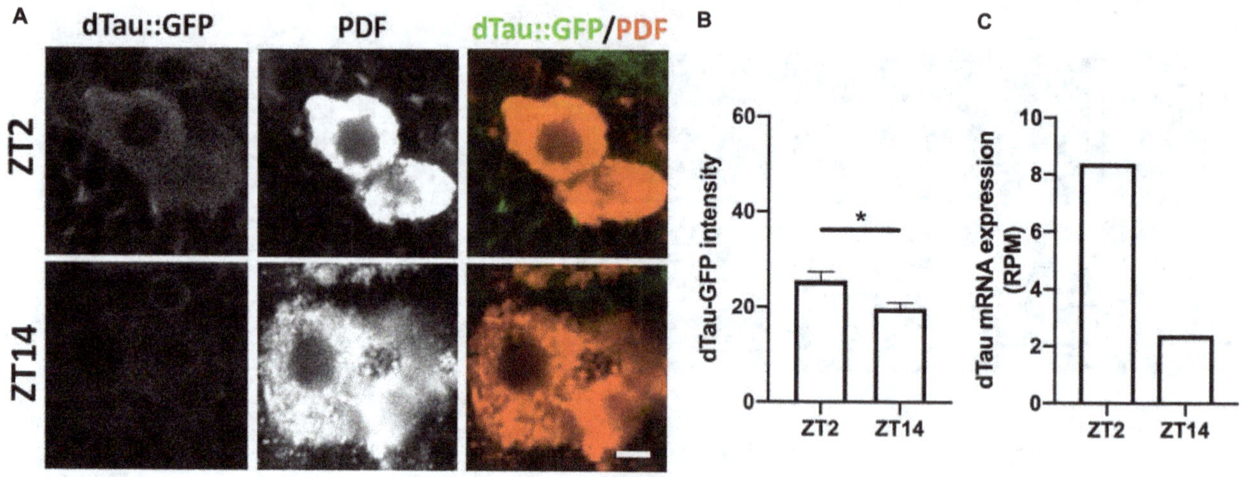

FIGURE 5 | Modulation of tau protein levels during daily rhythms. **(A)** Representative images of immunolabeled 7 day-old male dTau-GFP fly brains with anti-PDF antibody at ZT-2 and ZT-14 (early morning and early night time-points). Scale bar is 10 μm. **(B)** Plot representing absolute intensity values of dTau-GFP signal in LNv somas at ZT-2 and ZT-14. Results demonstrate a significant difference between dTau fluorescent signal at the studied Zeitgeber times, with intensity values higher at ZT-2 and lower at ZT-14. **(C)** Plot representing dTau mRNA levels resulting from PDF neurons RNA-seq analysis (Abruzzi et al., 2017). Results demonstrate a reduction in dTau transcript levels at ZT-14 in PDF neurons when compared to dTau mRNA levels at ZT-2. Data represent mean and SEM analyzed by non-parametric Mann–Whitney statistical test (*$p < 0.05$; $n = 12$–14 hemispheres).

During normal clock operation in *Drosophila*, levels of per and tim mRNA rise during the day. The two proteins start to accumulate, initially in the cytoplasm, and then around the middle of the night in the nucleus (Zheng and Sehgal, 2012). TIM stabilizes PER in the cytoplasm, and is required to transport it to the nucleus. Nuclear localization of the two proteins is also regulated by specific importins (Jang et al., 2015) and appears to be temporally regulated (Curtin et al., 1995; Meyer et al., 2006). Nuclear localization of PER and TIM coincides with the decline of their mRNA levels due to negative autoregulatory feedback by the proteins. PER and TIM cannot bind DNA, but regulate transcription by inhibiting their transcriptional activators, Clock and Cycle. We observed minimal but significant alterations in the core clock proteins in tau deficient flies (**Figure 3**). Alterations in tau proteostasis leading to detrimental loss-of-function effects have been shown in Alzheimer's disease and related tauopathies where pathogenic tau alters nucleocytoplasmic transport by interacting with components of the nuclear pore complex (Eftekharzadeh et al., 2018). Future studies would be necessary to rule out the role tau protein plays in modulating nucleocytoplasmic transport in clock neurons.

In *Drosophila,* rhythmic locomotor cycles rely on the activity of approximately 150 neurons grouped in seven clusters (Helfrich-Forster, 2003; Shafer et al., 2006; Dubowy and Sehgal, 2017). Work from many laboratories have pointed to the sLNvs as critical for circadian control of locomotor rhythmicity (Renn et al., 1999; Blanchardon et al., 2001; Grima et al., 2004; Stoleru et al., 2004, 2005). The sLNv neurons undergo circadian remodeling of their dorsal axonal projections allowing these circadian pacemaker neurons to change synaptic contacts across the day (Fernandez et al., 2008; Gorostiza et al., 2014). This plasticity is critical given the role sLNv neurons play in the Drosophila circuit connecting circadian clock neurons to sleep promoting neurons (Guo et al., 2018). Our results show that loss of tau impinges on circadian structural plasticity and temporal dynamics of the sLNv axonal projections (**Figure 4**). A similar effect of tau protein on structural plasticity has also been recently described in hippocampal granule neurons (Bolos et al., 2017). Structural alterations on terminal projections of sLNv could be promoted depending on tau protein's ability to interact with microtubules. In this regard, future studies are needed to further explore the role disease-associated hyperphosphorylated tau plays in structural plasticity and pathophysiology of clock neurons in Alzheimer's disease and related tauopathy. Additionally, disease-associated tau could play a crucial role in circadian disruption and sleep alterations observed in AD patients through interaction with the actin cytoskeleton in the terminal projections, altering circadian neuronal plasticity (Petsakou et al., 2015).

On the other hand, dysregulation of tau proteostasis could have implications beyond mere structural changes in terminal projections. Tau, through the regulation of cytoskeleton dynamics, could be modulating the biology of melatonin receptors, which play important roles in the sleep-wake cycle (Jarzynka et al., 2006, 2009).

We have found that dTau levels change during the day, presumably fulfilling the cytoskeletal demands during periods of structural remodeling, like the one observed for the dorsal projections of the sLNv neurons. However, it is unknown how tau levels are regulated in this context. Evidence is emerging for post-transcriptional clock regulators (Lim and Allada, 2013). As key regulators of mRNA stability and translation, microRNAs (miRNAs) are implicated in multiple aspects of time keeping. miRNAs are capable of binding to and silencing many target transcripts, providing an additional level of regulation that complements canonical transcriptional pathways. miR-219 and miR-132 were early miRNAs identified to regulate mammalian clocks (Cheng et al., 2007). Recently, it has been described that miR-219 dysregulation promotes neurodegeneration through posttranscriptional regulation of tau. Since miR-219 is the only conserved miRNA able to modulate tau across multiple species, it would be important, in future studies, to explore its mechanisms of regulating tau in clock neurons.

CONCLUSION

In conclusion, our results support the role tau protein plays in the regulation of circadian activity and sleep in *Drosophila*, presumably through the modulation of structural and temporal dynamics of the cytoskeleton in terminal projections of the circadian pacemaker neurons. This conclusion is based on the fact that tau deficiency disrupts the temporal dynamics of circadian pacemaker neurons. Our findings are also consistent with previously described observations on the possible role of tau on sleep regulation in mice. Therefore, further validation in mouse models and accompanying behavioral studies would be valuable. Further studies will provide a better understanding of the functions of tau and advance our understanding of the role it plays in circadian biology and sleep behavior.

AUTHOR CONTRIBUTIONS

MA, MEA, JC, and IS-M conceived and co-ordinated the study. IS-M and MA designed the experiments. MA, MEA, GL, and CK conducted the experiments and analyzed the data. IS-M wrote the first draft of the manuscript. CK and JJ contributed to the materials and critically revised the initial manuscript draft. All the authors discussed and commented on the final manuscript.

ACKNOWLEDGMENTS

We thank Dr. Linda Partridge for *Drosophila* stocks and Drs. Paul E. Hardin, Michael Rosbash, and Amita Segal for kindly sharing the antibodies against CWO, PER, and TIM, respectively.

REFERENCES

Abruzzi, K. C., Zadina, A., Luo, W., Wiyanto, E., Rahman, R., Guo, F., et al. (2017). RNA-seq analysis of drosophila clock and non-clock neurons reveals neuron-specific cycling and novel candidate neuropeptides. *PLoS Genet.* 13:e1006613. doi: 10.1371/journal.pgen.1006613

Aldrich, M. S., Foster, N. L., White, R. F., Bluemlein, L., and Prokopowicz, G. (1989). Sleep abnormalities in progressive supranuclear palsy. *Ann. Neurol.* 25, 577–581.

Blanchardon, E., Grima, B., Klarsfeld, A., Chelot, E., Hardin, P. E., Preat, T., et al. (2001). Defining the role of drosophila lateral neurons in the control of circadian rhythms in motor activity and eclosion by targeted genetic ablation and PERIOD protein overexpression. *Eur. J. Neurosci.* 13, 871–888. doi: 10.1046/j.0953-816x.2000.01450.x

Bolos, M., Pallas-Bazarra, N., Terreros-Roncal, J., Perea, J. R., Jurado-Arjona, J., Avila, J., et al. (2017). Soluble tau has devastating effects on the structural plasticity of hippocampal granule neurons. *Transl. Psychiatr.* 7:1267. doi: 10.1038/s41398-017-0013-6

Brandt, R., and Bakota, L. (2017). Microtubule dynamics and the neurodegenerative triad of alzheimer's disease: the hidden connection. *J. Neurochem.* 143, 409–417. doi: 10.1111/jnc.14011

Burnouf, S., Gronke, S., Augustin, H., Dols, J., Gorsky, M. K., Werner, J., et al. (2016). Deletion of endogenous Tau proteins is not detrimental in Drosophila. *Sci. Rep.* 6:23102. doi: 10.1038/srep23102

Cantero, J. L., Hita-Yanez, E., Moreno-Lopez, B., Portillo, F., Rubio, A., and Avila, J. (2010). Tau protein role in sleep-wake cycle. *J. Alzheimers Dis.* 21, 411–421. doi: 10.3233/JAD-2010-100285

Cantero, J. L., Moreno-Lopez, B., Portillo, F., Rubio, A., Hita-Yanez, E., and Avila, J. (2011). Role of tau protein on neocortical and hippocampal oscillatory patterns. *Hippocampus* 21, 827–834. doi: 10.1002/hipo.20798

Cheng, H. Y., Papp, J. W., Varlamova, O., Dziema, H., Russell, B., Curfman, J. P., et al. (2007). microRNA modulation of circadian-clock period and entrainment. *Neuron* 54, 813–829. doi: 10.1016/j.neuron.2007.05.017

Chiu, J. C., Low, K. H., Pike, D. H., Yildirim, E., and Edery, I. (2010). Assaying locomotor activity to study circadian rhythms and sleep parameters in Drosophila. *J. Vis. Exp.* 43:2157. doi: 10.3791/2157

Curtin, K. D., Huang, Z. J., and Rosbash, M. (1995). Temporally regulated nuclear entry of the Drosophila period protein contributes to the circadian clock. *Neuron* 14, 365–372. doi: 10.1016/0896-6273(95)90292-9

Dent, E. W. (2017). Of microtubules and memory: implications for microtubule dynamics in dendrites and spines. *Mol. Biol. Cell* 28, 1–8. doi: 10.1091/mbc.E15-11-0769

Donelson, N. C., Kim, E. Z., Slawson, J. B., Vecsey, C. G., Huber, R., and Griffith, L. C. (2012). High-resolution positional tracking for long-term analysis of drosophila sleep and locomotion using the "tracker" program. *PLoS One* 7:e37250. doi: 10.1371/journal.pone.0037250

Dubowy, C., and Sehgal, A. (2017). Circadian rhythms and sleep in *Drosophila melanogaster*. *Genetics* 205, 1373–1397. doi: 10.1534/genetics.115.185157

Eftekharzadeh, B., Daigle, J. G., Kapinos, L. E., Coyne, A., Schiantarelli, J., Carlomagno, Y., et al. (2018). Tau protein disrupts nucleocytoplasmic transport in alzheimer's disease. *Neuron* 99:e927.

Fernandez, M. P., Berni, J., and Ceriani, M. F. (2008). Circadian remodeling of neuronal circuits involved in rhythmic behavior. *PLoS Biol.* 6:e69. doi: 10.1371/journal.pbio.0060069

Gibson, E. M., Williams, W. P. III, and Kriegsfeld, L. J. (2009). Aging in the circadian system: considerations for health, disease prevention and longevity. *Exp. Gerontol.* 44, 51–56. doi: 10.1016/j.exger.2008.05.007

Gistelinck, M., Lambert, J. C., Callaerts, P., Dermaut, B., and Dourlen, P. (2012). Drosophila models of tauopathies: what have we learned? *Int. J. Alzheimers Dis.* 2012:970980. doi: 10.1155/2012/970980

Gorostiza, E. A., Depetris-Chauvin, A., Frenkel, L., Pirez, N., and Ceriani, M. F. (2014). Circadian pacemaker neurons change synaptic contacts across the day. *Curr. Biol.* 24, 2161–2167. doi: 10.1016/j.cub.2014.07.063

Grima, B., Chelot, E., Xia, R., and Rouyer, F. (2004). Morning and evening peaks of activity rely on different clock neurons of the drosophila brain. *Nature* 431, 869–873. doi: 10.1038/nature02935

Guo, F., Holla, M., Diaz, M. M., and Rosbash, M. (2018). A circadian output circuit controls sleep-wake arousal in *Drosophila. Neuron* 100, 624–635. doi: 10.1016/j.neuron.2018.09.002

Guo, T., Noble, W., and Hanger, D. P. (2017). Roles of tau protein in health and disease. *Acta Neuropathol.* 133, 665–704. doi: 10.1007/s00401-017-1707-9

Hafycz, J. M., and Naidoo, N. N. (2019). Sleep, aging, and cellular health: aged-related changes in sleep and protein homeostasis converge in neurodegenerative diseases. *Front. Aging Neurosci.* 11:140. doi: 10.3389/fnagi.2019.00140

Hardin, P. E. (2011). Molecular genetic analysis of circadian timekeeping in drosophila. *Adv. Genet.* 74, 141–173. doi: 10.1016/B978-0-12-387690-4.00005-2

Hastings, M. H., Reddy, A. B., and Maywood, E. S. (2003). A clockwork web: circadian timing in brain and periphery, in health and disease. *Nat. Rev. Neurosci.* 4, 649–661. doi: 10.1038/nrn1177

Heidary, G., and Fortini, M. E. (2001). Identification and characterization of the Drosophila tau homolog. *Mech. Dev.* 108, 171–178. doi: 10.1016/s0925-4773(01)00487-7

Helfrich-Forster, C. (2003). The neuroarchitecture of the circadian clock in the brain of *Drosophila melanogaster. Microsci. Res. Tech.* 62, 94–102. doi: 10.1002/jemt.10357

Hendricks, J. C., Finn, S. M., Panckeri, K. A., Chavkin, J., Williams, J. A., Sehgal, A., et al. (2000). Rest in drosophila is a sleep-like state. *Neuron* 25, 129–138. doi: 10.1016/s0896-6273(00)80877-6

Holth, J. K., Fritschi, S. K., Wang, C., Pedersen, N. P., Cirrito, J. R., Mahan, T. E., et al. (2019). The sleep-wake cycle regulates brain interstitial fluid tau in mice and CSF tau in humans. *Science* 363, 880–884. doi: 10.1126/science.aav2546

Homolak, J., Mudrovcic, M., Vukic, B., and Toljan, K. (2018). Circadian Rhythm and Alzheimer's Disease. *Med. Sci.* 6:52.

Jang, A. R., Moravcevic, K., Saez, L., Young, M. W., and Sehgal, A. (2015). Drosophila TIM binds importin alpha1, and acts as an adapter to transport PER to the nucleus. *PLoS Genet.* 11:e1004974. doi: 10.1371/journal.pgen.1004974

Jarzynka, M. J., Passey, D. K., Ignatius, P. F., Melan, M. A., Radio, N. M., Jockers, R., et al. (2006). Modulation of melatonin receptors and G-protein function by microtubules. *J. Pineal Res.* 41, 324–336. doi: 10.1111/j.1600-079x.2006.00371.x

Jarzynka, M. J., Passey, D. K., Johnson, D. A., Konduru, N. V., Fitz, N. F., Radio, N. M., et al. (2009). Microtubules modulate melatonin receptors involved in phase-shifting circadian activity rhythms: *in vitro* and *in vivo* evidence. *J. Pineal Res.* 46, 161–171. doi: 10.1111/j.1600-079X.2008.00644.x

Kolker, D. E., Fukuyama, H., Huang, D. S., Takahashi, J. S., Horton, T. H., and Turek, F. W. (2003). Aging alters circadian and light-induced expression of clock genes in golden hamsters. *J. Biol. Rhythms* 18, 159–169. doi: 10.1177/0748730403251802

Lim, C., and Allada, R. (2013). Emerging roles for post-transcriptional regulation in circadian clocks. *Nat. Neurosci.* 16, 1544–1550. doi: 10.1038/nn.3543

Logsdon, R. G., Teri, L., Mccurry, S. M., Gibbons, L. E., Kukull, W. A., and Larson, E. B. (1998). Wandering: a significant problem among community-residing individuals with Alzheimer's disease. *J. Gerontol. B Psychol. Sci. Soc. Sci.* 53, 294–299.

Matus, A. (1988). Microtubule-associated proteins: their potential role in determining neuronal morphology. *Annu. Rev. Neurosci.* 11, 29–44. doi: 10.1146/annurev.neuro.11.1.29

Meyer, P., Saez, L., and Young, M. W. (2006). PER-TIM interactions in living Drosophila cells: an interval timer for the circadian clock. *Science* 311, 226–229. doi: 10.1126/science.1118126

Musiek, E. S., Xiong, D. D., and Holtzman, D. M. (2015). Sleep, circadian rhythms, and the pathogenesis of Alzheimer disease. *Exp. Mol. Med.* 47:e148. doi: 10.1038/emm.2014.121

Niethard, N., Ngo, H. V., Ehrlich, I., and Born, J. (2018). Cortical circuit activity underlying sleep slow oscillations and spindles. *Proc. Natl. Acad. Sci. U.S.A.* 115, E9220–E9229. doi: 10.1073/pnas.1805517115

Petsakou, A., Sapsis, T. P., and Blau, J. (2015). Circadian rhythms in rho1 activity regulate neuronal plasticity and network hierarchy. *Cell* 162, 823–835. doi: 10.1016/j.cell.2015.07.010

Posluszny, A. (2014). The contribution of electrical synapses to field potential oscillations in the hippocampal formation. *Front. Neural. Circ.* 8:32. doi: 10.3389/fncir.2014.00032

Renn, S. C., Park, J. H., Rosbash, M., Hall, J. C., and Taghert, P. H. (1999). A pdf neuropeptide gene mutation and ablation of PDF neurons each cause severe abnormalities of behavioral circadian rhythms in drosophila. *Cell* 99, 791–802. doi: 10.1016/s0092-8674(00)81676-1

Rincon-Limas, D. E., Jensen, K., and Fernandez-Funez, P. (2012). Drosophila models of proteinopathies: the little fly that could. *Curr. Pharm Des.* 18, 1108–1122. doi: 10.2174/138161212799315894

Rodriguez, L., Mdzomba, J. B., Joly, S., Boudreau-Laprise, M., Planel, E., and Pernet, V. (2018). Human tau expression does not induce mouse retina neurodegeneration, suggesting differential toxicity of tau in brain vs. retinal neurons. *Front. Mol. Neurosci.* 11:293. doi: 10.3389/fnmol.2018.00293

Saleh, M., Reimer, J., Penn, R., Ojakangas, C. L., and Hatsopoulos, N. G. (2010). Fast and slow oscillations in human primary motor cortex predict oncoming behaviorally relevant cues. *Neuron* 65, 461–471. doi: 10.1016/j.neuron.2010.02.001

Shafer, O. T., Helfrich-Forster, C., Renn, S. C., and Taghert, P. H. (2006). Reevaluation of *Drosophila melanogaster's* neuronal circadian pacemakers reveals new neuronal classes. *J. Comp. Neurol.* 498, 180–193. doi: 10.1002/cne.21021

Shaw, P. J., Cirelli, C., Greenspan, R. J., and Tononi, G. (2000). Correlates of sleep and waking in *Drosophila melanogaster. Science* 287, 1834–1837. doi: 10.1126/science.287.5459.1834

Sholl, D. A. (1953). Dendritic organization in the neurons of the visual and motor cortices of the cat. *J. Anat.* 87, 387–406.

Shweiki, D. (1999). The physical imperative in circadian rhythm: a cytoskeleton-related physically resettable clock mechanism hypothesis. *Med. Hypotheses* 53, 413–420. doi: 10.1054/mehy.1998.0785

Stevanovic, K., Yunus, A., Joly-Amado, A., Gordon, M., Morgan, D., Gulick, D., et al. (2017). Disruption of normal circadian clock function in a mouse model of tauopathy. *Exp. Neurol.* 294, 58–67. doi: 10.1016/j.expneurol.2017.04.015

Stoleru, D., Peng, Y., Agosto, J., and Rosbash, M. (2004). Coupled oscillators control morning and evening locomotor behaviour of drosophila. *Nature* 431, 862–868. doi: 10.1038/nature02926

Stoleru, D., Peng, Y., Nawathean, P., and Rosbash, M. (2005). A resetting signal between Drosophila pacemakers synchronizes morning and evening activity. *Nature* 438, 238–242. doi: 10.1038/nature04192

Touitou, Y., and Haus, E. (2000). Alterations with aging of the endocrine and neuroendocrine circadian system in humans. *Chronobiol. Int.* 17, 369–390. doi: 10.1081/cbi-100101052

Tracy, T. E., and Gan, L. (2018). Tau-mediated synaptic and neuronal dysfunction in neurodegenerative disease. *Curr. Opin. Neurobiol.* 51, 134–138. doi: 10.1016/j.conb.2018.04.027

Van Swinderen, B., Nitz, D. A., and Greenspan, R. J. (2004). Uncoupling of brain activity from movement defines arousal states in drosophila. *Curr. Biol.* 14, 81–87. doi: 10.1016/s0960-9822(03)00987-4

Vitiello, M. V., and Borson, S. (2001). Sleep disturbances in patients with alzheimer's disease: epidemiology, pathophysiology and treatment. *CNS Drugs* 15, 777–796. doi: 10.2165/00023210-200115100-00004

Voelzmann, A., Okenve-Ramos, P., Qu, Y., Chojnowska-Monga, M., Del Cano-Espinel, M., Prokop, A., et al. (2016).). Tau and spectraplakins promote synapse formation and maintenance through Jun kinase and neuronal trafficking. *eLife* 5:e14694. doi: 10.7554/eLife.14694

Zheng, X., and Sehgal, A. (2012). Speed control: cogs and gears that drive the circadian clock. *Trends Neurosci.* 35, 574–585. doi: 10.1016/j.tins.2012.05.007

8

Role of Tau as a Microtubule-Associated Protein: Structural and Functional Aspects

Pascale Barbier[1], *Orgeta Zejneli*[2,3], *Marlène Martinho*[4], *Alessia Lasorsa*[2], *Valérie Belle*[4], *Caroline Smet-Nocca*[2], *Philipp O. Tsvetkov*[1], *François Devred*[1]* *and Isabelle Landrieu*[2]*

[1]Fac Pharm, Aix Marseille Univ., Centre National de la Recherche Scientifique (CNRS), Inst Neurophysiopathol (INP), Fac Pharm, Marseille, France, [2]Univ. Lille, Centre National de la Recherche Scientifique (CNRS), UMR 8576, Unité de Glycobiologie Structurale et Fonctionnelle (UGSF), Lille, France, [3]Univ. Lille, Institut National de la Santé et de la Recherche Médicale (INSERM), CHU-Lille, UMR-S 1172, Centre de Recherche Jean-Pierre AUBERT (JPArc), Lille, France, [4]Aix Marseille Univ., Centre National de la Recherche Scientifique (CNRS), UMR 7281, Bioénergétique et Ingénierie des Protéines (BIP), Marseille, France

***Correspondence:**
François Devred
francois.devred@univ-amu.fr
Isabelle Landrieu
isabelle.landrieu@univ-lille.fr

Microtubules (MTs) play a fundamental role in many vital processes such as cell division and neuronal activity. They are key structural and functional elements in axons, supporting neurite differentiation and growth, as well as transporting motor proteins along the axons, which use MTs as support tracks. Tau is a stabilizing MT associated protein, whose functions are mainly regulated by phosphorylation. A disruption of the MT network, which might be caused by Tau loss of function, is observed in a group of related diseases called tauopathies, which includes Alzheimer's disease (AD). Tau is found hyperphosphorylated in AD, which might account for its loss of MT stabilizing capacity. Since destabilization of MTs after dissociation of Tau could contribute to toxicity in neurodegenerative diseases, a molecular understanding of this interaction and its regulation is essential.

Keywords: post-translational modifications, biophysical methods, Alzheimer's disease, intrinsically disordered proteins, neurodegenerative diseases

INTRODUCTION

Tau is a microtubule-associated protein (MAP; Weingarten et al., 1975; Witman et al., 1976) that is abundant in the axons of neurons where it stabilizes microtubule (MT) bundles (Binder et al., 1985; Black et al., 1996). Together with other destabilizing MAPs, such as stathmin, Tau plays a central role in MT dynamics by regulating assembly, dynamic behavior and the spatial organization of MTs. Tau and other MAPs that bind to MTs are tightly regulated by a number of factors, including post-translational modifications (PTMs), to ensure the appropriate dynamics of the system (Lindwall and Cole, 1984; Mandelkow et al., 1995; Ramkumar et al., 2018). However, the exact mechanism of assembly and stabilization of MTs by Tau remains challenging to characterize

---

Abbreviations: AD, Alzheimer's Disease; EM, Electron Microscopy; EPR, Electron Paramagnetic Resonance spectroscopy; FRET, Förster Resonance Energy Transfer; FTD, Fronto-Temporal Dementia; GFP, Green Fluorescent Protein; HSQC, Heteronuclear Single Quantum Correlation; IDP, Intrinsically Disordered Protein; MAP, Microtubule Associated Protein; MS, Mass Spectrometry; MT, MicroTubule; NOE, Nuclear Overhauser Effect; NMR, Nuclear Magnetic Resonance spectroscopy; PHF6, Paired Helical Filament Hexapeptide; PRE, Paramagnetic Relaxation Enhancement; PTMs, Post-Translational Modifications; SLD, Stathmin-Like Domain; STD, Saturation Transfer Difference.

due to the inherent dynamics of the system and the disordered nature of Tau. The number of approaches that have been conducted so far to gain knowledge on this particular interaction is striking (Devred et al., 2010; Nouar et al., 2013; Di Maio et al., 2014; Tsvetkov et al., 2019). Tau is probably the most studied MAP because of its implication in a group of neurodegenerative diseases called tauopathies, associated with Tau aggregation into intraneuronal deposits (Brion et al., 1986), such as frontotemporal dementia (FTD), Alzheimer's disease (AD) and progressive supranuclear palsy.

Tau binding to MTs, as well as its propensity to aggregate, are affected by Tau mutations and by Tau PTMs, in particular, its hyper-phosphorylation (Alonso et al., 1994; LeBoeuf et al., 2008). These pathologically modified Tau molecules perturb MT function and axonal transport, contributing to neurodegeneration. Indeed, a reduction of MT density and fast axonal transport is observed in transgenic AD mouse models that exhibit hyperphosphorylated Tau inclusions in neurons (Cash et al., 2003). Furthermore, Tau mutations carried by FTD patients cause MT-mediated deformation of the nucleus, which in turn results in perturbation of the nucleocytoplasmic transport (Paonessa et al., 2019). In addition, mislocalized Tau in neurons of Tau-overexpressing transgenic mouse brain and of human AD brain directly interacts with the nucleoporins of the nuclear pore complex. This interaction disrupts the nuclear pore functions of nucleocytoplasmic transport and might contribute to Tau-related neurotoxicity (Eftekharzadeh et al., 2018).

Efforts for clinical intervention in the AD field have so far mainly focused on blocking the formation of extracellular amyloid β deposits, another type of aggregates observed in the brain of AD patients (Cummings et al., 2017). However, in the last several years, there has been an increase in studies aimed at the therapeutic targeting of Tau. An improved understanding of Tau functions could lead to the development of new strategies of therapeutic interventions (Mudher et al., 2017; Jadhav et al., 2019). This emphasizes the need to understand the finer details of structural and functional aspects of Tau/MTs interaction.

TUBULIN AND MTs

MTs are hollow cylinders composed of parallel protofilaments of α and β tubulin subunits (α/β tubulin heterodimer, here named tubulin) assembled head-to-tail, which form a pseudo helical lattice (Amos and Schlieper, 2005; **Figure 1**). During MT formation, tubulins self-assemble in their guanosine 5′ triphosphate (GTP)-bound state to form a sheet that closes into a 25 nm outside diameter tube (Chrétien et al., 1995). Whereas the MT core or lattice is constituted of guanosine 5′ diphosphate (GDP)-tubulin, a GTP cap forms at MT ends because of the delay between assembly and GTP hydrolysis at the tubulin inter-dimer interface (Carlier et al., 1989; Caplow and Shanks, 1990; Bowne-Anderson et al., 2015; Baas et al., 2016). This cap has been proposed to stabilize growing MTs since its loss induces MT depolymerization, with characteristic curled protofilaments at MT ends (Chrétien et al., 1995). MTs constantly undergo phases of assembly and disassembly in a process called "dynamic instability" (Mitchison and Kirschner, 1984). Due to these intrinsic dynamics of the system, MTs have been difficult to study from a structural point of view. During the past decades, numerous molecular models were used to simulate the mechanism of MT formation, resulting in a more nuanced model than the original GTP-cap one, which now accounts for the diverse regulatory activities of MAPs. In this model named "coupled-random model," GTP hydrolysis occurs with a constant rate for any tubulin in the MT lattice, except for the dimers at the very tip (Bowne-Anderson et al., 2015). GDP-tubulin does not assemble into MTs but forms double rings (Howard and Timasheff, 1986). It was thus originally considered that GTP would allosterically induce a straight conformation of tubulin capable of MT assembly and that GDP would induce a curved conformation favoring disassembly (Melki et al., 1989). It is now generally accepted that GTP-tubulin in solution is curved similarly to GDP-tubulin, based on the MT models derived from electron microscopy (EM) data, up to about 3.5 Å resolution (Zhang R. et al., 2015) and from X-ray crystallography up to 2 Å resolution (Nawrotek et al., 2011; Pecqueur et al., 2012) together with biochemical evidence (Barbier et al., 2010). Tubulin only straightens upon incorporation into MTs (Alushin et al., 2014). In addition to the GDP/GTP dual nature of tubulin, PTMs of tubulin, such as tyrosination and acetylation, modulate MT stability (Baas et al., 2016). In neurons, two MT regions are distinguished (**Figure 1**): a labile MT region mostly composed of tyrosinated and deacetylated GTP-tubulin, and a stable MT region (or lattice) mostly consisting of assembled detyrosinated and acetylated GDP-tubulin (Baas et al., 2016). These findings together with other recent studies of tubulin modifications—including phosphorylation, polyglycylation, deglutamylation and polyglutamylation—highlight the importance of these PTMs in regulating the different functions of MTs, generating a "tubulin code" (Gadadhar et al., 2017). Indeed, a defect of the deglutamylase CCP1, the enzyme responsible for tubulin deglutamylation, causes infantile-onset neurodegeneration (Shashi et al., 2018), while an excessive polyglutamylation of tubulin reduces the efficiency of neuronal transport in cultured hippocampal neurons (Magiera et al., 2018). Moreover, a default of acetylated tubulin is linked to abnormal axonal transport in several neurodegenerative diseases (Dompierre et al., 2007; Godena et al., 2014; Guo et al., 2017). Altogether, these studies suggest that enzymes responsible for tubulin PTMs could be promising therapeutic targets.

TAU PROTEIN

There are two major MAPs present in cells from the central nervous system, MAP2 and Tau. The expression of one or the other isoform is regulated during development, and their localizations differ. Tau is mainly found in the axonal compartment, while MAP2 is expressed specifically in cell bodies and dendrites (Melková et al., 2019). Both proteins exist as alternatively spliced isoforms, with some high-molecular weight isoforms for MAP2 (MAP2a and MAP2b). There are six isoforms

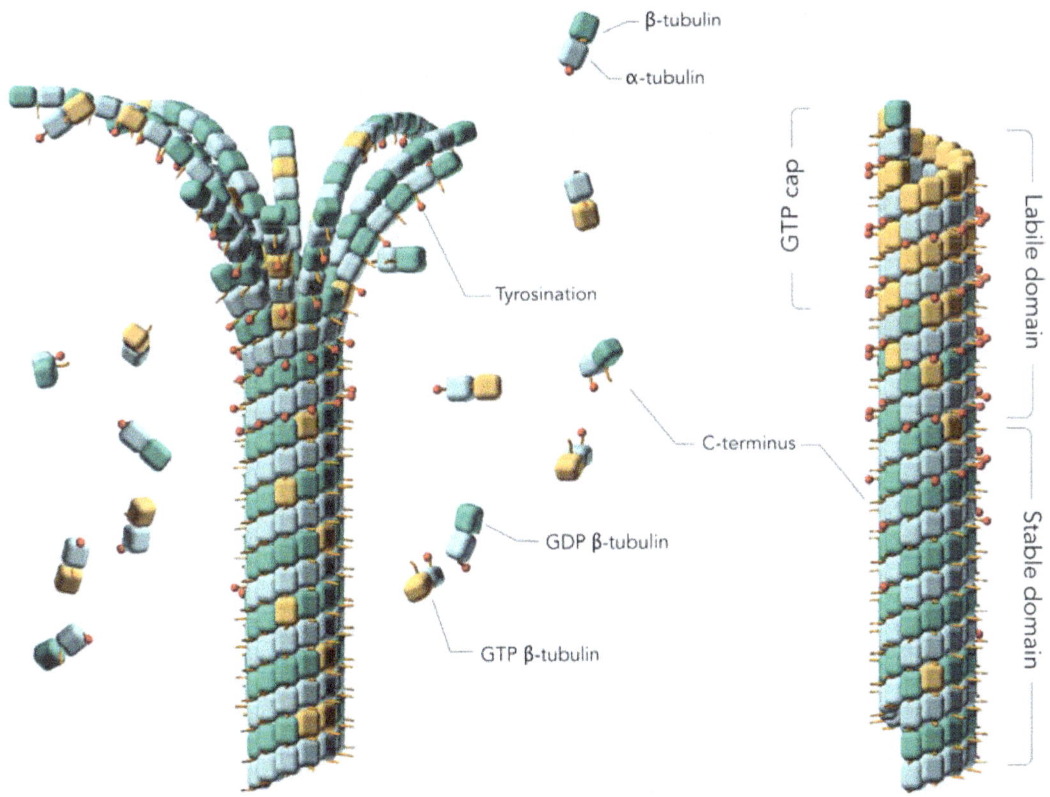

FIGURE 1 | Assembly of tubulins into Microtubules (MTs). Models of a depolymerizing (left) and polymerized (right) MTs. The guanosine 5′ triphosphate (GTP) cap or labile domain is composed mostly of tyrosinated GTP-tubulin. The stable domain is mostly composed of detyrosinated guanosine 5′ diphosphate (GDP)-tubulin. β-tubulin subunits are represented as orange cubes in their GTP-bound states and green cubes in their GDP-bound states. α-tubulin subunits are represented as blue cubes. Red sticks planted on the cubes represent the C-terminal tail of α- and β-tubulin subunits. Tyrosination is represented by a red dot on the C-terminal tail. Two MT regions are distinguished: a labile MT region mostly composed of tyrosinated GTP-tubulins, including the GTP cap, and a stable MT region mostly consisting of assembled detyrosinated GDP-tubulins. MT depolymerization is characterized by curled protofilaments at MT ends (*left*).

of Tau protein present in the central nervous system (ranging from 352 to 441 amino acid residues), resulting from mRNA alternative splicing of a single gene (Goedert et al., 1989; Himmler et al., 1989). Tau is divided into functional domains (numbering according to the longest isoform, **Figure 2**): an N-terminal projection domain Tau(1–165), a proline-rich region Tau(166–242) or PRR, a MT binding region Tau(243–367) or microtubule binding region (MTBR) and a C-terminal domain Tau(368–441). The MTBR consists of four partially repeated sequences R1(243–273), R2(274–304), R3(305–335), and R4(336–367; **Figure 2**). The isoforms differ by the presence, or not, of one/two insert(s) in the N-terminal domain (N1 and/or N2 presence or not), and three or four repeat sequences in the MTBR (R2 presence or not). Even though Tau is an intrinsically disordered protein (IDP), it has a tendency to form local secondary structures, in particular, β-strands in the MTBR and polyproline II helices in the PRR (Mukrasch et al., 2009; Sibille et al., 2012). It has been proposed that Tau N- and C-terminal domains fold back on the central PRR and MTBR domains due to contacts between the N- and C-termini of the protein (Jeganathan et al., 2006; Mukrasch et al., 2009). This model was initially built using distance measurements based on Förster Resonance Energy Transfer (FRET) detection between pairs of fluorophores attached to Tau (Jeganathan et al., 2006). Moreover, measurements of paramagnetic relaxation enhancement (PRE) by nuclear magnetic resonance spectroscopy (NMR) using paramagnetic centers attached at different positions along the Tau sequence, confirmed proximities of the N- and C-terminal domains with the central region of Tau (Mukrasch et al., 2009). Several co-factors were reported to enhance Tau structuration including ions such as Zinc (Roman et al., 2019), potentially regulating Tau functions.

MAP FUNCTION OF TAU

MT dynamics are regulated by proteins that stabilize or destabilize them (van der Vaart et al., 2009). The main role of Tau, one of the stabilizing MAPs, is to protect MTs against depolymerization by decreasing the dissociation of tubulin at both MT ends, resulting in an increased growth rate and decreased catastrophe frequency (Murphy et al., 1977; Trinczek et al., 1995). *In vitro*, Tau induces MT formation at 37°C and tubulin rings at 20°C under experimental conditions with no

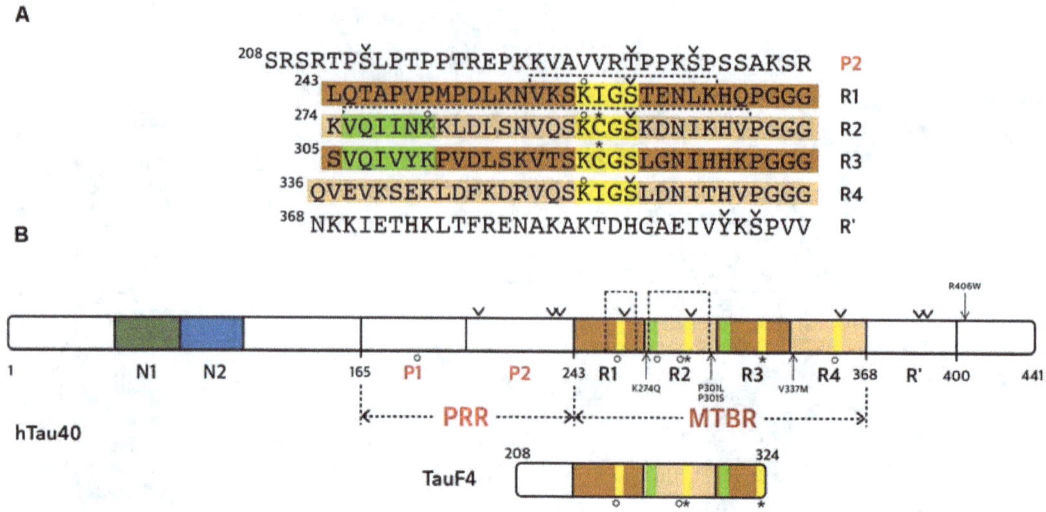

FIGURE 2 | Tau protein sequence and domain organization. The sequence numbering is according to the longest Tau isoform (441 amino acid residues). **(A)** Amino acid sequence of the microtubule binding region (MTBR) and flanking regions, P2 in the PRR and R' in the C-terminal domain. **(B)** General scheme of the full-length Tau protein and of TauF4 fragment. **(A,B)** The MTBR region of Tau consists of four partially repeated sequences, R1 to R4, highlighted in dark and light brown. PHF6* and PHF6 hexapeptides, in R1 and R2 repeats respectively, are highlighted in green and the KXGS motifs in yellow. Phosphorylation sites mentioned in the text are indicated with a v sign, cysteine residues with a star sign and acetylation with a circle. Segments of R1 and R2 shown in **Figure 3** are indicated with dashed lines.

self-assembly of tubulin alone, suggesting that Tau is a MT inducer in addition to being a MT stabilizer (Weingarten et al., 1975; Devred et al., 2004; Kutter et al., 2016).

Tau was proposed to bind preferentially to the GDP-tubulin from the lattice, in detriment of the GTP-tubulin from the plus-end cap, and in agreement with a stabilizing role of Tau (Duan et al., 2017). However, monitoring of Tau binding to MTs by FRET has shown Tau decoration on MT tips, as well as on the lattice (Breuzard et al., 2013). Furthermore, the capacity of Tau to induce *in vitro* MT formation is lost when GDP-tubulin is used (Devred et al., 2004). In agreement, Tau depletion in rat cortical neurons results in the loss of MT mass in the axon, predominantly from the labile domain containing tyrosinated tubulin, rather than the stable domain of MTs (Qiang et al., 2018). Green fluorescent protein (GFP)-tagged Tau was indeed observed to be more abundant on the labile domain of the MTs, or GTP-tubulin cap. Based on these observations obtained by quantitative immunofluorescence, the authors propose that Tau is not strictly a MT stabilizer, but rather allows the MTs to conserve long labile domains (Qiang et al., 2018; Baas and Qiang, 2019). However, a more likely explanation is that Tau is necessary to induce tubulin polymerization in the labile region.

Similar to many other IDPs, Tau can undergo phase-transition under *in vitro* conditions of molecular crowding, resulting in the formation of Tau liquid droplets similar to non-membrane compartments (Hernández-Vega et al., 2017). These Tau-rich drops have the capacity to concentrate tubulin 10 times or higher than the surrounding solution. Nucleation of MTs is observed inside the Tau drops, and MT bundle formation results in the elongation of the drops. This bundle formation could not be reproduced by mimicking the high concentration effect, in the absence of drops. This nucleation environment could support stabilization and provide sufficient plasticity for the formation of the long axonal MT bundles. Although it is not yet known whether this phenomenon is of physiological relevance, GFP-Tau droplets have been observed in transfected neurons (Wegmann et al., 2018).

STRUCTURAL ASPECTS OF TAU MTBR INTERACTION WITH MTs

Tau structure when bound to MTs has been the object of numerous investigations, leading to several models of Tau/MTs complex. *In vitro*, single-molecule FRET experiments showed that Tau bound to soluble tubulin adopts an open conformation (Melo et al., 2016), losing the global fold observed for Tau in solution (Jeganathan et al., 2006; Mukrasch et al., 2009; Schwalbe et al., 2014). However, FRET experiments in the cell, using a Tau protein labeled at its N- and C-termini with fluorophores (Di Primio et al., 2017) show that labeled-Tau bound to MTs displays a global folding, with the N- and C-termini in close proximity, as described for the "paperclip conformation" of free Tau in *in vitro* conditions (Jeganathan et al., 2006). This global fold is lost for unbound Tau, detached from the MTs. This discrepancy might be due to the fact that the cytoplasmic environment is much more complex than can be reproduced in *in vitro* experiments, and Tau might thus bind numerous other cellular partners that could influence its conformation (Di Primio et al., 2017).

Globally, tubulin-bound Tau retains its intrinsically disordered character, and forms a fuzzy complex with tubulin, which might be the reason why Tau binding mode accommodates more than one tubulin (Tompa and Fuxreiter, 2008; Martinho et al., 2018). In agreement, a combination of metal shadowing and cryo-electron microscopy (cryo-EM) revealed that Tau is randomly distributed on the MT surface (Santarella et al., 2004). FRET and fluorescence recovery after photo-bleaching in live cells similarly concluded to the distribution of the Tau/MTs interaction along the MTs, characterized by Tau diffusion coupled to binding phases (Breuzard et al., 2013). In-line with these observations, Tau was shown to diffuse along the MTs, bi-directionally and independently from active transport, in a manner described as kiss-and-hop interactions (Hinrichs et al., 2012). These interactions, observed by single molecule tracking in neurons, might explain why Tau does not seem to interfere with motor protein-mediated axonal transport along the MTs (Janning et al., 2014).

Early studies by peptide mapping allowed the first characterization of the interaction as an array of weakly interacting sites, defining the MTBR as the MT binding core, which contains the four highly homologous repeats R1–R4 (Butner and Kirschner, 1991; Goode et al., 2000). Recently, despite the challenges related to the dynamic and fuzzy nature of Tau/MTs interaction described above, the combination of cryo-EM at near-atomic resolution and Rosetta modeling generated models of the interaction. This breakthrough study highlights the crucial residues of Tau MTBR directly mediating the interaction and confirms the longitudinal mode of Tau binding on MTs (Kellogg et al., 2018). The complex used in the study consists of dynamic MTs without stabilizing agents other than Tau. Tau is found along the protofilaments, following the H11-H12 helices that form a ridge at the MT surface and that are close to the point of attachment of the C-terminal tails of tubulin (**Figure 3**). The observed density spans Tau residues 242–367, covering the MTBR, and is centered on the α-tubulin subunit while contacts with β-tubulin are detected on both sides. To obtain further details, artificial four R1 and four R2 constructs were used and showed that each repeat of the protein adopts an extended conformation that spans both intra- and inter-dimer interfaces, centered on α-tubulin and connecting three tubulin monomers.

A direct interaction of Tau peptides corresponding to residues 245–253 (in R1), 269–284 (in R2), and 300–313 (in R3) is proposed, based on the attenuation of Tau NMR signal upon addition of paclitaxel-stabilized MTs (Kadavath et al., 2015b). The described bound-motif in the R2 repeat closely matches the bound-stretch found in the EM structure of four R2 Tau repeats, but not the bound motif in the R1, for which the peptide 253–266 is rather proposed as the attachment point for R1 repeat (Kellogg et al., 2018). Additionally, the structure of the bound peptide Tau(267–312; a peptide overlapping R2-R3 repeats) was probed using transfer-NOEs NMR signals. Based on the NOE contacts, which detect spatial proximities, a family of converging conformers were calculated for residues 269–284 (R2) and 300–310 (R3). Both peptides fold into a hairpin-like structure, formed by the conserved PGGG motifs, upon binding to MTs (Kadavath et al., 2015b). However, it should be noted that the electron density in the EM structure models cannot accommodate this hairpin (Kellogg et al., 2018). The hexapeptides 275-VQIINK-280 in R2 (PHF6* or paired helical filament hexapeptide) and 306-VQIVYK-311 in R3 (PHF6; **Figure 2**) form an extended structure (Kadavath et al., 2015b), in agreement with the EM observation of an extended conformation for R2 (Kellogg et al., 2018). Both the EM and NMR models are incompatible with previous biochemical results, based on combined fluorescence correlation spectroscopy and acrylodan fluorescence screening, suggesting α-helical conformation of the bound-Tau repeats (Li et al., 2015).

The majority of structural data were obtained from the binding of Tau on MTs stabilized by exogenous agents such as Taxol, which facilitates the study by decreasing the dynamics of the system. Still, a number of studies show differences between Tau binding to Taxol pre-stabilized MTs, or to Tau-induced MTs, formed using Tau as an inducer. Kinetics analysis of Tau binding to Taxol-stabilized MTs in comparison with Tau-induced MTs suggests the existence of two different binding sites of Tau to tubulin (Makrides et al., 2004), one overlapping the Taxol binding site localized on β-tubulin in the inner surface of MTs, as previously suggested (Kar et al., 2003).

Site-directed spin labeling combined with electron-paramagnetic resonance spectroscopy (EPR) was used to compare Tau binding mode to Taxol-stabilized MTs and to tubulin when Tau is used as the sole inducer of the polymerization (Martinho et al., 2018). In these experiments, thiol-disulfide exchanges between Tau and tubulin or Taxol-stabilized MTs was observed by EPR measurements of paramagnetic labels linked by disulfide bridges to Tau two natural cysteines, or to single-cysteine Tau mutants. Differences in the kinetics of the label release were observed between preformed MTs and Tau-induced MTs, explained by the accessibility of cysteines of tubulin and MTs deduced from available structural data. Localization of the two putative binding sites of Tau on tubulin was proposed (**Figure 4**). The first one in proximity of Cys347 of α-tubulin subunit could interact with Cys291 of Tau in R2. The second one, located at the interface between two protofilaments, in proximity of Cys131 of β-tubulin subunit, could interact with Cys322 of Tau in R3. The first site is in agreement with models proposing that the R2-R3 would encompass the interface between tubulin (Kadavath et al., 2015a; Kellogg et al., 2018). Both sites are less accessible in Taxol-stabilized MTs, which might explain the much slower release of the disulfide-linked Tau label when Tau is in interaction with the Taxol-stabilized MTs.

ROLE OF THE REGULATORY REGIONS OUTSIDE OF TAU MTBR

A number of studies addressed the role of the regulatory regions outside the MTBR. The N-terminal projection domain of Tau modulates the formation of MT bundles (Chen et al., 1992; Rosenberg et al., 2008). This domain, described as a polyelectrolyte polymer brush, is proposed based on atomic force microscopy to exert a repulsive force (Mukhopadhyay and Hoh, 2001). In another model, the electrostatic zipper

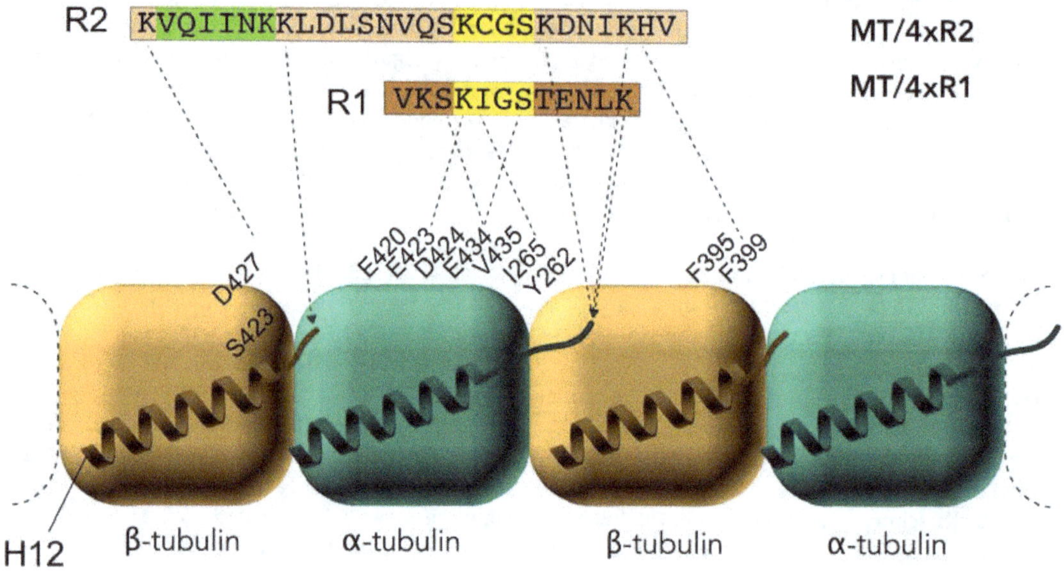

FIGURE 3 | Electron microscopy (EM) models of Tau/MTs interaction. α-tubulin subunit is represented as a blue cube and β-tubulin subunit as a brown cube. H12 C-terminal helix is schematized, the C-terminal tail prolongs the H12 helix. Model based on cryo-EM coupled to Rosetta modeling: contacts of the R1 repeat with the α-tubulin subunit, at the inter-dimer interface: S258 and S262 of R1 make hydrogen bonds with E434; K259 of R1 interacts with an acidic patch formed by E420, E423 and D424; I260 of R1 is in a hydrophobic pocket formed by residues I265, V435 and Y262; K267 of R1 is in contact with the acidic C-terminal tail. Additional contacts for the R2 repeat with β-tubulin subunit, at the intra-dimer interface: K274 of R2 interacts with an acidic patch formed by D427 and S423; K281 of R2 is in contact with the acidic C-terminal tail of β-tubulin subunit. The PHF6* peptide (highlighted green) is close to this tail and localize at the intra-dimer interface. Additional contacts for the R2 repeat with α-tubulin subunit: K294 and K298 are in contact with the acidic C-terminal tail of α-tubulin subunit. Finally, H299 of R2 is buried in a cleft formed by residues F395 and F399 of β-tubulin subunit.

model, Tau is proposed to organize MT spacing by dimerization of the projection domain and the PRR on adjacent MTs (Rosenberg et al., 2008). Both models might be valid but probably depend on the ionic strength of the solution (Donhauser et al., 2017). The N-terminal domain of Tau remains disordered and highly flexible upon tubulin binding, as seen by both NMR (Kadavath et al., 2015a) and smFRET studies (Melo et al., 2016).

Repeats in the MTBR are required for MT binding and assembly. However, as an isolated fragment, the MTBR is not as efficient in tubulin polymerization and in MT binding as full-length Tau. The regions directly flanking the MTBR, in the PRR and in the C-terminal region, are needed to enhance the binding (**Figure 2**). Several models have been proposed to describe the roles of MTBR and flanking regions. In the first one, termed the "jaws" model (Gustke et al., 1994; Trinczek et al., 1995; Preuss et al., 1997), the PRR, MTBR, and C-terminal extension domains bind very weakly, if at all, to MTs, and the binding is enhanced when two consecutive domains are associated in a single construct. An NMR study has determined the residues in the PRR and in the downstream repeats that constitute the "jaws" (Mukrasch et al., 2007). The second model proposes that the initial binding of Tau to MTs is mediated by an MTs-binding core within the MTBR, whereas the flanking regions are regulatory (Goode et al., 2000).

The interaction between full-length Tau and Taxol-stabilized MTs allowed mapping of the binding region on the Tau protein at the residue level (Sillen et al., 2007). In particular, both the MTBR and the flanking regions, namely the PRR and 10 amino acid residues located at the C-terminal end of the MTBR, were found to interact with the MTs. In both the PRR and the MTBR, the contribution of basic residues is important for Tau interaction with MTs (Goode et al., 1997; Kadavath et al., 2015b). Additionally, Tau proteolysis products interacting with tubulin were identified by using a complex named T_2R composed of two tubulins stabilized by the stathmin-like domain (SLD) of RB3 (Gigant et al., 2000; Fauquant et al., 2011). While the isolated fragments from the PRR and MTBR bind weakly to MTs, the Tau(208–324) construct, named TauF4, generated by combining two adjacent fragments included in the PRR and in the MTBR, binds strongly to MTs and stimulates MT assembly very efficiently (Fauquant et al., 2011). The MTBR included in TauF4 (R1, R2 and the N-terminal part of R3) mostly corresponds to the MT binding core initially proposed by Feinstein and co-workers (Goode et al., 2000). PRE experiments performed by introducing four cysteine mutations on the SLD, located along the protein in proximity of the interface of every tubulin subunit, indicated that TauF4 binds asymmetrically to the two tubulins, with the PRR preferentially located closer to the β tubulin subunits (intra-dimer interface). When bound to a single tubulin stabilized by an engineered SLD protein (TR'), a part of the R1 repeat of TauF4 adopts a turn-like conformation, which remains flexible, and thus not in direct contact with α-tubulin surface (Gigant et al., 2014). The turn-like structure is centered on the 260-IGSTENL-266 sequence (**Figure 5**). This peptide

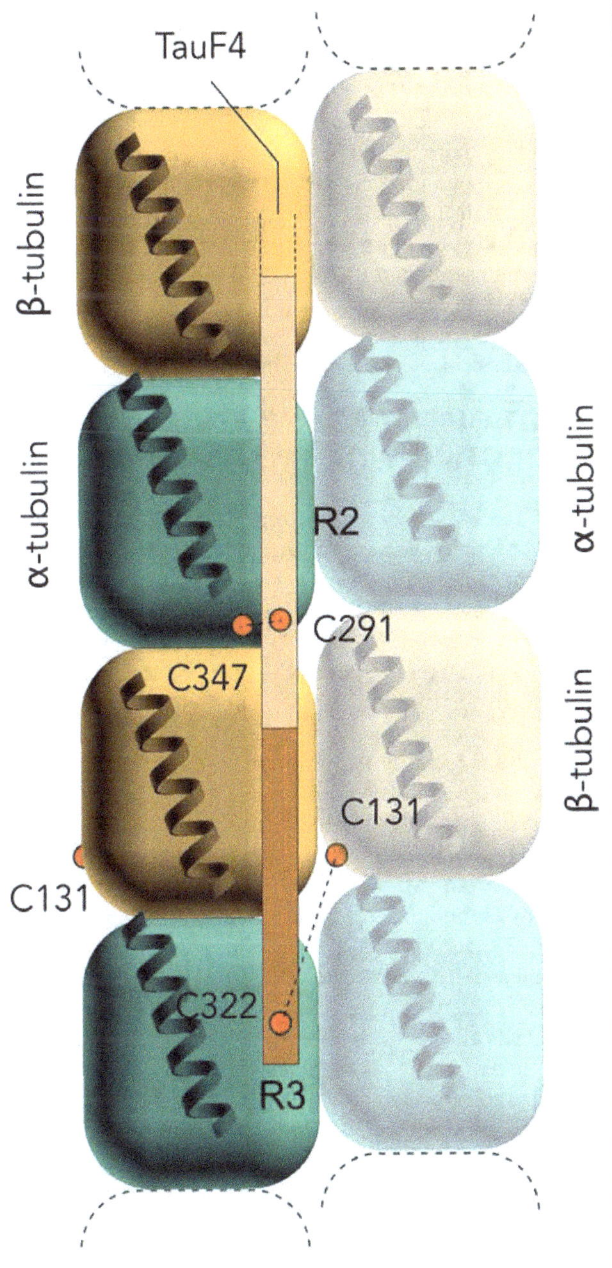

FIGURE 4 | Electron-paramagnetic resonance (EPR) models of the interaction of Tau F4 with MTs. C291 of Tau in R2 is proposed to interact with C347 of α-tubulin, and the C322 of Tau in R3 with C131 of β-subunit. Note that C322 could actually interact either with the β-subunit of the same protofilament or with the one of an adjacent protofilament (as depicted here).

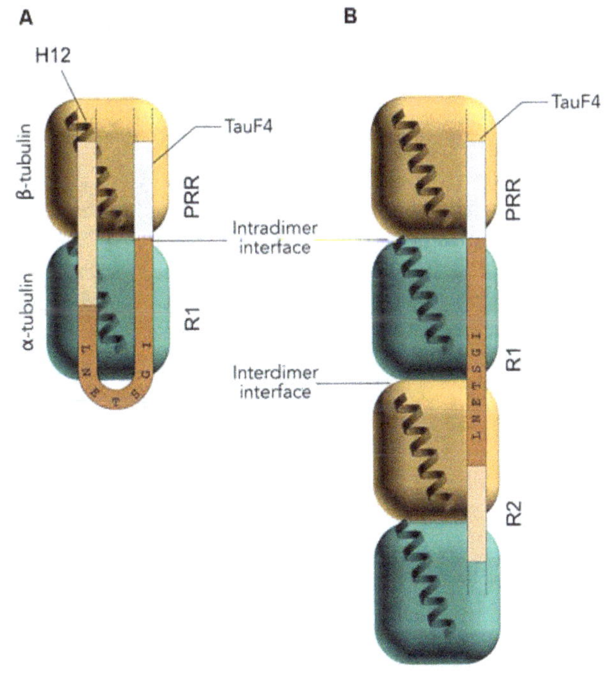

FIGURE 5 | Nuclear magnetic resonance (NMR) model of the interaction of TauF4 with stathmin-like domain (SLD)-stabilized tubulins. **(A)** In interaction with a single tubulin, the IGSTENL peptide of TauF4 is proposed to adopt a turn conformation and is not bound to tubulin. The PRR is mainly detected in proximity to the β-subunit. **(B)** In interaction with two tubulins, the IGSTENL peptide of TauF4 would be straight and overlapping two consecutive α- and β-subunits.

becomes immobilized in the T2R complex, as can now be explained by its position in the EM structure at the inter-dimer interface (Kellogg et al., 2018). The turn-like structure with a single tubulin present is not detected by smFRET (Melo et al., 2016), which is proposed to result from the different conditions of the experiments (large excess of tubulin for the smFRET or excess of Tau for the NMR experiments). The TauF4 fragment was further shown to bind, at least, at the inter-dimer interface as demonstrated by the competition between vinblastine binding and TauF4 for tubulin interaction (Kadavath et al., 2015a). The results of this study are in agreement with the stoichiometry of one Tau for the two tubulins suggested by others (Gigant et al., 2014).

Finally, the interaction between soluble tubulin and the flanking region downstream of the four Tau repeats was investigated by NMR. This region has sequence homology with the repeats and is often referred to as R' (**Figure 2**). By using saturation transfer difference (STD) NMR spectroscopy, two residue stretches centered on F378 and Y394 were identified in interaction with MTs (Kadavath et al., 2018).

IMPACT OF TAU PHOSPHORYLATION ON ITS INTERACTION WITH MTs

Tau-induced neurodegeneration is correlated with the appearance of Tau hyperphosphorylation, Tau aggregation into Paired Helical Filaments and/or the loss of Tau/MT binding (Hernández and Avila, 2007). Overall, phosphorylation is reported to decrease the affinity of Tau for the MTs, ensuring the dynamics of the system in healthy neurons (Lindwall and Cole, 1984; Mandelkow et al., 1995). Specific phosphorylation such as the phosphorylation of S214 (by PKA kinase) or of S262/356 (by MARK kinase) have been described to strongly decrease the affinity of Tau for MTs (Biernat et al., 1993; Scott et al., 1993; Sengupta et al., 1998;

Schneider et al., 1999). S262 makes hydrogen bonds with α-tubulin E434, thus explaining why phosphorylation of S262 residue strongly decreases MT binding (Kellogg et al., 2018). Since phosphorylation of S262 of the isolated R1 repeat peptide does not affect its affinity for MTs, it is likely that the consequences of S262 phosphorylation on Tau binding to tubulin are due to intramolecular rearrangements of the Tau protein (Devred et al., 2002). Interestingly, phosphorylation of S214 of Tau does not significantly affect the MT assembly capacity, despite the decreased affinity (Sillen et al., 2007). Phosphorylation of S214 could also have an indirect role *in vivo*, as this specific phosphorylation might play a role in the observed competition between MTs and the 14-3-3 proteins for Tau binding (Hashiguchi et al., 2000). Indeed, 14-3-3 protein binding to Tau is favored when S214 is phosphorylated (Tugaeva et al., 2017), which seems to result in neurite degeneration in neuronal cell cultures (Joo et al., 2015). The 14-3-3 protein family interacts mainly with phosphorylated protein partners and is especially abundant in brain tissue (Boston et al., 1982). The 14-3-3 proteins have been implicated in a variety of human diseases, including neurodegenerative diseases. Indeed, 14-3-3 proteins are abundant in the intraneuronal deposits of aggregated Tau (Layfield et al., 1996; Umahara et al., 2004; Qureshi et al., 2013).

When Tau is phosphorylated by the CDK2/CycA3 kinase *in vitro*, phosphorylation at S202/T205 and T231/S235 sites are identified by NMR. Even though these phosphorylations do not significantly affect Tau binding to MTs (Amniai et al., 2009), Tau loses its capacity to assemble tubulin into MTs when at least three out of four positions are phosphorylated. This data shows that a decreased capacity of Tau to assemble tubulin into MTs, such as observed for the CDK-phosphorylated Tau, cannot be explained solely by a decreased affinity for MT surface. Additional experiments, using the shortest Tau isoform (Tau 0N3R) with T231E and S235E mutations as pseudophosphorylations, confirmed that E231/E235 do not by themselves abolish the interaction of Tau with the MTs (Schwalbe et al., 2015). However, NMR signals corresponding to residues in the PRR were less attenuated upon addition of MTs to the mutated Tau 0N3R rather than to the wild-type Tau (Schwalbe et al., 2015). This indicates that the pseudophosphorylated Tau 0N3R was locally less tightly bound to the MTs. In addition, based on the models of the Tau(225–246) peptide phosphorylated on T231 and S235, issued from comprehensive calculations of NMR parameters (distances measurements and H-N orientations), the distances between the phosphate and the nitrogen in the directly preceding basic groups (R230 or K234, respectively) are less than 4.5Å, a distance compatible with the formation of a salt-bridge. The salt bridge proposed to link phosphorylated T231 and R230 side-chains of Tau could compete with a salt bridge formation with the MTs, participating in the effect of the phosphorylation of T231 (Schwalbe et al., 2015).

Finally, Pin1 peptidyl-prolyl cis/trans isomerase was proposed to restore the capacity of CDK-phosphorylated Tau to bind to the MTs and restore MT assembly (Lu et al., 1999). However, this model was recently challenged as Pin1 does not promote *in vitro* formation of phosphorylated Tau-induced MTs (Kutter et al., 2016).

For repeat R', the impact of phosphorylation on the binding affinity was assessed by means of STD NMR. Both phosphorylated Y394 and S396 were proved to weaken the interaction between Tau and MTs. However, by measuring residue-specific Kd values by STD, phosphorylation on S396 had a more pronounced effect than phosphorylation on Y394, despite the fact that they are only one residue apart (Kadavath et al., 2018).

Thus, Tau phosphorylation can have an effect on MT binding and assembly through several molecular mechanisms, including electrostatic perturbations, alteration/destabilization of Tau regions bound to the MTs, a disruption of hydrogen-bonds or salt-bridges and changes in structural parameters.

IMPACT OF TAU ACETYLATION ON ITS INTERACTION WITH MTs

Another Tau PTM reported to contribute to Tau pathology is lysine acetylation (Min et al., 2010, 2015); indeed, acetylated Tau is proposed as a marker of AD (Irwin et al., 2012, 2013). In this case, Lys residues are modified by the addition of an acetyl group on the NH_3 moiety of their side chains, neutralizing their positive charges and modifying their steric characteristics. Consequently, acetylation affects Tau binding to MTs and impairs MT assembly (Cohen et al., 2011). Mass spectrometry (MS) analysis revealed that 14 Lys residues, mainly located in the MTBR, were acetylated in Tau samples purified from healthy mice (Morris et al., 2015). Analysis of acetylation sites obtained by *in vitro* acetylation with recombinant p300 acetyl-transferase, by both MS and NMR (Kamah et al., 2014), identified as many as 23 modified-Lys residues. An acetylation mimicking mutation K274Q inhibits Tau tubulin polymerization ability and stimulates Tau aggregation *in vitro* (Rane et al., 2019). Interestingly, acetylation of K280 was detected in brain tissues from patients affected with AD and not in healthy brain tissues (Cohen et al., 2011). Similarly, Tau acetylation at K174 is reported as an early change in AD brain and in transgenic mice expressing Tau with the P301S mutation (PS19 transgenic mice; Min et al., 2015).

In addition, cross-talks between acetylation and phosphorylation modifications of Tau interplay in their regulatory role of MT dynamics (Carlomagno et al., 2017). Acetylation of K321 prevents the phosphorylation of S324, the latter being reported to inhibit Tau function of tubulin polymerization in *in vitro* assays (Carlomagno et al., 2017). Interestingly, this phosphorylation is one of the few modifications of Tau (among 63 modifications) specifically present in a human amyloid precursor protein transgenic AD mouse model when compared to a wild type mouse (Morris et al., 2015). Furthermore, phosphorylation of S324 is detected in post-mortem tissues of AD patients, but not in control samples (Carlomagno et al., 2017). Pseudo-phosphorylated mutants S324D and S324E have a diminished capacity to polymerize MTs from tubulin in *in vitro* assays. Similarly, acetylation of K259/K353 prevents phosphorylation of S262/S356 by the MARK kinase. Modulation of Tau acetylation could be a new strategy to inhibit Tau-mediated neurodegeneration.

Indeed, studies in mice suggest that this is a valid disease-modifying target. Increasing acetylation of Tau by deleting SIRT1 deacetylase in a TauP301S transgenic mouse model aggravates synapse loss, while SIRT1 overexpression limits Tau pathology propagation (Min et al., 2018). In the PS19 FTD transgenic mouse model, inhibition of p300 acetyltransferase activity lowers total Tau and K174-acetylated Tau levels. P300 inhibition prevents hippocampal atrophy and rescues memory deficits (Min et al., 2015). However, the complexity of the regulation of Tau function by PTMs has to be kept in mind. Acetylation can have both a direct inhibitory effect on Tau function and an indirect activation effect, by preventing phosphorylation in the KXGS motifs of the MTBR.

IMPACT OF TAU FTD MUTATIONS ON ITS INTERACTION WITH MTs

Tau protein is encoded by the *MAPT* gene located on chromosome 17. Pathogenic variants in this gene cause several related neurodegenerative diseases characterized by the presence of hyperphosphorylated Tau aggregates in the neurons (Wilhelmsen et al., 1994; D'Souza et al., 1999). Animal models with these mutations, such as P301L, have been extensively studied and are considered AD models (Lee et al., 2005). The FTD mutations of the *MAPT* gene alter Tau biochemical properties and/or the ratio of Tau isoforms (4R/3R ratio). Change in the isoform ratio has an indirect impact on MT assembly and the dynamics of the MT networks because the 3R Tau is known to have a lower capacity of MT stabilization and tubulin polymerization than the 4R Tau (Scott et al., 1991; Panda et al., 2003). The influence on Tau PTMs of the FTD mutations represents another indirect effect on Tau/MT interaction. The R406W Tau mutation is, for example, consistently reported to diminish Tau phosphorylation (Dayanandan et al., 1999; Matsumura et al., 1999; Delobel et al., 2002). However, almost all the FTD mutations also directly affect the ability of Tau to bind MTs and to promote tubulin assembly (Hasegawa et al., 1998; Hong et al., 1998). Tau with P301L, V337M or R406W mutations has a reduced binding to MTs and a decrease efficiency to initiate tubulin assembly. For P301L Tau, the initiation rate is decreased but the tubulin polymerization reaches the same extent in *in vitro* assays. Surprisingly, R406W Tau is reported to be the most affected, despite the fact that the mutation is not near the MTBR (Hong et al., 1998). This suggests that an alternative conformation might be involved. Later studies confirm the initial finding that FTD mutations affect the ability of Tau to bind MTs and to promote tubulin assembly in *in vitro* assays. However, there is no agreement on the extent of the specific effect of each of these mutations (Barghorn et al., 2000; DeTure et al., 2000; Combs and Gamblin, 2012). The effect of R5L, P301L, and R406W mutations of Tau differ in regard to their impact on Tau MT stabilizing capacity, not only based on their localization in Tau sequence, but also depending on the number of N-terminal inserts (0, 1 or 2 N isoforms), in the three considered 4R-Tau isoforms (Mutreja et al., 2019). In particular, Tau with the R5L mutation has a reduced ability to polymerize tubulin, with lower tubulin polymerization extent, lower rate, and longer lag time specifically for the 0N 4R Tau isoform, compared to the 1N and 2N that are behaving as the wild-type Tau (Mutreja et al., 2019). For the P301L mutation, the Tau-dependent defect in MTs seems to diminish with the removal of each N-terminal insert. This might be due to a differential effect of conformational changes induced by the mutations on the global hairpin-like conformation of Tau, which brings the N-terminal region close to the MTBR (Jeganathan et al., 2006). The impact of the FTD mutations on the MT stabilization capacity of Tau has been confirmed in intact cell context, with variable effect depending on the mutation (Delobel et al., 2002). Mammalian cells expressing Tau P301L show proportionally less Tau bound to MTs (Nagiec et al., 2001; Di Primio et al., 2017). However, a strong consensus on the impact of the FTD mutations in a cellular context has not yet been reached, since in neuroblastoma and CHO cells transfected with GFP-tagged Tau DNA constructs, the co-localization with MTs and generation of MT bundles were shown to be identical for both mutants and wild type Tau (DeTure et al., 2000). The site-dependent and isoform-dependent effect of the Tau mutations on MT stabilization were reproduced in COS cells transfected with 3R or 4R Tau isoforms (Sahara et al., 2000). For example, the V337M mutation has a significant effect when introduced in 3R Tau, but not in 4R Tau, showing disruption of the MT networks and diminished co-localization of Tau and tubulin. This isoform-specific effect of some of the mutations might explain part of the discrepancies reported on the impact of the FTD mutations of Tau on its MAP functions.

PERSPECTIVES

One of the proposed strategies in seeking AD treatment consists of compensating the loss of the MT-stabilizing Tau function (Cash et al., 2003; Brunden et al., 2009; Ballatore et al., 2011; Das and Ghosh, 2019). One path to this goal is to harness the therapeutic potential of MT-stabilizing agents, classically used in cancer therapies. This strategy to treat tauopathies was validated *in vivo* using Paclitaxel treatment in AD mouse models (Cash et al., 2003; Zhang B. et al., 2005) and in cell models (Brunden et al., 2011). Recently, Monacelli et al. (2017) provided an updated survey on the potential of repurposing cancer agents for AD. Besides its implication in neurodegenerative disease, Tau is also involved in regulatory mechanisms linked to cancer development. For example, Tau was shown to regulate the MT-dependent migration of cancer cells (Breuzard et al., 2019). Finally, similar to stathmin, Tau level of expression modulates clinical MT-targeting agent efficiencies, such as taxanes or vinca alkaloids (Rouzier et al., 2005; Li et al., 2013; Smoter et al., 2013; Malesinski et al., 2015; Lin et al., 2018).

MT stabilizing peptides are another option chosen to restore MT stability (Quraishe et al., 2016; Mondal et al., 2018). A peptide such as the PS3 octapeptide was designed from the taxol-binding pocket of β-tubulin (Mondal et al., 2018). The advantage of this peptide strategy is the moderate peptide affinity for MTs that preserves the MT dynamic capacity, which is crucial for synaptic plasticity and memory. Consequently, PS3 stimulates MT polymerization and increases expression of acetylated tubulin in PC12 neuron cell cultures but has much fewer toxic effects than taxol. Other neuroprotective peptides have MT stabilizing functions thanks to their ability for interactions with MT end-binding proteins, which protect MT from depolymerization (Oz et al., 2014). The NAP/SAL peptides, which interact with EB1 through a SIP motif, prevent and reverse MT breakdown and axonal transport deficits in a *Drosophila* model of tauopathy (Quraishe et al., 2013, 2016).

Finally, MTs could be stabilized not by mimicking MAP function, but by modulating MT PTMs, which have a crucial role in MT dynamics. Levels of total α-tubulin are reduced by approximately 65% in AD-patient brains compared to age-matched control brains but the relative ratio of acetylated tubulin is increased by approximately 31% compared to the controls (Zhang F. et al., 2015). This suggests a compensatory mechanism to counteract MT reduction due to a loss of Tau stabilization because this modification characterizes stable MTs with slow dynamics (Kull and Sloboda, 2014; Szyk et al., 2014). Inhibition of histone deacetylase 6 (HDAC6), the major tubulin deacetylase, is thus an alternative strategy to compensate for Tau MAP function. Indeed, in transgenic mouse models of AD, inhibition of HDAC6 improves memory (Kilgore et al., 2010; Govindarajan et al., 2013; Selenica (et al., 2014). Similarly, in *Drosophila*, HDAC6 null mutation rescues MT defects through increased tubulin acetylation Xiong et al., 2013).

Overall, Tau implication in neurodegenerative diseases, and other diseases where MTs play an important role, clearly shows the interest of the Tau/MTs interaction as a potential target for intervention (Pachima et al., 2016; Das and Ghosh, 2019). Many advances have been made in the understanding of Tau functions as a MAP, and in the structural aspects of the Tau/MTs interaction. On this basis, the importance of regulatory factors of the interaction, from PTMs to other endogenous cofactors such as Zinc (Fichou et al., 2019), can now be addressed. This will hopefully lead to new strategies targeting disease where MTs, and consequently Tau, are involved.

AUTHOR CONTRIBUTIONS

The content of the manuscript was drafted and edited by all authors.

REFERENCES

Alonso, A. C., Zaidi, T., Grundke-Iqbal, T., and Iqbal, K. (1994). Role of abnormally phosphorylated tau in the breakdown of microtubules in Alzheimer disease. *Proc Natl. Acad. Sci. U S A* 91, 5562–5566. doi: 10.1073/pnas.91.12.5562

Alushin, G. M., Lander, G. C., Kellogg, E. H., Zhang, R., Baker, D., and Nogales, E. (2014). High-resolution microtubule structures reveal the structural transitions in αβ-tubulin upon GTP hydrolysis. *Cell* 157, 1117–1129. doi: 10.1016/j.cell.2014.03.053

Amniai, L., Barbier, P., Sillen, A., Wieruszeski, J.-M., Peyrot, V., Lippens, G., et al. (2009). Alzheimer disease specific phosphoepitopes of Tau interfere with assembly of tubulin but not binding to microtubules. *FASEB J.* 23, 1146–1152. doi: 10.1096/fj.08-121590

Amos, L. A., and Schlieper, D. (2005). Microtubules and maps. *Adv. Protein Chem.* 71, 257–298. doi: 10.1016/S0065-3233(04)71007-4

Baas, P. W., and Qiang, L. (2019). Tau: it's not what you think. *Trends Cell Biol.* 29, 452–461. doi: 10.1016/j.tcb.2019.02.007

Baas, P. W., Rao, A. N., Matamoros, A. J., and Leo, L. (2016). Stability properties of neuronal microtubules. *Cytoskelet* 73, 442–460. doi: 10.1002/cm.21286

Ballatore, C., Brunden, K. R., Trojanowski, J. Q., Lee, V. M., Smith, A. B. III., and Huryn, D. M. (2011). Modulation of protein-protein interactions as a therapeutic strategy for the treatment of neurodegenerative tauopathies. *Curr. Top. Med. Chem.* 11, 317–330. doi: 10.2174/156802611794072605

Barbier, P., Dorléans, A., Devred, F., Sanz, L., Allegro, D., Alfonso, C., et al. (2010). Stathmin and interfacial microtubule inhibitors recognize a naturally curved conformation of tubulin dimers. *J. Biol. Chem.* 285, 31672–31681. doi: 10.1074/jbc.m110.141929

Barghorn, S., Zheng-Fischhöfer, Q., Ackmann, M., Biernat, J., von Bergen, M., Mandelkow, E. M., et al. (2000). Structure, microtubule interactions, and paired helical filament aggregation by tau mutants of frontotemporal dementias. *Biochemistry* 39, 11714–11721. doi: 10.1021/bi000850r

Biernat, J., Gustke, N., Drewes, G., Mandelkow, E. M., and Mandelkow, E. (1993). Phosphorylation of Ser262 strongly reduces binding of tau to microtubules: distinction between PHF-like immunoreactivity and microtubule binding. *Neuron* 11, 153–163. doi: 10.1016/0896-6273(93)90279-z

Binder, L. I., Frankfurter, A., and Rebhun, L. I. (1985). The distribution of tau in the mammalian central nervous system. *J. Cell Biol.* 101, 1371–1378. doi: 10.1083/jcb.101.4.1371

Black, M. M., Slaughter, T., Moshiach, S., Obrocka, M., and Fischer, I. (1996). Tau is enriched on dynamic microtubules in the distal region of growing axons. *J. Neurosci.* 16, 3601–3619. doi: 10.1523/JNEUROSCI.16-11-03601.1996

Boston, P. F., Jackson, P., and Thompson, R. J. (1982). Human 14-3-3 protein: radioimmunoassay, tissue distribution, and cerebrospinal fluid levels in patients with neurological disorders. *J. Neurochem.* 38, 1475–1482. doi: 10.1111/j.1471-4159.1982.tb07928.x

Bowne-Anderson, H., Hibbel, A., and Howard, J. (2015). Regulation of microtubule growth and catastrophe: unifying theory and experiment. *Trends Cell Biol.* 25, 769–779. doi: 10.1016/j.tcb.2015.08.009

Breuzard, G., Hubert, P., Nouar, R., De Bessa, T., Devred, F., Barbier, P., et al. (2013). Molecular mechanisms of Tau binding to microtubules and its role in microtubule dynamics in live cells. *J. Cell Sci.* 126, 2810–2819. doi: 10.1242/jcs.120832

Breuzard, G., Pagano, A., Bastonero, S., Malesinski, S., Parat, F., Barbier, P., et al. (2019). Tau regulates the microtubule-dependent migration of glioblastoma cells *via* the Rho-ROCK signaling pathway. *J. Cell Sci.* 132:jcs222851. doi: 10.1242/jcs.222851

Brion, J. P., Flament-Durand, J., and Dustin, P. (1986). Alzheimer's disease and tau proteins. *Lancet* 2:1098. doi: 10.1016/s0140-6736(86)90495-2

Brunden, K. R., Trojanowski, J. Q., and Lee, V. M. (2009). Advances in tau-focused drug discovery for Alzheimer's disease and related tauopathies. *Nat. Rev. Drug Discov.* 8, 783–793. doi: 10.1038/nrd2959

Brunden, K. R., Yao, Y., Potuzak, J. S., Ferrer, N. I., Ballatore, C., James, M. J., et al. (2011). The characterization of microtubule-stabilizing drugs as possible therapeutic agents for Alzheimer's disease and related tauopathies. *Pharmacol. Res.* 63, 341–351. doi: 10.1016/j.phrs.2010.12.002

Butner, K. A., and Kirschner, M. W. (1991). Tau protein binds to microtubules through a flexible array of distributed weak sites. *J. Cell Biol.* 115, 717–730. doi: 10.1083/jcb.115.3.717

Caplow, M., and Shanks, J. (1990). Mechanism of the microtubule GTPase reaction. *J. Biol. Chem.* 265, 8935–8941.

Carlier, M. F., Didry, D., Simon, C., and Pantaloni, D. (1989). Mechanism of GTP hydrolysis in tubulin polymerization: characterization of the kinetic intermediate microtubule-GDP-Pi using phosphate analogues. *Biochemistry* 28, 1783–1791. doi: 10.1021/bi00430a054

Carlomagno, Y., Chung, D.-E. C., Yue, M., Castanedes-Casey, M., Madden, B. J., Dunmore, J., et al. (2017). An acetylation-phosphorylation switch that regulates tau aggregation propensity and function. *J. Biol. Chem.* 292, 15277–15286. doi: 10.1074/jbc.M117.794602

Cash, A. D., Aliev, G., Siedlak, S. L., Nunomura, A., Fujioka, H., Zhu, X., et al. (2003). Microtubule reduction in Alzheimer's disease and aging is independent of tau filament formation. *Am. J. Pathol.* 162, 1623–1627. doi: 10.1016/s0002-9440(10)64296-4

Chen, J., Kanai, Y., Cowan, N. J., and Hirokawa, N. (1992). Projection domains of MAP2 and tau determine spacings between microtubules in dendrites and axons. *Nature* 360, 674–677. doi: 10.1038/360674a0

Chrétien, D., Fuller, S. D., and Karsenti, E. (1995). Structure of growing microtubule ends: two-dimensional sheets close into tubes at variable rates. *J. Cell Biol.* 129, 1311–1328. doi: 10.1083/jcb.129.5.1311

Cohen, T. J., Guo, J. L., Hurtado, D. E., Kwong, L. K., Mills, I. P., Trojanowski, J. Q., et al. (2011). The acetylation of tau inhibits its function and promotes pathological tau aggregation. *Nat. Commun.* 2:252. doi: 10.1038/ncomms1255

Combs, B., and Gamblin, T. C. (2012). FTDP-17 tau mutations induce distinct effects on aggregation and microtubule interactions. *Biochemistry* 51, 8597–8607. doi: 10.1021/bi3010818

Cummings, J., Lee, G., Mortsdorf, T., Ritter, A., and Zhong, K. (2017). Alzheimer's disease drug development pipeline: 2017. *Alzheimers Dement.* 3, 367–384. doi: 10.1016/j.trci.2017.05.002

D'Souza, I., Poorkaj, P., Hong, M., Nochlin, D., Lee, V. M., Bird, T. D., et al. (1999). Missense and silent tau gene mutations cause frontotemporal dementia with parkinsonism-chromosome 17 type, by affecting multiple alternative RNA splicing regulatory elements. *Proc. Natl. Acad. Sci. U S A* 96, 5598–5603. doi: 10.1073/pnas.96.10.5598

Das, G., and Ghosh, S. (2019). Why microtubules should be considered as one of the supplementary targets for designing neurotherapeutics. *ACS Chem. Neurosci.* 10, 1118–1120. doi: 10.1021/acschemneuro.9b00002

Dayanandan, R., Van Slegtenhorst, M., Mack, T. G., Ko, L., Yen, S. H., Leroy, K., et al. (1999). Mutations in tau reduce its microtubule binding properties in intact cells and affect its phosphorylation. *FEBS Lett.* 446, 228–232. doi: 10.1016/s0014-5793(99)00222-7

Delobel, P., Flament, S., Hamdane, M., Jakes, R., Rousseau, A., Delacourte, A., et al. (2002). Functional characterization of FTDP-17 tau gene mutations through their effects on Xenopus oocyte maturation. *J. Biol. Chem.* 277, 9199–9205. doi: 10.1074/jbc.M107716200

DeTure, M., Ko, L. W., Yen, S., Nacharaju, P., Easson, C., Lewis, J., et al. (2000). Missense tau mutations identified in FTDP-17 have a small effect on tau-microtubule interactions. *Brain Res.* 853, 5–14. doi: 10.1016/s0006-8993(99)02124-1

Devred, F., Barbier, P., Douillard, S., Monasterio, O., Andreu, J. M., and Peyrot, V. (2004) Tau induces ring and microtubule formation from αβ-tubulin dimers under nonassembly conditions. *Biochemistry* 43, 10520–10531. doi: 10.1021/bi0493160

Devred, F., Barbier, P., Lafitte, D., Landrieu, I., Lippens, G., and Peyrot, V. (2010). Microtubule and MAPs: thermodynamics of complex formation by AUC, ITC, fluorescence, and NMR. *Methods Cell Biol.* 95, 449–480. doi: 10.1016/S0091-679X(10)95023-1

Devred, F., Douillard, S., Briand, C., and Peyrot, V. (2002). First tau repeat domain binding to growing and taxol-stabilized microtubules and serine 262 residue phosphorylation. *FEBS Lett.* 523, 247–251. doi: 10.1016/s0014-5793(02)02999-x

Di Maio, I. L., Barbier, P., Allegro, D., Brault, C., and Peyrot, V. (2014). Quantitative analysis of tau-microtubule interaction using FRET. *Int. J. Mol. Sci.* 15, 14697–14714. doi: 10.3390/ijms150814697

Di Primio, C., Quercioli, V., Siano, G., Rovere, M., Kovacech, B., Novak, M., et al. (2017). The distance between N and C termini of Tau and of FTDP-17 mutants is modulated by microtubule interactions in living cells. *Front. Mol. Neurosci.* 10:210. doi: 10.3389/fnmol.2017.00210

Dompierre, J. P., Godin, J. D., Charrin, B. C., Cordelières, F. P., King, S. J., Humbert, S., et al. (2007). Histone deacetylase 6 inhibition compensates for the transport deficit in Huntington's disease by increasing tubulin acetylation. *J. Neurosci.* 27, 3571–3583. doi: 10.1523/JNEUROSCI.0037-07.2007

Donhauser, Z. J., Saunders, J. T., D'Urso, D. S., and Garrett, T. A. (2017). Dimerization and long-range repulsion established by both termini of the microtubule-associated protein Tau. *Biochemistry* 56, 5900–5909. doi: 10.1021/acs.biochem.7b00653

Duan, A. R., Jonasson, E. M., Alberico, E. O., Li, C., Scripture, J. P., Miller, R. A., et al. (2017). Interactions between Tau and different conformations of tubulin: implications for Tau function and mechanism. *J. Mol. Biol.* 429, 1424–1438. doi: 10.1016/j.jmb.2017.03.018

Eftekharzadeh, B., Daigle, J. G., Kapinos, L. E., Coyne, A., Schiantarelli, J., Carlomagno, Y., et al. (2018). Tau protein disrupts nucleocytoplasmic transport in Alzheimer's disease. *Neuron* 99, 925.e7–940.e7. doi: 10.1016/j.neuron.2018.07.039

Fauquant, C., Redeker, V., Landrieu, I., Wieruszeski, J. M., Verdegem, D., Laprevote, O., et al. (2011). Systematic identification of tubulin-interacting fragments of the microtubule-associated protein Tau leads to a highly efficient promoter of microtubule assembly. *J. Biol. Chem.* 286, 33358–33368. doi: 10.1074/jbc.m111.223545

Fichou, Y., Al-Hilaly, Y. K., Devred, F., Smet-Nocca, C., Tsvetkov, P. O., Verelst, J., et al. (2019). The elusive tau molecular structures: can we translate the recent breakthroughs into new targets for intervention? *Acta Neuropathol. Commun.* 7:31. doi: 10.1186/s40478-019-0682-x

Gadadhar, S., Bodakuntla, S., Natarajan, K., and Janke, C. (2017). The tubulin code at a glance. *J. Cell Sci.* 130, 1347–1353. doi: 10.1242/jcs.199471

Gigant, B., Curmi, P. A., Martin-Barbey, C., Charbaut, E., Lachkar, S., Lebeau, L., et al. (2000). The 4 A X-ray structure of a tubulin:stathmin-like domain complex. *Cell* 102, 809–816. doi: 10.1016/s0092-8674(00)00069-6

Gigant, B., Landrieu, I., Fauquant, C., Barbier, P., Huvent, I., Wieruszeski, J.-M., et al. (2014). Mechanism of Tau-promoted microtubule assembly as probed by NMR spectroscopy. *J. Am. Chem. Soc.* 136, 12615–12623. doi: 10.1021/ja504864m

Godena, V. K., Brookes-Hocking, N., Moller, A., Shaw, G., Oswald, M., Sancho, R. M., et al. (2014). Increasing microtubule acetylation rescues axonal transport and locomotor deficits caused by LRRK2 Roc-COR domain mutations. *Nat. Commun.* 5:5245. doi: 10.1038/ncomms6245

Goedert, M., Spillantini, M. G., Jakes, R., Rutherford, D., and Crowther, R. A. (1989). Multiple isoforms of human microtubule-associated protein tau: sequences and localization in neurofibrillary tangles of Alzheimer's disease. *Neuron* 3, 519–526. doi: 10.1016/0896-6273(89)90210-9

Goode, B. L., Chau, M., Denis, P. E., and Feinstein, S. C. (2000). Structural and functional differences between 3-repeat and 4-repeat tau isoforms. Implications for normal tau function and the onset of neurodegenetative disease. *J. Biol. Chem.* 275, 38182–38189. doi: 10.1074/jbc.m007489200

Goode, B. L., Denis, P. E., Panda, D., Radeke, M. J., Miller, H. P., Wilson, L., et al. (1997). Functional interactions between the proline-rich and repeat regions of tau enhance microtubule binding and assembly. *Mol. Biol. Cell* 8, 353–365. doi: 10.1091/mbc.8.2.353

Govindarajan, N., Rao, P., Burkhardt, S., Sananbenesi, F., Schlüter, O. M., Bradke, F., et al. (2013). Reducing HDAC6 ameliorates cognitive deficits in a mouse model for Alzheimer's disease. *EMBO Mol. Med.* 5, 52–63. doi: 10.1002/emmm.201201923

Guo, W., Naujock, M., Fumagalli, L., Vandoorne, T., Baatsen, P., Boon, R., et al. (2017). HDAC6 inhibition reverses axonal transport defects in motor neurons derived from FUS-ALS patients. *Nat. Commun.* 8:861. doi: 10.1038/s41467-017-00911-y

Gustke, N., Trinczek, B., Biernat, J., Mandelkow, E. M., and Mandelkow, E. (1994). Domains of tau protein and interactions with microtubules. *Biochemistry* 33, 9511–9522. doi: 10.1021/bi00198a017

Hasegawa, M., Smith, M. J., and Goedert, M. (1998). Tau proteins with FTDP-17 mutations have a reduced ability to promote microtubule assembly. *FEBS Lett.* 437, 207–210. doi: 10.1016/s0014-5793(98)01217-4

Hashiguchi, M., Sobue, K., and Paudel, H. K. (2000). 14-3-3ζ is an effector of tau protein phosphorylation. *J. Biol. Chem.* 275, 25247–25254. doi: 10.1074/jbc.m003738200

Hernández, F., and Avila, J. (2007). Tauopathies. *Cell. Mol. Life Sci.* 64, 2219–2233. doi: 10.1007/s00018-007-7220-x

Hernández-Vega, A., Braun, M., Scharrel, L., Jahnel, M., Wegmann, S., Hyman, B. T., et al. (2017). Local nucleation of microtubule bundles through tubulin concentration into a condensed Tau phase. *Cell Rep.* 20, 2304–2312. doi: 10.1016/j.celrep.2017.08.042

Himmler, A., Drechsel, D., Kirschner, M. W., and Martin, D. W. Jr. (1989). Tau consists of a set of proteins with repeated C-terminal microtubule-binding domains and variable N-terminal domains. *Mol. Cell. Biol.* 9, 1381–1388. doi: 10.1128/mcb.9.4.1381

Hinrichs, M. H., Jalal, A., Brenner, B., Mandelkow, E., Kumar, S., and Scholz, T. (2012). Tau protein diffuses along the microtubule lattice. *J. Biol. Chem.* 287, 38559–38568. doi: 10.1074/jbc.m112.369785

Hong, M., Zhukareva, V., Vogelsberg-Ragaglia, V., Wszolek, Z., Reed, L., Miller, B. I., et al. (1998). Mutation-specific functional impairments in distinct tau isoforms of hereditary FTDP-17. *Science* 282, 1914–1917. doi: 10.1126/science.282.5395.1914

Howard, W. D., and Timasheff, S. N. (1986). GDP state of tubulin: stabilization of double rings. *Biochemistry* 25, 8292–8300. doi: 10.1021/bi00373a025

Irwin, D. J., Cohen, T. J., Grossman, M., Arnold, S. E., McCarty-Wood, E., Van Deerlin, V. M., et al. (2013). Acetylated tau neuropathology in sporadic and hereditary tauopathies. *Am. J. Pathol.* 183, 344–351. doi: 10.1016/j.ajpath.2013.04.025

Irwin, D. J., Cohen, T. J., Grossman, M., Arnold, S. E., Xie, S. X., Lee, V. M., et al. (2012). Acetylated tau, a novel pathological signature in Alzheimer's disease and other tauopathies. *Brain* 135, 807–818. doi: 10.1093/brain/aws013

Jadhav, S., Avila, J., Schöll, M., Kovacs, G. G., Kövari, E., Skrabana, R., et al. (2019). A walk through tau therapeutic strategies. *Acta Neuropathol. Commun.* 7:22. doi: 10.1186/s40478-019-0664-z

Janning, D., Igaev, M., Sündermann, F., Brühmann, J., Beutel, O., Heinisch, J. J., et al. (2014). Single-molecule tracking of tau reveals fast kiss-and-hop interaction with microtubules in living neurons. *Mol. Biol. Cell* 25, 3541–3551. doi: 10.1091/mbc.e14-06-1099

Jeganathan, S., von Bergen, M., Brutlach, H., Steinhoff, H. J., and Mandelkow, E. (2006). Global hairpin folding of tau in solution. *Biochemistry* 45, 2283–2293. doi: 10.1021/bi0521543

Joo, Y., Schumacher, B., Landrieu, I., Bartel, M., Smet-Nocca, C., Jang, A., et al. (2015). Involvement of 14-3-3 in tubulin instability and impaired axon development is mediated by Tau. *FASEB J.* 29, 4133–4144. doi: 10.1096/fj.14-265009

Kadavath, H., Cabrales Fontela, Y., Jaremko, M., Jaremko, €., Overkamp, K., Biernat, J., et al. (2018). The binding mode of a Tau peptide with tubulin. *Angew. Chem. Int. Ed Engl.* 57, 3246–3250. doi: 10.1002/anie.201712089

Kadavath, H., Hofele, R. V., Biernat, J., Kumar, S., Tepper, K., Urlaub, H., et al. (2015a). Tau stabilizes microtubules by binding at the interface between tubulin heterodimers. *Proc. Natl. Acad. Sci. U S A* 112, 7501–7506. doi: 10.1073/pnas.1504081112

Kadavath, H., Jaremko, M., Jaremko, €., Biernat, J., Mandelkow, E., and Zweckstetter, M. (2015b). Folding of the Tau protein on microtubules. *Angew. Chem. Int. Ed Engl.* 54, 10347–10351. doi: 10.1002/anie.201501714

Kamah, A., Huvent, I., Cantrelle, F.-X., Qi, H., Lippens, G., Landrieu, I., et al. (2014). Nuclear magnetic resonance analysis of the acetylation pattern of the neuronal Tau protein. *Biochemistry* 53, 3020–3032. doi: 10.1021/bi500006v

Kar, S., Fan, J., Smith, M. J., Goedert, M., and Amos, L. A. (2003). Repeat motifs of tau bind to the insides of microtubules in the absence of taxol. *EMBO J.* 22, 70–77. doi: 10.1093/emboj/cdg001

Kellogg, E. H., Hejab, N. M. A., Poepsel, S., Downing, K. H., DiMaio, F., and Nogales, E. (2018). Near-atomic model of microtubule-tau interactions. *Science* 360, 1242–1246. doi: 10.1126/science.aat1780

Kilgore, M., Miller, C. A., Fass, D. M., Hennig, K. M., Haggarty, S. J., Sweatt, J. D., et al. (2010). Inhibitors of class 1 histone deacetylases reverse contextual memory deficits in a mouse model of Alzheimer's disease. *Neuropsychopharmacology* 35, 870–880. doi: 10.1038/npp.2009.197

Kull, F. J., and Sloboda, R. D. (2014). A slow dance for microtubule acetylation. *Cell* 157, 1255–1256. doi: 10.1016/j.cell.2014.05.021

Kutter, S., Eichner, T., Deaconescu, A. M., and Kern, D. (2016). Regulation of microtubule assembly by tau and not by Pin1. *J. Mol. Biol.* 428, 1742–1759. doi: 10.1016/j.jmb.2016.03.010

Layfield, R., Fergusson, J., Aitken, A., Lowe, J., Landon, M., and Mayer, R. J. (1996). Neurofibrillary tangles of Alzheimer's disease brains contain 14-3-3 proteins. *Neurosci. Lett.* 209, 57–60. doi: 10.1016/0304-3940(96)12598-2

LeBoeuf, A. C., Levy, S. F., Gaylord, M., Bhattacharya, A., Singh, A. K., Jordan, M. A., et al. (2008). FTDP-17 mutations in Tau alter the regulation of microtubule dynamics: an "alternative core" model for normal and pathological Tau action. *J. Biol. Chem.* 283, 36406–36415. doi: 10.1074/jbc.M803519200

Lee, V. M.-Y., Kenyon, T. K., and Trojanowski, J. Q. (2005). Transgenic animal models of tauopathies. *Biochim. Biophys. Acta* 1739, 251–259. doi: 10.1016/j.bbadis.2004.06.014

Li, X.-H., Culver, J. A., and Rhoades, E. (2015). Tau binds to multiple tubulin dimers with helical structure. *J. Am. Chem. Soc.* 137, 9218–9221. doi: 10.1021/jacs.5b04561

Li, Z.-H., Xiong, Q.-Y., Tu, J.-H., Gong, Y., Qiu, W., Zhang, H.-Q., et al. (2013). Tau proteins expressions in advanced breast cancer and its significance in taxane-containing neoadjuvant chemotherapy. *Med. Oncol.* 30:591. doi: 10.1007/s12032-013-0591-y

Lin, H., Zheng, L., Li, S., Xie, B., Cui, B., Xia, A., et al. (2018). Cytotoxicity of Tanshinone IIA combined with Taxol on drug-resist breast cancer cells MCF-7 through inhibition of Tau. *Phytother. Res.* 32, 667–671. doi: 10.1002/ptr.6014

Lindwall, G., and Cole, R. D. (1984). Phosphorylation affects the ability of tau protein to promote microtubule assembly. *J. Biol. Chem.* 259, 5301–5305.

Lu, P. J., Wulf, G., Zhou, X. Z., Davies, P., and Lu, K. P. (1999). The prolyl isomerase Pin1 restores the function of Alzheimer-associated phosphorylated tau protein. *Nature* 399, 784–788. doi: 10.1038/21650

Magiera, M. M., Bodakuntla, S., Žiak, J., Lacomme, S., Marques Sousa, P., Leboucher, S., et al. (2018). Excessive tubulin polyglutamylation causes neurodegeneration and perturbs neuronal transport. *EMBO J.* 37:e100440. doi: 10.15252/embj.2018100440

Makrides, V., Massie, M. R., Feinstein, S. C., and Lew, J. (2004). Evidence for two distinct binding sites for tau on microtubules. *Proc. Natl. Acad. Sci. U S A* 101, 6746–6751. doi: 10.1073/pnas.0400992101

Malesinski, S., Tsvetkov, P. O., Kruczynski, A., Peyrot, V., and Devred, F. (2015). Stathmin potentiates vinflunine and inhibits Paclitaxel activity. *PLoS One* 10:e0128704. doi: 10.1371/journal.pone.0128704

Mandelkow, E. M., Biernat, J., Drewes, G., Gustke, N., Trinczek, B., and Mandelkow, E. (1995). Tau domains, phosphorylation and interactions with microtubules. *Neurobiol. Aging* 16, 355–362; discussion 362–363. doi: 10.1016/0197-4580(95)00025-a

Martinho, M., Allegro, D., Huvent, I., Chabaud, C., Etienne, E., Kovacic, H., et al. (2018). Two Tau binding sites on tubulin revealed by thiol-disulfide exchanges. *Sci. Rep.* 8:13846. doi: 10.1038/s41598-018-32096-9

Matsumura, N., Yamazaki, T., and Ihara, Y. (1999). Stable expression in Chinese hamster ovary cells of mutated tau genes causing frontotemporal dementia and parkinsonism linked to chromosome 17 (FTDP-17). *Am. J. Pathol.* 154, 1649–1656. doi: 10.1016/s0002-9440(10)65420-x

Melki, R., Carlier, M. F., Pantaloni, D., and Timasheff, S. N. (1989). Cold depolymerization of microtubules to double rings: geometric stabilization of assemblies. *Biochemistry* 28, 9143–9152. doi: 10.1021/bi00449a028

Melková, K., Zapletal, V., Narasimhan, S., Jansen, S., Hritz, J., Škrabana, R., et al. (2019). Structure and functions of microtubule associated proteins tau and MAP2c: similarities and differences. *Biomolecules* 9:E105. doi: 10.3390/biom9030105

Melo, A. M., Coraor, J., Alpha-Cobb, G., Elbaum-Garfinkle, S., Nath, A., and Rhoades, E. (2016). A functional role for intrinsic disorder in the tau-tubulin complex. *Proc. Natl. Acad. Sci. U S A* 113, 14336–14341. doi: 10.1073/pnas.1610137113

Min, S.-W., Chen, X., Tracy, T. E., Li, Y., Zhou, Y., Wang, C., et al. (2015). Critical role of acetylation in tau-mediated neurodegeneration and cognitive deficits. *Nat. Med.* 21, 1154–1162. doi: 10.1038/nm.3951

Min, S. W., Cho, S. H., Zhou, Y., Schroeder, S., Haroutunian, V., Seeley, W. W., et al. (2010). Acetylation of tau inhibits its degradation and contributes to tauopathy. *Neuron* 67, 953–966. doi: 10.1016/j.neuron.2010.08.044

Min, S.-W., Sohn, P. D., Li, Y., Devidze, N., Johnson, J. R., Krogan, N. J., et al. (2018). SIRT1 deacetylates tau and reduces pathogenic tau spread in a mouse model of tauopathy. *J. Neurosci.* 38, 3680–3688. doi: 10.1523/jneurosci.2369-17.2018

Mitchison, T., and Kirschner, M. (1984). Dynamic instability of microtubule growth. *Nature* 312, 237–242. doi: 10.1038/312237a0

Monacelli, F., Cea, M., Borghi, R., Odetti, P., and Nencioni, A. (2017). Do cancer drugs counteract neurodegeneration? Repurposing for Alzheimer's disease. *J. Alzheimers Dis.* 55, 1295–1306. doi: 10.3233/jad-160840

Mondal, P., Das, G., Khan, J., Pradhan, K., and Ghosh, S. (2018). Crafting of neuroprotective octapeptide from taxol-binding pocket of β-tubulin. *ACS Chem. Neurosci.* 9, 615–625. doi: 10.1021/acschemneuro.7b00457

Morris, M., Knudsen, G. M., Maeda, S., Trinidad, J. C., Ioanoviciu, A., Burlingame, A. L., et al. (2015). Tau post-translational modifications in wild-type and human amyloid precursor protein transgenic mice. *Nat. Neurosci.* 18, 1183–1189. doi: 10.1038/nn.4067

Mudher, A., Brion, J.-P., Avila, J., Medina, M., and Buée, L. (2017). EuroTau: towing scientists to tau without tautology. *Acta Neuropathol. Commun.* 5:90. doi: 10.1186/s40478-017-0491-z

Mukhopadhyay, R., and Hoh, J. H. (2001). AFM force measurements on microtubule-associated proteins: the projection domain exerts a long-range repulsive force. *FEBS Lett.* 505, 374–378. doi: 10.1016/s0014-5793(01)02844-7

Mukrasch, M. D., Bibow, S., Korukottu, J., Jeganathan, S., Biernat, J., Griesinger, C., et al. (2009). Structural polymorphism of 441-residue tau at single residue resolution. *PLoS Biol.* 7:e34. doi: 10.1371/journal.pbio.1000034

Mukrasch, M. D., Markwick, P., Biernat, J., Bergen, M., Bernado, P., Griesinger, C., et al. (2007). Highly populated turn conformations in natively unfolded tau protein identified from residual dipolar couplings and molecular simulation. *J. Am. Chem. Soc.* 129, 5235–5243. doi: 10.1021/ja0690159

Murphy, D. B., Johnson, K. A., and Borisy, G. G. (1977). Role of tubulin-associated proteins in microtubule nucleation and elongation. *J. Mol. Biol.* 117, 33–52. doi: 10.1016/0022-2836(77)90021-3

Mutreja, Y., Combs, B., and Gamblin, T. C. (2019). FTDP-17 mutations alter the aggregation and microtubule stabilization propensity of tau in an isoform-specific fashion. *Biochemistry* 58, 742–754. doi: 10.1021/acs.biochem.8b01039

Nagiec, E. W., Sampson, K. E., and Abraham, I. (2001). Mutated tau binds less avidly to microtubules than wildtype tau in living cells. *J. Neurosci. Res.* 63, 268–275. doi: 10.1002/1097-4547(20010201)63:3<268::aid-jnr1020>3.0.co;2-e

Nawrotek, A., Knossow, M., and Gigant, B. (2011). The determinants that govern microtubule assembly from the atomic structure of GTP-tubulin. *J. Mol. Biol.* 412, 35–42. doi: 10.1016/j.jmb.2011.07.029

Nouar, R., Devred, F., Breuzard, G., and Peyrot, V. (2013). FRET and FRAP imaging: approaches to characterise tau and stathmin interactions with microtubules in cells. *Biol. Cell* 105, 149–161. doi: 10.1111/boc.201200060

Oz, S., Kapitansky, O., Ivashco-Pachima, Y., Malishkevich, A., Giladi, E., Skalka, N., et al. (2014). The NAP motif of activity-dependent neuroprotective protein (ADNP) regulates dendritic spines through microtubule end binding proteins. *Mol. Psychiatry* 19, 1115–1124. doi: 10.1038/mp.2014.97

Pachima, Y. I., Zhou, L., Lei, P., and Gozes, I. (2016). Microtubule-tau interaction as a therapeutic target for Alzheimer's disease. *J. Mol. Neurosci.* 58, 145–152. doi: 10.1007/s12031-016-0715-x

Panda, D., Samuel, J. C., Massie, M., Feinstein, S. C., and Wilson, L. (2003). Differential regulation of microtubule dynamics by three- and four-repeat tau: implications for the onset of neurodegenerative disease. *Proc. Natl. Acad. Sci. U S A* 100, 9548–9553. doi: 10.1073/pnas.1633508100

Paonessa, F., Evans, L. D., Solanki, R., Larrieu, D., Wray, S., Hardy, J., et al. (2019). Microtubules deform the nuclear membrane and disrupt nucleocytoplasmic transport in tau-mediated frontotemporal dementia. *Cell Rep.* 26, 582.e5–593.e5. doi: 10.1016/j.celrep.2018.12.085

Pecqueur, L., Duellberg, C., Dreier, B., Jiang, Q., Wang, C., Pluckthun, A., et al. (2012). A designed ankyrin repeat protein selected to bind to tubulin caps the microtubule plus end. *Proc. Natl. Acad. Sci. U S A* 109, 12011–12016. doi: 10.1073/pnas.1204129109

Preuss, U., Biernat, J., Mandelkow, E. M., and Mandelkow, E. (1997). The "jaws" model of tau-microtubule interaction examined in CHO cells. *J. Cell Sci.* 110, 789–800.

Qiang, L., Sun, X., Austin, T. O., Muralidharan, H., Jean, D. C., Liu, M., et al. (2018). Tau does not stabilize axonal microtubules but rather enables them to have long labile domains. *Curr. Biol.* 28, 2181.e4–2189.e4. doi: 10.1016/j.cub.2018.05.045

Quraishe, S., Cowan, C. M., and Mudher, A. (2013). NAP (davunetide) rescues neuronal dysfunction in a *Drosophila* model of tauopathy. *Mol. Psychiatry* 18, 834–842. doi: 10.1038/mp.2013.32

Quraishe, S., Sealey, M., Cranfield, L., and Mudher, A. (2016). Microtubule stabilising peptides rescue tau phenotypes *in vivo*. *Sci. Rep.* 6:38224. doi: 10.1038/srep38224

Qureshi, H. Y., Li, T., MacDonald, R., Cho, C. M., Leclerc, N., and Paudel, H. K. (2013). Interaction of 14-3-3ζ with microtubule-associated protein tau within Alzheimer's disease neurofibrillary tangles. *Biochemistry* 52, 6445–6455. doi: 10.1021/bi400442d

Ramkumar, A., Jong, B. Y., and Ori-McKenney, K. M. (2018). ReMAPping the microtubule landscape: how phosphorylation dictates the activities of microtubule-associated proteins. *Dev. Dyn.* 247, 138–155. doi: 10.1002/dvdy.24599

Rane, J. S., Kumari, A., and Panda, D. (2019). An acetylation mimicking mutation, K274Q, in tau imparts neurotoxicity by enhancing tau aggregation and inhibiting tubulin polymerization. *Biochem. J.* 476, 1401–1417. doi: 10.1042/bcj20190042

Roman, A. Y., Devred, F., Byrne, D., La Rocca, R., Ninkina, N. N., Peyrot, V., et al. (2019). Zinc induces temperature-dependent reversible self-assembly of tau. *J. Mol. Biol.* 431, 687–695. doi: 10.1016/j.jmb.2018.12.008

Rosenberg, K. J., Ross, J. L., Feinstein, H. E., Feinstein, S. C., and Israelachvili, J. (2008). Complementary dimerization of microtubule-associated tau protein: implications for microtubule bundling and tau-mediated pathogenesis. *Proc. Natl. Acad. Sci. U S A* 105, 7445–7450. doi: 10.1073/pnas.0802036105

Rouzier, R., Rajan, R., Wagner, P., Hess, K. R., Gold, D. L., Stec, J., et al. (2005). Microtubule-associated protein tau: a marker of paclitaxel sensitivity in breast cancer. *Proc. Natl. Acad. Sci. U S A* 102, 8315–8320. doi: 10.1073/pnas.0408974102

Sahara, N., Tomiyama, T., and Mori, H. (2000). Missense point mutations of tau to segregate with FTDP-17 exhibit site-specific effects on microtubule structure in COS cells: a novel action of R406W mutation. *J. Neurosci. Res.* 60, 380–387. doi: 10.1002/(sici)1097-4547(20000501)60:3<380::aid-jnr13>3.0.co;2-5

Santarella, R. A., Skiniotis, G., Goldie, K. N., Tittmann, P., Gross, H., Mandelkow, E.-M., et al. (2004). Surface-decoration of microtubules by human tau. *J. Mol. Biol.* 339, 539–553. doi: 10.1016/j.jmb.2004.04.008

Schneider, A., Biernat, J., von Bergen, M., Mandelkow, E., and Mandelkow, E. M. (1999). Phosphorylation that detaches tau protein from microtubules (Ser262, Ser214) also protects it against aggregation into Alzheimer paired helical filaments. *Biochemistry* 38, 3549–3558. doi: 10.1021/bi981874p

Schwalbe, M., Kadavath, H., Biernat, J., Ozenne, V., Blackledge, M., Mandelkow, E., et al. (2015). Structural impact of tau phosphorylation at threonine 231. *Structure* 23, 1448–1458. doi: 10.1016/j.str.2015.06.002

Schwalbe, M., Ozenne, V., Bibow, S., Jaremko, M., Jaremko, L., Gajda, M., et al. (2014). Predictive atomic resolution descriptions of intrinsically disordered hTau40 and α-synuclein in solution from NMR and small angle scattering. *Structure* 22, 238–249. doi: 10.1016/j.str.2013.10.020

Scott, C. W., Blowers, D. P., Barth, P. T., Lo, M. M., Salama, A. I., and Caputo, C. B. (1991). Differences in the abilities of human tau isoforms to promote microtubule assembly. *J. Neurosci. Res.* 30, 154–162. doi: 10.1002/jnr.490300116

Scott, C. W., Spreen, R. C., Herman, J. L., Chow, F. P., Davison, M. D., Young, J., et al. (1993). Phosphorylation of recombinant tau by cAMP-dependent protein kinase. Identification of phosphorylation sites and effect on microtubule assembly. *J. Biol. Chem.* 268, 1166–1173.

Selenica, M.-L., Benner, L., Housley, S. B., Manchec, B., Lee, D. C., Nash, K. R., et al. (2014). Histone deacetylase 6 inhibition improves memory and reduces total tau levels in a mouse model of tau deposition. *Alzheimers Res. Ther.* 6:12. doi: 10.1186/alzrt241

Sengupta, A., Kabat, J., Novak, M., Wu, Q., Grundke-Iqbal, I., and Iqbal, K. (1998). Phosphorylation of tau at both Thr 231 and Ser 262 is required for maximal inhibition of its binding to microtubules. *Arch. Biochem. Biophys.* 357, 299–309. doi: 10.1006/abbi.1998.0813

Shashi, V., Magiera, M. M., Klein, D., Zaki, M., Schoch, K., Rudnik-Schöneborn, S., et al. (2018). Loss of tubulin deglutamylase CCP1 causes infantile-onset neurodegeneration. *EMBO J.* 37:e100540. doi: 10.15252/embj.2018100540

Sibille, N., Huvent, I., Fauquant, C., Verdegem, D., Amniai, L., Leroy, A., et al. (2012). Structural characterization by nuclear magnetic resonance of the impact of phosphorylation in the proline-rich region of the disordered Tau protein. *Proteins* 80, 454–462. doi: 10.1002/prot.23210

Sillen, A., Barbier, P., Landrieu, I., Lefebvre, S., Wieruszeski, J. M., Leroy, A., et al. (2007). NMR investigation of the interaction between the neuronal protein tau and the microtubules. *Biochemistry* 46, 3055–3064. doi: 10.1021/bi061920i

Smoter, M., Bodnar, L., Grala, B., Stec, R., Zieniuk, K., Kozlowski, W., et al. (2013). Tau protein as a potential predictive marker in epithelial ovarian cancer patients treated with paclitaxel/platinum first-line chemotherapy. *J. Exp. Clin. Cancer Res.* 32:25. doi: 10.1186/1756-9966-32-25

Szyk, A., Deaconescu, A. M., Spector, J., Goodman, B., Valenstein, M. L., Ziolkowska, N. E., et al. (2014). Molecular basis for age-dependent microtubule acetylation by tubulin acetyltransferase. *Cell* 157, 1405–1415. doi: 10.1016/j.cell.2014.03.061

Tompa, P., and Fuxreiter, M. (2008). Fuzzy complexes: polymorphism and structural disorder in protein-protein interactions. *Trends Biochem. Sci.* 33, 2–8. doi: 10.1016/j.tibs.2007.10.003

Trinczek, B., Biernat, J., Baumann, K., Mandelkow, E. M., and Mandelkow, E. (1995). Domains of tau protein, differential phosphorylation and dynamic instability of microtubules. *Mol. Biol. Cell* 6, 1887–1902. doi: 10.1091/mbc.6.12.1887

Tsvetkov, P. O., La Rocca, R., Malesinski, S., and Devred, F. (2019). Characterization of microtubule-associated proteins (MAPs) and tubulin interactions by isothermal titration calorimetry (ITC). *Methods Mol. Biol.* 1964, 151–165. doi: 10.1007/978-1-4939-9179-2_12

Tugaeva, K. V., Tsvetkov, P. O., and Sluchanko, N. N. (2017). Bacterial co-expression of human Tau protein with protein kinase A and 14-3-3 for studies of 14-3-3/phospho-Tau interaction. *PLoS One* 12:e0178933. doi: 10.1371/journal.pone.0178933

Umahara, T., Uchihara, T., Tsuchiya, K., Nakamura, A., Iwamoto, T., Ikeda, K., et al. (2004). 14-3-3 proteins and ζ isoform containing neurofibrillary tangles in patients with Alzheimer's disease. *Acta Neuropathol.* 108, 279–286. doi: 10.1007/s00401-004-0885-4

van der Vaart, B., Akhmanova, A., and Straube, A. (2009). Regulation of microtubule dynamic instability. *Biochem. Soc. Trans.* 37, 1007–1013. doi: 10.1042/BST0371007

Wegmann, S., Eftekharzadeh, B., Tepper, K., Zoltowska, K. M., Bennett, R. E., Dujardin, S., et al. (2018). Tau protein liquid-liquid phase separation can initiate tau aggregation. *EMBO J.* 37:e98049. doi: 10.15252/embj.201798049

Weingarten, M. D., Lockwood, A. H., Hwo, S. Y., and Kirschner, M. W. (1975). A protein factor essential for microtubule assembly. *Proc. Natl. Acad. Sci. U S A* 72, 1858–1862. doi: 10.1073/pnas.72.5.1858

Wilhelmsen, K. C., Lynch, T., Pavlou, E., Higgins, M., and Nygaard, T. G. (1994). Localization of disinhibition-dementia-parkinsonism-amyotrophy complex to 17q21-22. *Am. J. Hum. Genet.* 55, 1159–1165.

Witman, G. B., Cleveland, D. W., Weingarten, M. D., and Kirschner, M. W. (1976). Tubulin requires tau for growth onto microtubule initiating sites. *Proc. Natl. Acad. Sci. U S A* 73, 4070–4074. doi: 10.1073/pnas.73.11.4070

Xiong, Y., Zhao, K., Wu, J., Xu, Z., Jin, S., and Zhang, Y. Q. (2013). HDAC6 mutations rescue human tau-induced microtubule defects in *Drosophila*. *Proc. Natl. Acad. Sci. U S A* 110, 4604–4609. doi: 10.1073/pnas.1207586110

Zhang, R., Alushin, G. M., Brown, A., and Nogales, E. (2015). Mechanistic origin of microtubule dynamic instability and its modulation by EB proteins. *Cell* 162, 849–859. doi: 10.1016/j.cell.2015.07.012

Zhang, B., Maiti, A., Shively, S., Lakhani, F., McDonald-Jones, G., Bruce, J., et al. (2005). Microtubule-binding drugs offset tau sequestration by stabilizing microtubules and reversing fast axonal transport deficits in a tauopathy model. *Proc. Natl. Acad. Sci. U S A* 102, 227–231. doi: 10.1073/pnas.0406361102

Zhang, F., Su, B., Wang, C., Siedlak, S. L., Mondragon-Rodriguez, S., Lee, H.-G., et al. (2015). Posttranslational modifications of α-tubulin in Alzheimer disease. *Transl. Neurodegener.* 4:9. doi: 10.1186/s40035-015-0030-4

9

Differences Between Human and Murine Tau at the N-Terminal End

Félix Hernández [1,2], Jesús Merchán-Rubira [2], Laura Vallés-Saiz [2], Alberto Rodríguez-Matellán [2] and Jesús Avila [1,2]*

[1]Network Center for Biomedical Research in Neurodegenerative Diseases (CIBERNED), Carlos III Institute of Health, Madrid, Spain, [2]Centro de Biología Molecular Severo Ochoa, Consejo Superior de Investigaciones Científicas (CSIC), Universidad Autonoma de Madrid (UAM), Madrid, Spain

Correspondence:
Félix Hernández
fhernandez@cbm.csic.es

Human tauopathies, such as Alzheimer's disease (AD), have been widely studied in transgenic mice overexpressing human tau in the brain. The longest brain isoforms of Tau in mice and humans show 89% amino acid identity; however, the expression of the isoforms of this protein in the adult brain of the two species differs. Tau 3R isoforms are not present in adult mice. In contrast, the adult human brain contains Tau 3R and also Tau 4R isoforms. In addition, the N-terminal sequence of Tau protein in mice and humans differs, a Tau peptide (residues 17–28) being present in the latter but absent in the former. Here we review the main published data on this N-terminal sequence that suggests that human and mouse Tau proteins interact with different endogenous proteins and also show distinct secretion patterns.

Keywords: Alzheimer's disease, human tau, murine tau, neurodegeneration, tauopathies

INTRODUCTION

The microtubule-associated protein Tau is mainly expressed in neurons (Weingarten et al., 1975; Drubin and Kirschner, 1986). Tau promotes the assembly and stabilization of microtubules (for a review, see Avila et al., 2004). However, it has recently been suggested that rather than stabilizing the microtubules, Tau allows them to have labile domains (Baas and Qiang, 2019). In addition, and taking into account the subcellular localizations of Tau outside the axonal compartment, new functions have been proposed for this protein in dendrites (involvement in synaptic plasticity and regulation of NMDA/AMPA receptors), the nucleus (regulation of heterochromatin stability and integrity of cytoplasmic and nuclear RNA) and the membrane (interaction con F-actin and membrane proteins; for a review, see Sotiropoulos et al., 2017).

The hyperphosphorylation and aggregation of Tau in neurons is a common pathological hallmark of several neurodegenerative diseases known as tauopathies, Alzheimer's disease (AD) being the most prevalent (Spillantini and Goedert, 2013). AD is characterized by the accumulation of extracellular plaques of β-amyloid peptide and intracellular neurofibrillary tangles (NFTs) formed by aggregated and hyperphosphorylated Tau protein. The amyloid cascade theory proposes that β-amyloid drives Tau phosphorylation and then Tau forms filaments and these filaments accumulate in NFTs (Selkoe and Hardy, 2016). The hypothesis suggests that β-amyloid accumulation precedes altered Tau metabolism. In addition, it has been demonstrated that a reduction of endogenous Tau ameliorates β-amyloid-induced deficits in AD (Rapoport et al., 2002; Santacruz et al., 2005; Roberson et al., 2007; Shipton et al., 2011). Under pathological conditions, the hyperphosphorylation of Tau protein prevents its binding to microtubules, resulting in its accumulation in the cytosol and consequent formation of intracellular NFTs. Aggregated Tau present in tauopathies does not seem to be the main toxic species. Instead, neuronal toxicity appears to be caused by smaller soluble aggregates or by specific conformations of Tau protein. In recent years, certain Tau conformations, called strains, have been linked to specific tauopathies (Sanders et al., 2014). Tau also accumulates in microglia and astrocytes in several of these conditions (Buée and Delacourte, 1999; Kovacs et al., 2016; Ferrer et al., 2018). The prion-like hypothesis proposes that Tau propagates from the entorhinal cortex and hippocampus to the cerebral cortex, thereby explaining in part the progression of AD (Braak and Braak, 1991). Tau is secreted and this extracellular form is taken up by neurons and glial cells (Gómez-Ramos et al., 2006; Calafate et al., 2015), thus contributing to the cell-to-cell spread of the protein (Holmes and Diamond, 2014; Medina and Avila, 2014).

Genetically altered mouse models have been widely used to study Tau metabolism (see https://www.alzforum.org/research-models) and have greatly contributed to our understanding of disease-related mechanisms. Furthermore, they are valuable for the evaluation of novel therapeutic approaches. Nevertheless, in addition to distinct splicing processes, mouse and human Tau protein show other differences. Here we focus on recent data suggesting that the N-terminal end of Tau protein explains why none of the murine models fully reproduces the complete spectrum of AD or related tauopathies.

DIFFERENCES BETWEEN HUMAN AND MURINE TAU GENE

Human *tau* (chromosome 17) spans 134 kb while murine *tau* (chromosome 11) stretches across 100 kb (for a review, see Poorkaj et al., 2001; **Figure 1A**). The genomic context for the microtubule-associated protein tau gene (MAPT) in humans and mice is similar (**Figure 1B**). MAPT through alternative splicing, give rise to distinct Tau isoforms in the central nervous system (CNS; Goedert et al., 1989; Andreadis et al., 1992). In the adult CNS, alternative splicing produces six distinct Tau isoforms, which differ in the presence or absence of exons 2, 3 and 10. While exon 2 can appear alone, exon 3 never appears independently of exon 2. Exon 10 encodes one of the four repeat sequences that form the microtubule-binding domain (MBD). Those isoforms that carry exon 10 result in Tau with four repeated microtubule-binding sequences (Tau 4R), while those without this exon have only three (Tau 3R; **Figure 1D**). The expression of these Tau isoforms is regulated by development. Tau 3R isoforms are present in early stages of development, while Tau 4R are found mainly in adults (for a review, see Avila et al., 2004; Wang and Mandelkow, 2016).

The main function of tau is to promote the polymerization of tubulins (Weingarten et al., 1975) and prevents their instability by its binding to microtubules (Drechsel et al., 1992). The Tau 4R isoform promotes microtubule assembly faster than Tau 3R (Goedert and Jakes, 1990). This observation suggests that the Tau 3R protein modulates brain development by decreasing the stability of microtubules. The expression of Tau 3R protein during development, as well as the absence of Tau 4R in the fetal human brain (Goedert et al., 1989; Kosik et al., 1989; Goedert and Jakes, 1990) support this notion. In the adult human brain, Tau 3R and Tau 4R isoforms are present in the same proportion (Avila et al., 2004). In addition to regulation through splicing, Tau phosphorylation is controlled during development, being higher in fetal neurons and decreasing with age (Brion et al., 1993). Tau phosphorylation during development correlates with the period of active neurite outgrowth, a process that requires a dynamic microtubule network.

The expression of Tau isoforms in the adult mice brain differs from humans. The Tau 3R isoform is not present in adult mice (Brion et al., 1993; Spillantini and Goedert, 1998). In this regard, adult hippocampal neurogenesis in mice is characterized by an unusual feature, namely Tau 3R is the main isoform present in newborn neurons in the hippocampal dentate gyrus (Bullmann et al., 2007) and in the subventricular zone (SVZ; Fuster-Matanzo et al., 2009). Doublecortin (DCX) is a microtubule-associated protein expressed in neural progenitor cells. DCX+ cells give rise to new neurons in the adult brain. DCX-positive neuroblasts express the Tau 3R isoform and Tau is also found in a phosphorylated form (Fuster-Matanzo et al., 2009). During the processes of differentiation to adult neurons, there is a progressive change towards Tau 4R in mature granule cells (Bullmann et al., 2007). These data support the notion that axonal outgrowth that takes place in these neuroblast DCX+ requires a dynamic microtubule network and that Tau protein contributes to this dynamic cytoskeleton. In this regard, neuronal polarity and axonal outgrowth take place during adult neurogenesis, microtubules express Tau isoforms with less affinity for microtubules as Tau 3R is hyperphosphorylated. Interestingly, it has been proposed that adult neurogenesis recapitulates neuronal development (Ming and Song, 2011) as Tau phosphorylation is higher in fetal neurons (Brion et al., 1993) and Tau 3R isoforms are found during early developmental stages (Avila et al., 2004).

In addition to the splicing differences between human and mouse Tau protein, intron 9 (between exon 9 and 10) of human *tau* has a region that can give rise to the expression of a protein known as saitohin (Conrad et al., 2002; **Figure 1B**). Saitohin is not present in mice. In this regard, although a homologous sequence is found in the mouse gene, the absence of an open reading frame in mice prevents Saitohin expression (Conrad et al., 2004).

DIFFERENCES BETWEEN HUMAN AND MURINE TAU PROTEIN

Tau of distinct origins shows some variability in primary sequence—variability in the N-terminal end being greatest (Nelson et al., 1996). Although mouse and human Tau

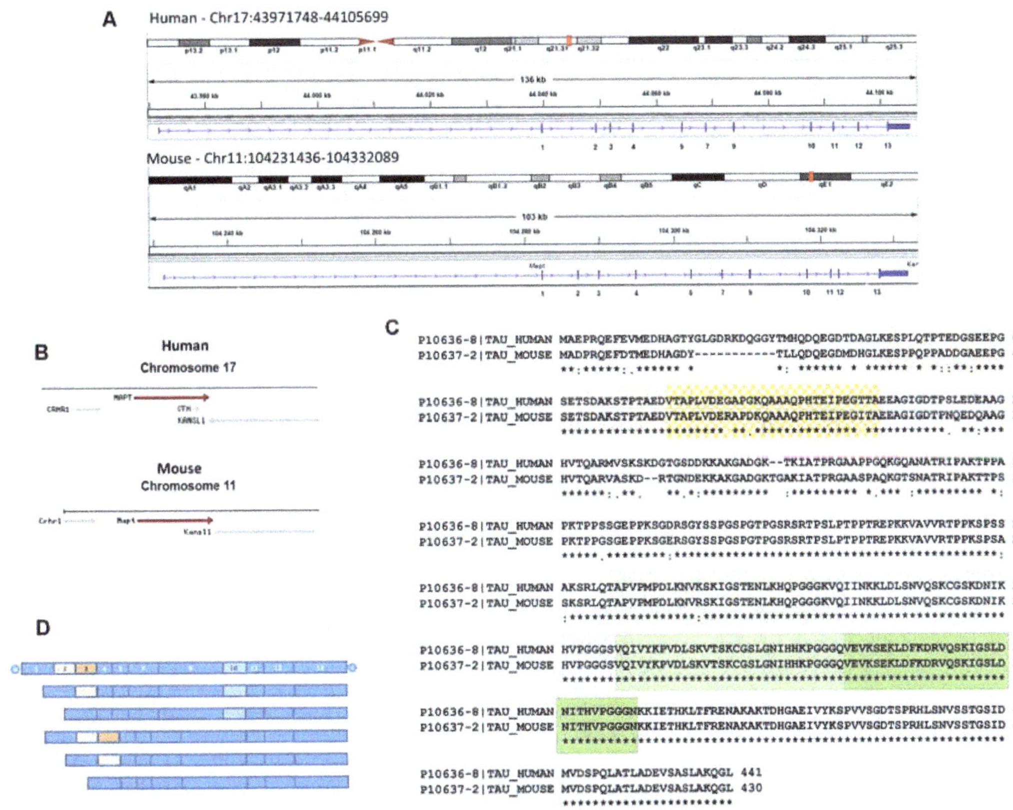

FIGURE 1 | (A) Human and murine *tau* organization. Integrative Genomics viewer (using Human19 and Mouse mm10 genome versions) has been used to show the longest central nervous system (CNS) splicing isoforms (Tau 4R). Exons are shown by a vertical bar. Distances between exons are proportional to the sizes of the introns. Exons that undergo alternative splicing in the CNS: 2, 3 and 10 are indicated. It should be noted that although human and murine *tau* are similar size in the figure, the former covers 134 kb while the latter extends across 100 kb. The chromosomic localizations (red boxes) are also shown. **(B)** The genomic context for microtubule-associated protein tau gene (MAPT) in human chromosome 17 and mouse chromosome 11 are shown using data from The National Center for Biotechnology Information (NCBI; https://www.ncbi.nlm.nih.gov/). KANSL1, KAT8 regulatory NSL complex subunit 1; CRHC1, corticotropin-releasing hormone receptor 1; MAPT, Tau; STH, saitohin. **(C)** Sequence alignment of human Tau (entry UniProt number P10636-8) and mouse Tau (entry UniProt number sequence P10637-2) using the Clustal Omega program from the UniProt website. N-terminal domains, as well as microtubule-binding domains (MBD), are shown. In the figure, the same amino acids (*), while conservative amino acids (:) or less conservative ones (.) are highlighted. **(D)** A scheme of Tau isoforms present in the CNS. Six main transcripts are generated from a single gene. These isoforms are generated by alternative splicing of exons 2, 3, and 10. Exon 3 never appears independently of exon 2. Exons 1, 4, 5, 7, 9, 11, 12 and 13 are constitutive. Alternative splices of exons 2 (light orange), 3 (orange), and 10 (light blue) are shown in panels **(C,D)**.

sequences are similar, the latter contains 11 amino acids in the N-terminal end that are absent in mice (**Figure 1C**). These amino acids probably affect some functions in which Tau is involved. Tau adopts the so-called "paperclip" folding in solution, and the N- and C-terminal domains fold onto the microtubule-binding repeat domains (Carmel et al., 1996; Jicha et al., 1997). The presence of residues 17–28 in humans, making the N-terminal end longer than in mice, could have implications for the intramolecular interaction between the N- and C-terminal ends of the protein and the microtubule-binding repeat domains. Given the difference in the N-terminal sequence of human and mouse Tau, it can be speculated that the latter would be less likely to adopt this pathological "paperclip" conformation, something that has been already proposed (Ando et al., 2011).

Figure 1C shows that the domain around tyrosine-18 differs between the two species. Tyrosine-18 is phosphorylated by Src-family non-receptor tyrosine kinase Fyn (Lee et al., 1998, 2004) and Tyrosine-18 phosphorylation modulates NMDA receptor in primary neuronal culture (Miyamoto et al., 2017). Interestingly, Tau mediates the targeting of Fyn to postsynaptic dendrites (Ittner et al., 2010). At present, it is not clear whether tyrosine-18 phosphorylation is increased or decreased in human Tau compared with the murine form of the protein. Given that the NMDA receptor may be necessary for the toxic effect of the β-amyloid peptide (Ittner et al., 2010), differences in tyrosine-18 phosphorylation in mouse and human tau could be relevant. Of note, proline residues Pro213, Pro216, and Pro219, which are important for the binding of Tau protein to Fyn (Lau et al., 2016), are present in both human and murine Tau (see **Figure 1**).

The N-terminal projection region of Tau protein, which protrudes around 19 nm from the microtubule surface (Hirokawa et al., 1988), allows interaction with other proteins. Several N-terminal Tau interaction partners have been identified. The first interaction described was with the neural plasma membrane through its N-terminal projection domain (Brandt et al., 1995), thereby suggesting that Tau was a mediator of microtubule-plasma membrane interactions and thus plays an important role in neuritic development. Recently, a study using a heterologous yeast system has revealed that Tau interacts with Annexin A2 in a Ca2+-dependent manner *via* the N-terminal projection domain (Gauthier-Kemper et al., 2018). This observation, therefore, suggests that Tau links microtubules to the axonal plasma membrane through this domain. The same study described that Tau also interacts with Annexin A6, which localizes to the axon initial segment (AIS), where the binding of Tau may lead to its retention in the axonal compartment (Gauthier-Kemper et al., 2018).

Another approach to study the function of the N-terminal end of Tau protein, specifically the role of amino acids 18–28 present in the human sequence (**Figure 1C**), involved removing these amino acids from the full length recombinant human protein and then performing glutathione-S transferase (GST) pull-down assays and mass spectrometry analysis. Thus, it was found that the human-specific N-terminal Tau motif interacts with neuronal proteins such as Synapsin-1 and Synaptotagmin-1 (proteins involved in synaptic transmission), proteins of the 14–3–3 family, and Annexin A5 (Stefanoska et al., 2018).

To test for proteins that specifically and only bind to human Tau residues 16–26 (not present in murine Tau), a column containing this peptide linked to Sepharose was used to study human brain proteins that bound to the resin from control subjects and from patients with Alzheimer disease. Creatine kinase-B (CK-B), gamma-enolase and glyceraldehyde 3-phosphate dehydrogenase were observed to bind to this human Tau peptide. Interestingly, CK-B from brain extracts taken from patients with AD did not bind to Tau (Hernández et al., 2019). This observation could be attributable to the oxidation of CK-B in this disease (Hernández et al., 2019). CK-B is a brain isoform that phosphorylates creatine in the presence of ATP (Wallimann et al., 1992), and enolase and glyceraldehyde 3-phosphate dehydrogenase are critical enzymes in the glycolytic pathway. These proteins are related to energetic processes and can have a high impact on neuronal functions that require energy. Moreover, the brain is highly susceptible to oxidative imbalance, and changes in the level of ATP may induce neurodegeneration (Wang et al., 2014). The CK-B/phosphocreatine complex may supply the ATP required for axonal transport under conditions in which this energy supply is interrupted (Wallimann et al., 2011). In fact, creatine protects cortical axons from energy depletion *in vitro* (Shen and Goldberg, 2012). Regarding the other proteins, enolase moves along the axon (Brady and Lasek, 1981) and glyceraldehyde 3-phosphate dehydrogenase has been implicated in rapid axonal transport (Zala et al., 2013). These data suggest that the presence of this domain (residues 16–26) in human Tau supports energy supply by glycolysis in times of low oxygen levels and may explain, at least in part, the decrease in glucose metabolism observed in AD due to altered Tau metabolism (Butterfield and Halliwell, 2019). Given that these studies have been carried out with the peptide that is present in human but not murine Tau, it is reasonable to propose that either these interactions do not take place in the latter or that the interaction of these proteins with murine Tau differs.

DIFFERENCES BETWEEN HUMAN AND MURINE TAU SECRETION

Tau is mainly an intracellular protein, although it is also present in brain interstitial fluid (for a review, see Yamada, 2017). Tau protein is secreted *in vivo*, and this process appears to be regulated in physiological conditions and modulated by neuronal activity (Pooler et al., 2013). The exact mechanism of Tau release is unclear. However, several studies have demonstrated the extracellular presence of vesicle-bound and soluble free Tau (Saman et al., 2012; Kanmert et al., 2015; Wang et al., 2017). Although it is not clear how Tau can localize at the cell membrane, several reports demonstrate its presence in this structure (Brandt et al., 1995; Arrasate et al., 2000). This localization may indeed favor its further secretion. In addition, it should be noted that neuronal death can result in the release of Tau into the extracellular space, thereby contributing to extracellular Tau in pathological conditions.

The abnormal accumulation of intracellular Tau can be mediated through the cell-to-cell propagation of seeds of the protein. This observation has given rise to the hypothesis of a prion-like transmission to explain the propagation of the main neuropathological hallmarks of AD (Goedert et al., 2010). This hypothesis suggests that pathology begins in a part of the brain and spreads through this organ over time, for example from the entorhinal cortex (Braak and Braak, 1991) or/and from the locus ceruleus (Braak and Del Tredici, 2011). The nature of the Tau species involved in secretion, spreading and uptake, as well as the apparent selectivity that could explain why certain neurons are affected while others are not, remains unclear. Greater knowledge of this process will contribute to the development of new therapeutic approaches focused on stopping the spread of the disease and of new approaches to facilitate early diagnosis. Interestingly, human Tau lacking N-terminal amino acids 18–28 is less efficiently secreted than full-length Tau upon overexpression in Cos7 cells (Sayas et al., 2019). That study demonstrated that the sequence containing human Tau residues 18–28 acts as a binding motif for End Binding proteins and that this interaction facilitates Tau secretion to the extracellular space (Sayas et al., 2019). Although a comparative study with murine Tau protein that lacks this sequence at the N-terminal end has not been carried out, differences with the human protein would be expected. However, this does not imply that murine Tau is not secreted since the protein is also found in the extracellular compartment of wild-type mice (Yamada et al., 2011).

CONCLUDING REMARKS

Given that decreased Tau expression is neuroprotective, strategies to achieve a reduction in its expression are among the most promising approaches for the development of AD therapeutic drugs (for a review, see Jadhav et al., 2019). In this regard, the evaluation of these strategies must first be validated in murine models. However, as shown in this mini-review, Tau metabolism in mice differs from that in humans, not only in the splicing process (presence of Tau 3R in adult humans but not in mice) but also in the primary sequence, mainly in the N-terminal end. These differences may limit the success of murine genetic models and explain why they do not fully reproduce the complete spectrum of AD pathology or related tauopathies.

AUTHOR CONTRIBUTIONS

All authors listed have made a substantial, direct and intellectual contribution to the work, and approved it for publication.

REFERENCES

Ando, K., Leroy, K., Heraud, C., Yilmaz, Z., Authelet, M., Suain, V., et al. (2011). Accelerated human mutant tau aggregation by knocking out murine tau in a transgenic mouse model. *Am. J. Pathol.* 178, 803–816. doi: 10.1016/j.ajpath.2010.10.034

Andreadis, A., Brown, W. M., and Kosik, K. S. (1992). Structure and novel exons of the human tau gene. *Biochemistry* 31, 10626–10633. doi: 10.1021/bi00158a027

Arrasate, M., Pérez, M., and Avila, J. (2000). Tau dephosphorylation at tau-1 site correlates with its association to cell membrane. *Neurochem. Res.* 25, 43–50. doi: 10.1023/a:1007583214722

Avila, J., Lucas, J. J., Perez, M., and Hernandez, F. (2004). Role of tau protein in both physiological and pathological conditions. *Physiol. Rev.* 84, 361–384. doi: 10.1152/physrev.00024.2003

Baas, P. W., and Qiang, L. (2019). Tau: it's not what you think. *Trends Cell Biol.* 29, 452–461. doi: 10.1016/j.tcb.2019.02.007

Braak, H., and Braak, E. (1991). Neuropathological stageing of Alzheimer-related changes. *Acta Neuropathol.* 82, 239–259. doi: 10.1007/bf00308809

Braak, H., and Del Tredici, K. (2011). The pathological process underlying Alzheimer's disease in individuals under thirty. *Acta Neuropathol.* 121, 171–181. doi: 10.1007/s00401-010-0789-4

Brady, S. T., and Lasek, R. J. (1981). Nerve-specific enolase and creatine phosphokinase in axonal transport: soluble proteins and the axoplasmic matrix. *Cell* 23, 515–523. doi: 10.1016/0092-8674(81)90147-1

Brandt, R., Léger, J., and Lee, G. (1995). Interaction of tau with the neural plasma membrane mediated by tau's amino-terminal projection domain. *J. Cell Biol.* 131, 1327–1340. doi: 10.1083/jcb.131.5.1327

Brion, J. P., Smith, C., Couck, A. M., Gallo, J. M., and Anderton, B. H. (1993). Developmental changes in tau phosphorylation: fetal tau is transiently phosphorylated in a manner similar to paired helical filament-tau characteristic of Alzheimer's disease. *J. Neurochem.* 61, 2071–2080. doi: 10.1111/j.1471-4159.1993.tb07444.x

Buée, L., and Delacourte, A. (1999). Comparative biochemistry of tau in progressive supranuclear palsy, corticobasal degeneration, FTDP-17 and Pick's disease. *Brain Pathol.* 9, 681–693. doi: 10.1111/j.1750-3639.1999.tb00550.x

Bullmann, T., de Silva, R., Holzer, M., Mori, H., and Arendt, T. (2007). Expression of embryonic tau protein isoforms persist during adult neurogenesis in the hippocampus. *Hippocampus* 17, 98–102. doi: 10.1002/hipo.20255

Butterfield, D. A., and Halliwell, B. (2019). Oxidative stress, dysfunctional glucose metabolism and Alzheimer disease. *Nat. Rev. Neurosci.* 20, 148–160. doi: 10.1038/s41583-019-0132-6

Calafate, S., Buist, A., Miskiewicz, K., Vijayan, V., Daneels, G., de Strooper, B., et al. (2015). Synaptic contacts enhance cell-to-cell tau pathology propagation. *Cell Rep.* 11, 1176–1183. doi: 10.1016/j.celrep.2015.04.043

Carmel, G., Mager, E. M., Binder, L. I., and Kuret, J. (1996). The structural basis of monoclonal antibody Alz50's selectivity for Alzheimer's disease pathology. *J. Biol. Chem.* 271, 32789–32795. doi: 10.1074/jbc.271.51.32789

Conrad, C., Vianna, C., Freeman, M., and Davies, P. (2002). A polymorphic gene nested within an intron of the tau gene: implications for Alzheimer's disease. *Proc. Natl. Acad. Sci. U S A* 99, 7751–7756. doi: 10.1073/pnas.112194599

Conrad, C., Vianna, C., Schultz, C., Thal, D. R., Ghebremedhin, E., Lenz, J., et al. (2004). Molecular evolution and genetics of the Saitohin gene and tau haplotype in Alzheimer's disease and argyrophilic grain disease. *J. Neurochem.* 89, 179–188. doi: 10.1046/j.1471-4159.2004.02320.x

Drechsel, D. N., Hyman, A. A., Cobb, M. H., and Kirschner, M. W. (1992). Modulation of the dynamic instability of tubulin assembly by the microtubule-associated protein tau. *Mol. Biol. Cell* 3, 1141–1154. doi: 10.1091/mbc.3.10.1141

Drubin, D. G., and Kirschner, M. W. (1986). Tau protein function in living cells. *J. Cell Biol.* 103, 2739–2746. doi: 10.1083/jcb.103.6.2739

Ferrer, I., Garcia, M. A., González, I. L., Lucena, D. D., Villalonga, A. R., Tech, M. C., et al. (2018). Aging-related tau astrogliopathy (ARTAG): not only tau phosphorylation in astrocytes. *Brain Pathol.* 28, 965–985. doi: 10.1111/bpa.12593

Fuster-Matanzo, A., de Barreda, E. G., Dawson, H. N., Vitek, M. P., Avila, J., and Hernandez, F. (2009). Function of tau protein in adult newborn neurons. *FEBS Lett.* 583, 3063–3068. doi: 10.1016/j.febslet.2009.08.017

Gauthier-Kemper, A., Suarez Alonso, M., Sundermann, F., Niewidok, B., Fernandez, M. P., Bakota, L., et al. (2018). Annexins A2 and A6 interact with the extreme N terminus of tau and thereby contribute to tau's axonal localization. *J. Biol. Chem.* 293, 8065–8076. doi: 10.1074/jbc.ra117.000490

Goedert, M., Clavaguera, F., and Tolnay, M. (2010). The propagation of prion-like protein inclusions in neurodegenerative diseases. *Trends Neurosci.* 33, 317–325. doi: 10.1016/j.tins.2010.04.003

Goedert, M., and Jakes, R. (1990). Expression of separate isoforms of human tau protein: correlation with the tau pattern in brain and effects on tubulin polymerization. *EMBO J.* 9, 4225–4230. doi: 10.1002/j.1460-2075.1990.tb07870.x

Goedert, M., Spillantini, M. G., Jakes, R., Rutherford, D., and Crowther, R. A. (1989). Multiple isoforms of human microtubule-associated protein tau: sequences and localization in neurofibrillary tangles of Alzheimer's disease. *Neuron* 3, 519–526. doi: 10.1016/0896-6273(89)90210-9

Gómez-Ramos, A., Díaz-Hernández, M., Cuadros, R., Hernández, F., and Avila, J. (2006). Extracellular tau is toxic to neuronal cells. *FEBS Lett.* 580, 4842–4850. doi: 10.1016/j.febslet.2006.07.078

Hernández, F., Cuadros, R., Ollá, I., García, C., Ferrer, I., Perry, G., et al. (2019). Differences in structure and function between human and murine tau. *Biochim. Biophys. Acta Mol. Basis Dis.* 1865, 2024–2030. doi: 10.1016/j.bbadis.2018.08.010

Hirokawa, N., Shiomura, Y., and Okabe, S. (1988). Tau proteins: the molecular structure and mode of binding on microtubules. *J. Cell Biol.* 107, 1449–1459. doi: 10.1083/jcb.107.4.1449

Holmes, B. B., and Diamond, M. I. (2014). Prion-like properties of Tau protein: the importance of extracellular Tau as a therapeutic target. *J. Biol. Chem.* 289, 19855–19861. doi: 10.1074/jbc.r114.549295

Ittner, L. M., Ke, Y. D., Delerue, F., Bi, M., Gladbach, A., van Eersel, J., et al. (2010). Dendritic function of tau mediates amyloid-β toxicity in Alzheimer's disease mouse models. *Cell* 142, 387–397. doi: 10.1016/j.cell.2010.06.036

Jadhav, S., Avila, J., Schöll, M., Kovacs, G. G., Kövari, E., Skrabana, R., et al. (2019). A walk through tau therapeutic strategies. *Acta Neuropathol. Commun.* 7:22. doi: 10.1186/s40478-019-0664-z

Jicha, G. A., Bowser, R., Kazam, I. G., and Davies, P. (1997). Alz-50 and MC-1, a new monoclonal antibody raised to paired helical filaments, recognize conformational epitopes on recombinant tau. *J. Neurosci. Res.* 48, 128–132. doi: 10.1002/(sici)1097-4547(19970415)48:2<128::aid-jnr5>3.0.co;2-e

Kanmert, D., Cantlon, A., Muratore, C. R., Jin, M., O'Malley, T. T., Lee, G., et al. (2015). C-terminally truncated forms of tau, but not full-length tau or its C-terminal fragments, are released from neurons independently of cell death. *J. Neurosci.* 35, 10851–10865. doi: 10.1523/JNEUROSCI.0387-15.2015

Kosik, K. S., Orecchio, L. D., Bakalis, S., and Neve, R. L. (1989). Developmentally regulated expression of specific tau sequences. *Neuron* 2, 1389–1397. doi: 10.1016/0896-6273(89)90077-9

Kovacs, G. G., Ferrer, I., Grinberg, L. T., Alafuzoff, I., Attems, J., Budka, H., et al. (2016). Aging-related tau astrogliopathy (ARTAG): harmonized evaluation strategy. *Acta Neuropathol.* 131, 87–102. doi: 10.1007/s00401-015-1509-x

Lau, D. H., Hogseth, M., Phillips, E. C., O'Neill, M. J., Pooler, A. M., Noble, W., et al. (2016). Critical residues involved in tau binding to fyn: implications for tau phosphorylation in Alzheimer's disease. *Acta Neuropathol. Commun.* 4:49. doi: 10.1186/s40478-016-0317-4

Lee, G., Newman, S. T., Gard, D. L., Band, H., and Panchamoorthy, G. (1998). Tau interacts with src-family non-receptor tyrosine kinases. *J. Cell Sci.* 111, 3167–3177.

Lee, G., Thangavel, R., Sharma, V. M., Litersky, J. M., Bhaskar, K., Fang, S. M., et al. (2004). Phosphorylation of tau by fyn: implications for Alzheimer's disease. *J. Neurosci.* 24, 2304–2312. doi: 10.1523/JNEUROSCI.4162-03.2004

Medina, M., and Avila, J. (2014). Is tau a prion-like protein? *J. Alzheimers Dis.* 40, S1–S3. doi: 10.3233/JAD-140755

Ming, G. L., and Song, H. (2011). Adult neurogenesis in the mammalian brain: significant answers and significant questions. *Neuron* 70, 687–702. doi: 10.1016/j.neuron.2011.05.001

Miyamoto, T., Stein, L., Thomas, R., Djukic, B., Taneja, P., Knox, J., et al. (2017). Phosphorylation of tau at Y18, but not tau-fyn binding, is required for tau to modulate NMDA receptor-dependent excitotoxicity in primary neuronal culture. *Mol. Neurodegener.* 12:41. doi: 10.1186/s13024-017-0176-x

Nelson, P. T., Stefansson, K., Gulcher, J., and Saper, C. B. (1996). Molecular evolution of tau protein: implications for Alzheimer's disease. *J. Neurochem.* 67, 1622–1632. doi: 10.1046/j.1471-4159.1996.67041622.x

Pooler, A. M., Phillips, E. C., Lau, D. H., Noble, W., and Hanger, D. P. (2013). Physiological release of endogenous tau is stimulated by neuronal activity. *EMBO Rep.* 14, 389–394. doi: 10.1038/embor.2013.15

Poorkaj, P., Kas, A., D'Souza, I., Zhou, Y., Pham, Q., Stone, M., et al. (2001). A genomic sequence analysis of the mouse and human microtubule-associated protein tau. *Mamm. Genome* 12, 700–712. doi: 10.1007/s00335-001-2044-8

Rapoport, M., Dawson, H. N., Binder, L. I., Vitek, M. P., and Ferreira, A. (2002). Tau is essential to β -amyloid-induced neurotoxicity. *Proc. Natl. Acad. Sci. U S A* 99, 6364–6369. doi: 10.1073/pnas.092136199

Roberson, E. D., Scearce-Levie, K., Palop, J. J., Yan, F., Cheng, I. H., Wu, T., et al. (2007). Reducing endogenous tau ameliorates amyloid β-induced deficits in an Alzheimer's disease mouse model. *Science* 316, 750–754. doi: 10.1126/science.1141736

Saman, S., Kim, W., Raya, M., Visnick, Y., Miro, S., Saman, S., et al. (2012). Exosome-associated tau is secreted in tauopathy models and is selectively phosphorylated in cerebrospinal fluid in early Alzheimer disease. *J. Biol. Chem.* 287, 3842–3849. doi: 10.1074/jbc.m111.277061

Sanders, D. W., Kaufman, S. K., DeVos, S. L., Sharma, A. M., Mirbaha, H., Li, A., et al. (2014). Distinct tau prion strains propagate in cells and mice and define different tauopathies. *Neuron* 82, 1271–1288. doi: 10.1016/j.neuron.2014.04.047

Santacruz, K., Lewis, J., Spires, T., Paulson, J., Kotilinek, L., Ingelsson, M., et al. (2005). Tau suppression in a neurodegenerative mouse model improves memory function. *Science* 309, 476–481. doi: 10.1126/science.1113694

Sayas, C. L., Medina, M., Cuadros, R., Ollá, I., García, E., Pérez, M., et al. (2019). Role of tau N-terminal motif in the secretion of human tau by End Binding proteins. *PLoS One* 14:e0210864. doi: 10.1371/journal.pone.0210864

Selkoe, D. J., and Hardy, J. (2016). The amyloid hypothesis of Alzheimer's disease at 25 years. *EMBO Mol. Med.* 8, 595–608. doi: 10.15252/emmm.201606210

Shen, H., and Goldberg, M. P. (2012). Creatine pretreatment protects cortical axons from energy depletion *in vitro*. *Neurobiol. Dis.* 47, 184–193. doi: 10.1016/j.nbd.2012.03.037

Shipton, O. A., Leitz, J. R., Dworzak, J., Acton, C. E., Tunbridge, E. M., Denk, F., et al. (2011). Tau protein is required for amyloid β-induced impairment of hippocampal long-term potentiation. *J. Neurosci.* 31, 1688–1692. doi: 10.1523/JNEUROSCI.2610-10.2011

Sotiropoulos, I., Galas, M. C., Silva, J. M., Skoulakis, E., Wegmann, S., Maina, M. B., et al. (2017). Atypical, non-standard functions of the microtubule associated Tau protein. *Acta Neuropathol. Commun.* 5:91. doi: 10.1186/s40478-017-0489-6

Spillantini, M. G., and Goedert, M. (1998). Tau protein pathology in neurodegenerative diseases. *Trends Neurosci.* 21, 428–433. doi: 10.1016/s0166-2236(98)01337-x

Spillantini, M. G., and Goedert, M. (2013). Tau pathology and neurodegeneration. *Lancet Neurol.* 12, 609–622. doi: 10.1016/S1474-4422(13)70090-5

Stefanoska, K., Volkerling, A., Bertz, J., Poljak, A., Ke, Y. D., Ittner, L. M., et al. (2018). An N-terminal motif unique to primate tau enables differential protein-protein interactions. *J. Biol. Chem.* 293, 3710–3719. doi: 10.1074/jbc.ra118.001784

Wallimann, T., Tokarska-Schlattner, M., and Schlattner, U. (2011). The creatine kinase system and pleiotropic effects of creatine. *Amino Acids* 40, 1271–1296. doi: 10.1007/s00726-011-0877-3

Wallimann, T., Wyss, M., Brdiczka, D., Nicolay, K., and Eppenberger, H. M. (1992). Intracellular compartmentation, structure and function of creatine kinase isoenzymes in tissues with high and fluctuating energy demands: the 'phosphocreatine circuit' for cellular energy homeostasis. *Biochem. J.* 281, 21–40. doi: 10.1042/bj2810021

Wang, Y., and Mandelkow, E. (2016). Tau in physiology and pathology. *Nat. Rev. Neurosci.* 17, 5–21. doi: 10.1038/nrn.2015.1

Wang, Y., Balaji, V., Kaniyappan, S., Krüger, L., Irsen, S., Tepper, K., et al. (2017). The release and trans-synaptic transmission of Tau *via* exosomes. *Mol. Neurodegener.* 12:5. doi: 10.1186/s13024-016-0143-y

Wang, X., Wang, W., Li, L., Perry, G., Lee, H. G., and Zhu, X. (2014). Oxidative stress and mitochondrial dysfunction in Alzheimer's disease. *Biochim. Biophys. Acta* 1842, 1240–1247. doi: 10.1016/j.bbadis.2013.10.015

Weingarten, M. D., Lockwood, A. H., Hwo, S. Y., and Kirschner, M. W. (1975). A protein factor essential for microtubule assembly. *Proc. Natl. Acad. Sci. U S A* 72, 1858–1862. doi: 10.1073/pnas.72.5.1858

Yamada, K. (2017). Extracellular tau and its potential role in the propagation of tau pathology. *Front. Neurosci.* 11:667. doi: 10.3389/fnins.2017.00667

Yamada, K., Cirrito, J. R., Stewart, F. R., Jiang, H., Finn, M. B., Holmes, B. B., et al. (2011). *In vivo* microdialysis reveals age-dependent decrease of brain interstitial fluid tau levels in P301S human tau transgenic mice. *J. Neurosci.* 31, 13110–13117. doi: 10.1523/jneurosci.2569-11.2011

Zala, D., Hinckelmann, M. V., Yu, H., Lyra da Cunha, M. M., Liot, G., Cordelieres, F. P., et al. (2013). Vesicular glycolysis provides on-board energy for fast axonal transport. *Cell* 152, 479–491. doi: 10.1016/j.cell.2012.12.029

10

A Novel Microtubule-Tau Association Enhancer and Neuroprotective Drug Candidate: Ac-SKIP

*Yanina Ivashko-Pachima and Illana Gozes**

Dr. Diana and Zelman Elton (Elbaum) Laboratory for Molecular Neuroendocrinology, Department of Human Molecular Genetics and Biochemistry, Sackler Faculty of Medicine, Sagol School of Neuroscience, Adams Super Center for Brain Studies, Tel Aviv University, Tel Aviv, Israel

Correspondence:
Illana Gozes
igozes@tauex.tau.ac.il;
igozes@post.tau.ac.il

Activity-dependent neuroprotective protein (ADNP) has been initially discovered through its eight amino acid sequence NAPVSIPQ, which shares SIP motif with SALLRSIPA – a peptide derived from activity-dependent neurotrophic factor (ADNF). Mechanistically, both NAPVSIPQ and SALLRSIPA contain a SIP motif that is identified as a variation of SxIP domain, providing direct interaction with microtubule end-binding proteins (EBs). The peptide SKIP was shown before to provide neuroprotection *in vitro* and protect against Adnp-related axonal transport deficits *in vivo*. Here we show, for the first time that SKIP enhanced microtubule dynamics, and prevented Tau-microtubule dissociation and microtubule disassembly induced by the Alzheimer's related zinc intoxication. Furthermore, we introduced, CH_3CO-SKIP-NH_2 (Ac-SKIP), providing efficacious neuroprotection. Since microtubule – Tau organization and dynamics is central in axonal microtubule cytoskeleton and transport, tightly related to aging processes and Alzheimer's disease, our current study provides a compelling molecular explanation to the *in vivo* activity of SKIP, placing SKIP motif as a central focus for MT-based neuroprotection in tauopathies with axonal transport implications.

Keywords: tau, microtubules, EBs, ADNP, SKIP

INTRODUCTION

Activity-dependent neuroprotective protein (ADNP) has been initially discovered through its eight amino acid sequence NAPVSIPQ (Bassan et al., 1999), which shares SIP motif with SALLRSIPA – a peptide derived from activity-dependent neurotrophic factor (ADNF) (Brenneman and Gozes, 1996; Zamostiano et al., 1999). ADNF, and then ADNP, have been originally found to mediate neuroprotective and neurotrophic activities of the vasoactive intestinal peptide (VIP) (Brenneman and Gozes, 1996; Brenneman et al., 1998). Subsequent studies have shown that ADNP is dysregulated in schizophrenia (Dresner et al., 2011; Merenlender-Wagner et al., 2015) and Alzheimer's disease (AD) (Yang et al., 2012; Malishkevich et al., 2016), and mutated in autism spectrum disorder (ASD) with 0.17% prevalence (together, these ASD cases are now identified as the ADNP syndrome) (Helsmoortel et al., 2014; Gozes et al., 2015). Importantly, it has been shown that ADNP is the only down-regulated protein in the serum of AD patients (Yang et al., 2012) and expression levels of ADNP in plasma/serum and lymphocyte is correlated with AD clinical progression, disease pathology and premorbid intelligence (Malishkevich et al., 2016). Animal studies with mice expressing *Adnp* from only one allele ($Adnp^{\pm}$) have shown that *Adnp* deficiency is associated with age-dependent neurodegeneration and cognitive impairment, coupled with tauopathy-like features such as an increase formation of tangle-like structures, defective axonal transport, and Tau hyperphosphorylation (Vulih-Shultzman et al., 2007).

Both peptides NAPVSIPQ (ADNP-derived) and SALLRSIPA (ADNF-derived) have shown neuroprotective activities against cognitive decline and peripheral neuropathy in various animal models (Shiryaev et al., 2011; Gozes et al., 2016). NAP biochemical activity has been broadly examined and found to be inextricably linked with microtubules (MTs) and MT-related cellular events: NAP increases MT elongation and dynamics (Ivashko-Pachima et al., 2017), augments axonal transport, in the face of MT deficiencies (Jouroukhin et al., 2013), and protects Tau-MT association under various insults (Oz et al., 2012; Ivashko-Pachima et al., 2017). Mechanistically, both NAPVSIPQ and SALLRSIPA contain a SIP motif that is identified as a variation of SxIP domain, providing direct interaction with MT end-binding proteins (EBs) (Honnappa et al., 2009). Our initial studies have shown a direct interaction of SIP- and SKIP-containing peptides with EB1 and EB3 proteins (Oz et al., 2014). We have further shown that four amino acid peptide SKIP docks to the EB3 binding site *in silico*, and stimulates axonal transport *in vivo*, which is reduced as a consequence of *Adnp* deficiency in Adnp$^{\pm}$ mice (Amram et al., 2016).

Here, we aimed to test the activity of SKIP and modified SKIP - CH_3CO-SKIP-NH_2 (Ac-SKIP) on MT dynamics and integrity, mediated by MT-associated proteins EB1 and Tau. EB proteins can directly influence MT dynamics (Komarova et al., 2009) and also enroll other MT-affecting proteins to the growing MT plus-ends (Honnappa et al., 2009). Tau is a broadly known MT-associated protein which stimulates MT assembly and Tau physiological and biochemical impairments are well-studied in a variety of neurodegenerative diseases, referred to tauopathies (Kneynsberg et al., 2017). Furthermore, it has been found that Tau directly associates with EB1 and EB3 proteins and modulates their location on the MTs (Sayas et al., 2015). Here, we tested different concentrations of SKIP and Ac-SKIP and found that at 10^{-9} M SKIP and Ac-SKIP exhibited consistent and significant activity: (1) increased elongation of freshly growing MT plus-ends; and prevented, (2) Tau-MT dissociation, and (3) MT disassembly, induced by extracellular zinc. Thus, our current study provided a molecular explanation to the previously observed effect of SKIP on MT-related functions: stimulation of axonal transport and normalization of social memory in Adnp ± mice. Furthermore, our results showed that Ac-SKIP provided surprisingly more efficacious neuroprotection and suggested that SKIP might be the shortest motif essential for MT-based neuroprotection, mediated by EB proteins and Tau.

MATERIALS AND METHODS

Cell Culture and Treatments

Mouse neuroblastoma N1E-115 cells (ATCC, Bethesda, MD, United States) were maintained in Dulbecco's modified Eagle's medium (DMEM), 10% fetal bovine serum (FBS), 2 mM glutamine and 100 U/ml penicillin, 100 mg/ml streptomycin (Biological Industries, Beit Haemek, Israel). Human neuroblastoma SH-SYS5 cells (ECACC, Public Health England, Porton Down, Salisbury, United Kingdom; passage numbers from 14 to 16) were maintained in Ham's F12: minimum essential media (MEM) Eagle (1:1), 2 mM Glutamine, 1% non-essential amino acids, 15% FBS and 100 U/ml penicillin, 100 mg/ml streptomycin (Biological Industries, Beit Haemek, Israel). Cells were incubated in 95% air/5% CO_2 in a humidified incubator at 37°C. Cells were differentiated with reduced FBS (2%) and DMSO (1.25%) containing medium (N1E-115 cells) or with retinoic acid at a concentration of 10 μM (SH-SY5Y cells) during 7 days before each experiment. Differentiated N1E-115 cells were treated for 2 or 4 h with SKIP/Ac-SKIP in final concentrations of 10^{-12} - 10^{-6} M, in the absence or presence of zinc (400 μM of $ZnCl_2$, stock solution - 0.1 M $ZnCl_2$ in water, Sigma, Rehovot, Israel).

Cell Viability Assay

A week before the experiment, N1E-115 cells were plated onto 96-well plates at a concentration of 5000 cells/well in 100 μl of the growth medium, which was replaced by differentiation medium a day after cell seeding. On an experimental day, cells were treated during 4 h with 400 μM of $ZnCl_2$ in the absence or presence of NAP (10^{-12} - 10^{-9} M). Cell survival was measured using XTT-based cell proliferation kit (Biological Industries, Beit Haemek, Israel), which was performed according to the manufacturer's instructions. The absorbance of the samples was measured with a spectrophotometer (ELISA reader) at wavelengths of 490/630 nm.

Time-Lapse Imaging of EB1 Comet-Like Structures

N1E-115 cells were plated on 35 mm dishes (81156, μ-Dish, Ibidi, Martinsried, Germany) at a concentration of 25000 cells/dish and then differentiated with reduced FBS, DMSO-containing medium during seven days. 48 h before live imaging, differentiated N1E-115 cells were transfected with 1 μg of EB1-RFP expressing plasmid. On an experimental day, N1E-115 cells were incubated at 37°C with a 5% CO_2/95% air mixture in a thermostatic chamber placed on the stage of a Leica TCS SP5 confocal microscope (objective ×100 (PL Apo) oil immersion, NA 1.4). Time-lapse images were automatically captured every 3 s during 2 min, using the Leica LAS AF software (Leica Microsystems, Wetzlar, Germany). Data were collected and analyzed by Imaris software (Bitplane, Concord, MA, United States).

Fluorescence Recovery After Photobleaching

Forty-eight hours before a fluorescence recovery after photobleaching (FRAP) experiment, differentiated N1E-115 cells were transfected with a 1 μg pmCherry-C1-Tau3R plasmid (Ivashko-Pachima et al., 2019). FRAP was performed using a Leica TCS SP5 confocal microscope [objective 100× (PL Apo) oil immersion, NA 1.4]. ROIs (regions of interest) for photobleaching were drawn in the proximal cell branches. mCherry-Tau molecules were bleached with argon laser during 15 s, and data about fluorescence recovery after bleaching were automatically collected (80 images every 0.74 s) by the Leica LAS AF software. Fluorescence intensities were measured by ImageJ Fiji (Schindelin et al., 2012), obtained data were normalized with easyFRAP software (Rapsomaniki et al., 2012). FRAP recovery results were fitted by a one-phase exponential association function and recovery curves were built using GraphPad Prism 6 (GraphPad Software, Inc., La Jolla, CA). Samples with $R^2 < 0.9$ were excluded.

Polymerized vs. Soluble Tubulin Quantification Assay

Quantification of tubulin polymerization was performed as previously (Oz et al., 2012; Ivashko-Pachima et al., 2017; Ivashko-Pachima and Gozes, 2018). Briefly, in order to extract soluble tubulin (S) differentiated N1E-115 cells were lysed with TritonX-100-containing MT-buffer (80 mM PIPES pH6.8, 1 mM $MgCl_2$, 2 mM EGTA, 5% Glycerol, with or without 0.5% TritonX-100) at room temperature for 5 min while centrifuging at 800 rcf; in order to collect the polymerized tubulin (P) pelleted cells were rinsed once again with equal volume of modified RIPA buffer (50 mM Tris–HCl pH7.4, 150 mM NaCl, 2 mM EGTA, 1% TritonX-100, 0.1% SDS, 0.1% sodium Deoxycholate, protease and phosphatase inhibitors: 1 mM phenylmethylsulphonyl-fluoride (PMSF), leupeptin 25 μg/ml, pepstatin 25 μg/ml, Na_3VO_4 1 mM, NaF 20 mM) on ice. The soluble and polymerized tubulin fractions were each mixed with the same amount of sample buffer (10 mM Tris–HCl, pH6.8, 1.5% SDS, 0.6% DTT and 6% (v/v) glycerol) and heated at 95°C for 5 min. An equal volume of each fraction was analyzed by immunoblotting with appropriate antibodies, and the results following ECL development (by a chemiluminescence kit, Pierce, Rockford, IL, United States) were quantified by densitometry (using GelQuant.NET software provided by biochemlabsolutions.com).

Co-immunoprecipitation Assay

Proteins were extracted from differentiated human neuroblastoma SH-SY5Y cells and Co-IP assay was performed as previously reported (Merenlender-Wagner et al., 2015; Ivashko-Pachima et al., 2017) using Co-IP kit according to the manufacture protocol (Pierce, Rockford, IL, United States). Briefly, 10 μg of antibodies of interest (EB1, ab53358, Abcam, Cambridge, United Kingdom; and total Tau antibody, AT-5004, MBL, Billerica, MA, United States) were cross-linked to the 30 μl of A/G PLUS-agarose beads (provided by the Co-IP kit). 2 μg of SKIP or Ac-SKIP, diluted into lysis buffer were added per sample (1 mg of cell lysate) for 2 h at room temperature. Flow-through, wash and elution fractions were then collected and analyzed by immunoblotting with appropriate antibodies, and the results following ECL (Pierce) development were quantified by densitometry (GelQuant.NET software provided by biochemlabsolutions.com).

Antibody List

Tubulin – monoclonal α-tubulin antibody (mouse IgG1 isotype, T6199, Sigma, Rehovot, Israel). Actin – mouse monoclonal actin antibody (Sigma, Rehovot, Israel). The secondary antibodies were peroxidase-conjugated AffiniPure goat anti-mouse IgG (Jackson ImmunoResearch, United States).

Statistical Analysis

Data are presented as the mean ± SEM from at least 3 independent experiments performed in triplicates. Statistical analysis of the data was performed by using one-way ANOVA test (followed by the Turkey or LSD *post hoc* test) by IBM SPSS Statistics software version 23 (IBM, Armonk, NY, United States). $^{*}P < 0.05$, $^{**}P < 0.01$, $^{***}P < 0.001$. Detailed statistical data are summarized in the **Supplementary File.**

RESULTS

The Protective Effect of SKIP and Ac-SKIP Against Cell Death Induced by Zinc Toxicity

A colorimetric method for cell viability (based on the tetrazolium salt – XTT) was used to assess the protective activity of SKIP and Ac-SKIP at different concentrations (10^{-12} – 10^{-9}M) against the cytotoxic effect of zinc in order to choose potent concentration for the further experiments. Differentiated neuroblastoma N1E-115 cells were treated with zinc alone or together with Ac-SKIP or SKIP for 4 h, and XTT-produced soluble dye was then measured by ELISA reader. Previously published data have shown a consistent and significant effect of zinc cytotoxicity at 400 μM (Sanchez-Martin et al., 2010; Oz et al., 2012; Ivashko-Pachima et al., 2017). Hence, here, we worked with 400 μM of zinc. Treatment with zinc caused a reduction of ~50% in cell viability, and peptide treatments showed significant protection against cell death, except for Ac-SKIP at 10^{-12} M. SKIP treatment at every examined concentration exhibited nearly equal ~20% protection that was found statistically significant. Ac-SKIP protective potency was found to be positively dependent on the peptide concentration: non-significant slight protection at 10^{-12} M; significant, a moderate effect at 10^{-11} M; and a ~100% protective effect at 10^{-10} M and 10^{-9} M. Ac-SKIP and SKIP exhibited the same protective potency at 10^{-11} M and significantly different magnitude of protective activity at 10^{-12} M (with a greater effect of SKIP), 10^{-10} M and 10^{-9} M (with a significantly greater effect of Ac-SKIP). For further experiments, we chose to work with 10^{-12} M and 10^{-9} M of Ac-SKIP/SKIP (**Figure 1**).

Ac-SKIP and SKIP Affect MT Dynamics

The direct interaction between SKIP and EB1/3 has been previously predicted by Pymol (Schrödinger, 2015), and peptides containing SxIP motif have displayed the association with EB1/3 in sulfolink columns. Here, we aimed to evaluate the effect of SKIP and Ac-SKIP on MT dynamics, mediated by direct interaction of these peptides with the EB1 protein. Differentiated

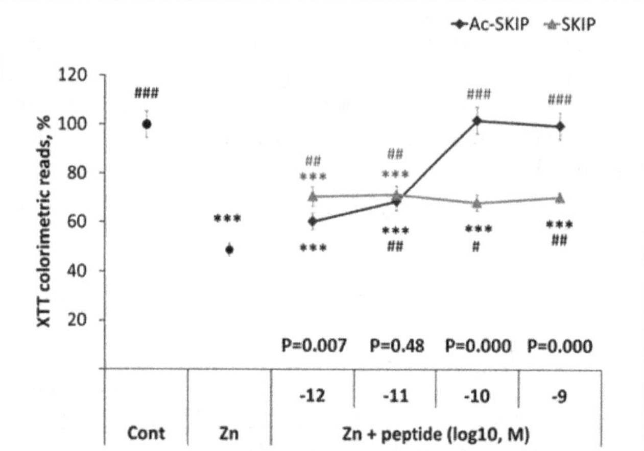

FIGURE 1 | SKIP and Ac-SKIP exhibit protective activity against zinc cytotoxicity in differentiated neuroblastoma N1E-115 cells. Results of mitochondrial activity were obtained by XTT colorimetric assay. "Cont" – cells without any treatment (n = 60); "Zn" – cells, exposed to 400 μM of zinc (n = 58); "Zn + peptide" – cells treated with zinc (400 μM) and different concentrations of Ac-SKIP or SKIP: 10^{-12} M Ac-SKIP (n = 22)/SKIP (n = 14), 10^{-11} M Ac-SKIP (n = 22)/SKIP (n = 14), 10^{-10} M Ac-SKIP (n = 22)/SKIP (n = 14), 10^{-9} M Ac-SKIP (n = 22)/SKIP (n = 14). Statistical analysis was performed by One-way ANOVA: $^{***}p < 0.001$, *post hoc* comparisons made in reference to "Cont" group; $\#p < 0.05$, $\#\#p < 0.01$, $\#\#\#p < 0.001$, *post hoc* comparisons made in reference to "Zn" group. Statistical analysis within the concentration group of peptides was done by the Student's t-test and P-values are displayed on the graph above concentration scale of peptides.

neuroblastoma cells were subjected to transient transfection with expression plasmid encoding to EB1 protein, tagged to RFP (**Figure 2A** and **Supplementary Figure S1**). Single-cell time-lapse imaging allowed the evaluation of the effect of the peptides on MT dynamics by tracking RFP-EB1 comet-like structures decorating newly polymerized MT plus-ends. Time-lapse imaging followed by the 4 h peptide treatment with Ac-SKIP or SKIP showed that both Ac-SKIP and SKIP at 10^{-9} M (but not at 10^{-12} M) significantly augmented the track length (**Figure 2B**) and velocity (**Figure 2C**) of the EB1 comets, reflecting the lengths of the MT growing events and the speed of MT assembly, respectively. Thus, both peptides had an impact on MT dynamics.

Protective Effect of Ac-SKIP and SKIP on Tau-MT Association, Disrupted by Zinc

In order to evaluate the protective activity of Ac-SKIP and SKIP against Tau-MT discharge we performed FRAP assay using zinc as Tau-MT dissociation agent (Craddock et al., 2012; Huang et al., 2014). Differentiated N1E-115 cells were transfected with a plasmid expressing mCherry-tagged Tau protein, and FRAP imaging (**Figure 3A** and **Supplementary Figure S2**) was performed after an hour of cell exposure to zinc alone or together with Ac-SKIP or SKIP (10^{-12} M, 10^{-9} M). MT regions decorated by mCherry-Tau were bleached (**Figure 3A**, marked squares, 0 s after bleaching) and recovery of mCherry fluorescence (**Figure 3A**, marked squares, 88 s after bleaching) resulted from interchange between MT-bound Tau (carrying bleached mCherry molecules) and previously unbound Tau proteins (carrying unbleached mCherry molecules). Thus, an unrecovered fraction of the initial mCherry fluorescence within a given bleached area indicated the immobile fraction mCherry-Tau proteins, reflecting Tau interaction with MTs. Subsequent analysis of the data obtained with a one-phase exponential association (**Figures 3B,C**) showed that zinc significantly abated Tau immobile fraction in comparison to the non-treated control (**Figures 3B,C**). Ac-SKIP and SKIP at both examined concentrations (10^{-12} M and 10^{-9} M) prevented excessive Tau release from MTs, induced by zinc, which was found statistically significant in comparison to zinc treatment alone (**Figures 3B,C**).

Ac-SKIP and SKIP Prevent MT Disassembly, Induced by Zinc Intoxication

Further, we aimed to determine the protective effect of Ac-SKIP and SKIP against MT disassembly induced by zinc as an MT disruptor. We examined the relative levels of polymerized and soluble tubulin pools in differentiated N1E-115 cells, exposed to extracellular zinc (400 μM) alone or together with Ac-SKIP or SKIP (10^{-12} M and 10^{-9} M). After treatment cells were lysed (as described in section "Materials and Methods" section) and the tubulin levels of polymerized and soluble fractions were evaluated by western blotting (**Figure 4A**, Tubulin panel, and **Supplementary Figure S3A**) followed by densitometric quantification (**Figure 4B**). Non-treated control cells exhibited a nearly equal distribution of tubulin between soluble (S) and polymerized (P) fractions, while zinc treatment significantly increased the ratio of soluble to polymerized tubulin content (**Figure 4A**, Tubulin panel; **Figure 4B**). Ac-SKIP or SKIP added together with zinc exhibited reduced the tubulin content in the soluble fraction compared to "zinc" group, which was found statistically significant for all peptide treatments, except for Ac-SKIP at 10^{-12} M (**Figure 4A**, Tubulin panel; **Figure 4B**).

There was no observed effect on the actin-microfilament pool following neither zinc nor Ac-SKIP/SKIP treatment (**Figure 4A**, Actin panel, and **Supplementary Figures S3B, S4**), suggesting that zinc/Ac-SKIP/SKIP had selective effects on the MT cytoskeleton.

SKIP/Ac-SKIP Enhance Tau-EB1 and Tau-Tubulin Interactions

To study the effect of SKIP and Ac-SKIP on the crosstalk between EB1-Tau and -tubulin, we performed co-immunoprecipitation (Co-IP) assays in differentiated human neuroblastoma SH-SY5Y cells as previously reported (Merenlender-Wagner et al., 2015; Ivashko-Pachima et al., 2017). We examined the effect of SKIP and Ac-SKIP on EB1-Tau interaction by protein complex immunoprecipitation (Co-IP) assays, using EB1 and Tau antibodies linked to agarose beads (**Figure 4C**, IP: EB1; **Figure 4D**, IP: Tau). The elution fractions, obtained from immunoprecipitations (IPs) performed with either anti-EB1 or anti-Tau, were analyzed by immunoblotting (IB) with EB1 and Tau antibodies (**Figure 4C**, IP: EB1 IB: Tau; **Figure 4D**, IP: Tau IB: EB1). Results showed that both SKIP and Ac-SKIP increased Tau-EB1 association, compared to the samples

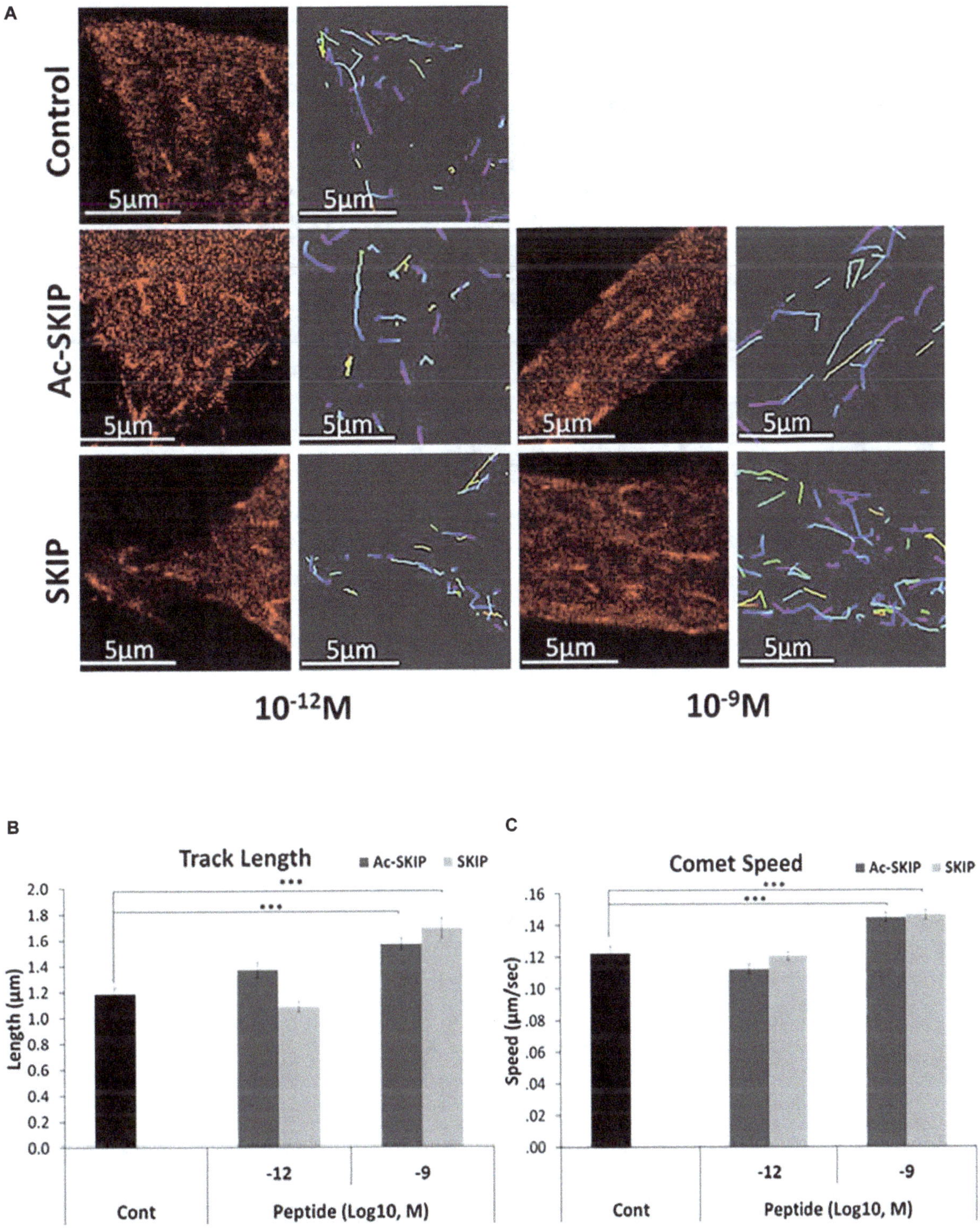

FIGURE 2 | SKIP and Ac-SKIP affect MT dynamics. **(A)** Live imaging of N1E-115 cells expressing EB1-RFP was performed after 4 h of treatment with Ac-SKIP or SKIP at 10^{-12} M and 10^{-9} M. Transfected cells without peptide treatment were used as a control group ("Control"). Time-lapse images were automatically captured every 3 s. during a 1 min using the Leica LAS AF software. Tracks of EB1 comet like structures presented as colored lines and were obtained by the Imaris software. Graphs represent quantification of the average track length **(B)** and comet speed **(C)**. Data were collected in unbiased fashion by the Imaris software, and statistical analysis of the data was performed by One-way ANOVA. Statistical significance is represented by $^{***}P < 0.001$. Comet length: Control, $n = 46$; Ac-SKIP 10^{-12} M, $n = 29$; SKIP 10^{-12} M, $n = 20$; Ac-SKIP 10^{-9} M, $n = 62$; SKIP 10^{-9} M, $n = 43$. Comet speed: Control, $n = 47$; Ac-SKIP 10^{-12} M, $n = 30$; SKIP 10^{-12} M, $n = 20$; Ac-SKIP 10^{-9} M, $n = 65$; SKIP 10^{-9} M, $n = 43$.

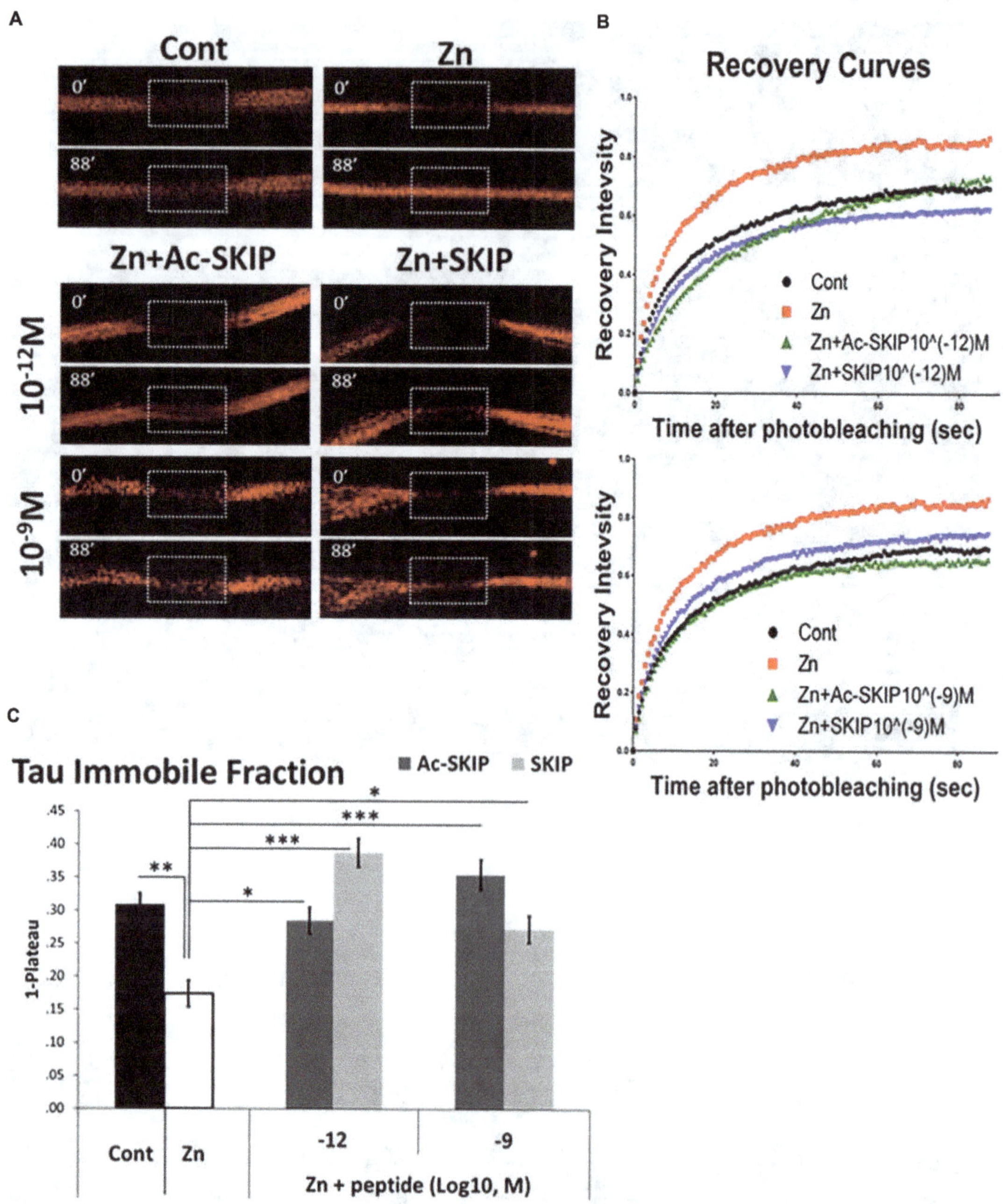

FIGURE 3 | Ac-SKIP and SKIP protective effect on Tau interaction with MTs, assessed by FRAP analysis. FRAP was performed on differentiated neuroblastoma N1E-115 cells after 2 h of treatment with extracellular zinc (400 μM) alone or together with Ac-SKIP or SKIP (10^{-12} M and 10^{-9} M). **(A)** Representative images of FRAP and fluorescence recovery of mCherry molecules conjugated to Tau. Marked squares represent the regions of bleaching immediately after photo-bleaching (0′–0 s after bleaching) and subsequent fluorescent recovery (88′–88 s after bleaching). **(B)** Obtained data of fluorescent recovery were normalized and recovery curves were built according to one-phase exponential association (see section "Materials and Methods"). **(C)** The graph represents the fitted data (by one-phase exponential association, see section "Materials and Methods") of immobile fractions (collected on 88 s after photobleaching). Statistical analysis was performed by One-way ANOVA with Tukey HSD. Statistical significance is presented by $^{*}P < 0.05$, $^{**}P < 0.01$, $^{***}P < 0.001$. Control, $n = 82$; Zn, $n = 43$; Zn + Ac-SKIP 10^{-12} M, $n = 44$; Zn + SKIP 10^{-12} M, $n = 79$; Zn + Ac-SKIP 10^{-9} M, $n = 76$; Zn + SKIP 10^{-9} M, $n = 81$.

incubated without these peptides (**Figure 4C**, IP: EB1 Cont – control, IB: Tau; **Figure 4D**, IP: Tau Cont IB: EB1). IP: EB1 IB: EB1 showed a significant increase in EB1-EB1 interaction (EB1 homodimer formation) following SKIP treatment and moderate non-significant increase following Ac-SKIP, compared to the control (**Figure 4C**, IP: EB1 Cont IB: EB1). IP: Tau IB: Tau did not show significant differences in Tau-Tau association following incubation with either SKIP or Ac-SKIP (**Figure 4D**). Further immunoblotting analysis with tubulin antibodies suggested increased Tau-tubulin, interaction following treatments with

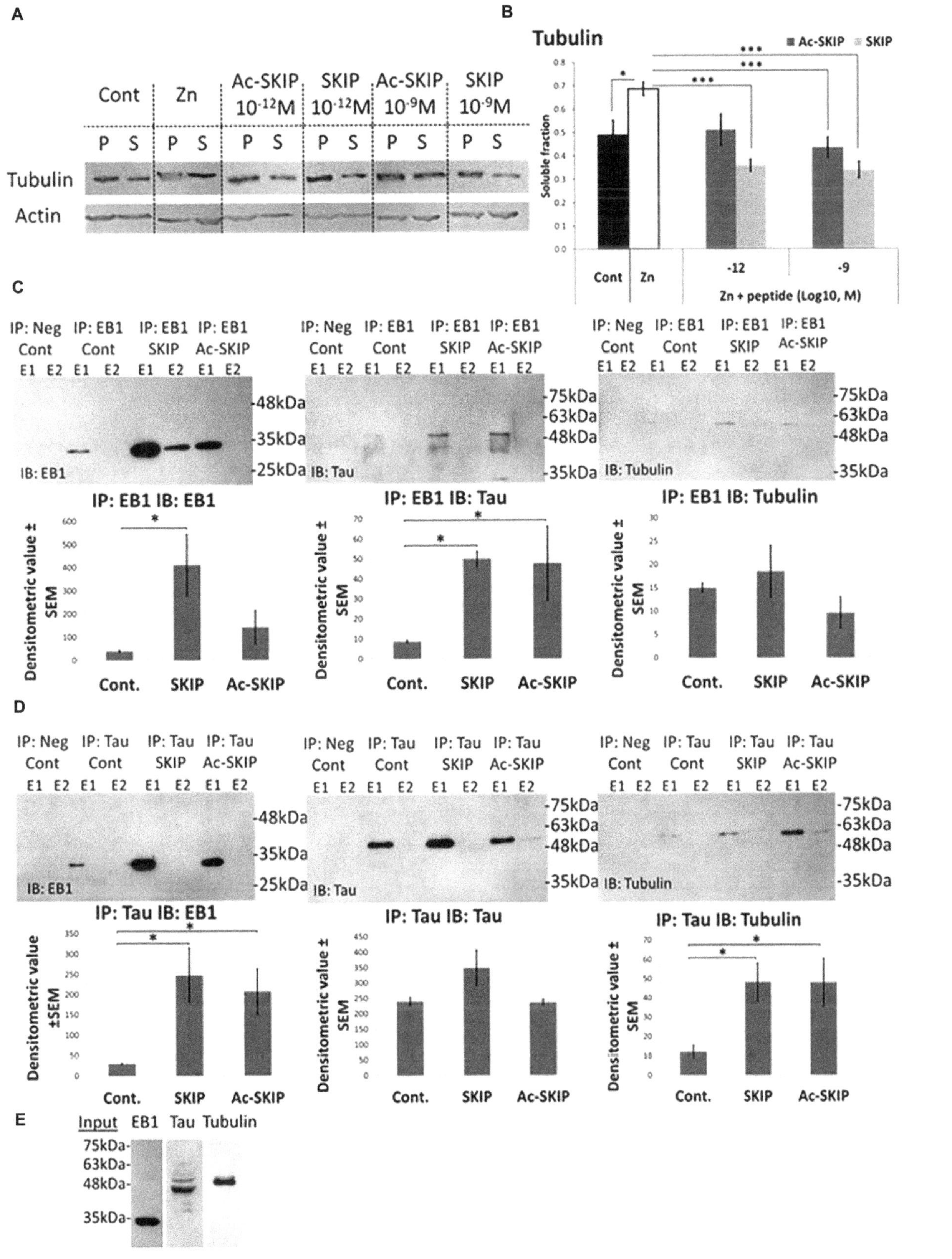

FIGURE 4 | Continued

FIGURE 4 | Ac-SKIP and SKIP effect on the polymerized vs. the soluble tubulin pool and the crosstalk between EB-Tau-tubulin. **(A)** Immunoblotting of polymerized (P) and soluble (S) protein fractions (obtained by polymerized vs. soluble tubulin assay, see section "Materials and Methods") with tubulin antibodies. Cells were treated with zinc (400 μM, 4 h) with or without Ac-SKIP or SKIP (10^{-12} M and 10^{-9} M, 4 h), non-treated cells served as controls. **(B)** The graph represents the densitometric quantification of soluble tubulin ratios. The intensity of each band was quantified by densitometry and the soluble protein ratio was calculated by dividing the densitometric value of soluble proteins by the total protein content (S/[S + P]). Statistical analysis was performed by One Way ANOVA with Tukey HSD. $^*P < 0.05$, $^{**}P < 0.01$, $^{***}P < 0.001$; Control, $n = 15$; Zn, $n = 18$; Zn + Ac-SKIP 10^{-12} M, $n = 15$; Zn + SKIP 10^{-12} M, $n = 9$; Zn + Ac-SKIP 10^{-9} M, $n = 18$; Zn + SKIP 10^{-9} M, $n = 11$. **(C,D)** A Co-IP assay was performed with EB1 or Tau antibodies, linked to agarose beads. SKIP (2 μg/sample) or Ac-SKIP (2 μg/sample), diluted into Pierce lysis buffer (see section "Materials and Methods") or the equal volume of lysis buffer w/o peptides (IP: EB1 Cont; IP: Tau Cont) were added to cell lysate of differentiated SH-SY5Y cells, 15 min before EB1 or Tau column application (IP: EB1; IP: Tau). Sequential IP elution fractions (E1, E2) were further analyzed by immunoblotting with EB1, Tau, and Tubulin antibodies (IB: EB1; IB: Tau; IB: Tubulin). In addition, columns with free agarose beads were used as negative controls (IP: Neg cont). The intensity of each band was quantified by densitometry. The bar graph shows the ratio of band intensities (densitometric value ± SEM) obtained upon SKIP and Ac-SKIP treatments as compared with non-treated cells (Cont). Statistical analysis was performed by One Way ANOVA with LSD HSD. Experiments were independently repeated three times. $^*P < 0.05$, $^{**}P < 0.01$, $^{***}P < 0.001$. **(E)** Cell lysates without column exposure were used as positive controls (Input). IP – immunoprecipitation, IB – immunoblot.

SKIP and Ac-SKIP (**Figure 4D**, IP: Tau IB: tubulin), while EB1-tubulin association remained without significant changes (**Figure 4C**, IP: EB1 IB: tubulin). Cell lysates without column exposure were used as positive controls (Input, **Figure 4E**) and flow-through and washing fractions were also collected and analyzed by immunoblotting with EB1 and Tau antibodies (**Supplementary Figure S5A**, IP: EB1 IB: EB1; **Supplementary Figure S5B**, IP: Tau IB: Tau).

DISCUSSION

Maintenance of axonal structure and transport underlies neuronal signal transduction and connectivity, and provide a proper brain function (Rasband, 2010). It has been well-established that axonal degeneration (axonopathy) is a central pathogenic feature common to numerous human tauopathies, including AD (Kneynsberg et al., 2017). Atrophy of axon-reach white matter is significant in patients with mild cognitive impairment and extends widely in advanced AD cases, while the degree of atrophy is associated with loss of cognitive functioning (Huang and Auchus, 2007). Furthermore, immunohistochemical analyses of AD brains have revealed that formation of neuropil threads (Tau inclusions within dystrophic neurites) are a prominent AD neuropathological feature that appears before neurofibrillary tangles (NFTs) (Kowall and Kosik, 1987). Mechanistically, a clear correlation between Tau lesions and axonopathy has been demonstrated by multiple models, linking aberrant phosphoregulation of Tau to alterations in axonal transport, and deficits in axonal transport to dying-back degeneration of neurons (Kanaan et al., 2011, 2012, 2013).

The functional repertoire of Tau includes, among other characteristics, regulation of EB protein localization on MTs (Sayas et al., 2015). EBs are MT plus-end tracking proteins that decorate growing MT ends and recruit a variety of other proteins that connect MTs to various cellular structures (Jiang et al., 2012) and control MT dynamics (Komarova et al., 2009). EB-binding proteins directly interact with EBs through a core SxIP motif (Honnappa et al., 2009).

We have previously shown that EB1/3-targeting SKIP ameliorates impaired axonal transport and social memory deficits in the face of *Adnp* deficiency (Adnp$^{\pm}$ mice) (Amram et al., 2016). Our current study focused on the molecular activity of SKIP and Ac-SKIP on the cellular compartment, relevant to the axonal transport – MTs, and MT-associated proteins Tau and EB1. We showed that SKIP and Ac-SKIP significantly increased the elongation and growth rate of MT plus-ends, mediated by EB1 proteins. Furthermore, the protective activity of SKIP and Ac-SKIP on Tau-MT interaction and MT integrity was assessed in the face of zinc intoxication. The well-established hypothesis of zinc dyshomeostasis in AD suggests aberrant zinc accumulation by Aβ-amyloid plaques, resulting in too low, or excessively high intracellular zinc concentrations (up to 1 mM) in zinc-enriched brain regions implicated in the cognitive functions and vulnerable to AD pathology (Deibel et al., 1996; Craddock et al., 2012; DeGrado et al., 2016). It has been suggested that high intracellular zinc concentrations (more than 100 μM) present adverse effects on nerve fibers during stimulation (Minami et al., 2006) and may lead to pathological implications and neuronal cell death (Frederickson et al., 2005; Sensi et al., 2009, 2011; Shuttleworth and Weiss, 2011). In addition, it has been shown that abnormally high concentrations (up to 250 μM) of zinc induce GSK-3β activation and Tau release from MTs (Boom et al., 2009). Neuronal loss has been observed when zinc levels reached 10–100 nM in the neuronal soma *in vitro* (Aizenman et al., 2000; Jiang et al., 2001; Bossy-Wetzel et al., 2004) and zinc influx of 300 μM causes ischemic neurodegeneration in rat brains and cortical cultures (Koh et al., 1996). It has also been found that NFTs and amyloid-beta (Aβ) plaques contain abnormally high levels of zinc (Bush et al., 1994a; Lee et al., 2018). Furthermore, it has been demonstrated that Aβ 1–40 (a major component of AD cerebral amyloid) specifically and in a saturable fashion binds zinc (Bush et al., 1994b) that could accelerate the Aβ plaques formation at 200 μM of zinc (Lee et al., 2018).

Here, we demonstrated an effect of SKIP and Ac-SKIP on the crosstalk between Tau, EB1, and MTs. In this respect, it has been previously shown that Tau directly interacts with EB proteins, modulating MT dynamics (Sayas et al., 2015). Based on the observed results, we suggest that the effect of SKIP and Ac-SKIP on MTs integrity and dynamics is mediated by increasing interaction between EB1 and Tau that is accompanied by the increased association of Tau with tubulin. In addition, SKIP and Ac-SKIP (the last with more moderate effect) enhance EB1 homodimer formation. EB proteins form homo- and heterodimers and play a master role in organizing dynamic protein networks in mammalian cells

(Akhmanova and Steinmetz, 2015). EB1 homodimers have a higher affinity to the p150^{glued} – N-terminal CAP-Gly domain of the dynactin (Honnappa et al., 2006; Bjelic et al., 2012), which in turn acts as a co-factor for the MT motor protein dynein. EB1-dependent ordered recruitment of dynactin to the MT plus-end is required for efficient initiation of retrograde axonal transport (Moughamian et al., 2013). Furthermore, actin-MT linkers – spectraplakins promote axonal growth in an EB1-dependent manner and stabilize MTs in the face of pharmacologically induced depolymerization (Alves-Silva et al., 2012). Thus, increased EB1 homodimer formation by SKIP/Ac-SKIP may have a direct effect on axonal retrograde transport, axonal growth, and neuroprotection.

The differential potency and efficacy of SKIP and Ac-SKIP might be attributed to potential steric hindrance of the modified SKIP at low concentration, and differential residence time at higher concentrations affecting cellular survival. Regardless, since MT organization and dynamics is central in axonal MT cytoskeleton and transport our current study provided a compelling molecular explanation to the *in vivo* activity of SKIP, placing SKIP motif as a central focus for MT-based neuroprotection in tauopathies with axonal transport implication. As MT reduction in AD and aging is independent of Tau filament formation (Cash et al., 2003), our studies implicate a paucity/dysregulation of EB-interacting endogenous proteins, like ADNP (Oz et al., 2014; Malishkevich et al., 2016) as a contributing mechanism and further provides hope with SKIP-containing drug candidates in future *in vivo* studies.

AUTHOR CONTRIBUTIONS

YI-P designed and performed the work and wrote the initial draft. IG inspired the project, guided the progress, provided all the required support, and finalized the manuscript.

ACKNOWLEDGMENTS

IG is the incumbent of the Lily and Avraham Gildor Chair for the Investigation of Growth Factors, and the Director of the Dr. Diana and Zelman Elton (Elbaum) Laboratory for Molecular Neuroendocrinology at Tel Aviv University. We thank Dr. Laura Sayas for her excellent collaboration and teaching us the microtubule dynamics methodology. This work is in partial fulfillment of the Ph.D. thesis requirements of Ms. Yanina Ivashko-Pachima and Ms. Alicia Koplowitz fellowship.

REFERENCES

Aizenman, E., Stout, A. K., Hartnett, K. A., Dineley, K. E., McLaughlin, B., and Reynolds, I. J. (2000). Induction of neuronal apoptosis by thiol oxidation: putative role of intracellular zinc release. *J. Neurochem.* 75, 1878–1888. doi: 10.1046/j.1471-4159.2000.0751878.x

Akhmanova, A., and Steinmetz, M. O. (2015). Control of microtubule organization and dynamics: two ends in the limelight. *Nat. Rev. Mol. Cell Biol.* 16, 711–726. doi: 10.1038/nrm4084

Alves-Silva, J., Sanchez-Soriano, N., Beaven, R., Klein, M., Parkin, J., Millard, T. H., et al. (2012). Spectraplakins promote microtubule-mediated axonal growth by functioning as structural microtubule-associated proteins and EB1-dependent +TIPs (tip interacting proteins). *J. Neurosci.* 32, 9143–9158. doi: 10.1523/JNEUROSCI.0416-12.2012

Amram, N., Hacohen-Kleiman, G., Sragovich, S., Malishkevich, A., Katz, J., Touloumi, O., et al. (2016). Sexual divergence in microtubule function: the novel intranasal microtubule targeting SKIP normalizes axonal transport and enhances memory. *Mol. Psychiatry* 21, 1467–1476. doi: 10.1038/mp.2015.208

Bassan, M., Zamostiano, R., Davidson, A., Pinhasov, A., Giladi, E., Perl, O., et al. (1999). Complete sequence of a novel protein containing a femtomolar-activity-dependent neuroprotective peptide. *J. Neurochem.* 72, 1283–1293. doi: 10.1046/j.1471-4159.1999.0721283.x

Bjelic, S., De Groot, C. O., Scharer, M. A., Jaussi, R., Bargsten, K., Salzmann, M., et al. (2012). Interaction of mammalian end binding proteins with CAP-Gly domains of CLIP-170 and p150(glued). *J. Struct. Biol.* 177, 160–167. doi: 10.1016/j.jsb.2011.11.010

Boom, A., Authelet, M., Dedecker, R., Frederick, C., Van Heurck, R., Daubie, V., et al. (2009). Bimodal modulation of tau protein phosphorylation and conformation by extracellular Zn2+ in human-tau transfected cells. *Biochim. Biophys. Acta* 1793, 1058–1067. doi: 10.1016/j.bbamcr.2008.11.011

Bossy-Wetzel, E., Talantova, M. V., Lee, W. D., Scholzke, M. N., Harrop, A., Mathews, E., et al. (2004). Crosstalk between nitric oxide and zinc pathways to neuronal cell death involving mitochondrial dysfunction and p38-activated K+ channels. *Neuron* 41, 351–365. doi: 10.1016/s0896-6273(04)00015-17

Brenneman, D. E., Glazner, G., Hill, J. M., Hauser, J., Davidson, A., and Gozes, I. (1998). VIP neurotrophism in the central nervous system: multiple effectors and identification of a femtomolar-acting neuroprotective peptide. *Ann. N. Y. Acad. Sci.* 865, 207–212. doi: 10.1111/j.1749-6632.1998.tb11180.x

Brenneman, D. E., and Gozes, I. (1996). A femtomolar-acting neuroprotective peptide. *J. Clin. Invest.* 97, 2299–2307. doi: 10.1172/JCI118672

Bush, A. I., Pettingell, W. H. Jr., de Paradis, M., Tanzi, R. E., and Wasco, W. (1994a). The amyloid beta-protein precursor and its mammalian homologues. Evidence for a zinc-modulated heparin-binding superfamily. *J. Biol. Chem.* 26618–26621.

Bush, A. I, Pettingell, W. H., Multhaup, G., d Paradis, M., Vonsattel, J. P., Gusella, J. F., et al. (1994b). Rapid induction of Alzheimer A beta amyloid formation by zinc. *Science* 265, 1464–1467. doi: 10.1126/science.8073293

Cash, A. D., Aliev, G., Siedlak, S. L., Nunomura, A., Fujioka, H., Zhu, X., et al. (2003). Microtubule reduction in Alzheimer's disease and aging is independent of tau filament formation. *Am. J. Pathol.* 162, 1623–1627.

Craddock, T. J., Tuszynski, J. A., Chopra, D., Casey, N., Goldstein, L. E., Hameroff, S. R., et al. (2012). The zinc dyshomeostasis hypothesis of Alzheimer's disease. *PLoS One* 7:e33552. doi: 10.1371/journal.pone.0033552

DeGrado, T. R., Kemp, B. J., Pandey, M. K., Jiang, H., Gunderson, T. M., Linscheid, L. R., et al. (2016). First PET imaging studies with 63Zn-zinc citrate in healthy human participants and patients with alzheimer disease. *Mol. Imaging* 15:1536012116673793. doi: 10.1177/1536012116673793

Deibel, M. A., Ehmann, W. D., and Markesbery, W. R. (1996). Copper, iron, and zinc imbalances in severely degenerated brain regions in Alzheimer's disease: possible relation to oxidative stress. *J. Neurol. Sci.* 143, 137–142. doi: 10.1016/s0022-510x(96)00203-1

Dresner, E., Agam, G., and Gozes, I. (2011). Activity-dependent neuroprotective protein (ADNP) expression level is correlated with the expression of the sister protein ADNP2: deregulation in schizophrenia. *Eur. Neuropsychopharmacol.* 21, 355–361. doi: 10.1016/j.euroneuro.2010.06.004

Frederickson, C. J., Koh, J. Y., and Bush, A. I. (2005). The neurobiology of zinc in health and disease. *Nat. Rev. Neurosci.* 6, 449–462. doi: 10.1038/nrn1671

Gozes, I., Helsmoortel, C., Vandeweyer, G., Van der Aa, N., Kooy, F., and Sermone, S. B. (2015). The compassionate side of neuroscience: tony sermone's undiagnosed genetic journey–ADNP mutation. *J. Mol. Neurosci.* 56, 751–757. doi: 10.1007/s12031-015-0586-586

Gozes, I., Sragovich, S., Schirer, Y., and Idan-Feldman, A. (2016). D-SAL and NAP: two peptides sharing a SIP domain. *J. Mol. Neurosci.* 59, 220–231. doi: 10.1007/s12031-015-0701-708

Helsmoortel, C., Vulto-van Silfhout, A. T., Coe, B. P., Vandeweyer, G., Rooms, L., van den Ende, J., et al. (2014). A SWI/SNF-related autism syndrome caused by de novo mutations in ADNP. *Nat. Genet.* 46, 380–384. doi: 10.1038/ng.2899

Honnappa, S., Gouveia, S. M., Weisbrich, A., Damberger, F. F., Bhavesh, N. S., Jawhari, H., et al. (2009). An EB1-binding motif acts as a microtubule tip localization signal. *Cell* 138, 366–376. doi: 10.1016/j.cell.2009.04.065

Honnappa, S., Okhrimenko, O., Jaussi, R., Jawhari, H., Jelesarov, I., Winkler, F. K., et al. (2006). Key interaction modes of dynamic +TIP networks. *Mol. Cell* 23, 663–671. doi: 10.1016/j.molcel.2006.07.013

Huang, J., and Auchus, A. P. (2007). Diffusion tensor imaging of normal appearing white matter and its correlation with cognitive functioning in mild cognitive impairment and Alzheimer's disease. *Ann. N. Y. Acad. Sci.* 1097, 259–264. doi: 10.1196/annals.1379.021

Huang, Y., Wu, Z., Cao, Y., Lang, M., Lu, B., and Zhou, B. (2014). Zinc binding directly regulates tau toxicity independent of tau hyperphosphorylation. *Cell Rep.* 8, 831–842. doi: 10.1016/j.celrep.2014.06.047

Ivashko-Pachima, Y., and Gozes, I. (2018). NAP protects against tau hyperphosphorylation through GSK3. *Curr. Pharm. Des.* 24, 3868–3877. doi: 10.2174/1381612824666181112105954

Ivashko-Pachima, Y., Maor-Nof, M., and Gozes, I. (2019). NAP (davunetide) preferential interaction with dynamic 3-repeat Tau explains differential protection in selected tauopathies. *PLoS One* 14:e0213666. doi: 10.1371/journal.pone.0213666

Ivashko-Pachima, Y., Sayas, C. L., Malishkevich, A., and Gozes, I. (2017). ADNP/NAP dramatically increase microtubule end-binding protein-Tau interaction: a novel avenue for protection against tauopathy. *Mol. Psychiatry* 22, 1335–1344. doi: 10.1038/mp.2016.255

Jiang, D., Sullivan, P. G., Sensi, S. L., Steward, O., and Weiss, J. H. (2001). Zn(2+) induces permeability transition pore opening and release of pro-apoptotic peptides from neuronal mitochondria. *J. Biol. Chem.* 276, 47524–47529. doi: 10.1074/jbc.M108834200

Jiang, K., Toedt, G., Montenegro Gouveia, S., Davey, N. E., Hua, S., van der Vaart, B., et al. (2012). A Proteome-wide screen for mammalian SxIP motif-containing microtubule plus-end tracking proteins. *Curr. Biol.* 22, 1800–1807. doi: 10.1016/j.cub.2012.07.047

Jouroukhin, Y., Ostritsky, R., Assaf, Y., Pelled, G., Giladi, E., and Gozes, I. (2013). NAP (davunetide) modifies disease progression in a mouse model of severe neurodegeneration: protection against impairments in axonal transport. *Neurobiol. Dis.* 56, 79–94. doi: 10.1016/j.nbd.2013.04.012

Kanaan, N. M., Morfini, G., Pigino, G., LaPointe, N. E., Andreadis, A., Song, Y., et al. (2012). Phosphorylation in the amino terminus of tau prevents inhibition of anterograde axonal transport. *Neurobiol. Aging* 33, e815–e830. doi: 10.1016/j.neurobiolaging.2011.06.006

Kanaan, N. M., Morfini, G. A., LaPointe, N. E., Pigino, G. F., Patterson, K. R., Song, Y., et al. (2011). Pathogenic forms of tau inhibit kinesin-dependent axonal transport through a mechanism involving activation of axonal phosphotransferases. *J. Neurosci.* 31, 9858–9868. doi: 10.1523/JNEUROSCI.0560-11.2011

Kanaan, N. M., Pigino, G. F., Brady, S. T., Lazarov, O., Binder, L. I., and Morfini, G. A. (2013). Axonal degeneration in Alzheimer's disease: when signaling abnormalities meet the axonal transport system. *Exp. Neurol.* 246, 44–53. doi: 10.1016/j.expneurol.2012.06.003

Kneynsberg, A., Combs, B., Christensen, K., Morfini, G., and Kanaan, N. M. (2017). Axonal degeneration in tauopathies: disease relevance and underlying mechanisms. *Front. Neurosci.* 11:572. doi: 10.3389/fnins.2017.00572

Koh, J. Y., Suh, S. W., Gwag, B. J., He, Y. Y., Hsu, C. Y., and Choi, D. W. (1996). The role of zinc in selective neuronal death after transient global cerebral ischemia. *Science* 272, 1013–1016. doi: 10.1126/science.272.5264.1013

Komarova, Y., De Groot, C. O., Grigoriev, I., Gouveia, S. M., Munteanu, E. L., Schober, J. M., et al. (2009). Mammalian end binding proteins control persistent microtubule growth. *J. Cell Biol.* 184, 691–706. doi: 10.1083/jcb.200807179

Kowall, N. W., and Kosik, K. S. (1987). Axonal disruption and aberrant localization of tau protein characterize the neuropil pathology of Alzheimer's disease. *Ann. Neurol.* 22, 639–643. doi: 10.1002/ana.410220514

Lee, M. C., Yu, W. C., Shih, Y. H., Chen, C. Y., Guo, Z. H., Huang, S. J., et al. (2018). Zinc ion rapidly induces toxic, off-pathway amyloid-beta oligomers distinct from amyloid-beta derived diffusible ligands in Alzheimer's disease. *Sci. Rep.* 8:4772. doi: 10.1038/s41598-018-23122-x

Malishkevich, A., Marshall, G. A., Schultz, A. P., Sperling, R. A., Aharon-Peretz, J., and Gozes, I. (2016). Blood-borne activity-dependent neuroprotective protein (ADNP) is correlated with premorbid intelligence, clinical stage, and alzheimer's disease biomarkers. *J. Alzheimers Dis.* 50, 249–260. doi: 10.3233/JAD-150799

Merenlender-Wagner, A., Malishkevich, A., Shemer, Z., Udawela, M., Gibbons, A., Scarr, E., et al. (2015). Autophagy has a key role in the pathophysiology of schizophrenia. *Mol. Psychiatry* 20, 126–132. doi: 10.1038/mp.2013.174

Minami, A., Sakurada, N., Fuke, S., Kikuchi, K., Nagano, T., Oku, N., et al. (2006). Inhibition of presynaptic activity by zinc released from mossy fiber terminals during tetanic stimulation. *J. Neurosci. Res.* 83, 167–176. doi: 10.1002/jnr.20714

Moughamian, A. J., Osborn, G. E., Lazarus, J. E., Maday, S., and Holzbaur, E. L. (2013). Ordered recruitment of dynactin to the microtubule plus-end is required for efficient initiation of retrograde axonal transport. *J. Neurosci.* 33, 13190–13203. doi: 10.1523/JNEUROSCI.0935-13.2013

Oz, S., Ivashko-Pachima, Y., and Gozes, I. (2012). The ADNP derived peptide, NAP modulates the tubulin pool: implication for neurotrophic and neuroprotective activities. *PLoS One* 7:e51458. doi: 10.1371/journal.pone.0051458

Oz, S., Kapitansky, O., Ivashco-Pachima, Y., Malishkevich, A., Giladi, E., Skalka, N., et al. (2014). The NAP motif of activity-dependent neuroprotective protein (ADNP) regulates dendritic spines through microtubule end binding proteins. *Mol. Psychiatry* 19, 1115–1124. doi: 10.1038/mp.2014.97

Rapsomaniki, M. A., Kotsantis, P., Symeonidou, I. E., Giakoumakis, N. N., Taraviras, S., and Lygerou, Z. (2012). easyFRAP: an interactive, easy-to-use tool for qualitative and quantitative analysis of FRAP data. *Bioinformatics* 28, 1800–1801. doi: 10.1093/bioinformatics/bts241

Rasband, M. N. (2010). The axon initial segment and the maintenance of neuronal polarity. *Nat. Rev. Neurosci.* 11, 552–562. doi: 10.1038/nrn2852

Sanchez-Martin, F. J., Valera, E., Casimiro, I., and Merino, J. M. (2010). Nerve growth factor increases the sensitivity to zinc toxicity and induces cell cycle arrest in PC12 cells. *Brain Res. Bull.* 81, 458–466. doi: 10.1016/j.brainresbull.2009.11.008

Sayas, C. L., Tortosa, E., Bollati, F., Ramirez-Rios, S., Arnal, I., and Avila, J. (2015). Tau regulates the localization and function of End-binding proteins 1 and 3 in developing neuronal cells. *J. Neurochem.* 133, 653–667. doi: 10.1111/jnc.13091

Schindelin, J., Arganda-Carreras, I., Frise, E., Kaynig, V., Longair, M., Pietzsch, T., et al. (2012). Fiji: an open-source platform for biological-image analysis. *Nat. Methods* 9, 676–682. doi: 10.1038/nmeth.2019

Schrödinger, L. (2015). *The PyMOL Molecular Graphics System, Version 2.0.*

Sensi, S. L., Paoletti, P., Bush, A. I., and Sekler, I. (2009). Zinc in the physiology and pathology of the CNS. *Nat. Rev. Neurosci.* 10, 780–791. doi: 10.1038/nrn2734

Sensi, S. L., Paoletti, P., Koh, J. Y., Aizenman, E., Bush, A. I., and Hershfinkel, M. (2011). The neurophysiology and pathology of brain zinc. *J. Neurosci.* 31, 16076–16085. doi: 10.1523/JNEUROSCI.3454-11.2011

Shiryaev, N., Pikman, R., Giladi, E., and Gozes, I. (2011). Protection against tauopathy by the drug candidates NAP (davunetide) and D-SAL: biochemical, cellular and behavioral aspects. *Curr. Pharm. Des.* 17, 2603–2612. doi: 10.2174/138161211797416093

Shuttleworth, C. W., and Weiss, J. H. (2011). Zinc: new clues to diverse roles in brain ischemia. *Trends Pharmacol. Sci.* 32, 480–486. doi: 10.1016/j.tips.2011.04.001

Vulih-Shultzman, I., Pinhasov, A., Mandel, S., Grigoriadis, N., Touloumi, O., Pittel, Z., et al. (2007). Activity-dependent neuroprotective protein snippet NAP reduces tau hyperphosphorylation and enhances learning in a novel transgenic mouse model. *J. Pharmacol. Exp. Ther.* 323, 438–449. doi: 10.1124/jpet.107.129551

Yang, M. H., Yang, Y. H., Lu, C. Y., Jong, S. B., Chen, L. J., Lin, Y. F., et al. (2012). Activity-dependent neuroprotector homeobox protein: a candidate protein identified in serum as diagnostic biomarker for Alzheimer's disease. *J. Proteomics* 75, 3617–3629. doi: 10.1016/j.jprot.2012.04.017

Zamostiano, R., Pinhasov, A., Bassan, M., Perl, O., Steingart, R. A., Atlas, R., et al. (1999). A femtomolar-acting neuroprotective peptide induces increased levels of heat shock protein 60 in rat cortical neurons: a potential neuroprotective mechanism. *Neurosci. Lett.* 264, 9–12. doi: 10.1016/s0304-3940(99)00168-8

11

Enhanced Tau Protein Translation by Hyper-Excitation

*Shunsuke Kobayashi[1], Toru Tanaka[1], Yoshiyuki Soeda[2] and Akihiko Takashima[2]**

[1] Department of Biochemistry, School of Pharmacy, Nihon University, Funabashi, Japan, [2] Laboratory for Alzheimer's Disease, Department of Life Science, Faculty of Science, Gakushuin University, Tokyo, Japan

Correspondence:
Akihiko Takashima
akihiko.takashima@gakushuin.ac.jp

Tau is a microtubule-associated protein, localizing mainly in the axon of mature neurons. Phenotypic analysis of *Tau* knockout mice has revealed an impairment of synaptic plasticity but without gross changes in brain morphology. Since we previously described the presence of tau mRNA in the somatodendritic compartment, including the postsynapse, and demonstrated that it could be locally translated in response to glutamate, it appears that the regulated translation of synaptic tau can have a direct impact on synaptic function. Using SH-SY5Y cells, we herein confirm that glutamate dose-dependently regulates the translation of tau protein without altering tau mRNA levels. This is supported by the finding that cycloheximide blocks glutamate-stimulated increases in tau protein levels. Our observation that neural excitation can directly upregulate tau mRNA translation helps explain the pathological accumulation of tau in the somatodendrite.

Keywords: tau, glutamate stimulation, translation, synapse, phosphorylation

INTRODUCTION

Intracellular inclusions of hyperphosphorylated tau protein (neurofibrillary tangles, NFTs) and extracellular deposits of amyloid β (Aβ) are prominent neuropathological features in the brains of Alzheimer disease patients (Selkoe, 2004). The propagation of NFTs from the entorhinal cortex to the neocortex, followed by neuronal and synapse loss, corresponds closely with the temporal and clinical manifestation of AD symptoms – from impaired memory to dementia (Braak and Braak, 1991; Gomez-Isla et al., 1997; Iqbal and Grundke-Iqbal, 2002). Thus, the formation and propagation of NFT is likely to contribute to AD symptomatology.

In the healthy brain, tau is an exclusively axonal protein, engaged in the assembly and stability of microtubules (Weingarten et al., 1975). In contrast, in the AD brain, tau is hyperphosphorylated and forms fibrils that appear as neuropil threads in dendrites and as NFTs in the somato-dendritic compartment and axons (Kowall and Kosik, 1987). Evidence showing that NFT formation is preceded by a pre-tangle stage where non-fibrillar and hyperphosphorylated tau accumulates in the soma and dendrites of neurons (Gotz et al., 1995; Uchihara et al., 2001; Braak and Del Tredici, 2013) indicates that tau hyperphosphorylation occurs in the somatodendrite before its fibrillation and the appearance of neurofibrilar lesions.

Tau has recently been ascribed with a role in synaptic function in physiological conditions. For example, we showed that tau is essential for the induction of long-term depression (LTD) (Kimura et al., 2014), a phenomenon that can be explained by its presence in the somatodendritic compartment: non-axonal tau is translated from tau mRNA that is transported to the post-synapse as a complex comprised of mRNA binding protein (mRNP) and MyosinIV (Kobayashi et al., 2017).

In line with previous work showing that neuronal excitation can trigger the local translation of other dendritic molecules implicated in synapse formation and plasticity (e.g., CaMKIIα, GluR, and Arc) (Steward and Halpain, 1999; Steward and Worley, 2002; Steward and Schuman, 2003; Bramham and Wells, 2007), we reported that glutamatergic stimulation enhances tau protein translation and the accumulation of hyperphosphorylated tau in somatodendrites of mouse hippocampal neurons (Kobayashi et al., 2017).

Our previous work (Kobayashi et al., 2017) was primarily based on immunohistochemical and immunoblotting analyses, approaches that allow visualization and quantitation of tau levels in neuronal dendrites, soma, and axons. The present experiments, performed on glutamate-stimulated human neuroblastoma SH-SY5Y cells, aimed at strengthening the evidence that accumulation of tau in somatodendritic compartment in disease states is due to enhancement of tau translation in response to glutamatergic stimulation.

RESULTS

Cell bodies and neurites of neural SH-SY5Y cells differentiated with retinoic acid (RA) displayed tau immunoreactivity when stained with a pan-tau antibody (**Figure 1A**). To confirm the interaction of dendritic mRNA-binding proteins with tau mRNA, whole-cell extracts of differentiated SH-SY5Y cells were immunoprecipitated using specific antibodies against the dendritic mRNA-binding proteins FMRP (Greenough et al., 2001), Staufen (Kiebler et al., 1999), ZBP1 (Tiruchinapalli et al., 2003), Pur α (Ohashi et al., 2000), and YB-1 (Funakoshi et al., 2003; Tanaka et al., 2010). After extraction of RNA from the immunoprecipitants, RT-PCR using specific primers for a common region in six tau mRNA isoforms was performed (**Figure 1B**). That analysis revealed that Tau mRNA interacts with all of the dendritic mRNA-binding proteins of interest. We also examined which tau mRNA – 3-repeat tau or 4-repeat tau – is expressed in the differentiated cytosolic fraction of SH-SY5Y cells (**Figure 1C**) by RT-PCR assays, using specific primers to detect the region encoding the microtubule-binding domains (MBDs). Only one RT-PCR product with a length corresponding to 3-repeat tau was detected, supporting an earlier report (Uberti et al., 1997).

Earlier work demonstrated that the excitotoxic effects of glutamate in SH-SY5Y only become manifest after extended (overnight) exposure to high doses of glutamate (Sun et al., 2010). This contrasts with the rapid (within 30 min) induction of translation of dendritic tau mRNA when hippocampal neurons are treated with 0.5 M of glutamate (Kobayashi et al., 2017). Here we show that neural activation with glutamate for 30 min

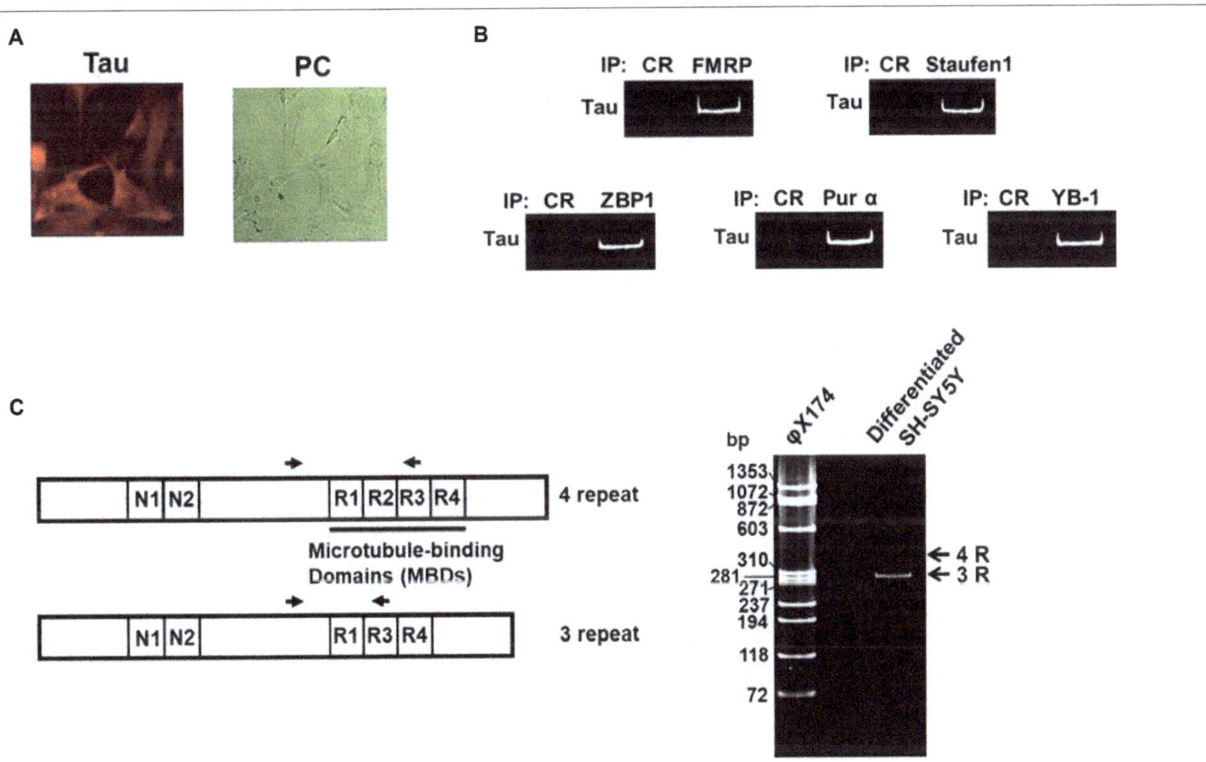

FIGURE 1 | Tau mRNA interacts with mRNA-binding proteins and is expressed in SH-SY5Y cells. **(A)** SH-SY5Y cells were treated with RA for 4 days and immunostained with anti-tau antibody (Alexa Fluor 555) (left-hand image); the right-hand image shows a phase contrast (PC). **(B)** The cytosolic fraction of differentiated SH-SY5Y cells was immunoprecipitated with specific antibodies directed against dendritic mRNA-binding proteins, or control IgG. RNA was extracted from the immune complex, and double-stranded tau cDNA was detected by RT-PCR. **(C)** RNA was extracted from the cytosolic fraction and RT-PCR was performed using specific primers to examine the presence of the 3- or 4-repeat regions. The primer positions are shown as opposed arrows. φX174: molecular marker.

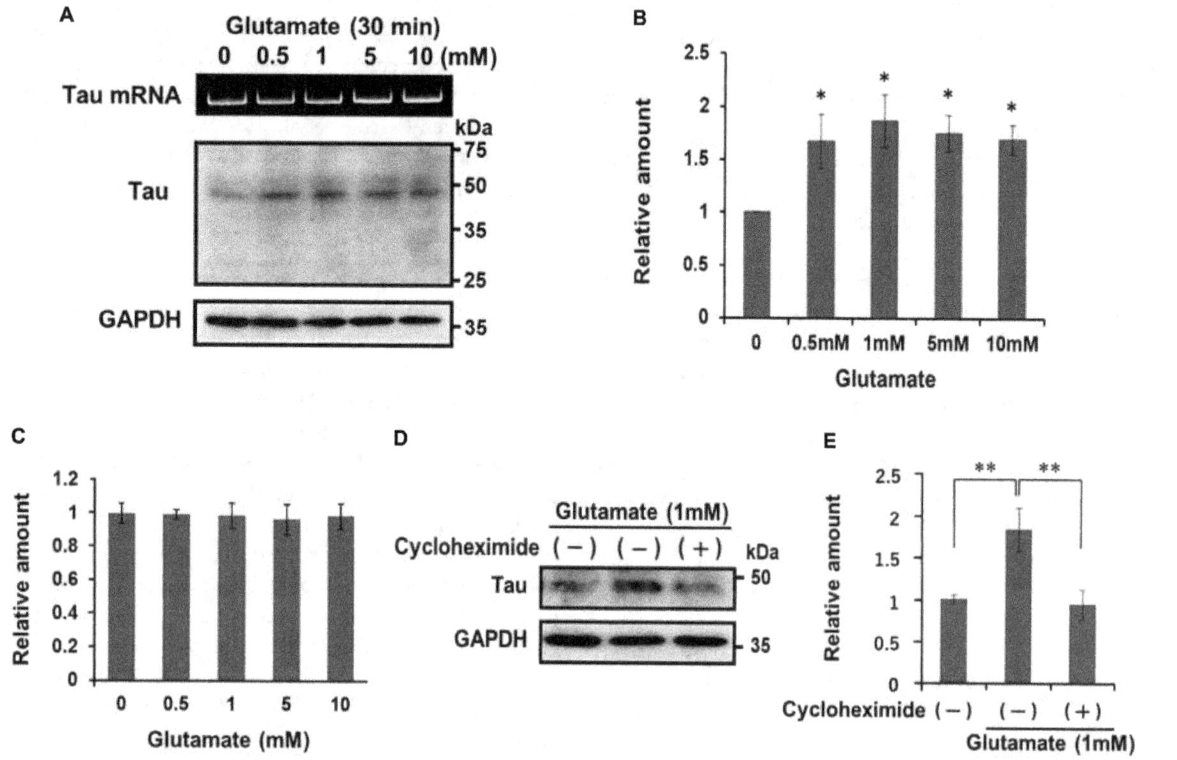

FIGURE 2 | Glutamate stimulates the translation of tau mRNA. **(A)** Differentiated SH-SY5Y cells were treated with various concentrations of glutamate for 30 min, and cell extracts were examined for tau protein content by Western blotting. GAPDH served as a control. RT-PCR data of tau mRNA is also shown. **(B)** The signal intensity of tau protein was normalized to that of GAPDH, and expressed as a relative amount. Each value represents the mean and standard error obtained from four independent experiments. $^*P < 0.05$ versus control (one-way ANOVA, followed by Tukey–Kramer *post hoc* test). **(C)** Quantitative RT-PCR of tau mRNA after exposure to various doses of glutamate concentration. **(D)** Differentiated SH-SY5Y cells were treated with glutamate (1 mM) for 30 min in the presence or absence of cycloheximide (20 μg/ml). Tau protein from each cell extract was analyzed by Western blotting. GAPDH was used as a loading control. **(E)** Levels of tau protein are expressed relative to that of GAPDH. Each value represents the mean and standard error obtained from four independent experiments. $^{**}P < 0.01$ versus control or in the presence of CHX (one-way ANOVA, followed by Tukey–Kramer *post hoc* test).

dose-dependently upregulates tau protein levels, as measured by quantitative Western blotting (**Figures 2A,B**); tau protein levels plateaued at glutamate doses >1 mM (**Figure 2B**). Glutamate treatment did not alter tau mRNA expression (**Figure 2C**) and importantly, the glutamate-induced increase in tau protein levels was abolished when the cells were co-incubated with cycloheximide (**Figures 2D,E**); the latter indicates that glutamate activates the translation of tau mRNA.

Subsequently, we undertook a detailed analysis of the time course of activity-dependent tau mRNA translation, using 1 mM glutamate (**Figures 3A–C**). Western blot analysis revealed that after peaking at 30 min after application of glutamate, tau protein levels declined gradually (**Figure 3B**). At no time point were the changes in tau protein accompanied by alterations in tau mRNA levels (**Figure 3C**). Another important observation from these experiments was that glutamate treatment resulted in a marked increase of phosphorylated tau bearing an AD-relevant epitope (detected by anti-tau pSer396 antibody) (**Figures 3D,E**). A significant upregulation of phosphorylated tau was also observable when results were normalized to total tau levels (**Figure 3F**), confirming that glutamate increases tau phosphorylation.

Together, these results demonstrate that glutamatergic stimulation leads to rapid *de novo* synthesis and phosphorylation of tau independently of tau mRNA transcription.

DISCUSSION

Regulation of Tau Translation

In healthy, mature neurons, tau is predominantly localized in axons, with only low levels of expression in dendrites (Kanai and Hirokawa, 1995; Hirokawa et al., 1996; Ittner and Ittner, 2018). In contrast, somatodendritic levels of tau are significantly increased in AD and other tauopathies (Kowall and Kosik, 1987; Hoover et al., 2010). While the mechanisms responsible for the differential distribution of tau in healthy vs. diseased neurons are still unclear, one plausible mechanism for somatodendritic accumulation of tau is through the transport of tau mRNA in association with mRNP to the somatodendritic compartment where tau protein is synthesized *de novo* upon neuronal activation, e.g., by glutamate (Kobayashi et al., 2017).

Using differentiated human SHSY5Y cells, we here confirmed our previous observation in primary mouse hippocampal

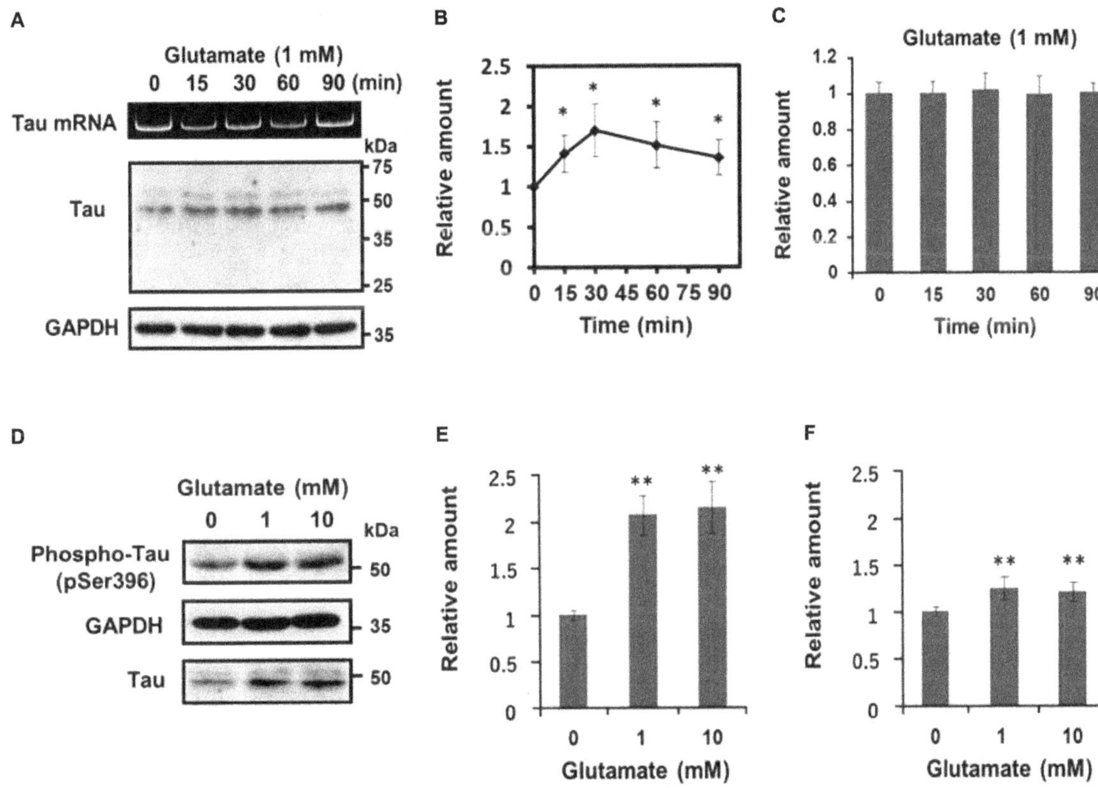

FIGURE 3 | Glutamate-responsive translational activation of tau mRNA is transient, but induces AD-relevant phosphorylation of the newly synthesized tau protein. **(A)** Time course analysis of the glutamate-dependent increase of tau protein levels. Differentiated SH-SY5Y cells were treated with 1 mM glutamate for the time indicated and tau protein from each cell extract was analyzed by Western blotting. GAPDH served as a loading control. RT-PCR analysis of tau mRNA is also shown. **(B)** The signal intensity of tau protein at each indicated time point was expressed relative to that of GAPDH. Each value represents the mean and standard error obtained from five independent experiments. $^{*}P < 0.05$ versus control (one-way ANOVA, followed by Tukey–Kramer *post hoc* test). **(C)** Quantitative RT-PCR of tau mRNA at each time point is shown. **(D)** Differentiated SH-SY5Y cells were treated with different concentrations of glutamate for 30 min, and total tau protein and phosphorylated tau (anti-tau pSer396) was detected by Western blotting. The amount of phosphorylated tau protein was expressed relative to that of GAPDH **(E)** or total tau **(F)**. Each value represents the mean and standard error obtained from four independent experiments. $^{**}P < 0.01$ versus control (one-way ANOVA, followed by Tukey–Kramer *post hoc* test).

neurons (Kobayashi et al., 2017) that tau mRNA associates with dendritic mRNA-binding proteins, such as FMRP (Greenough et al., 2001), Staufen (Kiebler et al., 1999), ZBP1 (Tiruchinapalli et al., 2003), Pur α (Ohashi et al., 2000), and YB-1 (Funakoshi et al., 2003; Tanaka et al., 2010); as in hippocampal neurons, tau protein was visualized in both the cell body and neurites of SHSY5Y cells. Further, glutamate was found to stimulate tau mRNA translation into tau protein in a dose-dependent manner; maximum levels of tau protein were detectable at 30 min after application of glutamate after which they declined gradually (**Figures 3A,B**). Proteasomal or autophagic activity are likely to be responsible for the latter reductions in dendritic tau protein (see Balaji et al., 2018).

Synaptic Tau

Although only transiently increased, it is highly plausible that the glutamate-stimulated translation of tau protein is of biological significance. Indeed, we previously reported that hippocampal LTD cannot be induced in mice lacking the *tau* gene (Kimura et al., 2014), suggesting a role for tau in synaptic plasticity and function. Furthermore, it has been reported that tau phosphorylation at Ser396 is required for LTD induction (Regan et al., 2015). Glutamate-induced phosphorylated tau in synapse may involve in synaptic plasticity.

While synaptic proteins, such as glutamate receptors and BDNF, are locally translated from their mRNA in the synaptic region (Kim et al., 2013; Leal et al., 2014), the origin of tau in synapses under physiological conditions has been somewhat controversial: although tau mRNA shares RNA binding proteins with synaptic protein mRNAs, and several authors reported the presence of presynaptic tau in human and animal brain tissue (Tai et al., 2012; Jadhav et al., 2015), other investigators failed to detect an overlap in immunolabeled endogenous mouse tau with dendritic proteins such as drebrin and microtubule-associated protein 2 (Kubo et al., 2019). Nonetheless, given the evidence that reducing tau levels has a major impact on synaptic function (Hoover et al., 2010; Kimura et al., 2014; Regan et al., 2015; Guo et al., 2017), a postsynaptic site of tau action seems highly likely. We suggest that synaptic tau may often elude detection because of its short lifespan.

Implications of Synaptic Tau for Neurodegeneration

Neurofibrillary tangles are a well-known pathological marker for neurodegeneration in AD and the other tauopathies and, conversely, correlate with cognitive decline. However, NFTs themselves do not induce neurotoxicity; rather, tau aggregation processes seem to be responsible for synaptic degradation and cognitive dysfunction (Santacruz et al., 2005; Kimura et al., 2010; Takashima, 2013). Since the shift in localization of tau from a predominantly axonal site to somatodendritic site occurs during early stages of neurodegeneration (Zempel et al., 2010; Zempel and Mandelkow, 2014), the consensus now holds that tau aggregates start to form from accumulations of phosphorylated tau in the somatodendritic compartment. Although it is still unclear as to how somatodendritic phosphorylated tau accumulation contributes to neurotoxicity, several hypotheses appear to be tenable. For example, we previously reported that granular tau oligomers appear before tau fibril formation and that an inhibitor of tau aggregation blocks the formation of granular tau and prevents neuronal loss in a mouse model of tauopathy (Soeda et al., 2015). These findings suggest that aggregates of granular tau oligomers are responsible for inducing neurotoxicity. Moreover, tau dimerization is known to be a crucial initiating step in the neurodegenerative process in tau-expressing cells; this, in turn, further enhances tau aggregation and the production of reactive oxygen species (ROS) and cytoplasmic Ca^{2+} which ultimately trigger cell death (Pickhardt et al., 2017). While any cytoplasmic tau can precipitate such neurotoxicity, it is worthwhile noting, in the context of this study, that tau aggregates in the synapse can impair clathrin-mediated endocytosis (Hoover et al., 2010; Yu et al., 2019). The loss of synaptic function through the aggregation of tau can potentially inhibit the endocytosis and homeostatic balance of excitatory synaptic receptors, thus disrupting synaptic plasticity and ultimately triggering cell death.

MATERIALS AND METHODS

Antibodies

Anti-tau (rabbit) antibody (catalog no. SC1996-R, lot no. B1213) was from Santa Cruz Biochemistry. Anti-tau pSer396 (rabbit) antibody (catalog no. BS4196, lot no. CJ36131) was from Bioworld Technology. Anti-FMRP (mouse) antibody (catalog no. MAB2160, lot no. 2137991, clone 1C3) was from Millipore. Rabbit anti-Staufen1 (catalog no. ab73478, Gr21579-1), mouse anti-Pur α (catalog no. ab77734, lot no. GR98153-2), and rabbit anti-YB-1 (catalog no. ab76149, GR221265-24, clone EP2708Y) antibodies were from Abcam. Anti-ZBP1/IMP1 (mouse) antibody (catalog no. RN001M, lot no. 001, clone 6H6) was from MBL Life Science. Alexa Fluor 555-conjugated goat anti-rabbit IgG (catalog no. A21428, lot no. 1937183) was purchased from Thermo Fisher Scientific. Horseradish peroxidase (HRP)-linked anti-rabbit IgG (donkey) (catalog no. NA934V. lot no. 377022) was from GE Healthcare Life Science.

Cell Culture and Immunocytochemistry

Human neuroblastoma SH-SY5Y cells were grown in Dulbecco's modified Eagle medium with 10% fetal bovine serum. Cells were differentiated by incubation with 33.3 μM RA for 4 days. For immunocytochemistry, the cells were fixed in 4% paraformaldehyde in phosphate-buffered saline (PBS) for 10 min, treated with 0.5% Triton X-100 in PBS for 15 min, and then incubated with anti-tau antibody in PBS containing 5% skimmed milk at room temperature for 2 h. After washing with PBS, specimens were incubated with Alexa Fluor 555-conjugated second antibody for 1 h, washed with PBS, and viewed with an Olympus inverted microscope linked to a DP-70 imaging system.

Western Blot Analysis

Cells were lysed in TKM buffer containing 50 mM triethanolamine (pH 7.8), 50 mM $MgCl_2$, 0.25 M sucrose, 1 mM phenylmethylsulfonyl fluoride (PMSF), 1 mM dithiothreitol (DTT), protease inhibitors (complete cocktail, Roche), 1× phosphatase inhibitor cocktail solution (Wako Pure Chemical Industries), and ribonuclease inhibitor (0.2 unit/μl, Takara Bio Inc.). The lysate was centrifuged at 3,000 rpm for 10 min and the supernatant was used as the cytosol fraction. Proteins were separated by SDS-PAGE and transferred to a Polyvinylidene difluoride (PVDF) membrane. After treatment with anti-tau antibody, the membrane was incubated with a secondary HRP-conjugated antibody. Protein signals were detected with an ECL kit (GE Healthcare Life Science) and assessed by densitometric analysis.

Immunoprecipitation and RT-PCR

Each antibody (2 μg) was bound to Dynabeads Protein G (Life Technologies) and incubated with cell lysate at 4°C for 4 h. The beads were washed with PBS containing 0.1% BSA and co-immunoprecipitated RNAs were extracted with SDS–phenol–chloroform and dissolved in water. First-strand cDNA was synthesized with Moloney Murine Leukemia Virus (MMLV) reverse transcriptase (Takara Bio Inc.) using an oligo (dT) primer. Double-stranded tau cDNA was synthesized using specific primers. The RT-PCR products were stained with ethidium bromide and analyzed using a gel documentation system (BioRad GelDoc XR Plus ImageLab). Primer pairs were: 5′-ACTGGCATCTCTGGAGTGTGTG-3′ (forward) and 5′-GCAGCTACAAGCTAGGGTGCAAG-3′ (reverse). To investigate which tau mRNA – 3-repeat tau or 4-repeat tau – is expressed in differentiated SH-SY5Y cells, RT-PCR was performed using specific primers with the following sequences: 5′-AGGTGAACCTCCAAAATCAGGGGATC-3′ (forward) and 5′-ACADTTGGAGGTCACTTTGCTC-3′ (reverse).

Quantitative RT-PCR (Real-Time qRT-PCR)

Total RNA was extracted with a mini-prep RNA extraction kit (QIAGEN) in accordance with the manufacturer's instructions, and first-strand cDNA was synthesized from 1.0 μg of total RNA using reverse transcriptase (Takara Bio Inc.) as described above. Aliquots of cDNA were used for qPCR with a StepOnePlus Real Time PCR system (Applied Biosystems) using PowerUp

SYBR Green Master Mix (Thermo Fisher Scientific). The level of tau mRNA expression was normalized to that of β-actin mRNA. The primer sequences used for double-stranded tau cDNA are given above. The primers for glyceraldehyde-3-phosphate dehydrogenase (GAPDH) mRNA were as follows: 5′-TGAGTACGTCGTGGAGTCCACTG-3′ (forward) and 5′-GGGATGATGTTCTGGAGAGC-3′ (reverse).

AUTHOR CONTRIBUTIONS

AT and SK made conception and design of this work. TT and YS collected and analyzed the data. SK drafted the manuscript. AT critically revised and finalized the manuscript.

REFERENCES

Balaji, V., Kaniyappan, S., Mandelkow, E., Wang, Y., and Mandelkow, E. M. (2018). Pathological missorting of endogenous MAPT/Tau in neurons caused by failure of protein degradation systems. *Autophagy* 14, 2139–2154. doi: 10.1080/15548627.2018.1509607

Braak, H., and Braak, E. (1991). Neuropathological stageing of Alzheimer-related changes. *Acta Neuropathol.* 82, 239–259. doi: 10.1007/bf00308809

Braak, H., and Del Tredici, K. (2013). Evolutional aspects of Alzheimer's disease pathogenesis. *J. Alzheimers Dis.* 33(Suppl. 1), S155–S161. doi: 10.3233/JAD-2012-129029

Bramham, C. R., and Wells, D. G. (2007). Dendritic mRNA: transport, translation and function. *Nat. Rev. Neurosci.* 8, 776–789. doi: 10.1038/nrn2150

Funakoshi, T., Kobayashi, S., Ohashi, S., Sato, T. A., and Anzai, K. (2003). Isolation and characterization of brain Y-box protein: developmentally regulated expression, polyribosomal association and dendritic localization. *Brain Res. Mol. Brain Res.* 118, 1–9. doi: 10.1016/s0169-328x(03)00328-0

Gomez-Isla, T., Hollister, R., West, H., Mui, S., Growdon, J. H., Petersen, R. C., et al. (1997). Neuronal loss correlates with but exceeds neurofibrillary tangles in Alzheimer's disease. *Ann. Neurol.* 41, 17–24. doi: 10.1002/ana.410410106

Gotz, J., Probst, A., Spillantini, M. G., Schafer, T., Jakes, R., Burki, K., et al. (1995). Somatodendritic localization and hyperphosphorylation of tau protein in transgenic mice expressing the longest human brain tau isoform. *EMBO J.* 14, 1304–1313. doi: 10.1002/j.1460-2075.1995.tb07116.x

Greenough, W. T., Klintsova, A. Y., Irwin, S. A., Galvez, R., Bates, K. E., and Weiler, I. J. (2001). Synaptic regulation of protein synthesis and the fragile X protein. *Proc. Natl. Acad. Sci. U.S.A.* 98, 7101–7106. doi: 10.1073/pnas.141145998

Guo, T., Noble, W., and Hanger, D. P. (2017). Roles of tau protein in health and disease. *Acta Neuropathol.* 133, 665–704. doi: 10.1007/s00401-017-1707-9

Hirokawa, N., Funakoshi, T., Sato-Harada, R., and Kanai, Y. (1996). Selective stabilization of tau in axons and microtubule-associated protein 2C in cell bodies and dendrites contributes to polarized localization of cytoskeletal proteins in mature neurons. *J. Cell Biol.* 132, 667–679. doi: 10.1083/jcb.132.4.667

Hoover, B. R., Reed, M. N., Su, J., Penrod, R. D., Kotilinek, L. A., Grant, M. K., et al. (2010). Tau mislocalization to dendritic spines mediates synaptic dysfunction independently of neurodegeneration. *Neuron* 68, 1067–1081. doi: 10.1016/j.neuron.2010.11.030

Iqbal, K., and Grundke-Iqbal, I. (2002). Neurofibrillary pathology leads to synaptic loss and not the other way around in Alzheimer disease. *J. Alzheimers Dis.* 4, 235–238. doi: 10.3233/jad-2002-4313

Ittner, A., and Ittner, L. M. (2018). Dendritic tau in Alzheimer's disease. *Neuron* 99, 13–27. doi: 10.1016/j.neuron.2018.06.003

Jadhav, S., Cubinkova, V., Zimova, I., Brezovakova, V., Madari, A., Cigankova, V., et al. (2015). Tau-mediated synaptic damage in Alzheimer's disease. *Transl. Neurosci.* 6, 214–226. doi: 10.1515/tnsci-2015-0023

Kanai, Y., and Hirokawa, N. (1995). Sorting mechanisms of tau and MAP2 in neurons: suppressed axonal transit of MAP2 and locally regulated microtubule binding. *Neuron* 14, 421–432. doi: 10.1016/0896-6273(95)90298-8

Kiebler, M. A., Hemraj, I., Verkade, P., Kohrmann, M., Fortes, P., Marion, R. M., et al. (1999). The mammalian staufen protein localizes to the somatodendritic domain of cultured hippocampal neurons: implications for its involvement in mRNA transport. *J. Neurosci.* 19, 288–297. doi: 10.1523/jneurosci.19-01-00288.1999

Kim, T. K., Sul, J. Y., Helmfors, H., Langel, U., Kim, J., and Eberwine, J. (2013). Dendritic glutamate receptor mRNAs show contingent local hotspot-dependent translational dynamics. *Cell Rep.* 5, 114–125. doi: 10.1016/j.celrep.2013.08.029

Kimura, T., Fukuda, T., Sahara, N., Yamashita, S., Murayama, M., Mizoroki, T., et al. (2010). Aggregation of detergent-insoluble tau is involved in neuronal loss but not in synaptic loss. *J. Biol. Chem.* 285, 38692–38699. doi: 10.1074/jbc.M110.136630

Kimura, T., Whitcomb, D. J., Jo, J., Regan, P., Piers, T., Heo, S., et al. (2014). Microtubule-associated protein tau is essential for long-term depression in the hippocampus. *Philos. Trans. R. Soc. Lond. B Biol. Sci.* 369:20130144. doi: 10.1098/rstb.2013.0144

Kobayashi, S., Tanaka, T., Soeda, Y., Almeida, O. F. X., and Takashima, A. (2017). Local somatodendritic translation and hyperphosphorylation of tau protein triggered by AMPA and NMDA receptor stimulation. *EBioMed.* 20, 120–126. doi: 10.1016/j.ebiom.2017.05.012

Kowall, N. W., and Kosik, K. S. (1987). Axonal disruption and aberrant localization of tau protein characterize the neuropil pathology of Alzheimer's disease. *Ann. Neurol.* 22, 639–643. doi: 10.1002/ana.410220514

Kubo, A., Misonou, H., Matsuyama, M., Nomori, A., Wada-Kakuda, S., Takashima, A., et al. (2019). Distribution of endogenous normal tau in the mouse brain. *J. Comp. Neurol.* 527, 985–998. doi: 10.1002/cne.24577

Leal, G., Comprido, D., and Duarte, C. B. (2014). BDNF-induced local protein synthesis and synaptic plasticity. *Neuropharmacology* 76(Pt C), 639–656. doi: 10.1016/j.neuropharm.2013.04.005

Ohashi, S., Kobayashi, S., Omori, A., Ohara, S., Omae, A., Muramatsu, T., et al. (2000). The single-stranded DNA- and RNA-binding proteins pur alpha and pur beta link BC1 RNA to microtubules through binding to the dendrite-targeting RNA motifs. *J. Neurochem.* 75, 1781–1790. doi: 10.1046/j.1471-4159.2000.0751781.x

Pickhardt, M., Biernat, J., Hubschmann, S., Dennissen, F. J. A., Timm, T., Aho, A., et al. (2017). Time course of Tau toxicity and pharmacologic prevention in a cell model of Tauopathy. *Neurobiol. Aging* 57, 47–63. doi: 10.1016/j.neurobiolaging.2017.04.022

Regan, P., Piers, T., Yi, J. H., Kim, D. H., Huh, S., Park, S. J., et al. (2015). Tau phosphorylation at serine 396 residue is required for hippocampal LTD. *J. Neurosci.* 35, 4804–4812. doi: 10.1523/JNEUROSCI.2842-14.2015

Santacruz, K., Lewis, J., Spires, T., Paulson, J., Kotilinek, L., Ingelsson, M., et al. (2005). Tau suppression in a neurodegenerative mouse model improves memory function. *Science* 309, 476–481. doi: 10.1126/science.1113694

Selkoe, D. J. (2004). Alzheimer disease: mechanistic understanding predicts novel therapies. *Ann. Intern. Med.* 140, 627–638.

Soeda, Y., Yoshikawa, M., Almeida, O. F., Sumioka, A., Maeda, S., Osada, H., et al. (2015). Toxic tau oligomer formation blocked by capping of cysteine residues with 1,2-dihydroxybenzene groups. *Nat. Commun.* 6:10216. doi: 10.1038/ncomms10216

Steward, O., and Halpain, S. (1999). Lamina-specific synaptic activation causes domain-specific alterations in dendritic immunostaining for MAP2 and CAM kinase II. *J. Neurosci.* 19, 7834–7845. doi: 10.1523/jneurosci.19-18-07834.1999

Steward, O., and Schuman, E. M. (2003). Compartmentalized synthesis and degradation of proteins in neurons. *Neuron* 40, 347–359. doi: 10.1016/s0896-6273(03)00635-4

Steward, O., and Worley, P. (2002). Local synthesis of proteins at synaptic sites on dendrites: role in synaptic plasticity and memory consolidation? *Neurobiol. Learn Mem.* 78, 508–527. doi: 10.1006/nlme.2002.4102

Sun, Z. W., Zhang, L., Zhu, S. J., Chen, W. C., and Mei, B. (2010). Excitotoxicity effects of glutamate on human neuroblastoma SH-SY5Y cells via oxidative damage. *Neurosci. Bull.* 26, 8–16. doi: 10.1007/s12264-010-0813-7

Tai, H. C., Serrano-Pozo, A., Hashimoto, T., Frosch, M. P., Spires-Jones, T. L., and Hyman, B. T. (2012). The synaptic accumulation of hyperphosphorylated tau oligomers in Alzheimer disease is associated with dysfunction of the ubiquitin-proteasome system. *Am. J. Pathol.* 181, 1426–1435. doi: 10.1016/j.ajpath.2012.06.033

Takashima, A. (2013). Tauopathies and tau oligomers. *J. Alzheimers Dis.* 37, 565–568. doi: 10.3233/JAD-130653

Tanaka, T., Ohashi, S., Funakoshi, T., and Kobayashi, S. (2010). YB-1 binds to GluR2 mRNA and CaM1 mRNA in the brain and regulates their translational levels in an activity-dependent manner. *Cell Mol. Neurobiol.* 30, 1089–1100. doi: 10.1007/s10571-010-9541-9

Tiruchinapalli, D. M., Oleynikov, Y., Kelic, S., Shenoy, S. M., Hartley, A., Stanton, P. K., et al. (2003). Activity-dependent trafficking and dynamic localization of zipcode binding protein 1 and beta-actin mRNA in dendrites and spines of hippocampal neurons. *J. Neurosci.* 23, 3251–3261. doi: 10.1523/jneurosci.23-08-03251.2003

Uberti, D., Rizzini, C., Spano, P. F., and Memo, M. (1997). Characterization of tau proteins in human neuroblastoma SH-SY5Y cell line. *Neurosci. Lett.* 235, 149–153. doi: 10.1016/s0304-3940(97)00715-5

Uchihara, T., Nakamura, A., Yamazaki, M., and Mori, O. (2001). Evolution from pretangle neurons to neurofibrillary tangles monitored by thiazin red combined with Gallyas method and double immunofluorescence. *Acta Neuropathol.* 101, 535–539.

Weingarten, M. D., Lockwood, A. H., Hwo, S. Y., and Kirschner, M. W. (1975). A protein factor essential for microtubule assembly. *Proc. Natl. Acad. Sci. U.S.A.* 72, 1858–1862. doi: 10.1073/pnas.72.5.1858

Yu, A., Fox, S. G., Cavallini, A., Kerridge, C., O'neill, M. J., Wolak, J., et al. (2019). Tau protein aggregates inhibit the protein-folding and vesicular trafficking arms of the cellular proteostasis network. *J. Biol. Chem.* 294, 7917–7930. doi: 10.1074/jbc.RA119.007527

Zempel, H., and Mandelkow, E. (2014). Lost after translation: missorting of tau protein and consequences for Alzheimer disease. *Trends Neurosci.* 37, 721–732. doi: 10.1016/j.tins.2014.08.004

Zempel, H., Thies, E., Mandelkow, E., and Mandelkow, E. M. (2010). Abeta oligomers cause localized Ca(2+) elevation, missorting of endogenous Tau into dendrites. *J. Neurosci.* 30, 11938–11950. doi: 10.1523/JNEUROSCI.2357-10.2010

12

Distinct Conformations, Aggregation and Cellular Internalization of Different Tau Strains

Thomas K. Karikari[1,2*†], David A. Nagel[3], Alastair Grainger[3], Charlotte Clarke-Bland[3], James Crowe[3], Eric J. Hill[3] and Kevin G. Moffat[1]

[1] School of Life Sciences, University of Warwick, Coventry, United Kingdom, [2] Midlands Integrative Biosciences Training Partnership, University of Warwick, Coventry, United Kingdom, [3] School of Life and Health Sciences, Aston University, Birmingham, United Kingdom

***Correspondence:**
Thomas K. Karikari
Thomas.Karikari@gu.se;
ohenekakari@gmail.com

†Present address:
Thomas K. Karikari,
Department of Psychiatry and Neurochemistry, Institute of Neuroscience and Physiology, The Sahlgrenska Academy at the University of Gothenburg, Gothenburg, Sweden

The inter-cellular propagation of tau aggregates in several neurodegenerative diseases involves, in part, recurring cycles of extracellular tau uptake, initiation of endogenous tau aggregation, and extracellular release of at least part of this protein complex. However, human brain tau extracts from diverse tauopathies exhibit variant or "strain" specificity in inducing inter-cellular propagation in both cell and animal models. It is unclear if these distinctive properties are affected by disease-specific differences in aggregated tau conformation and structure. We have used a combined structural and cell biological approach to study if two frontotemporal dementia (FTD)-associated pathologic mutations, V337M and N279K, affect the aggregation, conformation and cellular internalization of the tau four-repeat domain (K18) fragment. In both heparin-induced and native-state aggregation experiments, each FTD variant formed soluble and fibrillar aggregates with remarkable morphological and immunological distinctions from the wild type (WT) aggregates. Exogenously applied oligomers of the FTD tau-K18 variants (V337M and N279K) were significantly more efficiently taken up by SH-SY5Y neuroblastoma cells than WT tau-K18, suggesting mutation-induced changes in cellular internalization. However, shared internalization mechanisms were observed: endocytosed oligomers were distributed in the cytoplasm and nucleus of SH-SY5Y cells and the neurites and soma of human induced pluripotent stem cell-derived neurons, where they co-localized with endogenous tau and the nuclear protein nucleolin. Altogether, evidence of conformational and aggregation differences between WT and disease-mutated tau K18 is demonstrated, which may explain their distinct cellular internalization potencies. These findings may account for critical aspects of the molecular pathogenesis of tauopathies involving WT and mutated tau.

Keywords: tau protein, Alzheimer's disease, frontotemporal dementia, MAPT mutations, oligomer, nuclear tau, cellular internalization, induced pluripotent stem cell-derived neurons

---

Abbreviations: AD, Alzheimer's disease; ANOVA, analysis of variance; CBD, corticobasal degeneration; DPBS, Dulbecco's phosphate buffered saline; EDTA, ethylenediaminetetraacetic acid; FTD, frontotemporal dementia; hiPSC-derived neurons, human induced pluripotent stem cell-derived cortical neurons; LMW, low molecular weight; MT, microtubule; NFT, neurofibrillary tangle; PHF, paired helical filaments; PIPES, piperazine-N,N′-bis(2-ethanesulfonic acid); SF, straight filament; TCEP, tris(2-carboxyethyl)phosphine; TEM, transmission electron microscopy; WT, wild type.

INTRODUCTION

Tauopathies are characterized by the intracellular accumulation of NFTs composed of aggregated misfolded tau (Arriagada et al., 1992; Spillantini and Goedert, 2013). NFTs can be formed when tau proteins lose affinity for MTs and bind to themselves, forming insoluble aggregates that can subsequently develop into NFTs (Goedert, 2016). Although monomeric tau – the physiological form of the protein – is natively unfolded, it becomes progressively enriched in β-sheets through initial aggregation into soluble conformers and then into PHFs and NFTs (Barghorn et al., 2004; von Bergen et al., 2005). Although growing evidence indicates that tau dysfunction can cause neurodegeneration, the mechanisms involved are not well understood (Guo and Lee, 2014; Walsh and Selkoe, 2016). Many recent studies have shown that the typical temporal and spatial accumulation of tau inclusions in specific brain regions in AD and other tauopathies may be due to the propagation of aggregated tau between synaptically connected neurons (Frost et al., 2009; Guo and Lee, 2014; Usenovic et al., 2015). This inter-neuronal propagation of abnormal tau, often referred to as "spread," is understood to initiate the structural and functional differences observed in affected brain regions (Boluda et al., 2015; Usenovic et al., 2015). As a predominantly cytosolic protein, the spread of tau is expected to involve repeated cycles of the following steps: (i) secretion of tau, either in aggregated or soluble forms, from donor neurons; (ii) uptake of extracellular tau into specific neighboring neurons; (iii) induction of endogenous tau aggregation in the recipient neurons; and (iv) the secretion of at least part of this internalized tau-endogenous tau protein complex (Clavaguera et al., 2009; Frost et al., 2009; Guo and Lee, 2011; Lasagna-Reeves et al., 2012a; Michel et al., 2014). Nonetheless, the molecular mechanism governing this process is poorly understood (Walsh and Selkoe, 2016). As such, an improved understanding of the pathways involved in these diseases could lead to the development of new therapies.

The efficiency of the inter-cellular propagation of pathological tau appears to be influenced by the conformations of both the seed (internalized) and the seeded (recipient endogenous) proteins (Goedert et al., 2014; Sanders et al., 2014; Wegmann et al., 2015; Alonso et al., 2016; Kaufman et al., 2016). This has therefore led to the *tau strain hypothesis*, which proposes that different aggregated tau conformers (distinct strains) will have distinct pathology-initiating capacities because they interact with endogenous tau differently (Sanders et al., 2014; Gerson et al., 2016). This hypothesis is supported by several studies (Clavaguera et al., 2013; Sanders et al., 2014; Boluda et al., 2015; Kaufman et al., 2016; Narasimhan et al., 2017; Strang et al., 2017). For example, intracerebral introduction of human tauopathy brain isolates into brains of the non-filament-forming ALZ17 mice led to distinctions in the induction of tau inclusions, dependent on the source of homogenate (Clavaguera et al., 2013). Inclusions formed after injecting isolates from human AD, progressive supranuclear palsy, argyrophilic grain disease, CBD or tangle-only dementia propagated between neighboring brain regions. Conversely, propagation was not observed for aggregates formed in the case of Pick's disease. Importantly, these results were similar to those recorded after seeding WT mice with the same isolates, suggesting that the genetic background of the animals did not influence the outcome (Clavaguera et al., 2013). Similarly, intracerebral introduction of brain extracts from human CBD and AD cases into young tangle-forming PS19 mice brains resulted in the formation and propagation of tau inclusions and neuronal loss that appeared specific to selected cell types (Boluda et al., 2015). Extracts from CBD patients led to tau inclusions limited to oligodendrocytes of the fimbria and white matter around the injection site, while tau aggregates formed after introducing AD extracts were found in neuronal perikaya without obvious oligodendrocyte participation (Boluda et al., 2015). These results suggest that tau isolates from different sources can exhibit distinctions in their ability to induce tau inclusion formation in the recipient cell type, which may be due to conformational differences between the endogenous tau and the initiating tau seeds. Recently, both cell-type specificity and differential endogenous tau recruitment have been implicated as determinants of inter-cellular propagation of human tauopathy brain extracts (Narasimhan et al., 2017). Furthermore, recombinant full-length and truncated forms of tau, such as the four-repeat K18 region comprising residues 244–372 of full-length tau 441 (**Figure 1**), have been shown to initiate propagation by inducing endogenous tau aggregation (Guo and Lee, 2011; Iba et al., 2013; Michel et al., 2014; Falcon et al., 2015; Usenovic et al., 2015). This seeding capacity may be due to conformational similarities between some forms of recombinant tau applied as seeds and the endogenous tau, because these recombinant forms can take on endogenous tau conformation in some cell models (Falcon et al., 2015).

Whilst there is mounting data supporting the inter-cellular propagation of aggregated recombinant WT tau, we know little about FTD (Bodea et al., 2016). Many familial FTD cases are characterized by single point mutations in the *MAPT* gene, which encodes the tau protein. Specific FTD-associated *MAPT* mutations have been shown to alter the aggregation, β-sheet propensity, isoform ratio and MT binding properties of the WT tau (Hong et al., 1998; Barghorn et al., 2000; von Bergen et al., 2001; Combs and Gamblin, 2012; Kaniyappan et al., 2017). It is, however, unclear if aggregated tau proteins from FTD with *MAPT* mutations are conformationally distinct from WT tau, and if they have different cellular internalization behavior and co-localization dynamics with endogenous tau. Strang et al. (2017) recently demonstrated that the ability of exogenous WT tau K18 fibrils to induce aggregation in cells over-expressing tau carrying different FTD mutations is uniquely dependent on the specific mutation and its surrounding amino acid sequences. However, several questions remain, such as what structural features determine these distinct activities? Do the conformation and aggregation characteristics of tau variants influence their cellular internalization and endogenous tau interaction? Furthermore, it has been shown that the N279K variant of the tau 250–300 fragment localizes to the nucleus more efficiently that the WT when overexpressed in a mammalian cell line (Ritter et al., 2018). It is yet to be shown if exogenously applied aggregates of this and other FTD variants of tau can enter recipient cells and localize to the nucleus, in a process suggestive of

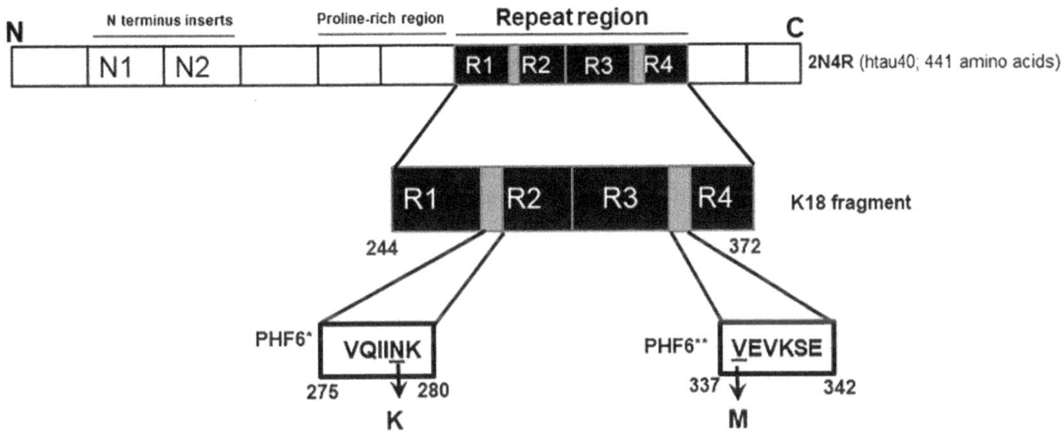

FIGURE 1 | Schematic illustration of the N279K and V337M mutations in tau. The K18 fragment used in this study was constructed based on the full-length human brain tau isoform (2N4R; htau40). The N279K mutation is located in the alternatively spliced second repeat region (R2), specifically within the hexapeptide motif at the start of R2 (PHF6*; gray). The V337M mutation can be found at the start of the fourth repeat domain, and falls within the third hexapeptide motif (PHF6**; second gray region).

cell-to-cell propagation. Answering these questions is critical to understanding the mechanisms by which AD and non-AD tauopathies develop, and will help to establish if selectivity is required in drug development for treating tauopathies.

In this study, we investigated the *in vitro* conformation and aggregation of tau K18-WT and two FTD variants, namely V337M and N279K. The N279K mutation is a part of the PHF6* hexapeptide motif (^{275}VQIINK^{280}) but the V337M mutation is located in the PHF6** hexapeptide motif (^{337}VEVKSE^{342}) (Li and Lee, 2006; Grüning et al., 2014). Since these motifs critically regulate tau aggregation and seeding behavior, amino acid mutations were hypothesized to alter these processes (von Bergen et al., 2000, 2001; Li and Lee, 2006; Grüning et al., 2014; Falcon et al., 2015). In addition, the N279K and V337M are located in the second and the fourth MT binding repeat regions, respectively (**Figure 1**). Thus, the characterization of these mutations should offer new understanding into the consequences of disease-related alterations in alternatively- and constitutively spliced domains. The mutations also have distinct pathological consequences in human brains (Hong et al., 1998), suggesting differential effects on tau aggregation and structure.

We have shown that the structural morphology and immunoreactivity of K18-WT aggregation products were distinctively altered in the presence of each mutation. Furthermore, internalization of exogenous structurally defined oligomers into SH-SY5Y cells was significantly increased in the presence of each FTD mutation. However, the sub-cellular localization and endogenous tau co-localization patterns were similar between the three protein variants, both in SH-SY5Y cells and differentiated human induced pluripotent stem cell (hiPSC)-derived neurons. This may suggest shared mechanisms of cellular uptake, but differences in the efficiency of uptake, between WT tau K18 and its V337M and N279K FTD variants. Together, the results give new insights into the structural and functional dynamics of WT and FTD tau. We hypothesize that the distinct conformation and aggregation behaviors of the tau K18 variants may influence their inter-cellular propagation characteristics. These findings may help to explain important aspects of similarities and heterogeneity in tauopathies involving WT and mutated tau.

MATERIALS AND METHODS

Materials

Heparin (#H3393), SH-SY5Y cells (#94030304), sodium chloride (#S/3160/60), sodium phosphate dibasic (#S9763-500 G), sodium phosphate monobasic dihydrate (#04269-1 KG), Triton X-100 (#X100-500 ML), Tween (#P9416-100 ML), F12 Ham (#51651C), L-Glutamine (#G7513), fetal bovine serum (#F2442) and antibiotic antimycotic acid (#A5955) were purchased from Sigma Aldrich, St. Louis, Missouri, United States. X1 Amersham Protran 0.45 μm electrochemiluminescence nitrocellulose membrane (#15259794) and Amersham electrochemiluminescence system (#RPN2108) were obtained from GE Healthcare, Buckinghamshire, United Kingdom. EDTA (#D/0700/53) was bought from Fisher Scientific, Loughborough, United Kingdom. PIPES (#A16090) was bought from Alfa Aesar, Heysham, United Kingdom, whilst DMSO (cell culture-grade; #P60-36720100) was from PAN-Biotech GmbH, Aidenbach, Germany. CL-XPosure Film (#34089) and ProLong Gold antifade mounting medium (#P36934) were purchased from Thermo Fisher Scientific, Rockford, Illinois, United States. CellMask® Deep Red plasma membrane stain (#C10046), Hoechst 33342 (#H21492) and Alexa Fluor® 488 C5-maleimide (#A10254) were bought from Molecular Probes, Eugene, Oregon, United States. Lactate dehydrogenase (LDH) cytotoxicity assay kit (#88954) was obtained from Pierce Biotechnology, Rockford, Illinois, United States. TCEP (#A2233,0001) was procured from Applichem GmbH, Damstadt, Germany. SynaptoRed™ C2 (FM4-64; #70021) was obtained from Biotium Hayward, California, United States. CellView™ dishes (#627975) were procured from Greiner Bio-One, Kremsmünster, Austria.

TABLE 1 | Antibodies used in this study.

Antibody	Epitope	Host species	Vendor	Dilution
Primary antibodies				
Polyclonal rabbit anti-human tau (#A0024)	The MT binding repeat of tau	Rabbit	Dako	1:1000
T22 oligomeric tau (#ABN454)	Tau MT binding domain	Rabbit	Merck	1:1000
HT7 anti-human tau (#MN1000)	Amino acid sequence ^{159}PPGQK^{163} of full length human tau 2N4R	Mouse	Thermo Scientific	1:100
Alexa Fluor® 647-conjugated anti-nucleolin (#ab198580)	Human nucleolin	Mouse	Abcam	1:500
Secondary antibodies				
Goat anti-rabbit IgG (#31460)	–	Goat	Thermo Fisher Scientific	1:1000
Alexa Fluor® 594-conjugated AffiniPure goat anti-mouse	–	Goat	Jackson ImmunoResearch	1:100

Formvar/carbon-coated 300-mesh copper grids (#S162) and mica (#G250-3) were purchased from Agar Scientific, Stansted, Essex, United Kingdom. Neural precursor cells (#ax0016), Axol neural maintenance medium kit (#ax0031), and Surebond reagent (#ax0041) were purchased from Axol Bioscience, Little Chesterford, Cambridge, United Kingdom. Marvel dried skimmed milk was obtained from Premier Foods Company, United Kingdom. Antibodies used have been described in **Table 1**.

Site Directed Mutagenesis, Protein Expression and Purification

Detailed description of the construction of the pProEx-HTa-Myc-K18 plasmid, and sequence-verified site-directed mutagenesis to create plasmid variants encoding the V337M and N279K mutations has been provided previously (Karikari et al., 2017). To prevent potential adverse functional effects of maleimide labeling, the native cysteines located in the central core of the MT binding region were each changed to alanine (C291A, C322A) and a new cysteine placed outside the central core of this region (I260C). These cysteine modifications were achieved by site-directed mutagenesis as described (Karikari et al., 2017). Several studies have used this approach, understood not to impact tau aggregation behavior, to study the biochemical properties and internalization of extracellular tau (Kumar et al., 2014; Michel et al., 2014; Shammas et al., 2015). The same cysteine-modified proteins were used in all experiments. Plasmids encoding N-terminal 6xHis-c-Myc K18-WT, K18-V337M and K18-N279K were expressed in BL21 (DE3)*pRosetta *Escherichia coli*, purified with immobilized metal affinity chromatography and quantified with the Bicinchoninic acid assay as described previously (Karikari et al., 2017).

Filament Assembly and Structural Characterization Using Negative-Stain Transmission Electron Microscopy (TEM)

K18-WT or its variants (38.5 μM) mixed with 125 μM heparin were incubated at 37°C without agitation for 4 or 45 days. Sodium phosphate buffer pH 7.4 was the diluent buffer used in all biochemical experiments unless otherwise indicated. All incubation was performed using an Eppendorf Mastercycler thermocycler, and aliquots removed for TEM. Five microliters of the indicated proteins were pipetted onto glow-discharged formvar/carbon-coated 300-mesh grids for 2 min, and filter paper strips used to remove unbound samples. Thereafter, 5 μl of 2% uranyl acetate was added for 2 min, and the excess removed as previously before imaging. Quantitative analyses of filament lengths and widths were performed using Image J.

Dot Blot Analysis of Protein Conformation

Protein variants at 55 μM were incubated at 37°C to promote aggregation. Aliquots removed at the given times were snap-frozen and stored at −80°C until needed. After diluting samples 1:2, 2 μl of the diluted samples were spotted onto 0.45-μm nitrocellulose membrane, air-dried, blocked for 30 min at room temperature with 10% non-fat milk in phosphate buffered saline (PBS), and washed five times using 10% Tris buffered saline-0.05% Tween. The membrane was incubated for 2 h in anti-tau #A0024 or T22, washed as previously, and incubated with anti-rabbit immunoglobulin G (**Table 1**) for a further 2 h. Each antibody was diluted 1:1000. The membrane was then washed five times, developed using electrochemiluminescence reagents (Amersham), imaged and analyzed as previously described (Karikari et al., 2017).

Preparation and Characterization of Labeled Oligomers

Proteins were treated with five times excess of TCEP for 1 h, and then treated with 4× Alexa Fluor 488-C5-maleimide in the presence of 1× BRB buffer (1 mM KCl, 80 mM PIPES, and 1 mM EDTA pH 6.8). Free fluorophore was dialyzed out against dialysis buffer (50 mM Tris HCl pH 7.5, 100 mM NaCl) in Slide-A-Lyzer MINI Dialysis Device (5 K MWCO; Thermo Fisher Scientific) with punctured buffer reservoirs placed in containers that can hold 2 L of dialysis buffer. The buffer was changed every 2 h with a total of five buffer replacements. Labeling was confirmed using non-denaturing sodium dodecyl sulfate-polyacrylamide gel electrophoresis followed by ultraviolet light exposure. The efficiency of labeling was routinely estimated using Beer's law and the molar extinction coefficient of 72,000/cm/M for Alexa Fluor 488-C5-maleimide.

SH-SY5Y Cell Culture

SH-SY5Y cells were cultured on 1:1 minimal essential medium/F12 Ham medium supplemented with 1% L-Glutamine, 15% fetal bovine serum, and 1% antibiotic antimycotic acid (10,000 units penicillin, 10 mg streptomycin and 25 μg amphotericin B). All experiments were performed using cells between passages two and ten. Cells were grown at a density of 200,000 cells/ml in CellView™ dishes, 10 μM labeled tau oligomers added to the medium, and incubated for 24 h at 37°C, 5% CO_2. After removing the used medium, the cells were washed with warm PBS and fresh medium with 2 μM Hoechst and 1:1000 dilution of CellMask Deep Red added before imaging.

hiPSC-Derived Neuronal Culture

Neural precursors – from cord blood CD34+ cells of a newborn female – that had been cultured for 21 days from iPSCs to neural precursor cells were bought from Axol Bioscience. Grade 12-well tissue culture plates (Corning, New York, United States) or plates containing plasma-cleaned and ethanol-sterilized 13 mm glass coverslips (Menzer, Thermo Fisher Scientific) were each pre-coated with 250 μl/cm^2 ReadySet reagent (Axol Bioscience) and kept at 37°C, 5% CO_2 for 45 min. The plates were then rinsed 4× with double-distilled water. Thereafter, Surebond reagent (Axol Bioscience) diluted in DPBS was added to the plates at 200 μl/cm^2 and kept at 37°C, 5% CO_2 for at least 1 h. Cells were seeded on plasma-cleaned 13 mm glass coverslips at 25,000 cells/cm^2 final density and stored at 37°C, 5% CO_2. The media was changed every other day for 14–16 days using the Axol Neural Maintenance Medium kit (#ax0031, Axol Bioscience). Phase contrast microscopy images taken periodically with the EVOS XL Core Imaging System (Life Technologies) and the expression of neuron-specific markers (data not shown) were used to monitor neuronal differentiation. Tau K18 oligomers diluted to 5 μM in neural maintenance medium were applied to cultured neurons and kept at 37°C, 5% CO_2 for 24 h, after which the used medium was carefully removed and the neurons washed with DPBS before the addition of fresh medium.

Immunocytochemistry

SH-SY5Y cells: the appropriate antibodies or dye were applied to the cells as described above and images taken with confocal microscopy without fixing. In internalization analysis, fresh media containing FM4-64 (2 μM) and Hoechst was added to cells after PBS wash as explained above. The cells were imaged after 30 min incubation at 37°C and 5% CO_2. Nucleolin co-localization was investigated by adding a 500× dilution of an Alexa Fluor-647-labeled anti-human nucleolin (**Table 1**) in tau-free medium to tau oligomer-treated cells after PBS wash as described above. Cells were imaged after 2 h incubation at 37°C and 5% CO_2. Cells were imaged without fixing.

hiPSC-derived neurons: Neurons were fixed with 4% paraformaldehyde for 30 min, twice washed with DPBS and then cleaned with permeabilizing solution (0.2% Triton in DPBS). Thereafter, the fixed neurons were stored in blocking buffer (DPBS containing 0.2% Triton and 2% BSA) for 1 h. Subsequently the cells were incubated with primary antibody and Hoechst for 1 h at 37°C and 5% CO_2. The fixed neurons were washed thrice, each for 5 min, with blocking buffer to remove unbound primary antibody and then incubated for 1 h with secondary antibody diluted in blocking buffer. After incubation with the secondary antibody, the wash steps were repeated. The prepared coverslips were rinsed with distilled water and slide-mounted with ProLong Gold antifade mounting medium. Slides were incubated in the dark for at least 24 h before imaging. Details of antibodies used are available in **Table 1**.

Confocal Microscopy

An LSM 710 (Leica) equipped with an C-Apochromat 63×/1.20 W Korr M27 objective lens was used to image SH-SY5Y cells. hiPSC-derived cortical neurons were imaged with the 63× objective of a Leica STP 6000 microscope. Images were analyzed with Image J. Internalization data are expressed as integrated density (area × mean fluorescent intensity). Identical imaging settings were used for each set of experiments (at least $n = 3$).

LDH Assay

The Pierce LDH cytotoxicity assay kit was used. SH-SY5Y cells were seeded at 20,000 cells/well in Falcon 96-well plates and the indicated oligomer concentrations added. Controls included spontaneous cytotoxicity (cells + 10 μl sterile water), media only (no cells) and maximum control (membrane lysed with a manufacturer-supplied reagent). Cells were incubated for 72 h at 37°C 5% CO_2. After incubation, lysis buffer was added to the maximum control wells and the plate incubated for a further 45 min. An aliquot (50 μl) of the sample mix in each well was transferred to a new 96-well plate and 50 μl reaction mix from the kit added to each well before incubation in the dark for 30 min. Stop solution (50 μl) was added and absorbance measured at 490 and 680 nm. Background readings at 680 nm were subtracted from corresponding 490 nm readings and LDH release (cytotoxicity) for each condition calculated by dividing that condition's LDH activity value by the value for the maximum LDH activity control, and subtracting the spontaneous LDH activity value from both the numerator and the denominator.

Statistics

Statistical analysis was done using Prism 6 (GraphPad Inc., CA, United States) at 95% confidence interval. The D'Agostino and Pearson test was used to test the datasets for normality. Whenever appropriate, parametric analysis was performed using one-way ANOVA with Tukey's *post hoc* test. Conversely, non-parametric datasets were analyzed using Kruskal-Wallis test with Dunn's *post hoc* test. Data are shown as mean ± standard error of the mean.

RESULTS

The K18 fragment consists of residues critical for tau aggregation and conformation, including the hexapeptide motifs at the beginning of repeat domains two (^{275}VQII<u>N</u>K^{280}), three (^{306}VQIVYK^{311}), and four (^{337}<u>V</u>EVKSE^{342}) (**Figure 1**). These motifs control aggregation by modulating tau-tau interactions that lead to conformational changes from random coil to cross β-sheet structures (von Bergen et al., 2000, 2005; Li and Lee, 2006; Grüning et al., 2014). Moreover, protomers comprising residues 306–378 form the core of tau filaments, with their differential packing mechanisms determining the type of aggregates formed

(Fitzpatrick et al., 2017). Furthermore, the protein's aggregation-seeding competence, partly responsible for its inter-cellular propagation, is held in the repeat region and its fragments consisting of specific motifs (Guo and Lee, 2011; Michel et al., 2014; Stöhr et al., 2017). As the repeat region contains residues that control tau aggregation, conformation and propagation, the K18 fragment was used to study potential effects of specific FTD mutations on these properties.

Familial FTD Mutations Alter the Ultra-Structure of Tau K18 Aggregates

Negative-stain TEM was used to study effects of the N279K and V337M mutations on tau K18 aggregation. Each sample was incubated with heparin at 37°C for four days (96 h) before TEM analysis. After this aggregation period, K18-WT mostly formed PHFs and, to a lesser degree, SFs. Both phenotypes of K18-WT have been reported previously (Barghorn and Mandelkow, 2002). The PHFs had different degrees of twisting, which increased up to ~45° (**Figure 2A** and **Supplementary Figure S1A**). Unlike the PHFs, the SFs had no obvious helical structures (**Figure 2Aiii**). Tau K18-V337M aggregates had two types of phenotypes: large amorphous aggregates (**Figure 2B** main image) and short filamentous aggregates (**Figure 2B** inset). On the other hand, K18-N279K formed thick bundles of filaments of various width and length (**Figure 2C**). **Supplementary Figure S1** is an extension of **Figure 2**, showing representative images from $n = 3$ independent experiments using different batches of purified proteins which further demonstrate the variety of aggregates formed by each tau K18 variant.

Filament length was significantly different when comparing all three proteins ($p < 0.0001$, Kruskal–Wallis test; mean lengths = 510.8 ± 42.3 nm, 106.6 ± 15.4 nm, and 534.8 ± 42.9 nm for WT, V337M, and N279K K18, respectively). Note that for K18-V337M, only the fibrils, but not the irregular amorphous structures, were analyzed. Filaments from both K18-WT and K18-N279K were significantly longer than those formed by K18-V337M ($p < 0.0001$, Kruskal–Wallis test with Dunn's *post hoc* test; **Figure 2D**). Filament length between K18-WT and K18-N279K were not significantly different to each other ($p > 0.9999$, Kruskal–Wallis test with Dunn's *post hoc* test). However, the three protein variants had significantly different filament widths ($p < 0.0001$, Kruskal–Wallis test; mean filament width = 27.9 ± 4.2 nm for K18-WT, 21.1 ± 0.8 nm for

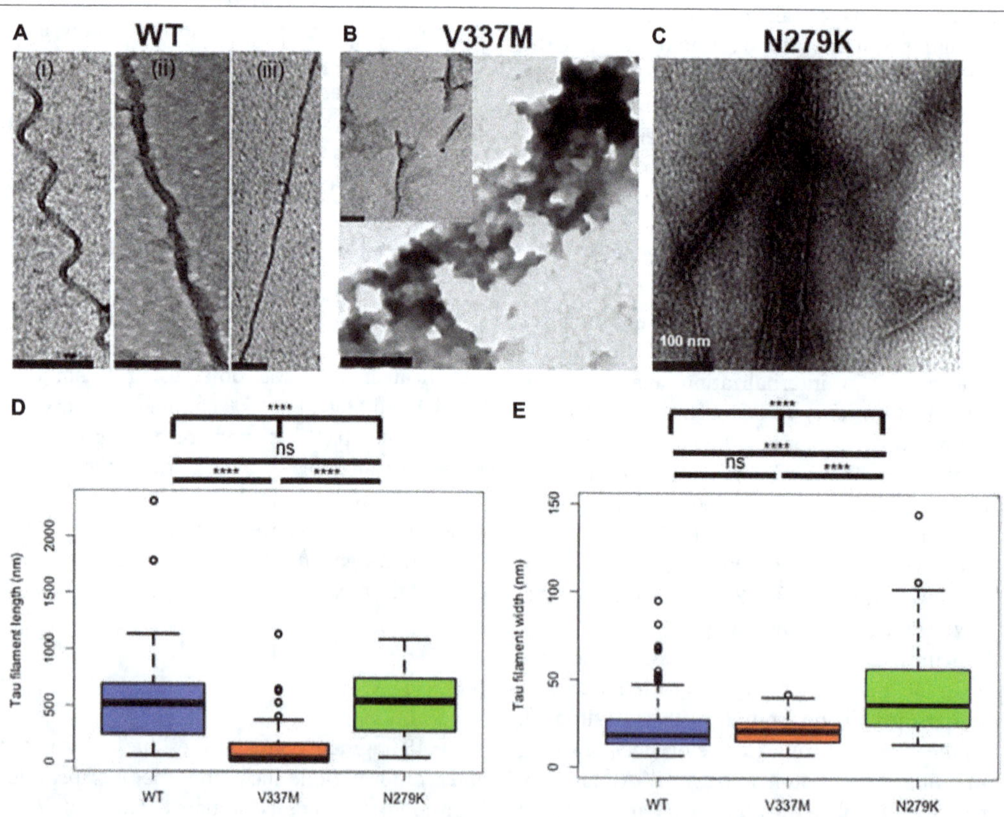

FIGURE 2 | Structural changes in tau K18 filaments formed in the presence of the V337M and N279K FTD mutations after 4 days of incubation. **(A)** Representative electron micrographs of K18-WT, showing PHFs and SFs. **(B)** Representative electron micrographs of K18-V337M, which formed amorphous aggregates and short filaments (examples shown in the main figure and inset, respectively). **(C)** Representative electron micrographs of K18-N279K, showing bundled filaments of different shapes and widths. Scale bar = 100 nm for all images. Extended examples of the tau aggregates shown here can be found in **Supplementary Figure S1**. **(D,E)** Box plots of filament lengths and widths, respectively for the tau K18 variants. The plots show the results of a total of 73, 112, and 47 analyzed fibrillar structures for K18-WT, K18-V337M, and K18-N279K, respectively across $n = 3$ independent experiments using different batches of purified proteins. Kruskal–Wallis test followed by Dunn's *post hoc* test; **** = $p < 0.0001$, ns, not significant.

K18-V337M, and 53.0 ± 8.3 nm for K18-N279K), with K18-WT and K18-V337M filaments being similar (p = 0.6698, Kruskal–Wallis test with Dunn's *post hoc* test; **Figure 2E**). K18-N279K filaments were significantly wider than those of K18-WT and K18-V337M (p < 0.0001 in both cases, Kruskal–Wallis test with Dunn's *post hoc* test; **Figure 2E**). Together, the morphology and structural properties of K18-WT aggregates significantly changed in the presence of the FTD mutations, causing a shift from PHFs and SFs to unstructured, amorphous aggregates and shorter but wider filaments for K18-V337M, with K18-N279K aggregating into bundled filaments of similar length to those of K18-WT but of increased width.

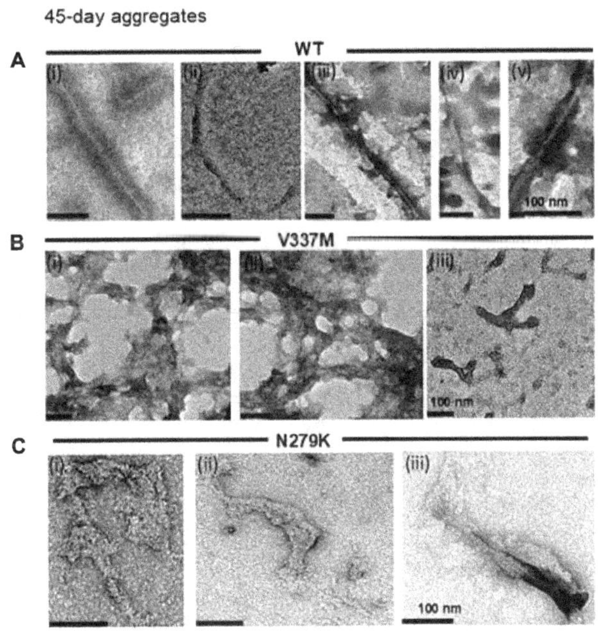

FIGURE 3 | The distinct structural phenotypes of tau K18 aggregates observed in the presence of the FTD mutations do not change with extended aggregation reactions. **(A)** K18-WT formed PHFs and SFs, similar to those recorded in the 4 days assay in **Figure 2A**. **(B)** K18-V337M formed amorphous aggregates in addition to short filaments, similar to those observed in the 4 days aggregation assay in **Figure 2B**. **(C)** K18-N279K formed thick filament bundles whose structural features shares major similarities with those in **Figure 2C**. Scale bar = 100 nm for all images. Three independent experiments each performed with a different batch of purified protein.

Phenotypes of Tau K18 Aggregates Do Not Change With Further Incubation

As aggregation and fracture are thought to modulate the aggregation of tau K18 (Meyer et al., 2016). incubation times were increased to ascertain if the structural properties identified after 4 days would be maintained following prolonged incubation. Because aggregate conformation is partly determined by soluble tau recruitment onto template conformers (Margittai and Langen, 2004; Guo and Lee, 2014), it is conceivable that multiple cycles of aggregation and fracture may favor the growth of minor conformers which would otherwise be undetected in shorter experiments (Meyer et al., 2014, 2016). The previously described TEM experimental setup was employed to image samples obtained from extended incubation periods (45 days). The aggregates formed had the same morphological phenotypes as those seen after 4 days for all protein variants (**Figure 3**), indicating that the conformation of K18-WT aggregates is changed by the N279K and V337M mutations, and that these conformations persist during extended incubation.

FTD Mutations Alter Immuno-Reactivity and Aggregation Products of Tau K18

The unique aggregation and structural properties of the FTD variants of K18 (**Figures 2–3**) are consistent with the hypothesis that they alter K18-WT conformation. In these experiments, heparin was added to accelerate the aggregation and filament formation process. However, the transient nature of heparin-treated tau aggregation can preclude the detection of important conformational changes. The tau proteins' propensity to self-aggregate into filaments in the heparin-free state and the conformations they adopt during this process were therefore, studied.

Reactivity to specific antibodies (total tau A0024 (K9JA) and T22 oligomer conformation-preferring) was used to test for any further indication of distinct conformations, since proteinopathic protein variants with different conformations can lead have differential immuno-reactivity profiles (Hatami et al., 2017). Incubation time was extended to 314 h without agitation to allow PHF formation. Incipient immuno-reactivity was analyzed by dot blotting (**Figure 4** and **Supplementary Figure S2**). K18-WT had the strongest immuno-reactivity to the total tau antibody A0024 at 0 h but this decreased over time (**Figures 4A,B**, upper panels). Similar immuno-reactivity, to A0024, of K18-N279K to that of K18-WT was observed, with the highest intensities recorded at early time points. However, K18-V337M had the lowest immuno-reactivity at each time point: the intensity at 0 h, the strongest recorded, was similar to the lowest intensity for K18-WT at 314 h (**Figures 4A,B**).

To gain insight into possible differences in oligomer conformation, reactivity to the oligomer-preferring T22 antibody was analyzed. Similar to its reactivity to A0024, K18-WT had its highest T22 immuno-reactivity at 0 h, which dropped sharply from 168 h onward (**Figures 4A,B**; lower panels). The reactivity of K18-V337M was low at all time points except at 24 h. K18-N279K had the least intensity to T22 at each time point (**Figures 4A,B**; lower panels and **Supplementary Figure S2**). This result implies that each protein variant folds differently with distinct epitope exposure during aggregation.

Dominant Aggregate Conformers of the Tau K18 Variants Are Unaffected by Seeded Aggregation

Mutations in tau K18 can cause preferential amplification of specific aggregate conformers (Meyer et al., 2014). However, it is unknown if the dominant tau K18 conformers are affected

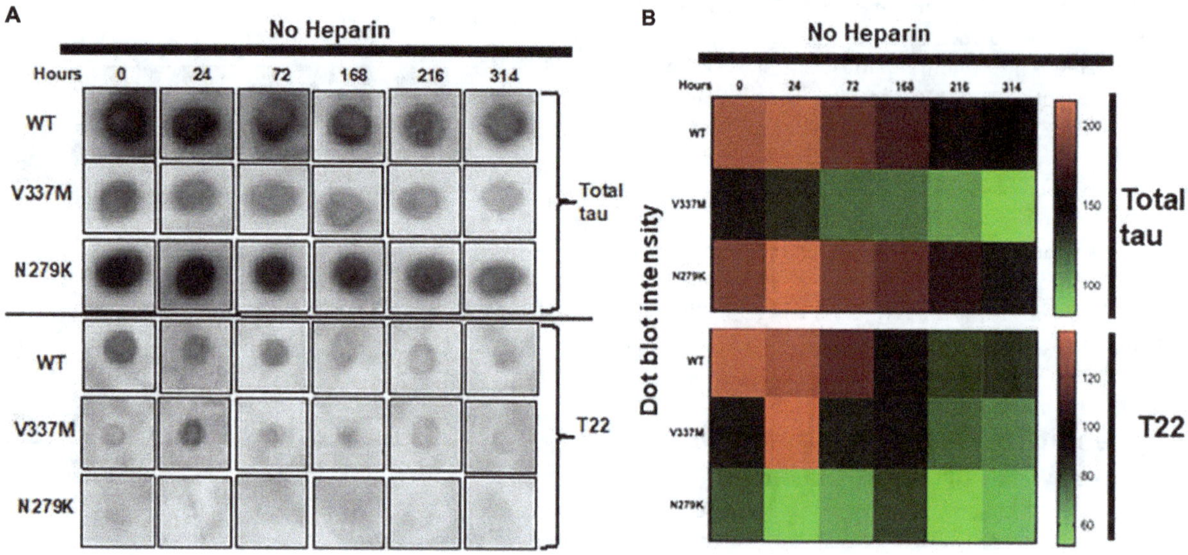

FIGURE 4 | The FTD mutations change the immuno-reactivity of tau K18. **(A)** Dot blots of K18-WT and its FTD variants aggregating in heparin-free conditions probed with two different tau antibodies; total tau (A0024 from Dako) and the oligomer-preferring T22. The dot blot data shown here were from identical experiments, with uncropped images shown in **Supplementary Figure S2**. **(B)** Semi-quantification of dot blot intensity using heat maps.

by seeded aggregation. We therefore, studied if the mutation-induced dominant conformations of the tau K18 variants are affected by the addition of aggregated seeds from different tau K18 variants. Using the same experimental setup as in **Figure 2**, we seeded monomers of tau K18 WT, V337M, and N279K each with 10% volume of 4 days preformed aggregates from each protein variant. Negative-stain TEM imaging showed that seeded reactions (**Supplementary Figures S3B–D**) resulted in aggregate structures with the same phenotypes as those in seed-free experiments (**Supplementary Figure S3A**, same as in **Figure 2**) irrespective of the seed identity. These results suggest that the conformations of the tau K18 aggregates are not only be distinct but may also be incompatible, and that the majority species preferentially aggregate even when seeded with other conformers.

Preparation and Characterization of Fluorescent K18 Oligomers for Functional Studies

Distinct structures of tau strains are thought to explain their divergent functional effects (Clavaguera et al., 2013; Boluda et al., 2015; Falcon et al., 2015; Narasimhan et al., 2017). We therefore, sought to take advantage of the conformational and aggregation differences of the tau K18 variants to investigate their possible influences on the cellular internalization of exogenously applied oligomers. To achieve this, Alexa Fluor-488-C5-maleimide-labeled oligomers were first prepared as detailed in section "Materials and Methods" and elsewhere (Karikari et al., 2019) before being used in *in vitro* cell culture assays. These stable oligomers were granular and non-fibrillar (**Supplementary Figure S4**).

FTD Mutations Enhance Tau K18 Oligomer Internalization in SH-SY5Y Cells

Increasing evidence suggests that the cellular internalization of tau oligomers is an initial trigger of tau pathology (Usenovic et al., 2015; Kolarova et al., 2017). It is, however, not known if FTD with tau mutations are characterized by the same or similar mechanism. To address this, fluorescently labeled oligomers of K18-WT, K18-V337M, and K18-N279K were applied exogenously to SH-SY5Y cells and their internalization dynamics investigated.

All three tau protein variants were internalized by SH-SY5Y cells (**Supplementary Figures S5–S8**). To account for both diffused and punctate phenotypes, we used integrated density (mean intensity x area occupied) to quantify internalized tau in experiments, where equal numbers of cells were seeded and treated with equimolar concentrations of each protein oligomers. The internalization data for each tau K18 variant was analyzed by normalizing the mean integrated density from representative images to the overall mean of the WT (**Figure 5**). Internalization was significantly different between the three protein variants (one-way ANOVA, p = 0.0007, F statistic = 10.08). The Tukey's multiple comparison *post hoc* test showed that internalization was significantly higher for both K18-V337M (p = 0.0122) and K18-N279K (p = 0.0006) against K18-WT but not significantly different between K18-V337M and K18-N279K (p = 0.4524, **Figure 5**).

Exogenous Tau K18 Oligomers Are Internalized by Endocytosis

Previous reports have suggested that K18-WT is internalized by endocytosis (Guo and Lee, 2011; Michel et al., 2014).

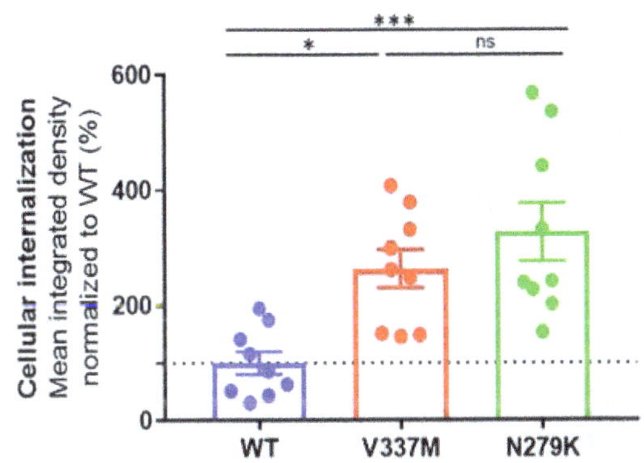

FIGURE 5 | Distinct internalization of K18-WT, K18-V337M, and K18-N279K oligomers in SH-SY5Y neuroblastoma cells. Plot of tau K18 oligomer internalization in SH-SY5Y cells. For each condition, the same number of cells was treated with 10 μM of each protein oligomers as explained in section "Materials and Methods." The graph shows % mean integrated density data normalized to WT. Internalization was significantly different between the tau K18 protein variants ($p = 0.0007$); significantly higher for both K18-V337M and K18-N279K against K18-WT ($p = 0.0122$ and $p = 0.0006$, respectively), using one-way ANOVA followed by Tukey's *post hoc* test. The dotted line shows the mean internalization data for the WT (100%) to which the rest of the data was compared. *Signs refer to significance levels as used in the figure.

However, the internalization mechanism of the FTD variants used in this study was not known. The endocytic marker FM4-64® (SynaptoRed) was used to stain SH-SY5Y cells during internalization, allowing a preliminary assessment of the localization of the internalized tau. Similar to K18-WT, internalized K18-V337M and K18-N279K oligomers co-localized with FM4-64, suggesting endocytic-dependent internalization (**Figures 6A–C**). As a control, incubating SH-SY5Y cells seeded with K18 oligomers at 4°C instead of 37°C blocked internalization (**Supplementary Figure S9**) as shown before for tau K18 and full-length tau 441 (Michel et al., 2014). We next tested if oligomer internalization in a more physiologically relevant cell model, hiPSC-derived neurons, also occurred by endocytosis. Tau taken up by neurons were ostensibly found in both neurites and soma, where they appeared to co-localize with FM4-64 in both compartments (**Figures 6D–F**). Together, these data suggest that tau K18 oligomers can be internalized by SH-SY5Y cells and hiPSC neurons at least partly through endocytosis.

Internalized Tau K18 Oligomers Co-localize With Endogenous Tau and the Nuclear Protein Nucleolin

The ability of internalized tau oligomers to interact with endogenous tau is a critical step in the inter-cellular propagation of tau (Lasagna-Reeves et al., 2012a; Michel et al., 2014; Usenovic et al., 2015). It is, however, unknown if tau variants of different conformations will interact with endogenous tau differently upon internalization. Internalized K18 oligomers were observed to co-localize with endogenous tau in hiPSC-derived neurons bearing the ^{159}PPGQK^{163} epitope (HT7 antibody). All three tau K18 variants co-localized with endogenous tau, occurring both in the neurites and the soma (**Figure 7**), suggestive of an interaction of internalized tau with endogenous tau.

The nuclear localization of both endogenous tau and tau overexpressed from genetic constructs has been reported in both the human and mouse brains (Rady et al., 1995; Liu and Götz, 2013) and cell culture models (Lu et al., 2014; Ritter et al., 2018). Nuclear tau staining is often predominantly apparent in the nucleolus, with tau signals co-localized with those of the nucleolar protein nucleolin (Sjöberg et al., 2006), although more diffuse nuclear staining for endogenous tau has been reported in response to cell stress (Sultan et al., 2011). In SH-SY5Y cells, the internalized tau was not generally detected in the nucleus. Although some association with nucleolin was observed, this was expected to result from the redistribution of the nucleolin protein during the different phases of the cell cycle in these dividing cells (data not shown). Cytoplasmic accumulation of internalized tau, as has been previously demonstrated, was recorded for both cell types. However, in contrast to the SH-SY5Y cells, tau-nucleolin co-localization was observed in hiPSC-derived neurons with nucleolar inclusion of internalized tau for both mutant and WT tau-K18 (**Figure 8**).

Internalized Tau K18 Oligomers Do Not Induce LDH-Dependent Cytotoxicity in SH-SY5Y Cells

Several studies have shown that internalized tau oligomers impair cell viability and/or induce cell death (Lasagna-Reeves et al., 2010; Guerrero-Muñoz et al., 2015) but others have reported the opposite (Kumar et al., 2014; Kaniyappan et al., 2017). However, the cytotoxicity potential of tau FTD variants is unknown. SH-SY5Y cells were therefore, treated with the respective oligomers and cytotoxicity studied by measuring LDH release. No significant differences in viability were observed between increasing concentrations of WT or mutant K18 oligomers (**Figure 9**), suggesting that the oligomers did not induce LDH-dependent cytotoxicity over 72 h.

DISCUSSION

Tau has important functions in the pathogenesis of AD and FTD (Ghetti et al., 2015; Wang and Mandelkow, 2016; Guo et al., 2017). Whilst several theories have been proposed toward understanding disease mechanisms, recent studies have pointed to possible involvement of an inter-neuronal transmission mechanism. Although this hypothesis has strong evidential support (Mohamed et al., 2013; Guo and Lee, 2014; Hu et al., 2016), it remains to be shown why tau isolates from different post-mortem tauopathy brains have distinct internalization and transmission capabilities. In this study, an integrated structural and cell biological approach was used to understand potential links between protein aggregation, conformation and cellular internalization. It was hypothesized that specific disease-associated *MAPT* mutations implicated in familial FTD will alter the structural features (conformation and aggregation) and cellular internalization of WT tau K18. It has been demonstrated that the N279K and V337M FTD-linked mutations do alter

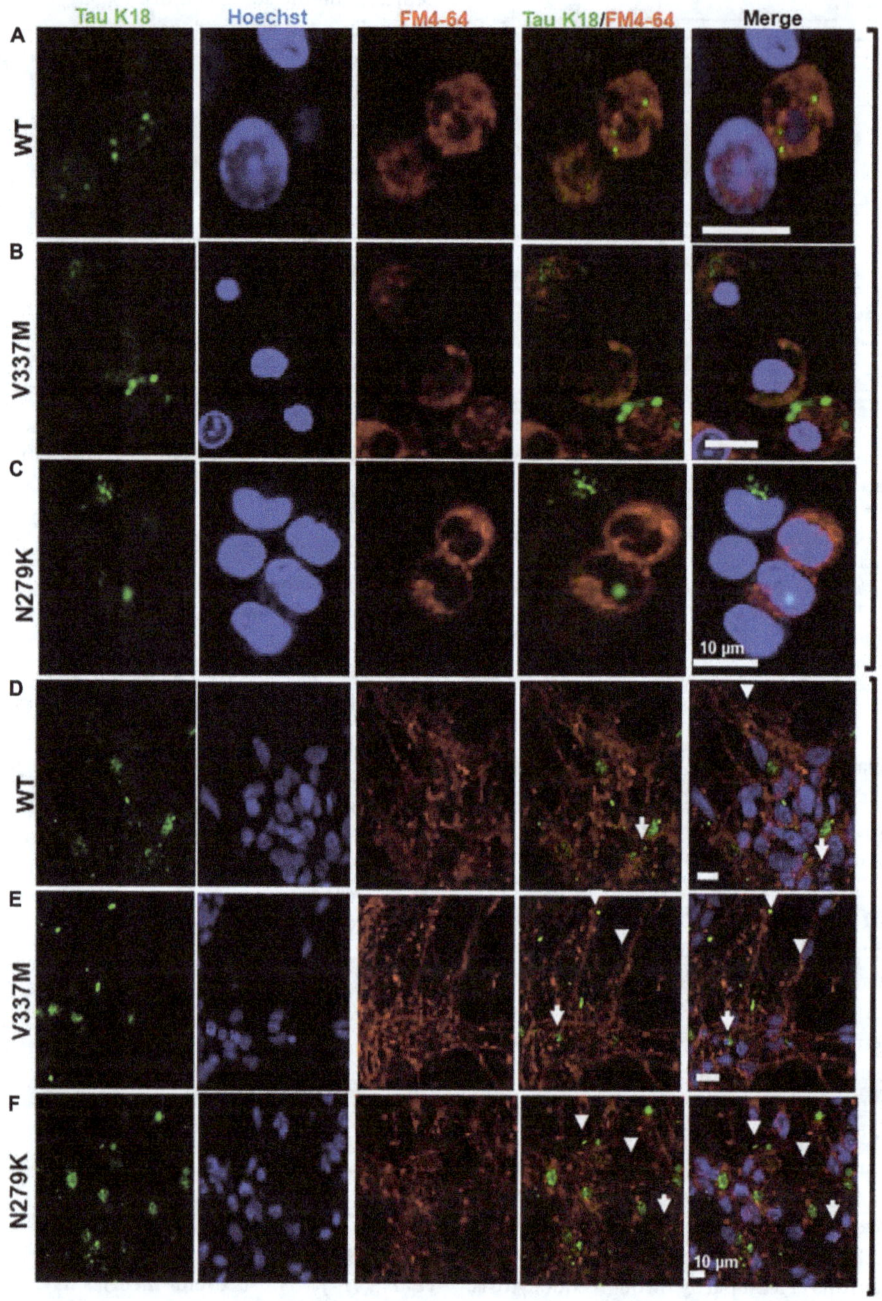

FIGURE 6 | Extracellular tau K18 oligomers are taken up by endocytosis, with the internalized soluble aggregates localizing to the neurites and soma of hiPSC-derived neurons. Panels **(A–C)**, respectively, show co-localization of oligomers of K18-WT, K18-V337M, and K18-N279K internalized by SH-SY5Y cells with the FM4-64 endocytosis marker. **(D–F)** Internalized exogenous oligomers of K18-WT, K18-V337M, and K18-N279K, respectively, co-localized with the FM4-64 endocytosis marker in hiPSC-derived neurons. Whilst some of the internalized oligomers of all three protein variants were found in the neurites (arrowheads), others appeared to be present in the soma (arrows). Scale bar = 10 μm for all images.

tau K18 aggregation and conformation. Moreover, the mutants had enhanced cellular internalization, yet all protein variants were internalized by endocytosis and had shared the same subcellular accumulation patterns. These data suggest that structural distinctions between tau variants may influence their cellular internalization properties, with potential implications for the molecular pathogenesis of tauopathies.

Previous studies of the V337M and N279K mutations did not identify any discernible effects on tau aggregation propensity (Barghorn et al., 2000; Combs and Gamblin, 2012). This may have been due to the use of thioflavin fluorescent reporter assays to quantify aggregation (Barghorn et al., 2000; Combs and Gamblin, 2012). Although commonly used to detect cross β-sheet-dependent aggregation (Lindberg et al., 2015), a major

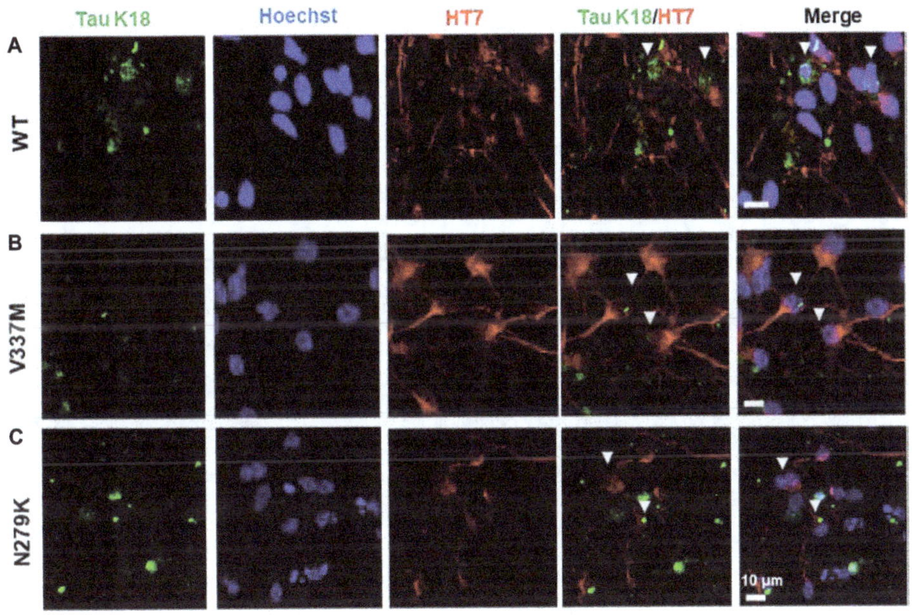

FIGURE 7 | Internalized tau K18 oligomers in hiPSC-derived neurons co-localize with endogenous tau bearing the HT7 (^{159}PPGQK^{163}) mid-region epitope. Extracellularly applied oligomers of tau K18-WT **(A)**, K18-V337M **(B)**, and K18-N279K **(C)** oligomers internalized in hiPSC-derived neurons co-localized with endogenous tau in the soma and the neurites. White arrowheads show sites of co-localization. Scale bar = 10 μm for all images. Figure extension in **Supplementary Figures S8A–C**.

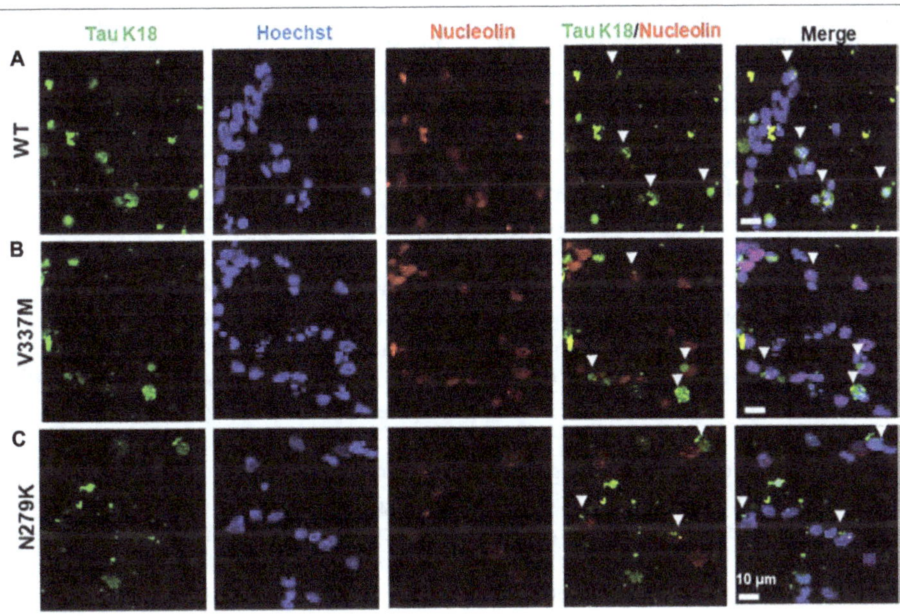

FIGURE 8 | Exogenous tau K18 oligomers internalized in the neurites of hiPSC-derived neurons co-localize with the nucleolar protein nucleolin. Panels **(A–C)** show the co-localization of internalized oligomers of WT, V337M, and N279K tau K18, respectively, with nucleolin. Scale bar = 10 μm for all images. Figure extension in **Supplementary Figures S8D–F**.

pitfall of thioflavin assays is that they appear to be probes of protein conformation instead of aggregation status since different folding behaviors can change the availability of different proteinopathic proteins to the binding sites of the dye (Coelho-Cerqueira et al., 2014; Wong et al., 2016; Hatami et al., 2017). For this reason, the ability of thioflavin dyes to distinguish between conformations of variants of the same protein can sometimes be complicated (Hatami et al., 2017). Although kinetics may remain apparently unaffected, our data using TEM to characterize aggregates suggest that both mutations

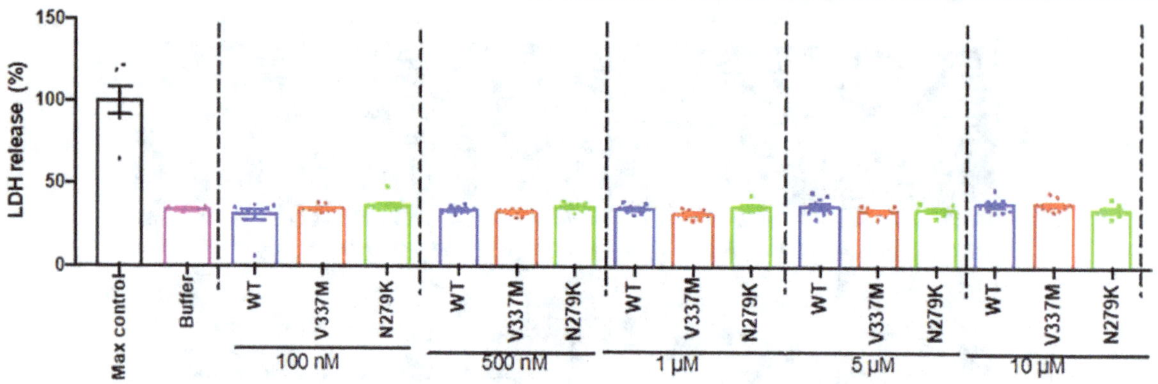

FIGURE 9 | Internalized tau K18 oligomers do not induce LDH-dependent cytotoxicity in SH-SY5Y cells. Increasing concentrations of oligomeric tau K18 variants were applied to SH-SY5Y cells for 72 h, and the cells analyzed for LDH release. We found no significant difference in LDH release between the controls (buffer only or maximum control) and the tau K18 variants at the concentrations studied (*n* = 3 each).

impact upon the aggregation of K18, a finding supported by atomic force microscopy analysis (data not shown). Immuno-reactivity data to probe conformation supported these findings. These complementary findings in multiple assays build a strong argument in support of the hypothesis that the mutations alter the aggregation and conformation of tau K18. Interestingly, similar profiles were observed for aggregation reactions carried out in the absence of the heparin aggregation inducer. Moreover, the FTD mutations altered the immuno-reactivity of aggregated K18-WT. K18-V337M had lower reactivity to both tau antibodies whilst the N279K mutation almost abolished reactivity to the oligomer-preferring T22 antibody but its reactivity to A0024 was comparable to that of K18-WT. Our results therefore, imply that each mutation shifts protein conformation which in turn dictates the pathway toward forming distinct aggregates. The consistent observation that each protein variant had distinct aggregate structures in several independent assays (both heparin-induced and native-state aggregation) additionally supports mutation-induced differences in protein aggregation and conformations, similar to that previously described for amyloid beta (Hatami et al., 2017). Two main reasons could account for the distinct T22 reactivity even at 0 h, where the samples were monomeric. Firstly, the T22 antibody is thought to selectively recognize an oligomeric conformational epitope. However, the antibody can also react with monomers which presumably share this same epitope (Lasagna-Reeves et al., 2012b). Secondly, the differential T22 binding to the tau K18 variants could also be due to the introduced mutations since the exact epitope of the antibody is unknown (it binds to the repeat domain region – amino acids 244–372 of full length tau 441). It is conceivable that the distinct aggregation and conformational dynamics of the protein variants would also lead to notable differences in epitope availability/recognition. Together, the data provided demonstrate that the V337M and N279K disease-associated mutations induce structural and conformational changes in tau K18 that are evident at distinct stages of aggregation, including oligomers and fibrils.

Tau oligomers are a potential sensitive biomarker for neurodegeneration (Sengupta et al., 2017) and can induce endogenous tau aggregation upon cellular internalization (Lasagna-Reeves et al., 2012a; Michel et al., 2014). Effects of the disease mutations on the cellular uptake of structurally characterized oligomers of tau K18 were therefore investigated. Differences in oligomer uptake were observed in respect to tau mutants. Irrespective of mutation, the uptake of K18 appeared to be endocytic. Uptake of all K18 forms tested highlight that different tau aggregates may each propagate disease by spreading into non-diseased cells. However, differences potentially mediated by aggregate conformation may provide critical insights into shared and distinct molecular mechanisms of tauopathies involving FTD and WT tau.

Consistent with previous reports that used recombinant or brain isolates of tau (Frost et al., 2009; Guo and Lee, 2011; Michel et al., 2014; Falcon et al., 2015; Ando et al., 2016; Calafate et al., 2016), the K18-WT oligomers were most likely internalized by endocytosis in both cell types, with same observed for the FTD variants. Whilst all protein variants appeared to be internalized by endocytosis, co-localized with endogenous tau and were found both in the cytoplasm and nucleus, the degree of internalization differed between the protein variants. We speculative that the new aggregation and/or conformation dynamics recorded in the presence of the FTD mutations may change tau K18 interaction with cell surface proteins that regulate endocytosis, resulting in altered cellular trafficking. In agreement, binding to heparan sulfate proteoglycans regulates the cellular internalization and inter-cellular propagation of aggregated tau, and that blocking the activity or expression of heparan sulfate proteoglycan prevents internalization (Holmes et al., 2013; Rauch et al., 2018). However, it is unknown if WT and mutant tau proteins bind heparan sulfate proteoglycans with the same or different affinities. Furthermore, dysfunctions in key steps in clathrin-mediated endocytosis have been implicated in tau propagation and inclusion formation in AD, FTD and other tauopathies (Ando et al., 2016; Calafate et al., 2016). It remains to be studied if mutation-induced conformational changes do modify tau internalization, propagation and toxicity in an *in vivo* model. However, with the *in vitro* evidence presented in the current study, we can speculate that the altered conformations of tau resulting from the FTD mutations leads to specific changes in the protein's vesicular uptake or receptor binding, resulting in altered uptake efficiency. Another possibility is that the FTD mutations alter the efficiency of degradation of internalized tau K18 in each cell line, resulting in differential amounts of internalized proteins. It is worth investigating if oligomers of WT and mutated tau are degraded through the same or different pathways, and if the mutations affect clearance efficiency. Previous studies have shown that internalized WT tau oligomers/aggregates and the internalized-endogenous tau aggregate complexes they form intracellularly may be cleared by autophagy (Wu et al., 2013; Usenovic et al., 2015). In agreement, treating hiPSC-derived neurons with rapamycin reduces the amount of internalized tau oligomers-endogenous tau aggregate complexes, suggesting that lysosomal elimination is a common degradation route for tau aggregates.

The ability of internalized exogenous tau aggregates to interact with endogenous tau is critical for the efficient inter-cellular propagation of tau aggregates and the associated neurotoxicity (Lasagna-Reeves et al., 2012a; Michel et al., 2014; Wegmann et al., 2015). The observed co-localization of all three protein variants with endogenous tau suggests that internalized tau K18 and the FTD variants can interact with endogenous tau, indicating the potential for propagation by inducing endogenous tau aggregation, possibly following a templated misfolding mechanism as described previously for tau K18 (Guo and Lee, 2011; Michel et al., 2014). As both the FTD mutants and WT K18 showed similar cellular distribution and localization, it would suggest the potential for prion-like propagation of the FTD mutant tau.

In hiPSC-derived neurons, the co-localization with nucleolin suggests that internalized tau can be taken up into the nucleus, and raises the possibility that internalized tau that gets into the nucleus may have functions in protein biosynthesis. Nuclear tau associates with nucleolin in AD brain, where reduced nuclear tau levels correlated with decreased amounts of nucleolin (Hernández-Ortega et al., 2016). Interaction of aggregated tau, both WT and disease-associated mutated variants, with specific ribosomal proteins can impair the protein synthesis machinery (Meier et al., 2016). Given that pathological tau can impair nucleocytoplasmic transport in AD brains and tau transgenic mice (Eftekharzadeh et al., 2018), and the overexpression of the N279K tau variant in a cell model is associated with increased nuclear localization (Ritter et al., 2018), the effect of tau on the protein synthesis machinery deserves further investigation.

Our findings that tau K18 oligomers, even at high concentrations, did not significantly induce LDH release was unexpected since some previous reports pointed to the contrary (Lasagna-Reeves et al., 2010, 2012a). Nonetheless, our present data is supported by other studies (Kumar et al., 2014; Tepper et al., 2014; Kaniyappan et al., 2017). The origin of these divergent data is unknown but could be explained by differences in oligomer concentrations, preparation methods and cytotoxicity assays. For example, 0.1–1 μM of full length tau-441 oligomers produced by seeding with oligomers from AD brain, amyloid β or α-synuclein were toxic to cells, as measured by the 3-(4,5-dimethylthiazol-2-yl)-5-(3-carboxymethoxyphenyl)-2-(4 sulfophenyl)-2H-tetrazolium (MTS) assay (Lasagna-Reeves et al., 2010, 2012a). On the other hand, applying 10 μM of tau K18 oligomers (recombinant or derived from Sf9 cells) to mouse primary cortical neurons or SH-SY5Y cells did not result in significant cytotoxicity within 3–72 h, as shown by the LDH or MTT (3-(4,5-dimethylthiazol-2-yl)-2,5-diphenyltetrazolium bromide) assays (Kumar et al., 2014; Tepper et al., 2014). Whether or not exogenous tau oligomers induce overt cytotoxicity, their most immediate toxic effect is likely to be an impairment of the structural and functional integrity of neurons and potentially other cell types. In support, internalized tau oligomers impair neural transmission, cause dendritic spine loss and increases in intracellular calcium levels and reactive oxygen species without evidence of overt changes to cell viability (Kumar et al., 2014; Tepper et al., 2014; Usenovic et al., 2015; Yin et al., 2016; Kaniyappan et al., 2017).

Together, these results demonstrate that specific disease-associated single nucleotide polymorphisms in tau can cause drastic changes in protein conformation and aggregation. These distinctive structural and conformational properties may be crucial determinants of the inter-cellular transmission efficiency of the oligomeric forms of these proteins. These findings may provide a molecular explanation as to why tau extracts obtained from different sources (including human tauopathy brains, tau transgenic mice brains, and recombinant preparations) have distinctive propagation potencies and endogenous tau aggregation abilities in both cellular and animal preclinical tauopathy models. Indeed, aggregated tau from transgenic mice brains and recombinant sources have been shown to have distinct conformations that can influence their seeding capabilities (Falcon et al., 2015). It can be argued that critical post-translational modifications such as phosphorylation and the *in vivo* environment in which this process occurs might have contributed to the conformational differences observed. As the recombinant tau proteins used in the present study were not phosphorylated, it can be said that phosphorylation and sites of phosphorylation *per se* may not be responsible for the conformational, structural and molecular activity differences previously observed for tau aggregates from diverse sources. The differential aggregation of the recombinant mutants reinforces the conclusion that specific amino acid modifications are sufficient to induce structural and functional differences in tau-K18. Such structural and functional differences may then be compounded by the differential phosphorylation of the mutant forms of tau or their differential recruitment of endogenous tau.

Importantly, these findings may help to understand why different tauopathies have distinct progression rates, neuropathological features, inclusion formation and types of inclusion (Delisle et al., 1999; Murrell et al., 1999; Sergeant et al., 2005; Ghetti et al., 2015). Furthermore, these results may pave the way for the development of more sensitive, disease- and mutation-specific platforms for early, more accurate diagnosis of tauopathies. Future studies should aim to ascertain if the findings described here are applicable to tau isolates from tauopathy brains: if their reported activity differences can be explained by structural and conformational distinctions.

AUTHOR CONTRIBUTIONS

TK, DN, EH, and KM conceived and co-ordinated the study. TK designed and conducted the experiments, analyzed the data, and wrote the first draft of the manuscript. AG, CC-B, and JC made significant contributions to hiPSC experiments, immunocytochemistry, and confocal microscopy. DN, EH, and KM contributed reagents and materials, made important contributions to data interpretation, and critically revised the initial manuscript draft. All authors discussed and commented on the final manuscript.

ACKNOWLEDGMENTS

The authors wish to thank Prof. Alison Rodger and Dr. Nikola Chmel of the Department of Chemistry, University of Warwick, for useful discussions and use of analytical biophysics facilities. The authors also thank Mr. Ian Hands-Portman (School of Life Sciences, University of Warwick) for training TK and providing him access to TEM facilities. TK acknowledges Drs. Mussa Quareshy and Greg Walkowiak for assistance with protein purification and microplate reader access, respectively. The authors acknowledge support from the Research Councils UK Block Grant at the University of Warwick for the payment of open access fee.

SUPPLEMENTARY MATERIAL

FIGURE S1 | The FTD mutations cause structural changes in the properties of tau K18 filaments. **(A)** Representative TEM images of K18-WT, showing PHFs and SFs. **(B)** Representative electron micrographs of K18-V337M, which formed amorphous aggregates [examples shown in (i), (ii), and (iii)] and short filaments [(iv) and (v)]. **(C)** Representative electron micrographs of K18-N279K, showing bundled filaments of varying shapes and widths. Scale bar = 100 nm for all images. $n = 3$ independent experiments for each protein. This figure is an extension of **Figure 2**.

FIGURE S2 | Uncropped dot blot data used for immuno-reactivity analysis in **Figure 4**. **(A)** Dot blot intensity data for K18-WT, K18-V337M, and K18-N279K following total tau A0024 reactivity. **(B)** T22 antibody reactivity profiles of K18-WT, K18-V337M, and K18-N279K. For better visualization, the sites of dot blotting are highlighted with black circles.

FIGURE S3 | Dominant aggregate conformers of the tau K18 variants are unaffected by seeded aggregation. Endpoint aggregates of K18 WT, V337M, and N279K from 4 days reactions were used to seed the aggregation of each protein in turn. The resulting product, after a further 4 days of incubation at room temperature, were analyzed by TEM imaging (**A**, unseeded; **B**, seeded with WT; **C**, seeded with V337M seeded; and **D**, seeded with N279K). Scale bars = 100 nm for all images.

FIGURE S4 | Structural characterization of fluorescently labeled oligomers of tau K18 and its FTD variants. **(A–C)** Representative TEM characterization of tau K18 oligomers labeled with Alexa Fluor 488 conjugated maleimide demonstrating the presence of granular structures for K18-WT, K18-V337M, and K18-N279K, respectively. Insets refer to higher magnification images. Scale bars for all images = 200 nm and 20 nm for insets. **(D)** Non-denaturing SDS PAGE image of labeled tau K18 oligomers.

FIGURE S5 | Uptake of extracellularly applied tau K18 oligomers into SH-SY5Y cells. Seeded cells were supplied with 10 μM tau K18 oligomers and incubated for 24 h at 37°C, 5% CO_2, following which the spent media were removed and the cells washed with warm 10 mM PBS before new tau-free media was added. Uptake of oligomers was demonstrated using confocal microscopy. Panels **(A–C)** show cellular internalization of K18-WT, K18-V337M, and K18-N279K oligomers, respectively. Scale bar = 10 μm for all images.

FIGURE S6 | Internalized oligomers of the tau K18 variants localize to the nuclei and cytoplasm of SH-SY5Y cells. Oligomeric aggregates of tau K18-WT **(A)**, K18-V337M **(B)**, and K18-N279K **(C)** internalized by the SH-SY5Y cells appeared to be distributed in the cytoplasm (open arrow heads) and nucleus (filled arrow heads). Scale bars = 10 μm for all images.

FIGURE S7 | Higher resolution images of internalized tau K18 oligomers in SH-SY5Y cells. The images here show AF-maleimide-labeled tau K18 oligomers (green) taken up mainly into the cytoplasm of K18-WT, K18-V337M, and K18-N279K (**A–C**, respectively). Scale bar = 10 μm for all images.

FIGURE S8 | Colocalization of tau K18 with endogenous tau and nucleolin at high intensity. These figures show digitally increased intensity of selected regions from the images in **Figures 7**, **8** to better demonstrate colocalization of tau K18 WT, V337M, and N279K with endogenous tau (**A–C**, respectively) or nucleolin (**D–F**, respectively). For better composite color appreciation, colocalization is shown in yellow - merger of red (endogenous tau or nucleolin) and green (tau K18) channels or white – merger of magenta (endogenous tau or nucleolin) and green (tau K18) channels. Arrows point to regions of colocalization.

FIGURE S9 | Incubation in cold conditions blocks the internalization of tau K18 oligomers by SH-SY5Y cells. **(A–C)** Oligomer uptake was significantly reduced for tau K18-WT, K18-V337M, and K18-N279K, respectively when SH-SY5Y cells were incubated at 4°C instead of 37°C (as shown in **Figure 6**).

REFERENCES

Alonso, A. D., Beharry, C., Corbo, C. P., and Cohen, L. S. (2016). Molecular mechanism of prion-like tau-induced neurodegeneration. *Alzheimers Dement.* 12, 1090–1097. doi: 10.1016/j.jalz.2015.12.014

Ando, K., Tomimura, K., Sazdovitch, V., Suain, V., Yilmaz, Z., Authelet, M., et al. (2016). Level of PICALM, a key component of clathrin-mediated endocytosis, is correlated with levels of phosphotau and autophagy-related proteins and is associated with tau inclusions in AD, PSP and Pick disease. *Neurobiol. Dis.* 94, 32–43. doi: 10.1016/j.nbd.2016.05.017

Arriagada, P. V., Growdon, J. H., Hedley-Whyte, E. T., and Hyman, B. T. (1992). Neurofibrillary tangles but not senile plaques parallel duration and severity of Alzheimer's disease. *Neurology* 42, 631–639.

Barghorn, S., Davies, P., and Mandelkow, E. (2004). Tau paired helical filaments from Alzheimer's Disease brain and assembled in vitro are based on β-structure in the core domain. *Biochemistry* 43, 1694–1703. doi: 10.1021/bi0357006

Barghorn, S., and Mandelkow, E. (2002). Toward a unified scheme for the aggregation of tau into Alzheimer paired helical filaments†. *Biochemistry* 41, 14885–14896. doi: 10.1021/bi026469j

Barghorn, S., Zheng-Fischhöfer, Q., Ackmann, M., Biernat, J., von Bergen, M., Mandelkow, E.-M., et al. (2000). Structure, microtubule interactions, and paired helical filament aggregation by tau mutants of frontotemporal dementias. *Biochemistry* 39, 11714–11721. doi: 10.1021/bi000850r

Bodea, L., Eckert, A., Ittner, L. M., Piguet, O., and Götz, J. (2016). Tau physiology and pathomechanisms in frontotemporal lobar degeneration. *J. Neurochem.* 138, 71–94. doi: 10.1111/jnc.13600

Boluda, S., Iba, M., Zhang, B., Raible, K. M., Lee, V. M.-Y., and Trojanowski, J. Q. (2015). Differential induction and spread of tau pathology in young PS19 tau transgenic mice following intracerebral injections of pathological tau from Alzheimer's disease or corticobasal degeneration brains. *Acta Neuropathol.* 129, 221–237. doi: 10.1007/s00401-014-1373-1370

Calafate, S., Flavin, W., Verstreken, P., and Moechars, D. (2016). Loss of bin1 promotes the propagation of tau pathology. *Cell Rep.* 17, 931–940. doi: 10.1016/j.celrep.2016.09.063

Clavaguera, F., Akatsu, H., Fraser, G., Crowther, R. A., Frank, S., Hench, J., et al. (2013). Brain homogenates from human tauopathies induce tau inclusions in mouse brain. *Proc. Natl. Acad. Sci. U.S.A.* 110, 9535–9540. doi: 10.1073/pnas.1301175110

Clavaguera, F., Bolmont, T., Crowther, R. A., Abramowski, D., Frank, S., Probst, A., et al. (2009). Transmission and spreading of tauopathy in transgenic mouse brain. *Nat. Cell Biol.* 11, 909–913. doi: 10.1038/ncb1901

Coelho-Cerqueira, E., Pinheiro, A. S., and Follmer, C. (2014). Pitfalls associated with the use of Thioflavin-T to monitor anti-fibrillogenic activity. *Bioorg. Med. Chem. Lett.* 24, 3194–3198. doi: 10.1016/j.bmcl.2014.04.072

Combs, B., and Gamblin, T. C. (2012). FTDP-17 tau mutations induce distinct effects on aggregation and microtubule interactions. *Biochemistry* 51, 8597–8607. doi: 10.1021/bi3010818

Delisle, M. B., Murrell, J. R., Richardson, R., Trofatter, J. A., Rascol, O., Soulages, X., et al. (1999). A mutation at codon 279 (N279K) in exon 10 of the Tau gene causes a tauopathy with dementia and supranuclear palsy. *Acta Neuropathol.* 98, 62–77. doi: 10.1007/s004010051052

Eftekharzadeh, B., Daigle, J. G., Kapinos, L. E., Coyne, A., Schiantarelli, J., Carlomagno, Y., et al. (2018). Tau protein disrupts nucleocytoplasmic transport in Alzheimer's Disease. *Neuron* 99, 925–940.e7. doi: 10.1016/j.neuron.2018.07.039

Falcon, B., Cavallini, A., Angers, R., Glover, S., Murray, T. K., Barnham, L., et al. (2015). Conformation Determines the seeding potencies of native and recombinant tau aggregates. *J. Biol. Chem.* 290, 1049–1065. doi: 10.1074/jbc.M114.589309

Fitzpatrick, A. W. P., Falcon, B., He, S., Murzin, A. G., Murshudov, G., Garringer, H. J., et al. (2017). Cryo-EM structures of tau filaments from Alzheimer's disease. *Nature* 547, 185–190. doi: 10.1038/nature23002

Frost, B., Jacks, R. L., and Diamond, M. I. (2009). Propagation of tau misfolding from the outside to the inside of a cell. *J. Biol. Chem.* 284, 12845–12852. doi: 10.1074/jbc.M808759200

Gerson, J. E., Mudher, A., and Kayed, R. (2016). Potential mechanisms and implications for the formation of tau oligomeric strains. *Crit. Rev. Biochem. Mol. Biol.* 51, 482–496. doi: 10.1080/10409238.2016.1226251

Ghetti, B., Oblak, A. L., Boeve, B. F., Johnson, K. A., Dickerson, B. C., and Goedert, M. (2015). Frontotemporal dementia caused by microtubule-associated protein tau gene (MAPT) mutations: a chameleon for neuropathology and neuroimaging. *Neuropathol. Appl. Neurobiol.* 41, 24–46. doi: 10.1111/nan.12213

Goedert, M. (2016). The ordered assembly of tau is the gain-of-toxic function that causes human tauopathies. *Alzheimers Dement.* 12, 1040–1050. doi: 10.1016/j.jalz.2016.09.001

Goedert, M., Falcon, B., Clavaguera, F., and Tolnay, M. (2014). Prion-like Mechanisms in the Pathogenesis of Tauopathies and Synucleinopathies. *Curr. Neurol. Neurosci. Rep.* 14:495. doi: 10.1007/s11910-014-0495-z

Grüning, C. S. R., Mirecka, E. A., Klein, A. N., Mandelkow, E., Willbold, D., Marino, S. F., et al. (2014). Alternative conformations of the tau repeat domain in complex with an engineered binding protein. *J. Biol. Chem.* 289, 23209–23218. doi: 10.1074/jbc.M114.560920

Guerrero-Muñoz, M. J., Gerson, J., and Castillo-Carranza, D. L. (2015). Tau oligomers: the toxic player at synapses in Alzheimer's Disease. *Front. Cell. Neurosci* 9:464. doi: 10.3389/fncel.2015.00464

Guo, J. L., and Lee, V. M. (2014). Cell-to-cell transmission of pathogenic proteins in neurodegenerative diseases. *Nat. Med.* 20, 130–138. doi: 10.1038/nm.3457

Guo, J. L., and Lee, V. M.-Y. (2011). Seeding of normal Tau by pathological Tau conformers drives pathogenesis of Alzheimer-like tangles. *J. Biol. Chem.* 286, 15317–15331. doi: 10.1074/jbc.M110.209296

Guo, T., Noble, W., and Hanger, D. P. (2017). Roles of tau protein in health and disease. *Acta Neuropathol.* 133, 665–704. doi: 10.1007/s00401-017-1707-1709

Hatami, A., Monjazeb, S., Milton, S., and Glabe, C. G. (2017). Familial Alzheimer's Disease Mutations within the Amyloid Precursor Protein Alter the Aggregation and Conformation of the Amyloid-β Peptide. *J. Biol. Chem.* 292, 3172–3185. doi: 10.1074/jbc.M116.755264

Hernández-Ortega, K., Garcia-Esparcia, P., Gil, L., Lucas, J. J., and Ferrer, I. (2016). Altered machinery of protein synthesis in Alzheimer's: from the nucleolus to the ribosome. *Brain Pathol.* 26, 593–605. doi: 10.1111/bpa.12335

Holmes, B. B., DeVos, S. L., Kfoury, N., Li, M., Jacks, R., Yanamandra, K., et al. (2013). Heparan sulfate proteoglycans mediate internalization and propagation of specific proteopathic seeds. *Proc. Natl. Acad. Sci.* 110, E3138–E3147. doi: 10.1073/pnas.1301440110

Hong, M., Zhukareva, V., Vogelsberg-Ragaglia, V., Wszolek, Z., Reed, L., Miller, B. I., et al. (1998). Mutation-specific functional impairments in distinct tau isoforms of hereditary FTDP-17. *Science* 282, 1914–1917. doi: 10.1126/science.282.5395.1914

Hu, W., Zhang, X., Tung, Y. C., Xie, S., Liu, F., and Iqbal, K. (2016). Hyperphosphorylation determines both the spread and the morphology of tau pathology. *Alzheimers Dement.* 12, 1066–1077. doi: 10.1016/j.jalz.2016.01.014

Iba, M., Guo, J. L., McBride, J. D., Zhang, B., Trojanowski, J. Q., and Lee, V. M.-Y. (2013). Synthetic Tau Fibrils Mediate Transmission of Neurofibrillary Tangles in a Transgenic Mouse Model of Alzheimer's-Like Tauopathy. *J. Neurosci.* 33, 1024–1037. doi: 10.1523/JNEUROSCI.2642-12.2013

Kaniyappan, S., Chandupatla, R. R., Mandelkow, E.-M., and Mandelkow, E. (2017). Extracellular low-n oligomers of tau cause selective synaptotoxicity without affecting cell viability. *Alzheimers Dement.* 13, 1270–1291. doi: 10.1016/j.jalz.2017.04.002

Karikari, T. K., Nagel, D. A., Grainger, A., Clarke-Bland, C., Hill, E. J., and Moffat, K. G. (2019). Preparation of stable tau oligomers for cellular and biochemical studies. *Anal. Biochem.* 566, 67–74. doi: 10.1016/j.ab.2018.10.013

Karikari, T. K., Turner, A., Stass, R., Lee, L. C. Y., Wilson, B., Nagel, D. A., et al. (2017). Expression and purification of tau protein and its frontotemporal dementia variants using a cleavable histidine tag. *Protein Expr. Purif.* 130, 44–54. doi: 10.1016/j.pep.2016.09.009

Kaufman, S. K., Sanders, D. W., Thomas, T. L., Ruchinskas, A. J., Vaquer-Alicea, J., Sharma, A. M., et al. (2016). Tau prion strains dictate patterns of cell pathology, progression rate, and regional vulnerability in vivo. *Neuron* 92, 796–812. doi: 10.1016/j.neuron.2016.09.055

Kolarova, M., Sengupta, U., Bartos, A., Ricny, J., and Kayed, R. (2017). Tau Oligomers in Sera of Patients with Alzheimer's Disease and Aged Controls. *J. Alzheimers Dis.* 58, 471–478. doi: 10.3233/JAD-170048

Kumar, S., Tepper, K., Kaniyappan, S., Biernat, J., Wegmann, S., Mandelkow, E.-M., et al. (2014). Stages and conformations of the tau repeat domain during aggregation and its effect on neuronal toxicity. *J. Biol. Chem.* 289, 20318–20332. doi: 10.1074/jbc.M114.554725

Lasagna-Reeves, C. A., Castillo-Carranza, D. L., Guerrero-Muñoz, M. J., Jackson, G. R., and Kayed, R. (2010). Preparation and characterization of neurotoxic tau oligomers. *Biochemistry* 49, 10039–10041. doi: 10.1021/bi1016233

Lasagna-Reeves, C. A., Castillo-Carranza, D. L., Sengupta, U., Guerrero-Munoz, M. J., Kiritoshi, T., Neugebauer, V., et al. (2012a). Alzheimer brain-derived tau oligomers propagate pathology from endogenous tau. *Sci. Rep.* 2:700. doi: 10.1038/srep00700

Lasagna-Reeves, C. A., Castillo-Carranza, D. L., Sengupta, U., Sarmiento, J., Troncoso, J., Jackson, G. R., et al. (2012b). Identification of oligomers at early stages of tau aggregation in Alzheimer's disease. *FASEB J.* 26, 1946–1959. doi: 10.1096/fj.11-199851

Li, W., and Lee, V. M.-Y. (2006). Characterization of Two VQIXXK Motifs for Tau Fibrillization in Vitro. *Biochemistry* 45, 15692–15701. doi: 10.1021/bi061422

Lindberg, D. J., Wranne, M. S., Gilbert Gatty, M., Westerlund, F., and Esbjörner, E. K. (2015). Steady-state and time-resolved Thioflavin-T fluorescence can report on morphological differences in amyloid fibrils formed by Aβ(1-40) and Aβ(1-42). *Biochem. Biophys. Res. Commun.* 458, 418–423. doi: 10.1016/j.bbrc.2015.01.132

Liu, C., and Götz, J. (2013). Profiling murine tau with 0N, 1N and 2N isoform-specific antibodies in brain and peripheral organs reveals distinct subcellular localization, with the 1N isoform being enriched in the nucleus. *PLoS One* 8:e84849. doi: 10.1371/journal.pone.0084849

Lu, J., Li, T., He, R., Bartlett, P. F., and Götz, J. (2014). Visualizing the microtubule-associated protein tau in the nucleus. *Sci. China Life Sci.* 57, 422–431. doi: 10.1007/s11427-014-4635-4630

Margittai, M., and Langen, R. (2004). Template-assisted filament growth by parallel stacking of tau. *Proc. Natl. Acad. Sci. U.S.A.* 101, 10278–10283. doi: 10.1073/pnas.0401911101

Meier, S., Bell, M., Lyons, D. N., Rodriguez-Rivera, J., Ingram, A., Fontaine, S. N., et al. (2016). Pathological tau promotes neuronal damage by impairing ribosomal function and decreasing protein synthesis. *J. Neurosci.* 36, 1001–1007. doi: 10.1523/JNEUROSCI.3029-15.2016

Meyer, V., Dinkel, P. D., Rickman Hager, E., and Margittai, M. (2014). Amplification of tau fibrils from minute quantities of seeds. *Biochemistry* 53, 5804–5809. doi: 10.1021/bi501050g

Meyer, V., Holden, M. R., Weismiller, H. A., Eaton, G. R., Eaton, S. S., and Margittai, M. (2016). Fracture and growth are competing forces determining the fate of conformers in tau fibril populations. *J. Biol. Chem.* 291, 12271–12281. doi: 10.1074/jbc.M116.715557

Michel, C. H., Kumar, S., Pinotsi, D., Tunnacliffe, A., George-Hyslop, P. S., Mandelkow, E., et al. (2014). Extracellular monomeric tau protein is sufficient to initiate the spread of tau protein pathology. *J. Biol. Chem.* 289, 956–967. doi: 10.1074/jbc.M113.515445

Mohamed, N.-V., Herrou, T., Plouffe, V., Piperno, N., and Leclerc, N. (2013). Spreading of tau pathology in Alzheimer's disease by cell-to-cell transmission. *Eur. J. Neurosci.* 37, 1939–1948. doi: 10.1111/ejn.12229

Murrell, J. R., Spillantini, M. G., Zolo, P., Guazzelli, M., Smith, M. J., Hasegawa, M., et al. (1999). Tau gene mutation G389R causes a tauopathy with abundant pick body-like inclusions and axonal deposits. *J. Neuropathol. Exp. Neurol.* 58, 1207–1226. doi: 10.1097/00005072-199912000-00002

Narasimhan, S., Guo, J. L., Changolkar, L., Stieber, A., McBride, J. D., Silva, L. V., et al. (2017). Pathological tau strains from human brains recapitulate the diversity of tauopathies in non-transgenic mouse brain. *J. Neurosci.* 37, 11406–11423. doi: 10.1523/JNEUROSCI.1230-17.2017

Rady, R. M., Zinkowski, R. P., and Binder, L. I. (1995). Presence of tau in isolated nuclei from human brain. *Neurobiol. Aging* 16, 479–486. doi: 10.1016/0197-4580(95)00023-28

Rauch, J. N., Chen, J. J., Sorum, A. W., Miller, G. M., Sharf, T., See, S. K., et al. (2018). Tau Internalization is Regulated by 6-O Sulfation on Heparan Sulfate Proteoglycans (HSPGs). *Sci. Rep.* 8:6382. doi: 10.1038/s41598-018-24904-z

Ritter, M. L., Avila, J., García-Escudero, V., Hernández, F., and Pérez, M. (2018). Frontotemporal dementia-associated N279K tau mutation localizes at the nuclear compartment. *Front. Cell. Neurosci.* 12:202. doi: 10.3389/fncel.2018.00202

Sanders, D. W., Kaufman, S. K., DeVos, S. L., Sharma, A. M., Mirbaha, H., Li, A., et al. (2014). Distinct Tau Prion Strains Propagate in Cells and Mice and Define Different Tauopathies. *Neuron* 82, 1271–1288. doi: 10.1016/j.neuron.2014.04.047

Sengupta, U., Portelius, E., Hansson, O., Farmer, K., Castillo-Carranza, D., Woltjer, R., et al. (2017). Tau oligomers in cerebrospinal fluid in Alzheimer's disease. *Ann. Clin. Transl. Neurol.* 4, 226–235. doi: 10.1002/acn3.382

Sergeant, N., Delacourte, A., and Buée, L. (2005). Tau protein as a differential biomarker of tauopathies. *Biochim. Biophys. Acta* 1739, 179–197. doi: 10.1016/j.bbadis.2004.06.020

Shammas, S. L., Garcia, G. A., Kumar, S., Kjaergaard, M., Horrocks, M. H., Shivji, N., et al. (2015). A mechanistic model of tau amyloid aggregation based on direct observation of oligomers. *Nat. Commun.* 6:7025. doi: 10.1038/ncomms8025

Sjöberg, M. K., Shestakova, E., Mansuroglu, Z., Maccioni, R. B., and Bonnefoy, E. (2006). Tau protein binds to pericentromeric DNA: a putative role for nuclear tau in nucleolar organization. *J. Cell Sci.* 119, 2025–2034. doi: 10.1242/jcs.02907

Spillantini, M. G., and Goedert, M. (2013). Tau pathology and neurodegeneration. *Lancet Neurol.* 12, 609–622. doi: 10.1016/S1474-4422(13)70090-70095

Stöhr, J., Wu, H., Nick, M., Wu, Y., Bhate, M., Condello, C., et al. (2017). A 31-residue peptide induces aggregation of tau's microtubule-binding region in cells. *Nat. Chem.* 9, 874–881. doi: 10.1038/nchem.2754

Strang, K. H., Croft, C. L., Sorrentino, Z. A., Chakrabarty, P., Golde, T. E., and Giasson, B. I. (2017). Distinct differences in prion-like seeding and aggregation between tau protein variants provide mechanistic insights into tauopathies. *J. Biol. Chem.* 293, 2408–2421. doi: 10.1074/jbc.M117.815357

Sultan, A., Nesslany, F., Violet, M., Bégard, S., Loyens, A., Talahari, S., et al. (2011). Nuclear Tau, a key player in neuronal DNA protection. *J. Biol. Chem.* 286, 4566–4575. doi: 10.1074/jbc.M110.199976

Tepper, K., Biernat, J., Kumar, S., Wegmann, S., Timm, T., Hübschmann, S., et al. (2014). Oligomer formation of tau protein hyperphosphorylated in cells. *J. Biol. Chem.* 289, 34389–34407. doi: 10.1074/jbc.M114.611368

Usenovic, M., Niroomand, S., Drolet, R. E., Yao, L., Gaspar, R. C., Hatcher, N. G., et al. (2015). Internalized tau oligomers cause neurodegeneration by inducing accumulation of pathogenic tau in human neurons derived from induced pluripotent stem cells. *J. Neurosci.* 35, 14234–14250. doi: 10.1523/JNEUROSCI.1523-15.2015

von Bergen, M., Barghorn, S., Biernat, J., Mandelkow, E.-M., and Mandelkow, E. (2005). Tau aggregation is driven by a transition from random coil to beta sheet structure. *Biochim. Biophys. Acta* 1739, 158–166. doi: 10.1016/j.bbadis.2004.09.010

von Bergen, M., Barghorn, S., Li, L., Marx, A., Biernat, J., Mandelkow, E.-M., et al. (2001). Mutations of tau protein in frontotemporal dementia promote aggregation of paired helical filaments by enhancing local β-structure. *J. Biol. Chem.* 276, 48165–48174. doi: 10.1074/jbc.m105196200

von Bergen, M., Friedhoff, P., Biernat, J., Heberle, J., Mandelkow, E.-M., and Mandelkow, E. (2000). Assembly of τ protein into Alzheimer paired helical filaments depends on a local sequence motif (306VQIVYK311) forming β structure. *Proc. Natl. Acad. Sci. U.S.A.* 97, 5129–5134. doi: 10.1073/pnas.97.10.5129

Walsh, D. M., and Selkoe, D. J. (2016). A critical appraisal of the pathogenic protein spread hypothesis of neurodegeneration. *Nat. Rev. Neurosci.* 17, 251–260. doi: 10.1038/nrn.2016.13

Wang, Y., and Mandelkow, E. (2016). Tau in physiology and pathology. *Nat. Rev. Neurosci.* 17, 22–35. doi: 10.1038/nrn.2015.1

Wegmann, S., Maury, E. A., Kirk, M. J., Saqran, L., Roe, A., DeVos, S. L., et al. (2015). Removing endogenous tau does not prevent tau propagation yet reduces its neurotoxicity. *EMBO J.* 34, 3028–3041. doi: 10.15252/embj.201592748

Wong, A. G., Wu, C., Hannaberry, E., Watson, M. D., Shea, J.-E., and Raleigh, D. P. (2016). Analysis of the amyloidogenic potential of pufferfish (takifugu rubripes) islet amyloid polypeptide highlights the limitations of thioflavin-T assays and the difficulties in defining amyloidogenicity. *Biochemistry* 55, 510–518. doi: 10.1021/acs.biochem.5b01107

Wu, J. W., Herman, M., Liu, L., Simoes, S., Acker, C. M., Figueroa, H., et al. (2013). Small misfolded Tau species are internalized via bulk endocytosis and anterogradely and retrogradely transported in neurons. *J. Biol. Chem.* 288, 1856–1870. doi: 10.1074/jbc.M112.394528

Yin, Y., Gao, D., Wang, Y., Wang, Z.-H., Wang, X., Ye, J., et al. (2016). Tau accumulation induces synaptic impairment and memory deficit by calcineurin-mediated inactivation of nuclear CaMKIV/CREB signaling. *Proc. Natl. Acad. Sci. U.S.A.* 113, E3773–E3781. doi: 10.1073/pnas.1604519113

13

Altered Levels and Isoforms of Tau and Nuclear Membrane Invaginations in Huntington's Disease

Marta Fernández-Nogales[1] *and José J. Lucas*[2,3]*

[1]*Instituto Neurociencias Alicante (CSIC-UMH), San Juan de Alicante, Spain,* [2]*Centro de Biología Molecular Severo Ochoa (CBMSO)(CSIC-UAM), Madrid, Spain,* [3]*Networking Research Center on Neurodegenerative Diseases (CIBERNED), Instituto de Salud Carlos III, Madrid, Spain*

***Correspondence:**
José J. Lucas
jjlucas@cbm.csic.es

Since the early reports of neurofibrillary Tau pathology in brains of some Huntington's disease (HD) patients, mounting evidence of multiple alterations of Tau in HD brain tissue has emerged in recent years. Such Tau alterations range from increased total levels, imbalance of isoforms generated by alternative splicing (increased 4R-/3R-Tau ratio) or by post-translational modifications such as hyperphosphorylation or truncation. Besides, the detection in HD brains of a new Tau histopathological hallmark known as Tau nuclear rods (TNRs) or Tau-positive nuclear indentations (TNIs) led to propose HD as a secondary Tauopathy. After their discovery in HD brains, TNIs have also been reported in hippocampal neurons of early Braak stage AD cases and in frontal and temporal cortical neurons of FTD-MAPT cases due to the intronic IVS10+16 mutation in the Tau gene (MAPT) which results in an increased 4R-/3R-Tau ratio similar to that observed in HD. TNIs are likely pathogenic for contributing to the disturbed nucleocytoplasmic transport observed in HD. A key question is whether correction of any of the mentioned Tau alterations might have positive therapeutic implications for HD. The beneficial effect of decreasing Tau expression in HD mouse models clearly implicates Tau in HD pathogenesis. Such beneficial effect might be exerted by diminishing the excess total levels of Tau or specifically by diminishing the excess 4R-Tau, as well as any of their downstream effects. In any case, since gene silencing drugs are under development to attenuate both Huntingtin (HTT) expression for HD and MAPT expression for FTD-MAPT, it is conceivable that the combined therapy in HD patients might be more effective than HTT silencing alone.

Keywords: huntington's disease, tau, tauopathy, tau nuclear rod (TNR), tau nuclear indentation (TNI)

INTRODUCTION

Huntington's Disease Overview

Huntington's disease (HD) is an autosomal dominant neurodegenerative disorder caused by a mutation in the gene that encodes for the protein Huntingtin (Htt). This mutation consists on an abnormal expansion of a CAG triplet (>35) in exon 1 of the gene that encodes for a stretch of polyglutamine (polyQ) in the N-terminal region of the protein (Gusella et al., 1993; MacDonald et al., 1993) and, thus, HD belongs to the group of the polyglutamine diseases (Zoghbi and Orr, 2000). Clinically, HD patients suffer multiple symptoms that include motor (involuntary body movements, chorea, dystonia, and gait abnormalities), cognitive (decreases in attention and mental flexibility) and psychiatric and/or behavioral impairment (apathy, irritability, impulsivity, depression and suicidal wishes) due to the affectation of different parts of the brain (Vonsattel and DiFiglia, 1998; Sturrock and Leavitt, 2010; Kim and Fung, 2014). Population without the disease has between 6 and 35 CAG triplets in the *HTT* gene, while individuals with expansions of 40 or more repeats develop HD. Carriers of 36–39 CAG repeats have lower penetrance and later onset of the disease (Andrew et al., 1993). There is a relationship between the length of CAG repeat and the onset and severity of the disease leading to a worse prognosis as the length increases [Snell et al., 1993; Genetic Modifiers of Huntington's Disease (GeM-HD) Consortium, 2019].

As in other polyglutaminopathies, illness is mainly due to a toxic gain of function of the expanded polyQ-containing protein and also of the expanded CAG-containing mRNA (Shieh and Bonini, 2011; Nalavade et al., 2013; Martí, 2016) rather than to a loss of function of mutant Htt (mHtt). Although the latter may also contribute to some of the HD-specific symptoms (Zuccato and Cattaneo, 2014). The Htt protein is expressed ubiquitously throughout the body with high levels in the brain and testes (Schulte and Littleton, 2011). It interacts with different partners that are implicated in cellular dynamics -like cytoskeleton, endocytosis, trafficking, and adhesion-, metabolism, protein turnover, transcription and RNA processing (Kaltenbach et al., 2007) and participates in vesicular transport, synaptic transmission and autophagy, playing a role in embryogenesis, signal transduction and cell adhesion (Schulte and Littleton, 2011; Smith-Dijak et al., 2019). The absence of Htt causes embryonic lethality while mice lacking one Htt allele do not show phenotypical changes (Nasir et al., 1995).

Regarding neuropathology, HD is characterized by neuronal death, primarily of medium-sized spiny neurons of the striatum producing a progressive atrophy of the basal ganglia (Hedreen and Folstein, 1995; Mitchell et al., 1999) but also in other structures that are related to cognition such as the cortex and hippocampus (Zheng and Diamond, 2012), which explains the different symptoms that patients suffer. Nowadays, there is no cure for HD and, normally, death takes place between 15 and 20 years after the onset of the symptoms.

Truncated N-terminal portions of mHtt can be generated through proteolytic cleavage by caspases, calpains or other endoproteases and this favors the agglomeration of mHtt—driven by the self-aggregation of polyQ. This process eventually leads to the formation of oligomers and globular intermediates that can interfere with multiple intracellular functions in the cytoplasm (such as organelle and mRNA transport, protein turnover, or mitochondrial function among others) and in the nucleus where gene expression can get altered (Graham et al., 2006). Besides, N-terminal fragments of mHtt are not only produced by proteolytic cleavage but also by aberrant splicing (Bates et al., 2015). Recently, it has been observed in a cohort of 56 HD patients a decrease in the levels of total Htt levels (using EM48 and CH00146 antibodies) and an increase in the levels of the N-terminal fragment without alteration in Htt mRNA levels. This is accompanied by an increase in Htt oligomers without changes in monomers according to Sarkosyl based protein fractionation, suggesting that abnormal translation and/or protein turnover is responsible for Htt misregulation in HD (St-Amour et al., 2018).

The aggregation of mHtt produces an histopathological mark in form of spherical inclusions that are detected in the nuclei and cytoplasm of neurons in HD patients (DiFiglia et al., 1997) but also in different transgenic animal models like mice (Davies et al., 1997) or *Drosophila* (Warrick et al., 1998). Inclusions can be detected using antibodies against Htt but also against other epitopes like polyQ or ubiquitin (DiFiglia et al., 1997; Sapp et al., 1997; Vonsattel et al., 2008). There is growing evidence that HD inclusions, in addition to mHtt, can nucleate other proteins like those that are characteristic of other neurodegenerative diseases, like α-synuclein -found in Parkinson's disease (Corrochano et al., 2012; Herrera and Outeiro, 2012; Tomas-Zapico et al., 2012), TDP-43 -found in amyotrophic lateral sclerosis- (Schwab et al., 2008; Coudert et al., 2019), or Tau -found in Tauopathies such as Alzheimer's disease (Fernández-Nogales et al., 2014; Vuono et al., 2015; St-Amour et al., 2018).

Tau Overview

Tau Gene and Isoforms Generated by Alternative Splicing

Tau is a microtubule-associated protein (MAP) that was first discovered in 1975 by Weingarten when it was co-purified along with tubulin (Weingarten et al., 1975). In humans, this protein is encoded by the gene *MAPT* that is located in the region q21.31 on chromosome 17 and contains 16 exons (Neve et al., 1986; Andreadis et al., 1992), while in mouse is located on chromosome 11. The human MAPT gene has two haplotypes, the more common H1 and the unusual H2 haplotype. The latter results from a large—approximately 970 kb—chromosomal inversion and a 238 bp deletion in intron 9 (Stefansson et al., 2005; Caillet-Boudin et al., 2015).

The MAPT gene is expressed at its highest levels in neurons in the central nervous system where it contributes to the maintenance of neuronal polarity by promoting microtubule assembly and stability.

Multiple Tau isoforms are generated by alternative splicing. The exons that are alternatively spliced in adult CNS are exons 2, 3 and 10, and their combinatorial usage generates six Tau isoforms in the adult human brain (Andreadis, 2005; Liu and Gong, 2008). On one hand, alternative splicing of exons 2 and 3 generates Tau isoforms that differ by the absence or the presence of an insert of 29 or 58 amino acids—corresponding to exons 2 or 2 and 3—in the N-terminal region. Thus, exon 2 can appear alone but exon 3 never appears independently of exon 2. This way the so-called 0N, 1N or 2N isoforms are generated (Andreadis et al., 1995). On the other hand, the exclusion or inclusion of exon 10—encoding a 31 amino acid sequence that provides one of the four possible tubulin-binding repeats in the C-terminal region of the protein—results in either 3R or 4R isoforms (Goedert and Spillantini, 2011).

The N-terminal region binds to plasma membrane components to regulate interactions while the C-terminal part of the protein binds microtubules (Derisbourg et al., 2015).

If we focus our attention in the C-terminal region, 4R-Tau isoforms bind microtubules with higher affinity and are more efficient at promoting microtubule assembly *in vitro* compared to 3R-Tau isoforms that have less affinity for microtubules (Lu and Kosik, 2001). More precisely, both 4R-Tau and 3R-Tau isoforms increase the growth rate of microtubules, but 3R-Tau shows less efficacy in protecting microtubules from disassembly than 4R Tau isoforms (Panda et al., 2003). During development, 0N3R isoform is the most abundant making 3R-Tau to predominate over 4R-Tau (Kosik et al., 1989). However, in healthy human adult brain, 3R-Tau and 4R-Tau are equally represented (Goedert et al., 1989). In the case of the adult mouse brain, 4R-Tau isoforms are predominant (Kosik et al., 1989; Takuma et al., 2003). The microtubule-binding repeats also comprise the paired-helical filament (PHF) core that is the primary structure of aggregated Tau filaments (Wischik et al., 1988) and dysregulation of the balance between 3R-Tau and 4R-Tau isoforms has been shown to contribute to neurodegeneration (Liu and Gong, 2008), as we are going to comment in more detail.

Functions of Tau

In healthy neurons, Tau is almost exclusively located in the axon (Wang and Mandelkow, 2016) where, as mentioned, it is implicated in microtubule assembly and stabilization. Microtubules are polar structures with a plus and a minus-end and they are formed from α and β-tubulin heterodimers. Tau binds both α and β-tubulin subunits and can promote microtubule growth (Witman et al., 1976; Kadavath et al., 2015). The assembly of microtubules consists of a phase of rapid polymerization and a steady-state, where no assembly occurs. Assembly occurs at the plus end while disassembly occurs at the minus end, keeping the overall length of the microtubule equal. Tau reduces the frequency of depolymerization by binding along the outer surface. Microtubule dynamics in the nervous system requires a high degree of stability. While the N-terminal region of Tau could contribute to the formation of microtubule bundles as it functions as a spacer in between them (Chen et al., 1992), the C-terminal region binds to microtubules to regulate their polymerization (Cleveland et al., 1977). In healthy conditions, due to its ability to modify microtubule dynamics (Trinczek et al., 1999; Dixit et al., 2008), Tau contributes to regulate different cellular functions such as transport of mRNA and proteins along the axons, as well as neurite extension. Accordingly, when Tau is knocked down, neurite formation is inhibited altering processes such as neuronal differentiation or synaptic plasticity (Caceres and Kosik, 1990; Kempf et al., 1996; Stamer et al., 2002; Spillantini and Goedert, 2013). Moreover, Tau is present in small amounts in dendrites and even in the nucleus where it can bind to DNA protecting it from damage (Wei et al., 2008; Violet et al., 2014). DNA binding of Tau takes place at both genic and intergenic regions (Benhelli-Mokrani et al., 2018) and results in modulation of gene expression (Siano et al., 2019). Interestingly, nuclear Tau has also been involved in nucleolar transcription (Maina et al., 2018) and the decrease in nuclear Tau (detected with Tau-100 antibody) that takes place in AD CA1 and dentate gyrus neurons along disease progression might be pathogenic by leading to decreased protein synthesis (Hernández-Ortega et al., 2016). Finally, different mutations that alter the proportion of Tau isoforms as well as post-translational modifications can modify the affinity of Tau for microtubules. The differential interaction of 4R-Tau and 3R-Tau with the microtubules may have important implications for neuronal diseases as the regulated expression of both isoforms is required for the correct function of the neurons. Therefore, in summary, both a loss of function of Tau and a toxic gain of function due to aggregate formation can contribute to neurodegeneration.

Post-translational Modifications of Tau

Tau protein can be modified after translation by phosphorylation, glycosylation, ubiquitination, acetylation or truncation, among others (Martin et al., 2011). Regarding phosphorylation of Tau, it can be phosphorylated in serine, threonine and tyrosine residues with 85 potential sites of phosphorylation, of which 45 have been validated (Wang and Mandelkow, 2016). The sites of phosphorylation can be divided depending on the kinases that can phosphorylate them: proline-directed kinases -like glycogen synthase kinase 3 (GSK-3), cyclin-dependent kinase 5 (CDK-5), cyclin-dependent kinase 1 (CDK-1), mitogen-activated protein kinase (p38), c-Jun N-terminal kinases (JNK), and other stress kinases—and non-proline-directed kinases—like protein kinase A (PKA), protein kinase C (PKC), calmodulin kinase II (CaMK-II), microtubule affinity regulating kinase (MARK) or casein kinase 2 (CK2).

Phosphorylation of Tau reduces its affinity for microtubule and different plasma membrane components, thus reducing microtubule stability. For example, phosphorylation on Ser-214 and Thr-231 promotes detaching of Tau from microtubules. Deregulation of Tau phosphorylation is deleterious for neurons and has been implicated in many diseases such as AD, where Tau hyperphosphorylation favors its detachment from the microtubules thus increasing the levels of soluble Tau available for self-aggregation leading to the formation of neurofibrillary tangles (NFT) and/or neuropil threads (NT; Wang and Mandelkow, 2016). GSK-3 is believed to play an important role in Tau hyperphosphorylation as it is able to phosphorylate the majority of the residues which are hyperphosphorylated in AD (Lovestone et al., 1994) and its levels are increased in AD brains (Pei et al., 1997). Apart from kinase hyperactivity, dysregulation of phosphatases can also lead to pathogenic hyperphosphorylation. Different phosphatases such as PP1, PP2A, PP2B (calcineurin) and PP2C can eliminate phosphates from Tau but only PP1, PP2A, and PP2B (Gong et al., 2004) have been shown to dephosphorylate abnormally hyperphosphorylated Tau.

Not only phosphorylation modulates Tau activity. Acetylation can also regulate its function as it has been observed that, *in vitro*, it can preclude microtubule assembly (Min et al., 2010; Cohen et al., 2011). Important sites of acetylation are K163, K274, K280, K281, and K369, with K281 and K274 being acetylated in AD patients (Tracy et al., 2016). Interestingly, when the levels of acetylated Tau are increased, its levels of phosphorylation are reduced (Min et al., 2010).

Other post-translational modifications that include N-glycosylation, truncation and isomerization stabilize PHFs. It has been described that N-glycosylation is related to Tau hyperphosphorylation and Tau aggregation (Ledesma et al., 1995). N-glycosylation stabilizes aggregated PHFs leading to tangle formation in AD. Phosphorylation on Ser-717 completely abolishes the O-GlcNAcylation on this site, while phosphorylation on Ser-713 and Ser-721 reduces O-GlcNAcylation. O-GlcNAcylation on Ser-717 decreases the phosphorylation on Ser-721 by about 41.5%. Truncation of Tau can also promote aggregation as Tau fragments have been found in the PHFs of AD patients (Wischik et al., 1988).

Finally, Tau can be ubiquitinated and this modification has mainly been found in aberrant aggregates such as the inclusion bodies found in Pick's or Parkinson's diseases or in PHFs in AD (Mayer et al., 1989; Morishima-Kawashima et al., 1993). PHF-Tau can be modified by three different forms of poly-ubiquitination, "Lys-48"-linked poly-ubiquitination is the major form but "Lys-6"-linked and "Lys-11"-linked poly-ubiquitination could also occur.

Tau Mutations and Tauopathies

The alteration of the amount and the structure of the Tau protein can disturb its localization and, as a consequence, its function producing different pathological effects. Tauopathies are a class of neurodegenerative disorders that are characterized by the aggregation and intracellular deposition of Tau in neurons and/or glial cells as a consequence of abnormal increase in the levels of phosphorylation, abnormal splicing of the mRNA or mutations in *MAPT* gene.

Tauopathies can be divided into: (a) primary Tauopathies that are a major class of Frontotemporal Lobar Degeneration (FTLD) neuropathology and can present clinically with several forms of Frontotemporal Dementia (FTD)—like Frontotemporal Dementia with parkinsonism linked to chromosome 17—(FTDP-17), progressive supranuclear palsy syndrome (PSP) or corticobasal degeneration (CBD); and (b) secondary or non-primary Tauopathies like Alzheimer's disease (AD) in which neurofibrillary Tau neuropathology occurs in addition to the amyloid-β (Aβ) plaques. The various Tauopathies affect different brain regions and cell types and they also show differences in the ratio of Tau isoforms present in the Tau filaments (Sergeant et al., 2005). In AD, there are similar levels of 3R-Tau and 4R-Tau in the PHFs (Goedert et al., 1995) while other Tauopathies like PSP or CBC show an increase in 4R-Tau isoforms and others like PiD show an increase in 3R-Tau isoforms (Arendt et al., 2016).

Missense, silent and intronic mutations in the MAPT gene have been directly related to different Tauopathies or constitute a risk factor for them (Goedert and Jakes, 2005). In 1998, it was discovered that mutations on the *MAPT* gene cause FTDP-17, confirming that Tau dysfunction is sufficient to cause neurodegeneration. These patients showed filamentous Tau inclusions in neurons and glia and atrophy of the frontal and temporal lobes (Hutton et al., 1998; Poorkaj et al., 1998; Spillantini et al., 1998). There are different missense mutations like ΔK280, P301L, G272V, V337M, R406W and N279K that reduce microtubule assembly contributing to PHFs stabilization and its aggregation forming NFTs (Barghorn et al., 2000). Regarding intronic mutations, they are located around exon 10 affecting its rate of inclusion and they lead to an imbalance of the ratio of 4R- and 3R-Tau isoforms (Liu and Gong, 2008).

TAU PATHOLOGY IN HUNTINGTON'S DISEASE

Along the last decades, many studies have demonstrated Tau alterations and Tau-positive histopathological hallmarks in HD patients as well as in animal models that could be contributing to the progression of the disease. Here, we aim to review these pieces of evidence to elucidate the role of Tau in the disease and to elaborate on whether this offers opportunities for therapeutic interventions to ameliorate HD prognosis.

Polymorphisms

It has been described that the MAPT H1 haplotype—that is the most abundant—could be a genetic risk factor for some Tauopathies like PSP or CBD (Houlden et al., 2001; Pittman et al., 2004). Also, H1 haplotype increases the expression of total MAPT transcript as well as specifically increases the inclusion of exon 10 and therefore the proportion of 4R-Tau isoforms (Myers et al., 2007). In HD, Tau polymorphisms have been linked to the progression of cognitive deficits. In a group of 960 HD patients that were genotyped for the H1 and H2 haplotypes-using the SNP rs9468, Vuono et al. (2015) reported that there is a correlation between increased number of CAG repeats and increased rate of cognitive decline in H2 carriers and that Tau H2 haplotype carriers show accelerated cognitive deterioration compared to H1/H1 homozygous carriers.

Tau Levels

Regarding Tau protein levels, a high increase in the levels of total Tau (Tau-5 antibody) was found in the cortex of HD patients and this is accompanied with the appearance of lower molecular weight (35 and 39 KD) bands (Fernández-Nogales et al., 2014), while no changes were found in the striatum (Fernández-Nogales et al., 2014). However, a more recent report has shown elevated Tau total mRNA levels in the putamen of HD patients (St-Amour et al., 2018). Importantly, the presence of an excess of Tau in HD brains most likely contributes to disease as Tau knock-down has been demonstrated to attenuate motor abnormalities in an HD mouse model (Fernández-Nogales et al., 2014).

Aberrant Splicing of Tau in HD

As previously commented, in some Tauopathies including PSP, CB, Pick's disease (PiD) and FTLD with Tau+ inclusions (FTLD-Tau), alteration of alternative splicing of exon 10 produces an imbalance in 4R-Tau and 3R-Tau isoforms (Park et al., 2016). Regarding HD, we demonstrated that patients (and mouse models of the disease, like the R6/1 and HD94 mice) show an increase in the ratio 4R-Tau/3R-Tau mRNA isoforms in cortex and striatum, accompanied by an increase of the levels of 4R-Tau protein. In the striatum, there also was a decrease in 3R-Tau protein (Fernández-Nogales et al., 2014). The imbalance of 4R-Tau/3R-Tau mRNA isoforms was corroborated by Vuono et al.

(2015) in the cortex and striatum of a cohort of 16 patients. More precisely, they detect 1N3R and 2N4R mRNA and protein isoforms and found an increase in 4R-Tau isoforms that leads to an altered ratio of isoforms. Recently, using putamen samples from a higher number of patients (St-Amour et al., 2018), it was shown a 2.5-fold increase in 4R-Tau/3R-Tau ratio at the protein level and a 1.8-fold increase at the mRNA level, due to an upregulation of 4R-Tau isoforms. The high number of samples analyzed in that study allowed them to conclude that the top increment takes place in grade 2 cases regarding the mRNA and in grade 3 cases regarding the protein, resulting in higher 0N4R and lower 1N3R isoforms (St-Amour et al., 2018). All these findings regarding altered isoform ratio in HD are very relevant in view of the fact that alteration in the ratio of 4R-Tau and 3R-Tau isoforms is sufficient to cause neurodegeneration (Hutton et al., 1998; Qian and Liu, 2014), as this might contribute *per se* to HD neurodegeneration independently of other deleterious effects of mHtt, thus becoming a therapeutic target for HD.

Alternative splicing of exon 10 is regulated by a system of factors that bind to the RNA regulating the splicing of the pre-mRNA itself. Among these factors, the family of the serine- and arginine-rich (SR) proteins participate on constitutive splicing while also regulating alternative splicing. Some members of this family promote the inclusion of exon 10, while others suppress it. Several studies have shown that SRSF1 (ASF/SF2), SRSF2 (SC35), SRSR6 (SRp55), and SRSF9 (SRp30c) promote exon 10 inclusion, while SRSF3, SRSF4, SRSF7, and SRSF11 suppress its inclusion (Qian and Liu, 2014).

It was bioinformatically predicted (Sathasivam et al., 2013) and biochemically confirmed (Schilling et al., 2019) that the splicing factor SRSF6 can bind CAG RNA repeats and this leads to incomplete splicing of Htt RNA and to production of a small form of Htt known as exon 1-Htt (Sathasivam et al., 2013). Besides, SRSF6 was indeed found altered in the striatum of HD patients and in the R6/1 mouse model of the disease, as it gets sequestered into mHtt inclusions (Fernández-Nogales et al., 2014). The activity and localization of SR proteins could be modulated by post-translational modifications such as phosphorylation of their multiple serine and threonine residues, and such phosphorylation is required, in general, for the translocation of SR proteins from the cytoplasm to the nucleus. In this regard, it has been shown an increase in the levels of phosphorylation of SRSF6 in the striatum and cortex of HD patients and R6/1 mice (Fernández-Nogales et al., 2014) which may favor dissociation from nuclear speckles (Yin et al., 2012; Naro and Sette, 2013). This, together with the sequestration of SRSF6 into mHtt inclusions, suggests a decrease in SRSF6 activity that could explain the modulation observed of exon 10 splicing in HD. Moreover, SRSF6 not only modulates alternative splicing of MAPT, as it also modulates alternative splicing of MAP2, another MAP whose alternative splicing is altered in HD (Cabrera and Lucas, 2017).

Recently, it has been proposed the splicing factor proline- and glutamine-rich (SFPQ) could also be responsible for the 4R-Tau/3R-Tau imbalance as it has been shown to modulate exon 10 splicing and to interact with FUS, one major component of mHtt inclusions (Fujioka et al., 2013; Ishigaki et al., 2017). Although no association was apparent between SFPQ nuclear signal intensity and presence or absence of HD-associated intranuclear inclusions in striatal and cortical neurons of seven HD cases (Baskota et al., 2019), the reduced nuclear availability of free FUS in HD and, as a consequence, a decreased interaction with SFPQ, might affect 4R-Tau/3R-Tau ratio.

More recently, St-Amour et al. (2018) have explored the alternative splicing that affects exon 2 and 3 on the MAPT gene. It has been observed an increase of 1.7 fold-change in the isoforms that do not contain exons 2 and 3 (0N-Tau) at mRNA level and a 0.5 fold-change in the isoforms that only contain exon 2 (St-Amour et al., 2018). Further investigation is required to know the effect of the alteration in the ratio of these isoforms in the progression of the disease as the N-terminal region of Tau participates in the interaction with different membrane components.

Tau Phosphorylation in HD

As previously described, Tau functions are modulated by site-specific phosphorylation and its alteration produce a toxic loss of function as the microtubule-binding ability is decreased, but also a toxic gain of function as it generates deposits as a result of its aggregation. There are multiple studies showing Tau hyperphosphorylation in HD that could contribute to the disease. The first evidence of Tau hyperphosphorylation in HD patients was obtained by immunohistochemistry with the AT8 antibody which revealed positive staining -with or without NTs in 13 of 27 analyzed patients (Jellinger, 1998). In good agreement, a recent study on 16 cases including young HD cases (26 and 40 years) has shown AT-8 positive neuronal inclusions with different shapes and conformations like ring-like perinuclear, flame-shaped and globular inclusions in the cortex and striatum as well as astrocytic plaques, NT, dots and nuclear rods (Gratuze et al., 2015; Vuono et al., 2015). Using antibodies other than AT-8, an increase in Tau phosphorylation at Ser396/Ser404/Ser199 and Thr205 epitopes, while no changes in epitopes Ser235/Ser262/Ser356, has been observed in the putamen of a cohort of 56 patients (St-Amour et al., 2018). Recently, hyperphosphorylated Tau (detected with antibodies AT8, CP13, AT180b and PHF-1) has been detected in fetal tissue transplanted into cortex and striatum of two HD cases (Cisbani et al., 2017).

There is some controversy regarding the presence of hyperphosphorylated Tau in the Sarkosyl-insoluble fraction obtained from HD brains. While Vuono et al. (2015) found elevated AT-8 Tau in this fraction, two different studies failed to replicate this. More precisely, we did not detect hyperphosphorylated Tau (with AT-8 or with PHF-1) in this insoluble fraction of HD brains (Fernández-Nogales et al., 2014) and neither did the more recent study by St-Amour et al. (2018) which analyzed a much higher number of HD cases. Interestingly, in the latter, they report that multiple antibodies against Tau phospho-epitopes were below detection levels in the Sarkosyl-insoluble fraction.

Regarding cellular and animal models of HD, mHtt expression promotes Tau hyperphosphorylation at Ser396 as evidenced in cells in which Tau was co-transfected with mHtt, in contrast to what happens when Tau is co-transfected with wild type Htt in which the levels of phosphorylation are maintained stable (Blum et al., 2015). The Q111 striatal knock-in cellular model that mimics the polyglutamine expansion shows Tau hyperphosphorylation when there is pharmacological inhibition of PP2B/calcineurin in comparison with Q7 cells (Gratuze et al., 2015).

In animal models of HD, there are plenty of demonstrations of Tau hyperphosphorylation. Thus, Gratuze et al. (2015) showed increased Tau hyperphosphorylation at PHF-1 epitope in presymptomatic R6/2 whereas symptomatic R6/2 mice displayed Tau hyperphosphorylation at multiple Tau phospho-epitopes like AT-8, CP13, PT205 and PHF1 in the hippocampus. Besides, the zQ175 knock-in mice show increased phosphorylation with PS199. Similarly, Blum et al. (2015) showed that R6/2 and KI140 mice display increased phosphorylation in Ser404 and Ser396 by western blot and also by immunofluorescence with the pSer396 antibody in KI140 mice. Besides, they also detected a decrease in Tau1 (unphosphorylated Tau) in R6/2 and KI140 mice.

The phosphorylation of Tau is a balance between the activity of its kinases and phosphatases (Sergeant et al., 2008). One of the main kinases that phosphorylates Tau is GSK-3 which has been shown to mediate Tau phosphorylation in Alzheimer's disease (Hernandez et al., 2013) and bipolar disorder (Beaulieu et al., 2004; Li et al., 2010). However, there is a dramatic decrease in GSK-3 levels and activity in the striatum and cortex from HD patients (Lim et al., 2014; Fernández-Nogales et al., 2015) as well as in R6/1 mouse model (Saavedra et al., 2010; Fernández-Nogales et al., 2015), while an increase in active pGSK-3β-Tyr^{216} does take place in hippocampus of HD patients and R6/2 mice (L'Episcopo et al., 2016). It has been reported that GSK-3β, CamKII, AKT, JNK, p38, ERk or CDK-5 are not activated in R6/2 and Q175 mice and there is even increased Ser9 phosphorylation of GSK-3β (resulting in the inactive form of the kinase) and reduced phosphorylation and levels of CamKII, as well as reduced cdk5 and ERK expression in the cortex of R6/2 and KI140 mice (Deckel et al., 2002; Blum et al., 2015; Gratuze et al., 2015). Together, all these results do not fit with the Tau hyperphosphorylation observed in HD. In contrast, and regarding the phosphatases implicated in Tau dephosphorylation, it has been shown a decrease in PP1, PP2A and PP2B expression in R6/2 mouse model and a significant reduction in Calcineurin/PP2B expression in KI140 (Blum et al., 2015; Gratuze et al., 2015) which may explain the hyperphosphorylation phenotype.

Tau Truncation in HD

As mentioned, Tau truncation may be relevant to neurodegeneration as it may alter the Tau function and favor the formation of Tau aggregates. There are different truncated forms of Tau depending on the protease responsible for the cleavage. The ΔTau314 has been demonstrated to be generated by Casp2 and to cause synaptic dysfunction and cognitive deficits in cellular and transgenic mouse models of FTDP-17 (Zhang et al., 2014). Recently, it has been reported that both Casp2 and ΔTau314 proteins are higher in the striatum (caudate nucleus) and prefrontal cortex (Brodmann's area 8/9) of HD patients as compared non-HD individuals (Liu et al., 2019).

TAU-POSITIVE NUCLEAR MEMBRANE INVAGINATIONS AND OTHER HISTOPATHOLOGICAL MARKS IN HD

For decades, there have been numerous histopathological reports of HD patients in whom the presence of NFT—the histopathological hallmark characteristic of different Tauopathies such as Alzheimer's disease—has been detected (McIntosh et al., 1978; Myers et al., 1985; Reyes and Gibbons, 1985; Moss et al., 1988; Caparros-Lefebvre et al., 2009). More systematic studies using larger patient cohorts have detected Tau pathology in 60% (16/27; Jellinger, 1998) or 80% (9/11; Davis et al., 2014) of HD cases. Due to the growing evidence of the presence of Tau pathology in HD patients and in an attempt to understand how it may or may not contribute to the pathology of the disease, different studies in which animal models and patients are used have tried to systematically analyze this question.

mHtt and Tau Co-localization

Different approaches have been attempted to study if mHtt and Tau are directly or indirectly related to understand the mechanism of the confluence of both proteinopathies in HD patients. Some co-localization between mHtt aggregates (evidenced with EM48 antibody) and Tau deposits stained with antibodies that recognize 3R-Tau, 4R-Tau or pathologically phosphorylated Tau (AT-8 and pS199) has been detected in cortical and striatal sections of HD patients (Vuono et al., 2015). In contrast, other studies have failed to detect Tau within HD inclusions. For instance, Tau (Ht-7 antibody) could not be found in mHtt inclusions (evidenced with ubiquitin antibody) by immunofluorescence in cortical tissue of HD patients (Fernández-Nogales et al., 2014). Similarly, in animal models, no co-localization of both proteins could be found by confocal immunofluorescence using Tau pSer396 and mHtt (2B4 or EM48) antibodies in KI140 mice (Blum et al., 2015).

To clarify if there is or not an authentic co-localization between both proteins, different co-immunoprecipitation studies have been performed. In human tissue, no co-immunoprecipitation between both proteins was observed using the Tau 5 antibody that detects total Tau and the EM-48 in striatal homogenates of HD patients (Fernández-Nogales et al., 2014). No co-immunoprecipitation between both proteins was achieved either with cortical samples of KI140 mice nor was Tau detected in cortical Sarkosyl-insoluble protein fractions from R6/2 mice (Blum et al., 2015). Interestingly, in BIFC experiments *in vitro* with constructs with 25Q (wt) or 103Q mHtt and Tau fused with non-fluorescence halves of a fluorescence reporter protein, Blum et al. (2015) observed that when they put together 103Q and Tau, 103QHtt is recruited in the microtubular cytoskeleton network. Besides, Tau is hyperphosphorylated and, although its subcellular distribution is altered and its aggregation

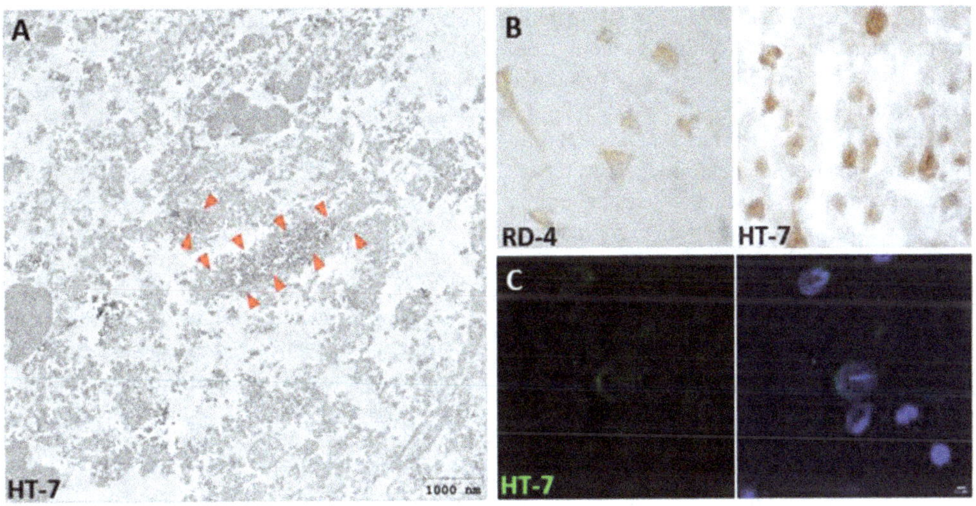

FIGURE 1 | Presence of Tau nuclear indentations (TNIs) in Huntington's disease (HD) brains. **(A)** Immunoelectron microscopy analysis of HD neurons with HT-7 positive nuclear indentations. Red arrows indicate the diaminobenzidine precipitate. **(B)** Immunohistochemistry with RD4 and Ht-7 antibodies in neurons of HD brain. **(C)** HT-7 immunofluorescence (green) with DAPI (blue) counterstaining in HD striatal neurons.

favored, it is not obvious the existence of a toxic interaction of both proteins and further studies are needed to clarify that.

Tau-Positive Cytoplasmic Aggregates

In view of the abnormal Tau "processing" that we initially detected in HD brains (Fernández-Nogales et al., 2014) that leads to an alteration of 4R-Tau/3R-Tau ratio in favor of 4R-Tau isoforms (similar to that seen in some FTD forms caused by intronic Tau mutations), we explored the possibility of Tau deposits in HD brains. We detected granular cytoplasmic Tau deposits which often form perinuclear rings in cortical and striatal neurons (Fernández-Nogales et al., 2014) by immunohistochemistry with antibodies that recognize 4R-Tau isoforms (RD4), 3R-Tau isoforms (RD-3) or Total Tau (Tau-5 and HT-7), but not with anti-phospho-Tau antibodies. Vuono et al. (2015) detected similar Tau deposits like perinuclear rings, flame-shaped and globular inclusions as well as astrocytic plaques in striatum and cortex of HD subjects but, in this case, with an antibody against phosphorylated Tau (AT-8). Similarly, in a more recent study, Cisbani et al. (2017) also detected AT-8 positive neuronal inclusions—apart from NFTs and NTs—in striatum and cortex of HD patients.

Tau-Positive Nuclear Membrane Invaginations

Interestingly, we also described for the first time the presence of Tau nuclear indentations (TNIs) also known as Tau Nuclear Rods (TNRs) in the striatum and cortex of HD patients (Fernández-Nogales et al., 2014). We detected TNIs using antibodies that recognize 4R-Tau isoforms (RD4), 3R-Tau isoforms (RD-3), Total Tau (Tau-5 and HT-7) or Tau oligomers (T22), but not with antibodies against phosphorylated Tau (such as AT-8 or PHF-1; Fernández-Nogales et al., 2014). Immuno-electron microscopy with HT-7 antibody revealed that this structure has an ordered filamentous ultrastructure immunopositive for Tau that fills neuronal invaginations of the nuclear envelope that partially or totally span the neuronal nuclear space (Fernández-Nogales et al., 2014). This new Tau histopathological hallmark thus seems to fill the previously reported neuronal nuclear membrane invaginations detected in ultrastructural analyses and whose incidence is higher in striatum of HD patients than in control subjects (Bots and Bruyn, 1981; Roos and Bots, 1983). Examples of TNIs evidenced by IHC, IF and immuno-EM are shown in **Figure 1**. The presence of TNIs in HD brains was confirmed in an independent study with a higher number of HD patient samples (Vuono et al., 2015) although, in this case, using the AT-8 antibody against phosphorylated Tau. In contrast, a recent study on samples from seven HD cases (Vonsattel grades 3 and 4), failed to detect TNIs (Baskota et al., 2019) and they reasoned that this may be due to technical features because the variety of antibodies they used did not detect neurons with cytoplasmic Tau staining, which are the ones displaying TNIs in the above-mentioned studies which do detect them. In HD mouse models, TNIs have also has been detected with Tau-5 and RD4 antibodies in the R6/1 and HD94 mice although with much lower abundance than in human HD tissue (Fernández-Nogales et al., 2014).

Interestingly, TNIs can be found in brain tissue of other neurodegenerative diseases. More precisely, in two Tauopathies: AD and FTD. Thus, we detected TNIs in the hippocampus of different Braak stage AD patients using the RD4 antibody (Fernández-Nogales et al., 2014). More recently, TNIs have also been detected in frontal and temporal cortex samples from two independent cohorts of patients with FTD-MAPT due to the MAPT intronic IVS10+16 mutation (Paonessa et al., 2019). Such mutation increases exon 10 inclusion and, therefore, increases the 4R-Tau/3R-Tau ratio in favor of 4R-Tau isoforms (similar to what we have described in HD brains).

Paonessa et al. (2019) also detected increased incidence of TNIs in IPSC-neurons derived from FTD-MAPT cases due to the MAPT IVS10+16 mutation and also, but to a lower extent, from FTD-MAPT cases due to missense P301L mutation that produces an aggregation-prone form of Tau.

Regarding the possible pathogenic relevance of TNIs, lamin dysfunction and neuronal nuclear indentations in AD have been linked to the improper cytoskeletal/nucleoskeletal coupling that was suggested as a novel mediator of neurotoxicity in Tauopathies (Frost et al., 2016) and more recently, pathological Tau has been shown to impair nucleocytoplasmic transport in Tau-overexpressing mice and AD brain tissue (Eftekharzadeh et al., 2018) which has been further confirmed recently (Paonessa et al., 2019). In this regard, nuclear integrity and nucleocytoplasmic transport have also been reported altered in Huntington's disease (Gasset-Rosa et al., 2017; Grima et al., 2017).

Regarding the mechanism by which TNIs get formed, analysis of a transgenic mouse model that overexpresses human 4R-Tau with a FTLD with the P301S Tau point mutation revealed that Tau alteration is sufficient for TNI formation/detection (Fernández-Nogales et al., 2017). Similarly, a *Drosophila* model with pan-neuronal expression of a disease-causing mutant form of human Tau, Tau^{R406W}, produces nuclear invagination that co-localizes with phosphorylated Tau (Cornelison et al., 2019). These observations raised the question of whether increased Tau (either total Tau or 4R-Tau regardless of point mutations) fills nuclear invaginations formed by Tau-independent mechanisms or whether the incidence of nuclear envelope invaginations increases upon Tau alteration, for instance, because it stabilizes microtubule bundles that deform the nucleus. The latter is precisely what Paonessa et al. (2019) demonstrate in human iPSC-derived neurons with MAPT P301L and MAPT IVS16+10 mutations as treatment with nocodazole significantly reduced the proportion of neurons with nuclear invaginations and restored round nuclear morphology. This is in contrast with the fact that the number of nuclear indentations in hippocampal neurons of P301S mice is not higher than in wild type mice (Fernández-Nogales et al., 2017). In case the induction of nuclear envelope invagination upon Tau alteration occurred only in culture, TNI detection in histopathological analysis still emerges as an efficient way to screen for brains with altered Tau (levels, isoform ratio, or simply function). Additional work will be needed to clarify this.

PATHOGENIC AND THERAPEUTIC IMPLICATIONS: FUTURE DIRECTIONS

Here we have shown multiple alterations of Tau in HD brain tissue which range from increased total levels, imbalance of alternative splicing-generated isoforms, hyperphosphorylation and truncation, to the formation of Tau-positive cytoplasmic aggregates and nuclear envelope invaginations. The likely pathogenic role of the latter—through interference of nuclear envelope function—and the possible mechanisms by which TNIs are formed are also discussed. A key question is whether correction of any of these tau alterations and of this Tau histopathological hallmark might have positive therapeutic implications for the disease.

Regarding the therapeutic implications of the current knowledge of the involvement of Tau in HD pathogenesis, a convincing evidence supporting that Tau contributes to HD pathogenesis originates from the beneficial effect of decreasing Tau expression in HD mouse models by combining with Tau knock-out mice—even partial reduction in heterozygous knock-out background (Fernández-Nogales et al., 2014). This beneficial effect might be due to the attenuation of the excess total levels of Tau in the cortex of HD mice or by attenuation specifically of the excess 4R-Tau observed both in striatum and cortex. But in any case, since gene silencing drugs are under development to attenuate both HTT expression for HD and to attenuate MAPT expression for FTD-MAPT (Mullard, 2019), it is conceivable that the combined therapy in HD patients might be more effective than HTT silencing alone.

ETHICS STATEMENT

Brain specimens reviewed in this study from frontal cortex and striatum of HD subjects and controls were provided by Institute of Neuropathology (HUB-ICO-IDIBELL) Brain Bank (Hospitalet de Llobregat, Spain), the Neurological Tissue Bank of the IDIBAPS Biobank (Barcelona, Spain), the Banco de Tejidos Fundación Cien (BT-CIEN, Madrid, Spain) and the Netherlands Brain Bank (Amsterdam, The Netherlands). Written informed consent for brain removal after death for diagnostic and research purposes was obtained from brain donors and/or next of kin. Procedures, information and consent forms have been approved by the Bioethics Subcommittee of Centro Superior de Investigaciones Científicas (Madrid, Spain).

AUTHOR CONTRIBUTIONS

Both authors (MF-N and JL) revised the literature and wrote the manuscript.

ACKNOWLEDGMENTS

We thank Felix Hernández, Ivó H. Hernández and María Santos-Galindo for suggestions and critical reading of the manuscript.

REFERENCES

Andreadis, A. (2005). Tau gene alternative splicing: expression patterns, regulation and modulation of function in normal brain and neurodegenerative diseases. *Biochim. Biophys. Acta* 1739, 91–103. doi: 10.1016/j.bbadis.2004.08.010

Andreadis, A., Broderick, J. A., and Kosik, K. S. (1995). Relative exon affinities and suboptimal splice site signals lead to non-equivalence of two cassette exons. *Nucleic Acids Res.* 23, 3585–3593. doi: 10.1093/nar/23.17.3585

Andreadis, A., Brown, W. M., and Kosik, K. S. (1992). Structure and novel exons of the human tau gene. *Biochemistry* 31, 10626–10633. doi: 10.1021/bi00158a027

Andrew, S. E., Goldberg, Y. P., Kremer, B., Telenius, H., Theilmann, J., Adam, S., et al. (1993). The relationship between trinucleotide (CAG) repeat length and clinical features of Huntington's disease. *Nat. Genet.* 4, 398–403. doi: 10.1038/ng0893-398

Arendt, T., Stieler, J. T., and Holzer, M. (2016). Tau and tauopathies. *Brain Res. Bull* 126, 238–292. doi: 10.1016/j.brainresbull.2016.08.018

Barghorn, S., Zheng-Fischhofer, Q., Ackmann, M., Biernat, J., von Bergen, M., Mandelkow, E. M., et al. (2000). Structure, microtubule interactions, and paired helical filament aggregation by tau mutants of frontotemporal dementias. *Biochemistry* 39, 11714–11721. doi: 10.1021/bi000850r

Baskota, S. U., Lopez, O. L., Greenamyre, J. T., and Kofler, J. (2019). Spectrum of tau pathologies in Huntington's disease. *Lab. Invest.* 99, 1068–1077. doi: 10.1038/s41374-018-0166-9

Bates, G. P., Dorsey, R., Gusella, J. F., Hayden, M. R., Kay, C., Leavitt, B. R., et al. (2015). Huntington disease. *Nat. Rev. Dis. Primers* 1:15005. doi: 10.1038/nrdp.2015.5

Beaulieu, J. M., Sotnikova, T. D., Yao, W. D., Kockeritz, L., Woodgett, J. R., Gainetdinov, R. R., et al. (2004). Lithium antagonizes dopamine-dependent behaviors mediated by an AKT/glycogen synthase kinase 3 signaling cascade. *Proc. Natl. Acad. Sci. U S A* 101, 5099–5104. doi: 10.1073/pnas.0307921101

Benhelli-Mokrani, H., Mansuroglu, Z., Chauderlier, A., Albaud, B., Gentien, D., Sommer, S., et al. (2018). Genome-wide identification of genic and intergenic neuronal DNA regions bound by Tau protein under physiological and stress conditions. *Nucleic Acids Res.* 46, 11405–11422. doi: 10.1093/nar/gky929

Blum, D., Herrera, F., Francelle, L., Mendes, T., Basquin, M., Obriot, H., et al. (2015). Mutant huntingtin alters Tau phosphorylation and subcellular distribution. *Hum. Mol. Genet.* 24, 76–85. doi: 10.1093/hmg/ddu421

Bots, G. T., and Bruyn, G. W. (1981). Neuropathological changes of the nucleus accumbens in Huntington's chorea. *Acta Neuropathol.* 55, 21–22. doi: 10.1007/bf00691525

Cabrera, J. R., and Lucas, J. J. (2017). MAP2 splicing is altered in Huntington's disease. *Brain Pathol.* 27, 181–189. doi: 10.1111/bpa.12387

Caceres, A., and Kosik, K. S. (1990). Inhibition of neurite polarity by tau antisense oligonucleotides in primary cerebellar neurons. *Nature* 343, 461–463. doi: 10.1038/343461a0

Caillet-Boudin, M. L., Buee, L., Sergeant, N., and Lefebvre, B. (2015). Regulation of human MAPT gene expression. *Mol. Neurodegener.* 10:28. doi: 10.1186/s13024-015-0025-8

Caparros-Lefebvre, D., Kerdraon, O., Devos, D., Dhaenens, C. M., Blum, D., Maurage, C. A., et al. (2009). Association of corticobasal degeneration and Huntington's disease: can Tau aggregates protect Huntingtin toxicity? *Mov. Disord.* 24, 1089–1090. doi: 10.1002/mds.22204

Chen, J., Kanai, Y., Cowan, N. J., and Hirokawa, N. (1992). Projection domains of MAP2 and tau determine spacings between microtubules in dendrites and axons. *Nature* 360, 674–677. doi: 10.1038/360674a0

Cisbani, G., Maxan, A., Kordower, J. H., Planel, E., Freeman, T. B., and Cicchetti, F. (2017). Presence of tau pathology within foetal neural allografts in patients with Huntington's and Parkinson's disease. *Brain* 140, 2982–2992. doi: 10.1093/brain/awx255

Cleveland, D. W., Hwo, S. Y., and Kirschner, M. W. (1977). Purification of tau, a microtubule-associated protein that induces assembly of microtubules from purified tubulin. *J. Mol. Biol.* 116, 207–225. doi: 10.1016/0022-2836(77)90213-3

Cohen, T. J., Guo, J. L., Hurtado, D. E., Kwong, L. K., Mills, I. P., Trojanowski, J. Q., et al. (2011). The acetylation of tau inhibits its function and promotes pathological tau aggregation. *Nat. Commun.* 2:252. doi: 10.1038/ncomms1255

Cornelison, G. L., Levy, S. A., Jenson, T., and Frost, B. (2019). Tau-induced nuclear envelope invagination causes a toxic accumulation of mRNA in *Drosophila*. *Aging Cell* 18:e12847. doi: 10.1111/acel.12847

Corrochano, S., Renna, M., Carter, S., Chrobot, N., Kent, R., Stewart, M., et al. (2012). α-Synuclein levels modulate Huntington's disease in mice. *Hum. Mol. Genet.* 21, 485–494. doi: 10.1093/hmg/ddr477

Coudert, L., Nonaka, T., Bernard, E., Hasegawa, M., Schaeffer, L., and Leblanc, P. (2019). Phosphorylated and aggregated TDP-43 with seeding properties are induced upon mutant Huntingtin (mHtt) polyglutamine expression in human cellular models. *Cell. Mol. Life Sci.* 76, 2615–2632. doi: 10.1007/s00018-019-03059-8

Davies, S. W., Turmaine, M., Cozens, B. A., DiFiglia, M., Sharp, A. H., Ross, C. A., et al. (1997). Formation of neuronal intranuclear inclusions underlies the neurological dysfunction in mice transgenic for the HD mutation. *Cell* 90, 537–548. doi: 10.1016/s0092-8674(00)80513-9

Davis, M. Y., Keene, C. D., Jayadev, S., and Bird, T. (2014). The co-occurrence of Alzheimer's disease and Huntington's disease: a neuropathological study of 15 elderly Huntington's disease subjects. *J. Huntingtons Dis.* 3, 209–217. doi: 10.3233/jhd-140111

Deckel, A. W., Elder, R., and Fuhrer, G. (2002). Biphasic developmental changes in Ca2+/calmodulin-dependent proteins in R6/2 Huntington's disease mice. *Neuroreport* 13, 707–711. doi: 10.1097/00001756-200204160-00034

Derisbourg, M., Leghay, C., Chiappetta, G., Fernandez-Gomez, F. J., Laurent, C., Demeyer, D., et al. (2015). Role of the Tau N-terminal region in microtubule stabilization revealed by new endogenous truncated forms. *Sci. Rep.* 5:9659. doi: 10.1038/srep09659

DiFiglia, M., Sapp, E., Chase, K. O., Davies, S. W., Bates, G. P., Vonsattel, J. P., et al. (1997). Aggregation of huntingtin in neuronal intranuclear inclusions and dystrophic neurites in brain. *Science* 277, 1990–1993. doi: 10.1126/science.277.5334.1990

Dixit, R., Ross, J. L., Goldman, Y. E., and Holzbaur, E. L. (2008). Differential regulation of dynein and kinesin motor proteins by tau. *Science* 319, 1086–1089. doi: 10.1126/science.1152993

Eftekharzadeh, B., Daigle, J. G., Kapinos, L. E., Coyne, A., Schiantarelli, J., Carlomagno, Y., et al. (2018). Tau protein disrupts nucleocytoplasmic transport in Alzheimer's disease. *Neuron* 99, 925.e7–940.e7. doi: 10.1016/j.neuron.2018.07.039

Fernández-Nogales, M., Cabrera, J. R., Santos-Galindo, M., Hoozemans, J. J., Ferrer, I., Rozemuller, A. J., et al. (2014). Huntington's disease is a four-repeat tauopathy with tau nuclear rods. *Nat. Med.* 20, 881–885. doi: 10.1038/nm.3617

Fernández-Nogales, M., Hernández, F., Miguez, A., Alberch, J., Ginés, S., Peréz-Navarro, E., et al. (2015). Decreased glycogen synthase kinase-3 levels and activity contribute to Huntington's disease. *Hum. Mol. Genet.* 24, 5040–5052. doi: 10.1093/hmg/ddv224

Fernández-Nogales, M., Santos-Galindo, M., Merchán-Rubira, J., Hoozemans, J. J. M., Rábano, A., Ferrer, I., et al. (2017). Tau-positive nuclear indentations in P301S tauopathy mice. *Brain Pathol.* 27, 314–322. doi: 10.1111/bpa.12407

Frost, B., Bardai, F. H., and Feany, M. B. (2016). Lamin dysfunction mediates neurodegeneration in tauopathies. *Curr. Biol.* 26, 129–136. doi: 10.1016/j.cub.2015.11.039

Fujioka, Y., Ishigaki, S., Masuda, A., Iguchi, Y., Udagawa, T., Watanabe, H., et al. (2013). FUS-regulated region- and cell-type-specific transcriptome is associated with cell selectivity in ALS/FTLD. *Sci. Rep.* 3:2388. doi: 10.1038/srep02388

Gasset-Rosa, F., Chillon-Marinas, C., Goginashvili, A., Atwal, R. S., Artates, J. W., Tabet, R., et al. (2017). Polyglutamine-expanded huntingtin exacerbates age-related disruption of nuclear integrity and nucleocytoplasmic transport. *Neuron* 94, 48.e4–57.e4. doi: 10.1016/j.neuron.2017.03.027

Genetic Modifiers of Huntington's Disease (GeM-HD) Consortium. (2019). CAG repeat not polyglutamine length determines timing of Huntington's disease onset. *Cell* 178, 887.e14–900.e14. doi: 10.1016/j.cell.2019.06.036

Goedert, M., and Jakes, R. (2005). Mutations causing neurodegenerative tauopathies. *Biochim. Biophys. Acta* 1739, 240–250. doi: 10.1016/j.bbadis.2004.08.007

Goedert, M., and Spillantini, M. G. (2011). Pathogenesis of the tauopathies. *J. Mol. Neurosci.* 45, 425–431. doi: 10.1007/s12031-011-9593-4

Goedert, M., Spillantini, M. G., Jakes, R., Crowther, R. A., Vanmechelen, E., Probst, A., et al. (1995). Molecular dissection of the paired helical filament. *Neurobiol. Aging* 16, 325–334. doi: 10.1016/0197-4580(95)00017-9

Goedert, M., Spillantini, M. G., Jakes, R., Rutherford, D., and Crowther, R. A. (1989). Multiple isoforms of human microtubule-associated protein tau: sequences and localization in neurofibrillary tangles of Alzheimer's disease. *Neuron* 3, 519–526. doi: 10.1016/0896-6273(89)90210-9

Gong, C. X., Liu, F., Wu, G., Rossie, S., Wegiel, J., Li, L., et al. (2004). Dephosphorylation of microtubule-associated protein tau by protein phosphatase 5. *J. Neurochem.* 88, 298–310. doi: 10.1111/j.1471-4159.2004.02147.x

Graham, R. K., Deng, Y., Slow, E. J., Haigh, B., Bissada, N., Lu, G., et al. (2006). Cleavage at the caspase-6 site is required for neuronal dysfunction and degeneration due to mutant huntingtin. *Cell* 125, 1179–1191. doi: 10.1016/j.cell.2006.04.026

Gratuze, M., Noël, A., Julien, C., Cisbani, G., Milot-Rousseau, P., Morin, F., et al. (2015). Tau hyperphosphorylation and deregulation of calcineurin in mouse models of Huntington's disease. *Hum. Mol. Genet.* 24, 86–99. doi: 10.1093/hmg/ddu456

Grima, J. C., Daigle, J. G., Arbez, N., Cunningham, K. C., Zhang, K., Ochaba, J., et al. (2017). Mutant huntingtin disrupts the nuclear pore complex. *Neuron* 94, 93.e6–107.e6. doi: 10.1016/j.neuron.2017.03.023

Gusella, J. F., MacDonald, M. E., Ambrose, C. M., and Duyao, M. P. (1993). Molecular genetics of Huntington's disease. *Arch. Neurol.* 50, 1157–1163. doi: 10.1001/archneur.1993.00540110037003

Hedreen, J. C., and Folstein, S. E. (1995). Early loss of neostriatal striosome neurons in Huntington's disease. *J. Neuropathol. Exp. Neurol.* 54, 105–120. doi: 10.1097/00005072-199501000-00013

Hernández-Ortega, K., Garcia-Esparcia, P., Gil, L., Lucas, J. J., and Ferrer, I. (2016). Altered machinery of protein synthesis in Alzheimer's: from the nucleolus to the ribosome. *Brain Pathol.* 26, 593–605. doi: 10.1111/bpa.12335

Hernandez, F., Lucas, J. J., and Avila, J. (2013). GSK3 and tau: two convergence points in Alzheimer's disease. *J. Alzheimers Dis.* 33, S141–S144. doi: 10.3233/jad-2012-129025

Herrera, F., and Outeiro, T. F. (2012). α-synuclein modifies huntingtin aggregation in living cells. *FEBS Lett.* 586, 7–12. doi: 10.1016/j.febslet.2011.11.019

Houlden, H., Baker, M., Morris, H. R., MacDonald, N., Pickering-Brown, S., Adamson, J., et al. (2001). Corticobasal degeneration and progressive supranuclear palsy share a common tau haplotype. *Neurology* 56, 1702–1706. doi: 10.1212/wnl.56.12.1702

Hutton, M., Lendon, C. L., Rizzu, P., Baker, M., Froelich, S., Houlden, H., et al. (1998). Association of missense and 5'-splice-site mutations in tau with the inherited dementia FTDP-17. *Nature* 393, 702–705. doi: 10.1038/31508

Ishigaki, S., Fujioka, Y., Okada, Y., Riku, Y., Udagawa, T., Honda, D., et al. (2017). Altered tau isoform ratio caused by loss of FUS and SFPQ function leads to FTLD-like phenotypes. *Cell Rep.* 18, 1118–1131. doi: 10.1016/j.celrep.2017.01.013

Jellinger, K. A. (1998). Alzheimer-type lesions in Huntington's disease. *J. Neural Transm.* 105, 787–799. doi: 10.1007/s007020050095

Kadavath, H., Hofele, R. V., Biernat, J., Kumar, S., Tepper, K., Urlaub, H., et al. (2015). Tau stabilizes microtubules by binding at the interface between tubulin heterodimers. *Proc. Natl. Acad. Sci. U S A* 112, 7501–7506. doi: 10.1073/pnas.1504081112

Kaltenbach, L. S., Romero, E., Becklin, R. R., Chettier, R., Bell, R., Phansalkar, A., et al. (2007). Huntingtin interacting proteins are genetic modifiers of neurodegeneration. *PLoS Genet.* 3:e82. doi: 10.1371/journal.pgen.0030082

Kempf, M., Clement, A., Faissner, A., Lee, G., and Brandt, R. (1996). Tau binds to the distal axon early in development of polarity in a microtubule- and microfilament-dependent manner. *J. Neurosci.* 16, 5583–5592. doi: 10.1523/JNEUROSCI.16-18-05583.1996

Kim, S. D., and Fung, V. S. (2014). An update on Huntington's disease: from the gene to the clinic. *Curr. Opin. Neurol.* 27, 477–483. doi: 10.1097/WCO.0000000000000116

Kosik, K. S., Orecchio, L. D., Bakalis, S., and Neve, R. L. (1989). Developmentally regulated expression of specific tau sequences. *Neuron* 2, 1389–1397. doi: 10.1016/0896-6273(89)90077-9

Ledesma, M. D., Bonay, P., and Avila, J. (1995). Tau protein from Alzheimer's disease patients is glycated at its tubulin-binding domain. *J. Neurochem.* 65, 1658–1664. doi: 10.1046/j.1471-4159.1995.65041658.x

L'Episcopo, F., Drouin-Ouellet, J., Tirolo, C., Pulvirenti, A., Giugno, R., Testa, N., et al. (2016). GSK-3β-induced Tau pathology drives hippocampal neuronal cell death in Huntington's disease: involvement of astrocyte-neuron interactions. *Cell Death Dis.* 7:e2206. doi: 10.1038/cddis.2016.104

Li, X., Liu, M., Cai, Z., Wang, G., and Li, X. (2010). Regulation of glycogen synthase kinase-3 during bipolar mania treatment. *Bipolar Disord.* 12, 741–752. doi: 10.1111/j.1399-5618.2010.00866.x

Lim, N. K., Hung, L. W., Pang, T. Y., McLean, C. A., Liddell, J. R., Hilton, J. B., et al. (2014). Localized changes to glycogen synthase kinase-3 and collapsin response mediator protein-2 in the Huntington's disease affected brain. *Hum. Mol. Genet.* 23, 4051–4063. doi: 10.1093/hmg/ddu119

Liu, F., and Gong, C. X. (2008). Tau exon 10 alternative splicing and tauopathies. *Mol. Neurodegener.* 3:8. doi: 10.1186/1750-1326-3-8

Liu, P., Smith, B. R., Huang, E. S., Mahesh, A., Vonsattel, J. P. G., Petersen, A. J., et al. (2019). A soluble truncated tau species related to cognitive dysfunction and caspase-2 is elevated in the brain of Huntington's disease patients. *Acta Neuropathol. Commun.* 7:111. doi: 10.1186/s40478-019-0764-9

Lovestone, S., Reynolds, C. H., Latimer, D., Davis, D. R., Anderton, B. H., Gallo, J. M., et al. (1994). Alzheimer's disease-like phosphorylation of the microtubule-associated protein tau by glycogen synthase kinase-3 in transfected mammalian cells. *Curr. Biol.* 4, 1077–1086. doi: 10.1016/s0960-9822(00)00246-3

Lu, M., and Kosik, K. S. (2001). Competition for microtubule-binding with dual expression of tau missense and splice isoforms. *Mol. Biol. Cell* 12, 171–184. doi: 10.1091/mbc.12.1.171

MacDonald, M. E., Ambrose, C. M., Duyao, M. P., Myers, R. H., Lin, C., Srinidhi, L., et al. (1993). A novel gene containing a trinucleotide repeat that is expanded and unstable on Huntington's disease chromosomes. *Cell* 72, 971–983. doi: 10.1016/0092-8674(93)90585-e

Maina, M. B., Bailey, L. J., Wagih, S., Biasetti, L., Pollack, S. J., Quinn, J. P., et al. (2018). The involvement of tau in nucleolar transcription and the stress response. *Acta Neuropathol. Commun.* 6:70. doi: 10.1186/s40478-018-0565-6

Martí, E. (2016). RNA toxicity induced by expanded CAG repeats in Huntington's disease. *Brain Pathol.* 26, 779–786. doi: 10.1111/bpa.12427

Martin, L., Latypova, X., and Terro, F. (2011). Post-translational modifications of tau protein: implications for Alzheimer's disease. *Neurochem. Int.* 58, 458–471. doi: 10.1016/j.neuint.2010.12.023

Mayer, A., Siegel, N. R., Schwartz, A. L., and Ciechanover, A. (1989). Degradation of proteins with acetylated amino termini by the ubiquitin system. *Science* 244, 1480–1483. doi: 10.1126/science.2544030

McIntosh, G. C., Jameson, H. D., and Markesbery, W. R. (1978). Huntington disease associated with Alzheimer disease. *Ann. Neurol.* 3, 545–548. doi: 10.1002/ana.410030616

Min, S. W., Cho, S. H., Zhou, Y., Schroeder, S., Haroutunian, V., Seeley, W. W., et al. (2010). Acetylation of tau inhibits its degradation and contributes to tauopathy. *Neuron* 67, 953–966. doi: 10.1016/j.neuron.2010.08.044

Mitchell, I. J., Cooper, A. J., and Griffiths, M. R. (1999). The selective vulnerability of striatopallidal neurons. *Prog. Neurobiol.* 59, 691–719. doi: 10.1016/s0301-0082(99)00019-2

Morishima-Kawashima, M., Hasegawa, M., Takio, K., Suzuki, M., Titani, K., and Ihara, Y. (1993). Ubiquitin is conjugated with amino-terminally processed tau in paired helical filaments. *Neuron* 10, 1151–1160. doi: 10.1016/0896-6273(93)90063-w

Moss, R. J., Mastri, A. R., and Schut, L. J. (1988). The coexistence and differentiation of late onset Huntington's disease and Alzheimer's disease. A case report and review of the literature. *J. Am. Geriatr. Soc.* 36, 237–241. doi: 10.1111/j.1532-5415.1988.tb01807.x

Mullard, A. (2019). Pioneering antisense drug heads into pivotal trials for Huntington disease. *Nat. Rev. Drug Discov.* 18, 161–163. doi: 10.1038/d41573-019-00018-7

Myers, A. J., Pittman, A. M., Zhao, A. S., Rohrer, K., Kaleem, M., Marlowe, L., et al. (2007). The MAPT H1c risk haplotype is associated with increased expression of tau and especially of 4 repeat containing transcripts. *Neurobiol. Dis.* 25, 561–570. doi: 10.1016/j.nbd.2006.10.018

Myers, R. H., Sax, D. S., Schoenfeld, M., Bird, E. D., Wolf, P. A., Vonsattel, J. P., et al. (1985). Late onset of Huntington's disease. *J. Neurol. Neurosurg. Psychiatry* 48, 530–534. doi: 10.1136/jnnp.48.6.530

Nalavade, R., Griesche, N., Ryan, D. P., Hildebrand, S., and Krauss, S. (2013). Mechanisms of RNA-induced toxicity in CAG repeat disorders. *Cell Death Dis.* 4:e752. doi: 10.1038/cddis.2013.276

Naro, C., and Sette, C. (2013). Phosphorylation-mediated regulation of alternative splicing in cancer. *Int. J. Cell Biol.* 2013:151839. doi: 10.1155/2013/151839

Nasir, J., Floresco, S. B., O'Kusky, J. R., Diewert, V. M., Richman, J. M., Zeisler, J., et al. (1995). Targeted disruption of the Huntington's disease gene results in embryonic lethality and behavioral and morphological changes in heterozygotes. *Cell* 81, 811–823. doi: 10.1016/0092-8674(95)90542-1

Neve, R. L., Harris, P., Kosik, K. S., Kurnit, D. M., and Donlon, T. A. (1986). Identification of cDNA clones for the human microtubule-associated protein tau and chromosomal localization of the genes for tau and microtubule-associated protein 2. *Brain Res.* 387, 271–280. doi: 10.1016/0169-328x(86)90033-1

Panda, D., Samuel, J. C., Massie, M., Feinstein, S. C., and Wilson, L. (2003). Differential regulation of microtubule dynamics by three- and four-repeat tau: implications for the onset of neurodegenerative disease. *Proc. Natl. Acad. Sci. U S A* 100, 9548–9553. doi: 10.1073/pnas.1633508100

Paonessa, F., Evans, L. D., Solanki, R., Larrieu, D., Wray, S., Hardy, J., et al. (2019). Microtubules deform the nuclear membrane and disrupt nucleocytoplasmic transport in tau-mediated frontotemporal dementia. *Cell Rep.* 26, 582.e585–593.e585. doi: 10.1016/j.celrep.2018.12.085

Park, S. A., Ahn, S. I., and Gallo, J. M. (2016). Tau mis-splicing in the pathogenesis of neurodegenerative disorders. *BMB Rep.* 49, 405–413. doi: 10.5483/bmbrep.2016.49.8.084

Pei, J. J., Tanaka, T., Tung, Y. C., Braak, E., Iqbal, K., and Grundke-Iqbal, I. (1997). Distribution, levels and activity of glycogen synthase kinase-3 in the Alzheimer disease brain. *J. Neuropathol. Exp. Neurol.* 56, 70–78. doi: 10.1097/00005072-199701000-00007

Pittman, A. M., Myers, A. J., Duckworth, J., Bryden, L., Hanson, M., Abou-Sleiman, P., et al. (2004). The structure of the tau haplotype in controls and in progressive supranuclear palsy. *Hum. Mol. Genet.* 13, 1267–1274. doi: 10.1093/hmg/ddh138

Poorkaj, P., Bird, T. D., Wijsman, E., Nemens, E., Garruto, R. M., Anderson, L., et al. (1998). Tau is a candidate gene for chromosome 17 frontotemporal dementia. *Ann. Neurol.* 43, 815–825. doi: 10.1002/ana.410430617

Qian, W., and Liu, F. (2014). Regulation of alternative splicing of tau exon 10. *Neurosci. Bull.* 30, 367–377. doi: 10.1007/s12264-013-1411-2

Reyes, M. G., and Gibbons, S. (1985). Dementia of the Alzheimer's type and Huntington's disease. *Neurology* 35, 273–277. doi: 10.1212/wnl.35.2.273

Roos, R. A., and Bots, G. T. (1983). Nuclear membrane indentations in Huntington's chorea. *J. Neurol. Sci.* 61, 37–47. doi: 10.1016/0022-510x(83)90053-9

Saavedra, A., Garcia-Martinez, J. M., Xifro, X., Giralt, A., Torres-Peraza, J. F., Canals, J. M., et al. (2010). PH domain leucine-rich repeat protein phosphatase 1 contributes to maintain the activation of the PI3K/Akt pro-survival pathway in Huntington's disease striatum. *Cell Death Differ.* 17, 324–335. doi: 10.1038/cdd.2009.127

Sapp, E., Schwarz, C., Chase, K., Bhide, P. G., Young, A. B., Penney, J., et al. (1997). Huntingtin localization in brains of normal and Huntington's disease patients. *Ann. Neurol.* 42, 604–612. doi: 10.1002/ana.410420411

Sathasivam, K., Neueder, A., Gipson, T. A., Landles, C., Benjamin, A. C., Bondulich, M. K., et al. (2013). Aberrant splicing of HTT generates the pathogenic exon 1 protein in Huntington disease. *Proc. Natl. Acad. Sci. U S A* 110, 2366–2370. doi: 10.1073/pnas.1221891110

Schilling, J., Broemer, M., Atanassov, I., Duernberger, Y., Vorberg, I., Dieterich, C., et al. (2019). Deregulated splicing is a major mechanism of RNA-induced toxicity in Huntington's disease. *J. Mol. Biol.* 431, 1869–1877. doi: 10.1016/j.jmb.2019.01.034

Schulte, J., and Littleton, J. T. (2011). The biological function of the Huntingtin protein and its relevance to Huntington's disease pathology. *Curr. Trends Neurol.* 5, 65–78.

Schwab, C., Arai, T., Hasegawa, M., Yu, S., and McGeer, P. L. (2008). Colocalization of transactivation-responsive DNA-binding protein 43 and huntingtin in inclusions of Huntington disease. *J. Neuropathol. Exp. Neurol.* 67, 1159–1165. doi: 10.1097/nen.0b013e31818e8951

Sergeant, N., Bretteville, A., Hamdane, M., Caillet-Boudin, M. L., Grognet, P., Bombois, S., et al. (2008). Biochemistry of Tau in Alzheimer's disease and related neurological disorders. *Expert Rev. Proteomics* 5, 207–224. doi: 10.1586/14789450.5.2.207

Sergeant, N., Delacourte, A., and Buée, L. (2005). Tau protein as a differential biomarker of tauopathies. *Biochim. Biophys. Acta* 1739, 179–197. doi: 10.1016/j.bbadis.2004.06.020

Shieh, S. Y., and Bonini, N. M. (2011). Genes and pathways affected by CAG-repeat RNA-based toxicity in *Drosophila*. *Hum. Mol. Genet.* 20, 4810–4821. doi: 10.1093/hmg/ddr420

Siano, G., Varisco, M., Caiazza, M. C., Quercioli, V., Mainardi, M., Ippolito, C., et al. (2019). Tau modulates VGluT1 expression. *J. Mol. Biol.* 431, 873–884. doi: 10.1016/j.jmb.2019.01.023

Smith-Dijak, A. I., Sepers, M. D., and Raymond, L. A. (2019). Alterations in synaptic function and plasticity in Huntington disease. *J. Neurochem.* 150, 346–365. doi: 10.1111/jnc.14723

Snell, R. G., MacMillan, J. C., Cheadle, J. P., Fenton, I., Lazarou, L. P., Davies, P., et al. (1993). Relationship between trinucleotide repeat expansion and phenotypic variation in Huntington's disease. *Nat. Genet.* 4, 393–397. doi: 10.1038/ng0893-393

Spillantini, M. G., Bird, T. D., and Ghetti, B. (1998). Frontotemporal dementia and Parkinsonism linked to chromosome 17: a new group of tauopathies. *Brain Pathol.* 8, 387–402. doi: 10.1111/j.1750-3639.1998.tb00162.x

Spillantini, M. G., and Goedert, M. (2013). Tau pathology and neurodegeneration. *Lancet Neurol.* 12, 609–622. doi: 10.1016/S1474-4422(13)70090-5

Stamer, K., Vogel, R., Thies, E., Mandelkow, E., and Mandelkow, E. M. (2002). Tau blocks traffic of organelles, neurofilaments and APP vesicles in neurons and enhances oxidative stress. *J. Cell Biol.* 156, 1051–1063. doi: 10.1083/jcb.200108057

St-Amour, I., Turgeon, A., Goupil, C., Planel, E., and Hebert, S. S. (2018). Co-occurrence of mixed proteinopathies in late-stage Huntington's disease. *Acta Neuropathol.* 135, 249–265. doi: 10.1007/s00401-017-1786-7

Stefansson, H., Helgason, A., Thorleifsson, G., Steinthorsdottir, V., Masson, G., Barnard, J., et al. (2005). A common inversion under selection in Europeans. *Nat. Genet.* 37, 129–137. doi: 10.1038/ng1508

Sturrock, A., and Leavitt, B. R. (2010). The clinical and genetic features of Huntington disease. *J. Geriatr. Psychiatry Neurol.* 23, 243–259. doi: 10.1177/0891988710383573

Takuma, H., Arawaka, S., and Mori, H. (2003). Isoforms changes of tau protein during development in various species. *Brain Res. Dev. Brain Res.* 142, 121–127. doi: 10.1016/s0165-3806(03)00056-7

Tomas-Zapico, C., Diez-Zaera, M., Ferrer, I., Gomez-Ramos, P., Moran, M. A., Miras-Portugal, M. T., et al. (2012). α-Synuclein accumulates in huntingtin inclusions but forms independent filaments and its deficiency attenuates early phenotype in a mouse model of Huntington's disease. *Hum. Mol. Genet.* 21, 495–510. doi: 10.1093/hmg/ddr507

Tracy, T. E., Sohn, P. D., Minami, S. S., Wang, C., Min, S. W., Li, Y., et al. (2016). Acetylated tau obstructs kibra-mediated signaling in synaptic plasticity and promotes tauopathy-related memory loss. *Neuron* 90, 245–260. doi: 10.1016/j.neuron.2016.03.005

Trinczek, B., Ebneth, A., Mandelkow, E. M., and Mandelkow, E. (1999). Tau regulates the attachment/detachment but not the speed of motors in microtubule-dependent transport of single vesicles and organelles. *J. Cell Sci.* 112, 2355–2367.

Violet, M., Delattre, L., Tardivel, M., Sultan, A., Chauderlier, A., Caillierez, R., et al. (2014). A major role for Tau in neuronal DNA and RNA protection *in vivo* under physiological and hyperthermic conditions. *Front. Cell. Neurosci.* 8:84. doi: 10.3389/fncel.2014.00084

Vonsattel, J. P., and DiFiglia, M. (1998). Huntington disease. *J. Neuropathol. Exp. Neurol.* 57, 369–384. doi: 10.1097/00005072-199805000-00001

Vonsattel, J. P., Del Amaya, M. P., and Keller, C. E. (2008). Twenty-first century brain banking. Processing brains for research: the Columbia University methods. *Acta Neuropathol.* 115, 509–532. doi: 10.1007/s00401-007-0311-9

Vuono, R., Winder-Rhodes, S., de Silva, R., Cisbani, G., Drouin-Ouellet, J., REGISTRY Investigators of the European Huntington's Disease Network, et al. (2015). The role of tau in the pathological process and clinical expression of Huntington's disease. *Brain* 138, 1907–1918. doi: 10.1093/brain/awv107

Wang, Y., and Mandelkow, E. (2016). Tau in physiology and pathology. *Nat. Rev. Neurosci.* 17, 5–21. doi: 10.1038/nrn.2015.1

Warrick, J. M., Paulson, H. L., Gray-Board, G. L., Bui, Q. T., Fischbeck, K. H., Pittman, R. N., et al. (1998). Expanded polyglutamine protein forms nuclear inclusions and causes neural degeneration in *Drosophila*. *Cell* 93, 939–949. doi: 10.1016/s0092-8674(00)81200-3

Wei, Y., Qu, M. H., Wang, X. S., Chen, L., Wang, D. L., Liu, Y., et al. (2008). Binding to the minor groove of the double-strand, tau protein prevents DNA from damage by peroxidation. *PLoS One* 3:e2600. doi: 10.1371/journal.pone.0002600

Weingarten, M. D., Lockwood, A. H., Hwo, S. Y., and Kirschner, M. W. (1975). A protein factor essential for microtubule assembly. *Proc. Natl. Acad. Sci. U S A* 72, 1858–1862. doi: 10.1073/pnas.72.5.1858

Wischik, C. M., Novak, M., Thogersen, H. C., Edwards, P. C., Runswick, M. J., Jakes, R., et al. (1988). Isolation of a fragment of tau derived from the core of the paired helical filament of Alzheimer disease. *Proc. Natl. Acad. Sci. U S A* 85, 4506–4510. doi: 10.1073/pnas.85.12.4506

Witman, G. B., Cleveland, D. W., Weingarten, M. D., and Kirschner, M. W. (1976). Tubulin requires tau for growth onto microtubule initiating sites. *Proc. Natl. Acad. Sci. U S A* 73, 4070–4074. doi: 10.1073/pnas.73.11.4070

Yin, X., Jin, N., Gu, J., Shi, J., Zhou, J., Gong, C. X., et al. (2012). Dual-specificity tyrosine phosphorylation-regulated kinase 1A (Dyrk1A) modulates serine/arginine-rich protein 55 (SRp55)-promoted Tau exon 10 inclusion. *J. Biol. Chem.* 287, 30497–30506. doi: 10.1074/jbc.m112.355412

Zhang, Z., Song, M., Liu, X., Kang, S. S., Kwon, I. S., Duong, D. M., et al. (2014). Cleavage of tau by asparagine endopeptidase mediates the neurofibrillary pathology in Alzheimer's disease. *Nat. Med.* 20, 1254–1262. doi: 10.1038/nm.3700

Zheng, Z., and Diamond, M. I. (2012). Huntington disease and the huntingtin protein. *Prog. Mol. Biol. Transl. Sci.* 107, 189–214. doi: 10.1016/B978-0-12-385883-2.00010-2

Zoghbi, H. Y., and Orr, H. T. (2000). Glutamine repeats and neurodegeneration. *Annu. Rev. Neurosci.* 23, 217–247. doi: 10.1146/annurev.neuro.23.1.217

Zuccato, C., and Cattaneo, E. (2014). Huntington's disease. *Handb. Exp. Pharmacol.* 220, 357–409. doi: 10.1007/978-3-642-45106-5_14

14

The Evolution of Tau Phosphorylation and Interactions

Nataliya I. Trushina[1], *Lidia Bakota*[1], *Armen Y. Mulkidjanian*[2,3,4] *and Roland Brandt*[1,5,6*]

[1]Department of Neurobiology, University of Osnabrück, Osnabrück, Germany, [2]Department of Physics, University of Osnabrück, Osnabrück, Germany, [3]School of Bioengineering and Bioinformatics, Lomonosov Moscow State University, Moscow, Russia, [4]A.N. Belozersky Institute of Physico-Chemical Biology, Lomonosov Moscow State University, Moscow, Russia, [5]Center for Cellular Nanoanalytics, University of Osnabrück, Osnabrück, Germany, [6]Institute of Cognitive Science, University of Osnabrück, Osnabrück, Germany

***Correspondence:**
Roland Brandt
brandt@biologie.uni-osnabrueck.de

Tau is a neuronal microtubule-associated protein (MAP) that is involved in the regulation of axonal microtubule assembly. However, as a protein with intrinsically disordered regions (IDRs), tau also interacts with many other partners in addition to microtubules. Phosphorylation at selected sites modulates tau's various intracellular interactions and regulates the properties of IDRs. In Alzheimer's disease (AD) and other tauopathies, tau exhibits pathologically increased phosphorylation (hyperphosphorylation) at selected sites and aggregates into neurofibrillary tangles (NFTs). By bioinformatics means, we tested the hypothesis that the sequence of tau has changed during the vertebrate evolution in a way that novel interactions developed and also the phosphorylation pattern was affected, which made tau prone to the development of tauopathies. We report that distinct regions of tau show functional specialization in their molecular interactions. We found that tau's amino-terminal region, which is involved in biological processes related to "membrane organization" and "regulation of apoptosis," exhibited a strong evolutionary increase in protein disorder providing the basis for the development of novel interactions. We observed that the predicted phosphorylation sites have changed during evolution in a region-specific manner, and in some cases the overall number of phosphorylation sites increased owing to the formation of clusters of phosphorylatable residues. In contrast, disease-specific hyperphosphorylated sites remained highly conserved. The data indicate that novel, non-microtubule related tau interactions developed during evolution and suggest that the biological processes, which are mediated by these interactions, are of pathological relevance. Furthermore, the data indicate that predicted phosphorylation sites in some regions of tau, including a cluster of phosphorylatable residues in the alternatively spliced exon 2, have changed during evolution. In view of the "antagonistic pleiotropy hypothesis" it may be worth to take disease-associated phosphosites with low evolutionary conservation as relevant biomarkers into consideration.

Keywords: disorder, microtubule-associated protein, phosphorylation, tau, tauopathy

---

Abbreviations: aa, amino acid; AD, Alzheimer's disease; BP, biological process; CNS, central nervous system; CTR, carboxy-terminal region; GO, Gene Ontology; IDP, intrinsically disordered protein; IDR, intrinsically disordered region; MAP, microtubule-associated protein; MBR, microtubule-binding region; MCI, mild cognitive impairment; MT, microtubule; NFT, neurofibrillary tangle; NTR, amino-terminal region; PHF, paired helical filament; PKA, cAMP-dependent protein kinase; PRR, proline-rich region; PTM, posttranslational modification.

INTRODUCTION

The microtubule-associated protein (MAP) tau is involved in the regulation of neuronal microtubule (MT) assembly. Together with the closely related MAP2, it has arisen in evolution after a duplication of an ancestral gene of ancient cyclostomes (Sündermann et al., 2016). Tau and MAP2 contain a similar C-terminal region (CTR) with a highly conserved microtubule-binding region (MBR), while their amino-terminal sequences vary (Dehmelt and Halpain, 2005). It has been proposed that this variance plays a role in the differential localization and function of these proteins in cells, as tau is enriched in the axon, whereas MAP2 is localized to the somato-dendritic compartment (Weissmann et al., 2009).

Tau is encoded by a single gene, which, in the human genome, is located on chromosome 17q21 (Andreadis et al., 1992). In the human central nervous system (CNS) tau is expressed in several alternatively spliced isoforms, of which the longest isoform is encoded by 11 exons and contains 441 amino acids (aa); three of the exons (exons 2, 3 and 10) are alternatively spliced to generate six different CNS isoforms (Bakota et al., 2017). Tau is also subject to many posttranslational modifications (PTMs) including phosphorylation, O-glycosylation, ubiquitination, methylation, acetylation, sumoylation and proteolytic cleavage, which, together with the different splice variants, generates many proteoforms that may exhibit different localization and functional specialization (Heinisch and Brandt, 2016; Guo et al., 2017). The best-studied PTM of tau is phosphorylation since tau belongs to the major phosphoproteins in the brain.

Tau can aggregate into neurofibrillary tangles (NFTs), which are a hallmark of several neurodegenerative diseases collectively called "tauopathies" (Arendt et al., 2016). The most common tauopathy is Alzheimer's disease (AD), where intracellular NFTs are joined by the presence of extracellular amyloid plaques containing aggregated amyloid-β (Aβ). Analysis of the histopathological changes in patients with AD has shown that tau inclusions correlate much better with cognitive impairment than amyloid plaques (Nelson et al., 2012) suggesting a major role of changes in tau expression and phosphorylation for disease development. NFTs are composed of tau proteins with increased phosphorylation ("hyperphosphorylation") in paired helical filaments (PHFs) or straight filaments (Crowther, 1991). Dysregulation of tau splicing resulting in the expression of longer tau isoforms at the expense of shorter ones has been shown to be associated with the development of tauopathies and tau aggregation (Goedert et al., 1998). Indeed, increased expression of longer tau isoforms containing exon 10 without a change in total tau induced pathological changes in human tau-expressing mice including increased tau phosphorylation and a shift towards oligomeric tau (Schoch et al., 2016).

Structurally, tau belongs to the class of intrinsically disordered proteins (IDPs), which are known to interact with many binding partners and are considered to be involved in various signaling and regulation processes (Brandt and Leschik, 2004; Uversky, 2015). As an IDP, tau contains intrinsically disordered regions (IDRs), which lack well-defined, three-dimensional structures at physiological conditions, provide a larger interaction surface area and exhibit conformational flexibility. IDRs differ in amino acid composition from regions with defined secondary structures, which allows predicting the presence of IDRs by bioinformatics means. In particular, IDRs contain higher numbers of hydrophilic amino acids and fewer hydrophobic ones (Dyson and Wright, 2005). They may also have more proline and serine residues, which are considered to be disorder-promoting (Atkins et al., 2015). IDRs also bear diverse PTMs, which, in many cases, were shown to have functional importance (Babu et al., 2011; Bah and Forman-Kay, 2016; Darling and Uversky, 2018). As argued by Darling and Uversky, IDRs appear to be the main targets of PTM-catalyzing enzymes (Darling and Uversky, 2018). The available crystal structures of complexes between protein-modifying enzymes (kinases, phosphatases, deacetylases, methyltransferases, glycosyltransferases) and peptides derived from their protein targets show the same mechanism of interaction where the extended, unfolded peptide fits into a narrow grove of the enzyme (Darling and Uversky, 2018). It appears that even the structured protein regions should transiently unfold to be modified. After the very existence of IDRs was postulated (Dunker et al., 2001), many well-studied sites of PTMs were mapped to IDRs of respective proteins (Darling and Uversky, 2018). Although the functional consequences from PTMs of IDRs are extensively described in recent comprehensive reviews (Bah and Forman-Kay, 2016; Darling and Uversky, 2018), it is not possible to predict the impact of a PTM on a particular interaction, i.e., to say whether the PTM will strengthen the interaction or, in contrast, make it weaker. The reason for this ambiguity is that the mechanism of interaction between IDRs and their protein partners is poorly understood (Darling and Uversky, 2018). In the absence of a general understanding, case-by-case studies appear to be the main option.

Based on sequence and functional properties, four regions of tau can be differentiated (**Figure 1A**; Bakota et al., 2017). These are the N-terminal projection region (NTR), which protrudes from the MT surface when tau interacts with MTs, the MBR, and the proline-rich region (PRR) and CTR, which flank the MBR amino-terminally and carboxy-terminally, respectively. The carboxy-terminal half of tau containing the MBR and CTR is highly conserved in mammals, birds, reptiles and bony fish and is also present in other members of the MAPT/MAP2/MAP4 family of MAPs. This region contains several repeats of a highly similar motif with a length of 18 amino acids (Niewidok et al., 2016) and encompasses the main microtubule-interacting sites (Kadavath et al., 2015; Kellogg et al., 2018). The NTR and PRR are much less conserved and may represent regions, where compartment-specific, non-microtubule related interactions of tau developed during evolution. These regions may also have contributed to tau's malfunction during the development of tauopathies, which occur in higher vertebrates. In fact, the NTR and PRR contain IDRs, which may play diverse roles in the modulation and control of the functions of many different binding partners (Uversky, 2015; Trushina et al., 2019). Alternatively spliced exons of tau CNS isoforms code for regions that are located

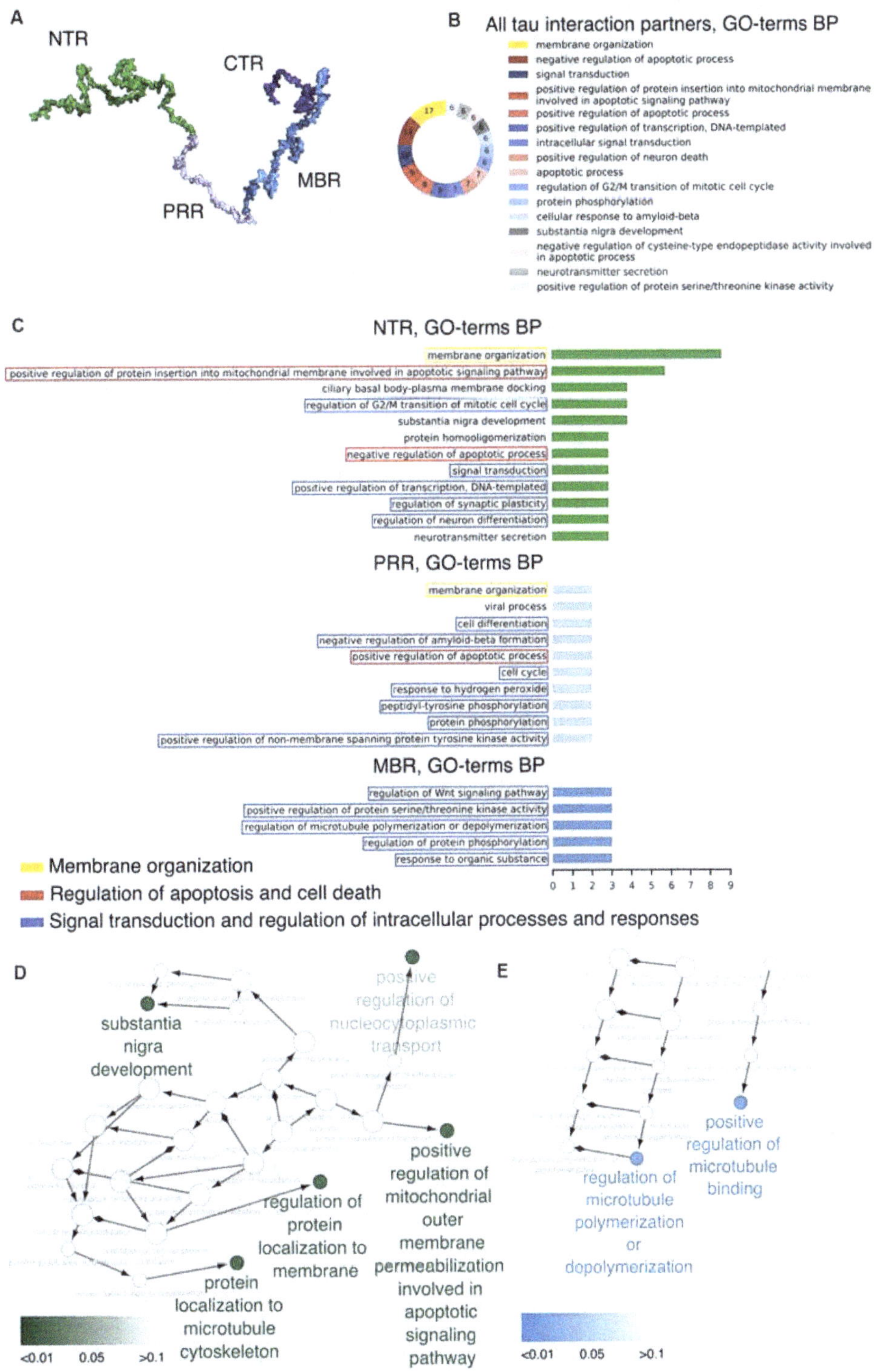

FIGURE 1 | Distinct regions of tau show functional specialization in their molecular interactions. **(A)** A potential 3D structure of tau [441 amino acid (aa) central nervous system (CNS) isoform] generated by the Random Coil Generator (RCG; Jha et al., 2005) is shown. Tau's region organization was mapped onto the model and regions were color-coded as follows: amino-terminal region (NTR, 1–171)—green; proline-rich region (PRR, 172–243)—light blue; microtubule-binding region (MBR, 244–368)—blue; carboxy-terminal region (CTR, 369–441)—dark blue. **(B)** Most common Gene Ontology (GO)-terms for biological processes (BP) of tau's interaction partners are shown. **(C)** Bar plots indicate most frequent GO-terms for BP associated with interaction partners of tau, which have been mapped to interact with the NTR, PRR and MBP. Processes associated with membrane organization are shown in yellow boxes, with apoptosis and cell death-related processes in red boxes, and with signaling and complex regulation processes in blue boxes. **(D,E)** GO-term enrichment analysis for genes identified as interaction partners of tau's NTR **(D)** and MBR **(E)** was performed. Enriched GO-terms for BP are presented in the graph. Enrichment analysis was performed for *Homo sapiens* genes.

in the NTR (exon 2 and 3) and in the MBR (exon 10); exon 10 codes for an additional microtubule-interacting site (**Figure 4B**).

We have previously provided evidence that evolutionary changes in tubulin-structure proteins, MT-binding proteins and tubulin-sequestering proteins are prominent drivers for the development of increased neuronal complexity (Trushina et al., 2019). We also provided evidence that tau displays an increase in disorder extent during evolution. However, potential consequences with respect to the different functional interactions of tau remained open and changes in sites for PTMs during evolution were not addressed. In this study, we examined published results of tau's interactions by bioinformatics means to extract information about potential functional specialization of individual regions of tau protein. We determined changes in disorder of individual regions of tau with the help of multiple disorder prediction algorithms and examined changes in the number of predicted phosphorylated residues throughout evolution. In addition, we examined the distribution and conservation of potentially disease-associated tau phosphorylation sites.

MATERIALS AND METHODS

GO-Term Analysis

Uniprot[1] IDs for some of tau's interaction partners were retrieved for the respective human proteins; their QuickGO[2] annotations were searched for Gene Ontology (GO)-terms corresponding to Biological Process (BP). Different cut-off values for the number of proteins associated with most frequent GO-terms were selected (six for all interaction partners regardless of the region, three for NTR and MBR and two for PRR, as it had the lowest number of annotated interaction partners). Data analysis and visualization were performed with Cytoscape 3.7.1 (Shannon et al., 2003), GO-term enrichment was performed using ClueGO plug-in (Shannon et al., 2003; Bindea et al., 2009).

Modeling Tau 3D Structure

A potential structural model of the longest human CNS tau isoform (441 aa isoform) was generated by the Random Coil Generator (RCG) software (Jha et al., 2005) with side-chain conformation predicted by Scwrl4 with standard parameters (Krivov et al., 2009). The random coil model is frequently used to generate conformational ensembles of IDPs. The structure was represented as a surface; visualization and structure rendering was performed using PyMOL[3]. Tau's region organization was mapped onto the model with the following color-code: NTR—green, PRR—light blue, MBR—blue and CTR—dark blue. The surface of residues that were shown to be phosphorylated was colored red and major phosphorylation sites were colored yellow.

[1] uniprot.org, release 04/2019
[2] ebi.ac.uk/QuickGO
[3] pymol.org

Selecting Tau Sequences From Various Species

MAPT sequences were retrieved from Uniprot[1] and RefSeq Release 93[4] databases; we also used the sequences that were manually cured for previous work in our laboratory (Sündermann et al., 2016). The best represented higher taxons in our analysis were bony fish (13 sequences), reptiles and birds (2 and 11 sequences, respectively) and mammals (16 sequences). We also included into our analysis sequences from cyclostomes—hagfish (*Eptatretus burgeri*) and lamprey (*Petromyzon marinus*), cartilaginous fish (*Callorhinchus milii*), coelacanth (*Latimeria chalumnae*) and amphibian (*Xenopus tropicalis*). The selected organisms were grouped according to higher taxons (Cyclostomata, Chondrichthyes, Actinopterygii, Coelacanthiformes, Amphibia, Sauropsida, Mammalia) and were color-coded from light yellow to orange in the respective order. The following estimated divergence times between mammals and other groups of vertebrates were obtained from TimeTree[5]: Cyclostomata—615 MYA (million years ago), Chondrichthyes—473, Actinopterygii—435, Coelacanthiformes—413, Amphibia—352, Sauropsida—312 and Mammalia as 0 (Kumar et al., 2017). We included hagfish and lampreys as they are considered to be at the origin of all vertebrates and to have diverged shortly after the separation of cyclostomes (Kuraku and Kuratani, 2006).

Disorder Prediction

The following disorder prediction algorithms were used to analyze disorder of different tau regions: (1) IUPred2A (long, short); predicts structural disorder based on a biophysical model and optimized for different length disordered regions (Dosztányi et al., 2005). (2) PONDR® (VLXT, VL3-BA and VSL2); mostly neural networks that were trained on different datasets of ordered and disordered proteins to predict disorder for analyzed sequences (Romero et al., 2001; Peng et al., 2006). (3) SLIDER; gives the score resembling how likely a protein has long disorder segment (Peng et al., 2014). (4) Espritz (N—NMR, X—X-ray and D—Disprot); networks that were trained on different datasets, e.g., NMR mobility data, X-ray crystallography of short disorder and Disprot data for long disorder (Walsh et al., 2012).

Phosphorylation Database Use and Phosphorylation Prediction

We used the following phosphorylation databases and prediction software: (1) PhosphoSitePlus®[6]-PTM database containing information on experimentally observed modifications (Hornbeck et al., 2015); (2) NetPhos[7] (Blom et al., 1999) for prediction of phosphorylation sites.

Alignment and Disorder Mapping

Alignment of selected sequences was performed with Tcoffee (Notredame et al., 2000) and further edited manually. To map

[4] ncbi.nlm.nih.gov/refseq
[5] timetree.org
[6] phosphosite.org/
[7] cbs.dtu.dk/services/NetPhos/

the predicted disorder scores onto the alignment the predictions from IUPred2A were used.

Statistical Analysis

Two-sided Mann–Whitney U test was used to analyze the differences between most represented groups of vertebrates' predicted disorder and phosphorylation. Significance levels were defined as follows: $^{*}p \leq 0.05$, $^{**}p \leq 0.01$, $^{***}p \leq 0.001$, $^{****}p \leq 0.0001$. Linear regression analysis was used to evaluate the changes throughout tau sequences of all selected species.

RESULTS

The longest isoform of tau (often called "big tau"; Goedert et al., 1992) is produced specifically in the peripheral nervous system (PNS) and is encoded by 14 exons generating a protein with an apparent molecular mass of about 110 kDa. However, due to the involvement of tau in pathologies of the CNS, most functional and structural studies concentrated on tau isoforms expressed from the MAPT gene in CNS neurons; thus, we will restrict our analysis to the longest CNS tau isoform containing 441 amino acids (aa) in humans, which is encoded by 11 exons (Andreadis et al., 1992) including the three exons, which are alternatively spliced in the CNS (exon 2, 3 and 10; **Figure 4B**).

Distinct Regions of Tau Show Functional Specialization in Their Molecular Interactions

To determine potential functionally relevant interactions of different regions of tau protein with cellular binding partners, we first performed a literature search for cellular components, which have been reported to interact with tau. All together the search revealed about 60 different interaction partners. About one-third of the interactions were reported to be sensitive to phosphorylation. **Table 1.1** shows a summary of the results for tau binding partners, whose interactions have been mapped to specific regions of tau protein. **Table 1.2** displays additional partners, whose interaction sites have not been mapped. Genes and Uniprot IDs for the respective human genes coding for the interaction partners are shown in **Supplementary Table S1**.

The data indicate that tau interacts with a variety of different proteins and cellular components, which appear to be different for the NTR, the PPR and the MBR, respectively. None of the interaction partners was specific for the CTR. Interestingly, many interaction partners of tau appeared to be structurally unrelated to each other, which may be due to tau's intrinsic disorder properties that is associated with the presence of multiple interactions with relatively low affinity (Babu et al., 2011). To determine potentially common functional features of the interaction partners, we analyzed GO-terms associated with biological processes (BP) for the interacting partners (**Figure 1B**). Most GO-terms of the interaction partners (**Tables 1.1, 1.2, Supplementary Table S1**) were related to "membrane organization," "regulation of apoptotic processes" and "signal transduction." When the most frequent GO-terms were grouped for the individual tau regions, we observed that "membrane organization" and "regulation of apoptotic processes" were among the GO-terms, which were specific for the amino-terminal part of tau (NTR and PRR), while all common GO-terms for the MBR were "signal transduction and regulation of intracellular processes and responses" (**Figure 1C**).

GO-term enrichment analysis for genes identified as interaction partners of tau's NTR and MBR, respectively, confirmed the functional specialization of these two regions (**Figures 1D,E**). We observed a strong enrichment for "regulation of protein localization to membrane" and "involvement in apoptotic signaling pathway" for the NTR, while the MBR was particularly specialized for "regulation of MT polymerization."

Thus, the data indicate that the highly conserved MBR on one side and the much less conserved N-terminal region on the other side show specific functional specialization. The data also suggest that in particular tau's potential functions with respect to membrane organization and regulation of apoptotic processes are mediated *via* the NTR and PRR. Until to date, no interaction partners have been identified, which specifically interact with sequences encoded by the three alternatively spliced exons in CNS tau (exons 2, 3 and 10). However, experiments using recombinant tau fragments have provided evidence that segments encoded by exons 2 and 10 promoted tau aggregation, whereas the segment encoded by exon 3 depressed it (Zhong et al., 2012). Thus, sequences that are encoded by exons 2, 3 and 10 may modulate tau-tau interaction rather than contributing additional interactions. This is in line with data showing that an increase in isoforms containing exon 10 leads to the formation of abnormal tau filaments in patients with tauopathies (Spillantini et al., 1998) and that carriers of the MAPT H2 haplotype, which express more tau containing exons 2/3 than H1 carriers, appear to be more protected from neurodegeneration (Caffrey et al., 2008). It has also been reported that the peptide NAP (davunetide, CP201), which has been tested in clinical trials for the treatment of tauopathies, preferentially interacts with tau isoforms lacking exon 10 suggesting that some interactions may also be specific for shorter tau isoforms (Ivashko-Pachima et al., 2019).

Tau's Amino-Terminal, Non-microtubule Binding Region Exhibits a Strong Evolutionary Increase in Disorder

Previously, we reported a tendency of increased disorder of tau protein structure during evolution, a feature, which tau shared with MAP6 protein, which is involved in stabilization of axonal microtubules (Tortosa et al., 2017). In contrast, we did not observe a similar increase in disorder in the structure of the somatodendritic MAP2 protein (Trushina et al., 2019). Since IDRs provide a larger interaction surface area and are known to be hubs for cellular interactions, different tau regions may differ in their extent of disorder. Furthermore, evolutionary changes in the extent of disorder of particular regions of tau could indicate, which type of interactions may have evolved during evolutionary development.

IDRs are characterized by the presence of low sequence complexity and amino acid compositional bias (Dyson and

TABLE 1.1 | Tau binding partners, whose interactions have been mapped to specific regions of tau protein.

Protein	Gene name (*H. sapiens*)	Selected references	Potential physiological function
N-terminal projection region (NTR)			
End-binding proteins	MAPRE1, MAPRE3	Sayas et al. (2019)	regulation of microtubule dynamics
Annexin A2	ANXA2	Gauthier-Kemper et al. (2018)	contribution to tau's axonal localization
Annexin A6	ANXA6	Gauthier-Kemper et al. (2018)	contribution to tau's axonal localization
Annexin A5	ANXA5	Stefanoska et al. (2018)	
14–3–3β, 14–3–3β	YWHAB, YWHAH	Stefanoska et al. (2018)	modulation of cell signaling
Synapsin-1	SYN1	Stefanoska et al. (2018)	modulation of transmitter release
Synaptotagmin-1	SYT1	Stefanoska et al. (2018)	modulation of transmitter release
14–3–3ε, γ, ζ, and σ	YWHAE, YWHAG, YWHAZ, SFN	Tugaeva et al. (2017)	modulation of ell signaling
Synaptic vesicles	VAMP2	Zhou et al. (2017)	modulation of transmitter release
Prion protein (PrP)	PRNP	Wang et al. (2008)	
Dynactin complex	DCTN1	Magnani et al. (2007)	modulation of organelle transport
Heparin	NA	Sibille et al. (2006)	
Glycogen synthase kinase-3β	GSK3B	Sun et al. (2002)	modulation of axonal phosphorylation
Membrane cortex	ACTB	Brandt et al. (1995) and Maas et al. (2000)	contribution to tau's axonal localization
Proline-rich region (PRR)			
Bridging integrator-1 (BIN1)	BIN1	Malki et al. (2017) and Sottejeau et al. (2015)	
14–3–3σ	SFN	Joo et al. (2015)	modulation of cell signaling
DNA	NA	Qi et al. (2015)	transcriptional regulation
Protein phosphatase PP2A/Bα	PPP2R2A	Sontag et al. (2012)	modulation of axonal phosphorylation
Src-family non-receptor tyrosine kinases fyn	FYN	Lee et al. (1998) and Usardi et al. (2011)	modulation of cell signaling
Heparin	NA	Sibille et al. (2006)	
Peptidyl prolyl cis/trans-isomerase Pin1	PIN1	Smet et al. (2004)	
Src-family non-receptor tyrosine kinases src	SRC	Lee et al. (1998)	modulation of cell signaling
Microtubule-binding region (MBR)			
Heat shock cognate 71 kDa protein (Hsc70)	HSPA8	Taylor et al. (2018) and Sarkar et al. (2008)	
Small heat shock protein HspB1/heat shock protein 27 (Hsp27)	HSPB1	Freilich et al. (2018)	
End-binding proteins (EBs)	MAPRE1, MAPRE3	Ramirez-Rios et al. (2016)	regulation of microtubule dynamics
14–3–3σ	SFN	Joo et al. (2015)	modulation of cell signaling
DNA	NA	Qi et al. (2015)	transcriptional regulation
Amyloid β (Aβ)	APP	Pérez et al. (2004) and Manczak and Reddy (2013)	
Protein disulfide isomerase (PDI)	P4HB	Xu et al. (2013)	
Protein phosphatase PP2A/Bα	PPP2CA	Sontag et al. (2012)	modulation of axonal phosphorylation
Heparin	NA	Zhu et al. (2010) and Sibille et al. (2006)	
Histone deacetylase 6	HDAC6	Ding et al. (2008)	transcriptional regulation
Prion protein (PrP)	PRNP	Wang et al. (2008)	
Phosphatase 2A (PP2A) isoform ABalphaC	PPP2CA	Sontag et al. (1999) and Eidenmuller et al. (2000)	modulation of axonal phosphorylation
Tau (tau-tau interaction)	MAPT	Pérez et al. (1996)	
Actin filaments	ACTB	Correas et al. (1990), Moraga et al. (1993) and Selden and Pollard (1986)	regulation of cytoskeletal interactions
Microtubules	NA	Butner and Kirschner (1991), Lee et al. (1989) and Gustke et al. (1992)	regulation of microtubule dynamics
Calmodulin	CALM1	Padilla et al. (1990)	modulation of cell signaling
C-terminal region (CTR)			
Microtubules	NA	Kadavath et al. (2015)	regulation of microtubule dynamics
Heparin	NA	Sibille et al. (2006)	

Interactions, which have been reported to be sensitive to phosphorylation, are indicated in red color.

Wright, 2005; Atkins et al., 2015), which allows predicting the presence of IDRs by bioinformatics means. To determine the level of disorder within the tau protein and potential changes during evolution, we employed disorder predicting algorithms to determine disorder scores for tau sequences of selected species. Since all of the individual algorithms have constraints because the predictors were trained on different training sets and take into account certain factors while neglecting others, we decided to employ a set of various prediction algorithms and determine average scores.

The species were grouped by divergence times between mammals and other taxonomy groups of vertebrates (cyclostomes or jawless fishes—615 MYA, cartilaginous fishes—473 MYA, bony fishes—435 MYA, coelacanths—413 MYA, amphibians—352 MYA, reptiles and birds—312 MYA and mammals as a 0 value) and the relation of

TABLE 1.2 | Additional binding partners, whose interactions have not been mapped to tau specific regions.

Protein	Gene name (*H. sapiens*)	Selected references	Potential physiological function
Additional interactions (not mapped)			
α-synuclein	SNCA	Yan et al. (2018) and Esposito et al. (2007)	modulation of transmitter release
DEAD box RNA helicase DDX6	DDX	Chauderlier et al. (2018)	
Heat shock protein 90 (Hsp90)	HSP90AB1	Radli and Rüdiger (2018)	
Voltage dependent anion channel (VDAC) proteins	VDAC1	Magri and Messina (2017)	
Transferrin	TF	Jahshan et al. (2016)	
Ferritin	FTH1	Jahshan et al. (2016)	
FK506-binding protein 4 (FKBP52)	FKBP4	Kamah et al. (2016)	
RNA-Binding Protein TIA1	TIA1	Vanderweyde et al. (2016)	modification of stress response
Death-associated protein kinase 1 (DAPK1)	DAPK1	Pei et al. (2015)	
Leucine-rich repeat kinase 2 (LRRK2)	LRRK2	Shanley et al. (2015)	
Clusterin (apolipoprotein J)	CLU	Zhou et al. (2014)	
14–3–3zeta	YWHAZ	Qureshi et al. (2013), Sluchanko et al. (2011) and Sluchanko et al. (2009)	
Dynamin-related protein (Drp1)	DNM1L	Manczak and Reddy (2012)	
Phospholipid membranes	NA	Künze et al. (2012)	
Synaptic proteins	SYN1, SYT1, VAMP2	Mondragón-Rodríguez et al. (2012)	modulation of transmitter release
C-Jun N-terminal kinase-interacting protein 1 (JIP1)	MAPK8IP1	Ittner et al. (2009)	
Golgi membranes	NA	Farah et al. (2006)	
Fe65 protein	APBB1	Barbato et al. (2005)	
Rb binding protein Che-1	AATF	Barbato et al. (2003)	
Alu-derived domain	NA	Hoenicka et al. (2002)	
S100b	S100B	Baudier and Cole (1988) and Yu and Fraser (2001)	
Cdc2-like protein kinase	CDK2	Sobue et al. (2000)	modulation of axonal phosphorylation
Presenilin 1	PSEN1	Takashima et al. (1998)	
Apolipoprotein E	APOE	Richey et al. (1995) and Fleming et al. (1996)	
Phosphatidylinositol	NA	Surridge and Burns (1994)	
Spectrin	SPTAN1	Carlier et al. (1984)	regulation of cytoskeletal interactions

Interactions, which have been reported to be sensitive to phosphorylation, are indicated in red color.

predicted disorder values and divergence times were analyzed with linear regression model. An example of a respective representation of the change in the level of disorder of different tau regions through vertebrate evolution with one disorder predicting algorithm is shown in **Figure 2A**. To increase the reliability of the disorder prediction, we determined the average disorder prediction slope for full-length tau and the different regions from nine different disorder predicting algorithms (**Figure 2B**; see "Materials and Methods" section). The disorder extent of full-length tau increased during evolution as judged from most prediction programs (**Figure 2B**; the prediction of the individual algorithms are shown in **Supplementary Figure S1**). The increase in protein disorder during vertebrate evolution was highest in the NTR followed by the PRR. In contrast, the MBR and CTR showed a negative trend. In addition, we determined the evolutionary changes in disorder for NTR lacking the alternatively spliced exons 2/3 and 3 (**Figure 2C**) and for MBR lacking exon 10 (**Figure 2D**). Interestingly, no significant increase in protein disorder of the NTR was observed in sequence lacking exon 2/3, while lack of exon 3 alone did not change the evolutionary increase in the extent of disorder of the NTR. A lack of exon 10 did not lead to any change.

Thus, the data indicate that in particular tau's amino-terminal region (NTR and PRR) with a noticeable contribution of the alternatively spliced exon 2 exhibits a strong evolutionary increase in disorder, which suggests that novel interactions in addition to tau's microtubule-related activities developed during evolution. As discussed before, this may, in particular, involve biological processes related to "membrane organization" and "regulation of apoptotic processes" which are both mediated by this region.

The Number of Predicted Phosphorylation Sites Changes During Evolution in a Region-Specific Manner and Evolves in the NTR and PRR in an Opposite Manner

Phosphorylation is a common PTM, which regulates the function of many proteins and is also thought to modulate the conformational flexibility and interactions of IDRs. Tau is subject to many phosphorylation events and changes in the pattern, the stoichiometry and the dynamics of phosphorylation have been associated with functional changes of tau during physiological and pathological conditions.

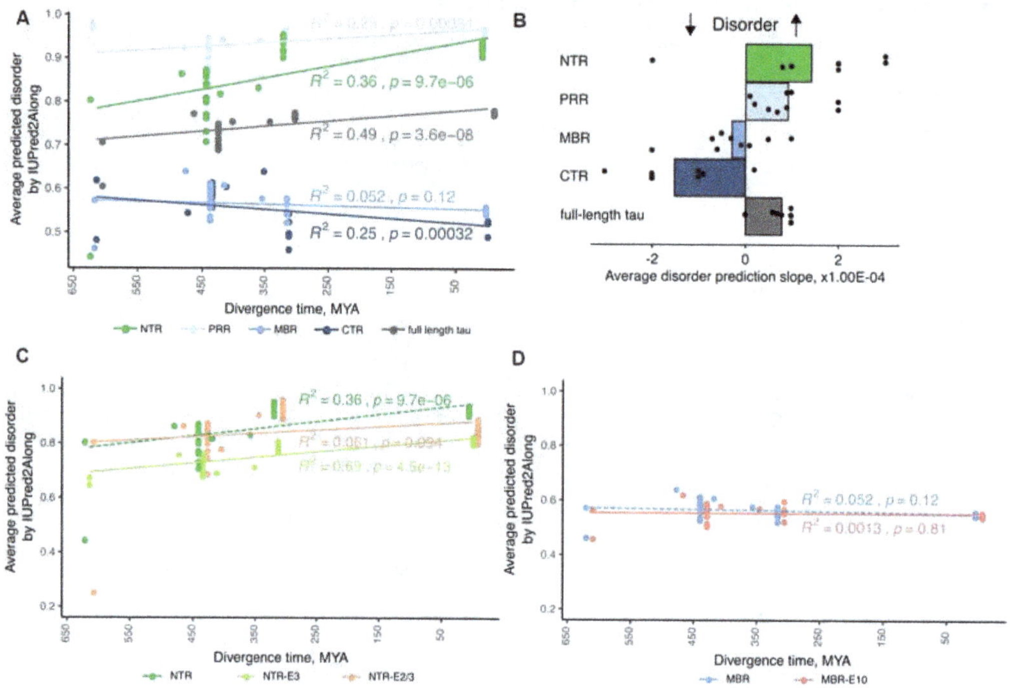

FIGURE 2 | Tau's amino-terminal, non-microtubule binding region exhibits a strong evolutionary increase in disorder. **(A)** An exemplary plot of disorder prediction by IUPred2A long is shown. Species are grouped by divergence times between their higher taxons and mammals [cyclostomes or jawless fishes—615 million years ago (MYA), cartilaginous fishes—473 MYA, bony fishes—435 MYA, coelacanths—413 MYA, amphibians—352 MYA, reptiles and birds—312 MYA and mammals as a 0 value]. R squared and *p*-value characterizing the linear fit to the data are presented close to each respective fitting line. **(B)** Average values of slopes based on linear regression analysis of predicted disorder values from all selected algorithms for full-length tau and all selected regions (NTR—green, PRR—light blue, MBR—blue and CTR—dark blue) are shown. Black dots represent values for measured slopes for the individual prediction algorithms while bars show average values. Note, that NTR and PRR show an increase in disorder, while the CTR shows a decrease. **(C,D)** Plots of disorder prediction by IUPred2A for NTR lacking exon 2/3 or exon 3 **(C)** and MBR lacking exon 10 **(D)** are shown. Full-length NTR and MBR as also presented in **(A)** are indicated by dashed lines. Species are grouped as described before. R squared and *p*-value characterizing the linear fit to the data are presented close to each respective fitting line.

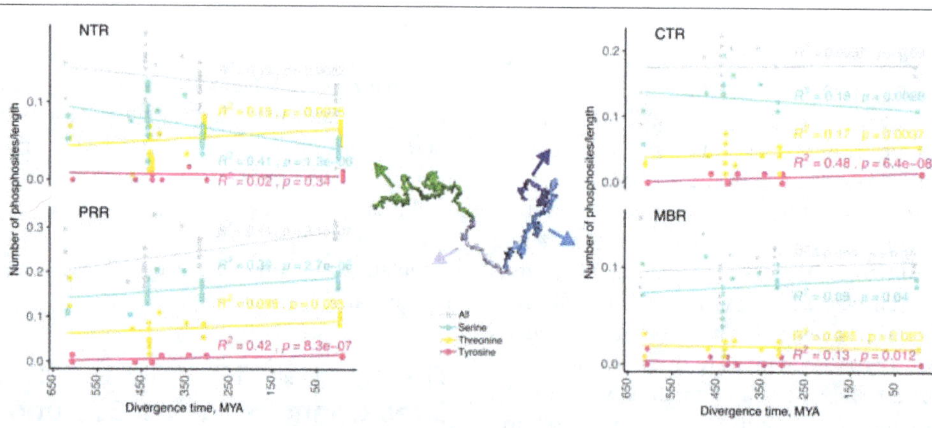

FIGURE 3 | The number of predicted phosphorylation sites changes during evolution in a region-specific manner. Predicted phosphorylation sites for the different regions of tau (NTR, PRR, MBR and CTR) are shown. The numbers of predicted sites were normalized by the length of the analyzed regions. Selected species were grouped by divergence times between mammals and other groups of vertebrates. Coefficients of determination and *p*-values for the linear regression model are presented near the line fits. Fits with *p*-values higher than 0.05 are considered to show no significant relationship between divergence times and normalized numbers of predicted phosphorylation sites. Note, that the PRR is the only region where overall phosphorylation increases during evolution.

Phosphorylation occurs at three different residues, serine, threonine and tyrosine. To determine potential changes in phosphorylation during evolution, we used the NetPhos3 phosphorylation prediction server to obtain numbers of sites that could be phosphorylated with high confidence. After normalization to the number of residues we analyzed

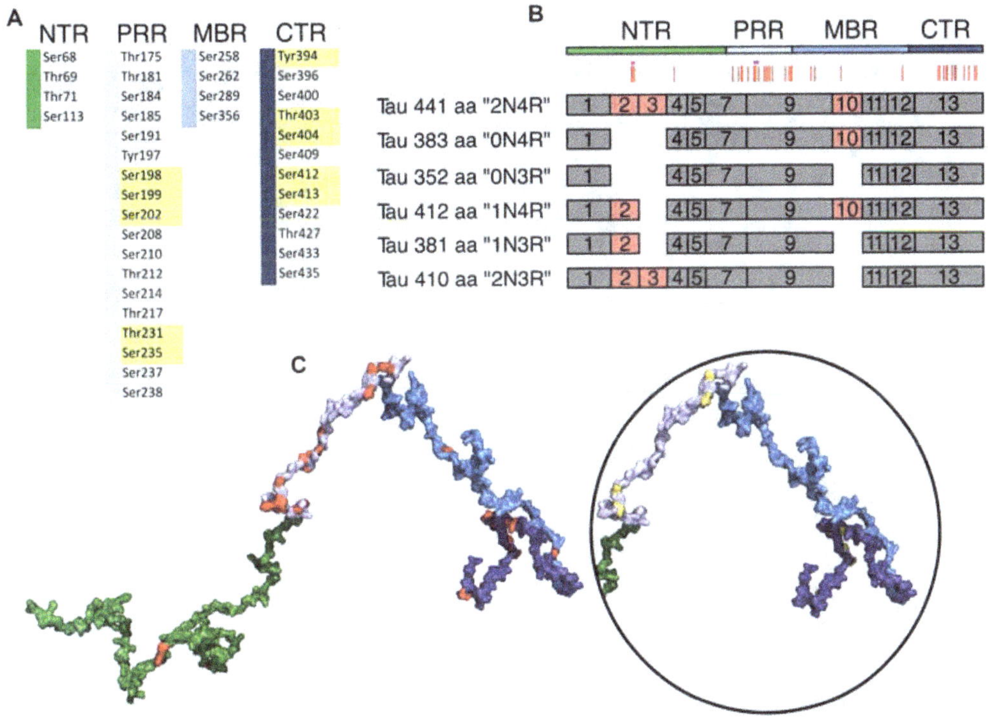

FIGURE 4 | Schematic representation of disease-associated phosphorylation sites in tau. **(A)** The distribution of tau phosphorylation sites as they have been determined by mass spectroscopy of PHF tau from brains of Alzheimer's disease (AD) patients is shown (based on Hanger et al., 2007). The different tau regions are indicated in green (NTR), gray (PRR), light blue (MBR) and dark blue (CTR). Numbers are based on tau from *Homo sapiens* (441 aa CNS isoform). Major phosphorylation sites, are shown in yellow (based on Morishima-Kawashima et al., 1995). **(B)** Schematic representation of splice isoforms of tau in the CNS. Alternatively, spliced exons are indicated as red boxes. Vertical red lines on top represent the phosphorylation sites listed in **(A)**. The STPT site and the YSSPGS motif are shown by pink and violet horizontal lines, respectively. **(C)** Location of the phosphorylation on one of the potential 3D structures of tau (441 aa isoform) generated by the RCG (Jha et al., 2005) is shown. The sites from **(A)** are indicated in red. In the circle, the positions of the 10 major phosphorylation sites, which are clustered in the PRR and CTR, are indicated.

the changes in overall phosphosite number and the numbers of serine, threonine and tyrosine phosphosites from different tau regions throughout evolution (**Figure 3**). The PRR was the only region where overall phosphorylation sites increased, which was due to increased number of serine and threonine phosphorylation sites with divergence time. In contrast, the NTR showed a strong decrease in serine phosphosites, while threonine phosphosites increased. No major changes were observed in the MBR and CTR. Comparison between fish, birds and mammals also revealed a steady increase in overall phosphorylation sites in the PRR, which was mainly due to an increased number of threonine residues and a decrease of serine phosphorylation sites in the NTR (**Supplementary Figure S3**). In many cases, the overall phosphorylation sites increased owing to the formation of clusters of phosphorylatable residues. Specifically, the STPT site in human tau corresponds to a single potential phosphosite in *Xenopus tropicalis* and simpler organisms (**Figures 4B, 5A**, pink line). Interestingly, the STPT site is located in the alternatively spliced exon 2. Since inclusion of exon 2 has been shown to promote tau aggregation (Zhong et al., 2012), a change in the phosphorylation pattern within this region may affect tau-tau binding and thus be of pathological relevance. A similar increase in the number of clustered phosphorylatable residues in the course of evolution is seen in the case of the human YSSPGS motif in the PRR (**Figures 4B, 5A**, violet line).

The data indicates that changes in the number of phosphorylation sites during evolution occurred mainly in the N-terminal part of tau (NTR and PRR), while the number of phosphorylatable residues in the C-terminus (MBR and CTR) remained unaltered. This is in line with the observation that the C-terminus, in general, is evolutionary much more conserved. Interestingly, the NTR and PRR showed opposite changes. While the number of phosphorylation sites in the NTR decreased, which was mostly due to decreased number of serine residues, the number of phosphosites in the PRR showed a strong increase with divergence time.

Disease-Associated Tau Hyperphosphorylation Sites Are Highly Conserved While Many Phosphosites in the NTR and PRR Exhibit a Lower Degree of Evolutionary Conservation

Pathological changes in tau phosphorylation are thought to induce tau-mediated toxicity and affect tau aggregation (Fath et al., 2002; Noble et al., 2003; Bakota and Brandt, 2016). In

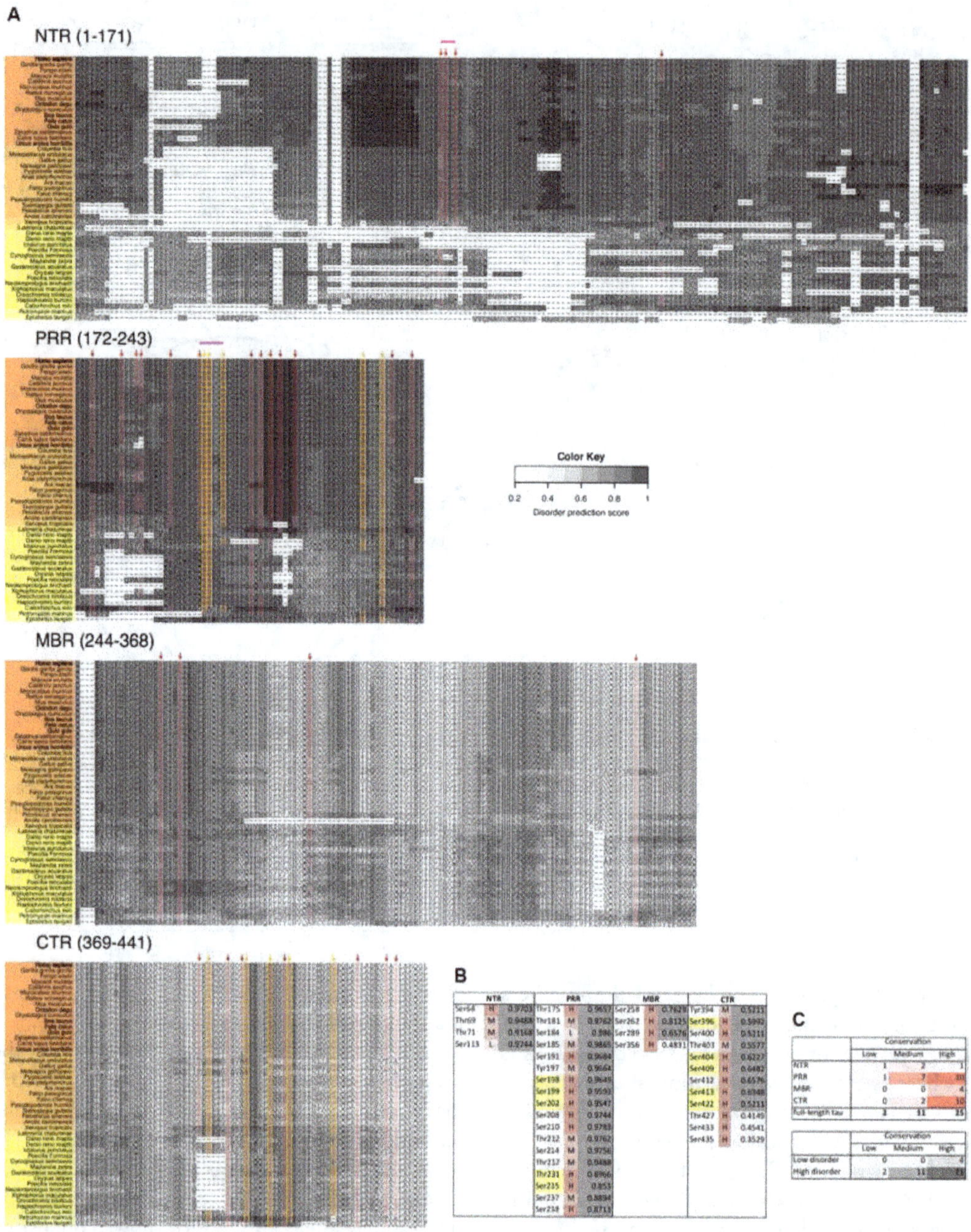

FIGURE 5 | Disease-associated tau hyperphosphorylation sites are highly conserved while many phosphosites in the NTR and PRR exhibit a lower degree of evolutionary conservation. **(A)** Comparison of tau sequences from 47 different species is shown. The selected organisms are grouped according to higher taxons (Cyclostomata, Actinopterygii, Coelacanthiformes, Amphibia, Sauropsida, Mammalia) and are color-coded from yellow (lower vertebrates) to orange (higher vertebrates). The extent of disorder (as predicted by IUPred2A) is indicated by the gray value according to the color key. The position of disease-associated phosphorylation sites as they have been shown in **Figure 4** are indicated by red arrows, major phosphorylation sites by yellow arrows. The STPT site and the YSSPGS motif in the human sequence, which show an increase in the number of clustered phosphorylatable residues is shown by pink and violet lines, respectively. **(B)** Level of conservation of the disease-associated phosphorylation sites is shown (H: high conservation—present in >66% of species; M: medium conservation—present in 33%–66% of species; L: low conservation—present <33% of species). The extent of disorder (as predicted by IUPred2A) is also shown. Light gray indicates disorder <0.5, dark gray >0.5. **(C)** Summary representation of the level of conservation of the phosphorylation sites with respect to the region of tau (top), and the extent of disorder (bottom).

most studies, changes in tau phosphorylation in different species have been studied using phosphorylation-sensitive antibodies such as the AT8 antibody, which detects phosphorylated sites at Ser202/Thr205 in the PRR, or the PHF1 antibody, which is specific for a phosphorylated epitope in the CTR (Ser396/Ser404). To avoid bias, which is caused by the availability of antibodies against certain phosphosites but not others and a potential influence of additional phosphorylation events in antibody reactivity (e.g., pSer208 for the reactivity of the AT8 antibody; Malia et al., 2016) or crossreactivity to other epitopes (e.g., cross-reactivity of AT8 to two doubly phosphorylated motifs containing either serines 199 and 202 or serines 205 and 208 of the human tau sequence; Porzig et al., 2007), we restricted our analysis to reports, which have employed mass spectrometry to systematically determine the pattern of phosphorylation.

In tau from PHFs, which have been isolated from patients with AD, a total of 38 phosphorylated sites have been identified by mass spectrometry (Hanger et al., 2007). Ten of the sites represent major phosphorylation sites and may, therefore, qualify as being "hyperphosphorylated" (Morishima-Kawashima et al., 1995). **Figure 4** shows the distribution of these sites with respect to the four different regions of tau protein. The majority of the sites and all of the 10 major phosphorylation sites (**Figure 4A**, yellow boxes) are concentrated in the PRR and the CTR, which flank the MBR on both sides. Additional sites, which are phosphorylated to a lower extent, are also present in the other regions. One can see that in many cases the disease-associated phosphosites shown in **Figures 4B, 5A** belong to the aforementioned clusters of phosphorylatable residues.

To determine, whether the presence of the phosphosites changed during evolution, we determined the level of conservation of the respective phosphosites by comparing tau sequences across species (**Figure 5A**). We found that all of the 10 major phosphorylation sites were highly (>66%) conserved across species (**Figure 5B**). Two sites (Ser113 in the NTR and Ser184 in the PRR) showed a particularly low degree of conservation. In many species, Ser113 was replaced by asparagine and Ser184 by glycine or alanine, i.e., nonpolar amino acids.

The data suggest that most disease-associated phosphorylation events are concentrated in two regions, which flank the MBR on both sites. Also, all of the major phosphorylation sites (hyperphosphorylated sites) are present in these two regions. In general, the disease-associated phosphorylation sites with low conservation are present in the NTR and PRR. All phosphorylation sites in regions of low disorder are highly conserved, whereas about 40% of phosphorylation sites in high disorder regions displayed lower conservation (**Figure 5C**), which is in line with the observation that IDRs changed during evolution.

Evolutionary Changes of Specific Tau Phosphorylation Sites of Pathological Relevance

Specific phosphosites of tau may be of particular importance during disease development and may be different from those, which have been identified in tau isolated from PHFs. Recent profiling of phosphorylated tau peptides in cerebrospinal fluid (CSF) by mass spectrometry has revealed 11 sites that are increased by at least 40% in the CSF of patients with AD compared to controls (Russell et al., 2017). A summary of the sites together with their localization in different tau regions and the level of conservation is shown in **Figure 6**. One of the sites is Thr181, an established core biomarker for AD in CSF (Vanmechelen et al., 2000), which has also been detected in PHF tau. Thr181 is one of three sites, which shows only a moderate conservation during evolution. Another site of potential interest is Thr205; phosphorylation of Thr205 has been shown to decrease Aβ-induced toxicity (Ittner et al., 2016) and is therefore the only phosphorylation site, which has been reported to have a protective rather than toxicity-promoting effect. This site is highly conserved but has not yet been identified in tau from PHFs. It should also be noted that two of the CSF-sites are located in the NTR and none of them had been identified in PHFs.

Site	Conservation	Disorder
Ser46	M	0.9703
Ser61	H	0.986
Thr181	M	0.9762
Ser199	H	0.9593
Thr205	H	0.9308
Thr212	M	0.9762
Thr231	H	0.8966
Ser235	H	0.853
Ser238	H	0.8713
Ser262	H	0.8125
Ser396	H	0.5992

FIGURE 6 | Evolutionary changes of specific tau phosphorylation sites of pathological relevance. Summary representation showing phosphorylation sites that have been reported to be significantly enriched in cerebrospinal fluid (CSF) from AD patients compared to controls (based on Russell et al., 2017). The different tau regions are indicated in green (NTR), gray (PRR), light blue (MBR) and dark blue (CTR). The level of conservation is indicated as described in the legend of **Figure 5**. The extent of disorder is color-coded from light to dark grey with darker colors showing higher disorder. Thr205 is shown in light-green as its phosphorylation has been shown to decrease Aβ-induced toxicity (Ittner et al., 2016).

The data show that only partial overlap exists between phosphorylated sites that have been identified in PHF tau and in CSF samples from AD patients. With respect to the identification of phosphorylation sites that may have made tau prone for the development of tauopathies, it may be informative to further analyze those sites that are present in regions which changed during evolution and may have developed novel functions (i.e., NTR and PRR) and which exhibit moderate conservation.

DISCUSSION

We tested the hypothesis that the sequence of tau has changed during vertebrate evolution in a way that novel interactions developed. We also tested the hypothesis that tau phosphorylation may have been affected by evolutionary changes, which made tau prone for the development of tauopathies. We show that: (1) distinct regions of tau show functional specialization in their molecular interactions; (2) tau's amino-terminal, non-microtubule binding region exhibits a strong evolutionary increase in protein disorder; and (3) the number of predicted phosphorylation sites changes during evolution in a region-specific manner, while disease-specific hyperphosphorylated sites are highly conserved.

Our data indicate that the highly conserved MBR on one side and the much less conserved N-terminal region on the other side show specific functional specialization. Since the MT-associated proteins tau, MAP2 and MAP4 contain a similar CTR with multiple highly conserved microtubule-binding repeats, tau's N-terminal region may provide the tau-specific interactions, which may also be involved in its unique subcellular localization with an enrichment in the axonal compartment, which occurs early during neuronal development (Kempf et al., 1996). In fact, GO-terms associated with biological processes for the interaction partners of tau showed a strong enrichment for "regulation of protein localization to membranes" for the NTR, which was clearly different from the MBR, which was mostly associated with "regulation of microtubule polymerization." Thus, the data suggest that the involvement of tau's N-terminus in membrane organization is responsible for tau's axonal enrichment. This is an agreement with previous results that overexpression of tau's extreme N-terminus interferes with the axonal enrichment of endogenous tau protein in primary neurons (Gauthier-Kemper et al., 2018). Since the MAPT and MAP2 genes are the result of a gene duplication event at the dawn of the vertebrates (Sündermann et al., 2016) it is also likely that the functions related to tau's localization to the membrane were responsible for the compartment-specific separation of tau and MAPs in the axonal (tau) and somatodendritic (MAP2) compartment.

Interestingly, several interaction partners of the NTR and PRR were also associated with regulation of apoptotic processes, while this was not the case for the MBR and CTR. Current data with respect to an involvement of tau in neuronal survival and regulation of apoptosis are contradictory. On one side it has been reported that overexpression of tau renders cells more resistant to apoptosis, which has been induced by pro-apoptotic factors (Li et al., 2007; Wang et al., 2010). Similarly, accumulation of highly phosphorylated tau, specifically in the cones of primates, has shown to make these cells resilient to apoptosis (Aboelnour et al., 2017). On the other side, tau expression has been shown to be essential for stress-induced brain pathology (Lopes et al., 2016) and reduction of tau ameliorated Aβ induced deficits in a mouse model of AD (Roberson et al., 2007). In one study, anti-apoptotic activity of tau has been located in tau's amino-terminal region (residues 1–230; Amadoro et al., 2004). In fact, GO-term analysis for biological processes has also identified "negative regulation of apoptotic processes" in the NTR and "positive regulation of apoptotic processes" in the adjacent PRR, which may indicate that different regions of tau may have antagonistic effects with respect to the regulation of neurodegenerative processes, which might be differentially regulated by region-specific phosphorylation.

Tau's NTR and PRR exhibited an evolutionary increase in disorder, which was particularly strong for the NTR. In contrast, the MBR and CTR exhibited no increase or even a decrease in disorder. Many IDPs and proteins with a substantial extent of IDRs have multiple interaction partners (Uversky, 2015). Thus, an increase in IDRs during evolution may provide a mechanism for increased binding promiscuity and improved ability to adapt to changes in the environment. This suggests that in particular tau's potential functions with respect to membrane organization and regulation of apoptotic processes, which are both predominantly mediated *via* the NTR, were beneficial for the development of a complex nervous system, which is paralleled by an increased ability of the microtubule system for regulated interactions (Trushina et al., 2019). The involvement of IDPs such as tau in neurodegenerative diseases of mammals could then be interpreted in the context of the "antagonistic pleiotropy hypothesis," as it was first proposed by Williams (1957). In such a view, increased disorder of tau could be beneficial for the organism's fitness by providing increased ability for regulated interactions, while it would be detrimental at higher age due to increased propensity for miss-regulation and aggregation.

Intrinsically disordered proteins are thought to develop spread wide structures, which are maintained by networks of weak bonds that become disrupted at higher temperature (Uversky, 2009; Langridge et al., 2014); thus, the body temperature of the respective organisms may influence to what extent disordered regions developed during evolution. Therefore, we determined the changes of the extent of disorder between the tau proteins of poikilotherms (e.g., fishes), which operate at lower temperatures than those of homeotherms (e.g., mammals). As a further comparison we included birds, which belong to the homeotherms but generally operate at higher temperature levels (~41°C) than mammals (Prinzinger et al., 1991). Indeed we observed an increase in disorder as judged from most prediction programs for full-length tau and the NTR from fish to birds but a decrease from birds to mammals (**Supplementary Figures S2A,B**). For the PRR, we observed a continuous increase from fish to birds to mammals. The results could suggest that the evolutionary increase in disorder for the NTR is influenced by the different body temperature of the organisms in a way that the predicted disorder is highest for species with the highest body temperature. It should also be noted that there are mammalian species, which do change their body temperature at certain seasons. These are the hibernating animals, which show an activity and metabolic depression. These animals regulate this process also by hibernation-state dependent tau phosphorylation in various brain regions. Interestingly, the phosphorylation sites that are undergoing changes in phosphorylation extent and kinetics are overlapping with sites that are stoichiometrically highly phosphorylated during tauopathies (Stieler et al., 2011). This may provide an additional way of modulating the disordered state of tau protein.

We observed that the number of predicted phosphorylation sites changes during evolution in a region-specific manner. Again, changes were most prominent in the amino-terminal part of tau (NTR and PRR). Interestingly, however, the NTR and PRR showed opposite changes in the number of predicted phosphorylation sites during evolution. While the number of predicted phosphorylation sites in the NTR decreased, the PRR showed a strong increase with divergence time and also when fish, birds and mammals were compared. Thus, the data suggest that the propensity of regulation by phosphorylation evolved in an opposite manner in the PRR and the NTR. While it increased in the PRR, it decreased in the NTR. This could also be of relevance for the regulation of apoptotic processes, where the PRR and NTR had an antagonistic effect, which might be differentially regulated by region-specific phosphorylation. Of note, changes in tau phosphorylation during evolution can also be caused by changes in the number and regulation of kinases and phosphatases. Eukaryotic protein kinases regulate almost every biological process and have evolved as dynamic molecular switches (Taylor et al., 2019). However, due to the presence of several subunits in many kinases, which provide high diversity in function and specificity, general statements about the alteration of the activity of kinases towards specific target proteins during evolution are difficult to draw. Attempts are therefore mainly focusing on the analysis of the catalytic subunits. With respect to one of the best-studied kinase, cAMP-dependent protein kinase (PKA) the catalytic subunit isoforms *PRKACA* and *PRKACB* are highly conserved paralogous genes, which result from a gene duplication event around the evolution of the first vertebrate species (Søberg et al., 2013); this is approximately at the same time, when tau has arisen after a duplication of an ancestral gene of ancient cyclostomes (Sündermann et al., 2016). PKA is of particular interest because it modulates GSK3β- and cdk5-catalyzed phosphorylation of tau (Liu et al., 2006). On the other hand, the cyclin-dependent kinases and their regulatory cyclin proteins were evolving much earlier at the level of metazoans, which also indicates their involvement in a much more conserved function, like cell cycle regulation (Cao et al., 2014). Phosphatases are often also composed of several subunits. Furthermore, some need adaptor proteins, which provide phosphatase specificity and pathway insulation in signaling networks (Rowland et al., 2015). Therefore, it is also difficult to follow evolutionary trends that would affect one specific target protein.

The data indicated that most disease-associated phosphorylation events are concentrated in two regions, which flank the MBR on both sites. Also, all of the major phosphorylation sites ("hyperphosphorylated" sites) were present in these two regions. The sequence comparison revealed that all of the hyperphosphorylated sites are highly conserved and thus have the potential to be phosphorylated in most species. Comparison of the occurrence of NFTs in various animal species indicates that certain species such as degu (*Octodon degu*), and domestic cat *(Felis catus)* develop NFTs, while closely related species such as rat (*Rattus norvegicus*) or the domestic dog *(Canis lupus familiaris)* do not (Youssef et al., 2016; **Figure 5A**). Thus, it appears that the simple presence of these sites cannot explain why NFTs develop in certain species but not in others. With respect to the development of potentially new mechanisms of regulation, which may also become mis-regulated during pathological processes, it may, therefore, be worth to also take phosphosites with lower evolutionary conservation and later development during evolution as relevant biomarkers into consideration. In this context it is interesting to note that tau phosphorylated at the moderately conserved threonine residue 181 (pThr181) is an established core biomarker for AD (Vanmechelen et al., 2000), which shows a significant increase in phosphorylation in the CSF of patients with AD compared to controls (Russell et al., 2017). Furthermore, it has also been shown that pThr181 has a potential to serve as a predictor during differential diagnosis while it showed a significant increase in phosphorylation in the CSF of patients with mild cognitive impairment (MCI), whose diseases progresses to AD, compared to patients with MCI showing stable cognitive function. It has also been shown that several non-AD type dementias exhibit a significant lower phosphorylation level at Thr181 compared to CSF samples from AD patients (Kang et al., 2013).

Noteworthy, some of the highly conserved phosphorylation sites are not having exclusively a disease relation but are also highly phosphorylated during development as it was shown in the hippocampus of kittens where phosphorylation of tau at Ser202/Thr205 disappeared from axons above 1 month of age (Riederer et al., 2001) or human hippocampal biopsy samples where the number of Ser199 immunoreactive neuronal cells were counted high at very young age and were steeply declining during aging in healthy individuals (Maurage et al., 2001).

The observed increase in the number of clustered phosphorylatable residues in the course of evolution (**Figure 5A**) strongly resembles duplications of functionally important aspartate residues in case of the apoptotic protease activating factor 1 (Apaf-1). In the intrinsic apoptotic cascade, cytochrome c, when released from damaged mitochondria, binds between the tryptophan (W) and aspartate (D)-rich WD-8 and WD-7 domains of Apaf-1. This binding causes a major conformational change that eventually could lead to the assembly of apoptosome. Molecular modeling predicted that cytochrome c binds owing to the interaction of its lysine residues with conserved Asp residues of Apaf-1 (Shalaeva et al., 2015). The recently resolved apoptosome structure confirmed the involvement of conserved Asp residues in cytochrome c binding (Zhou et al., 2015). In four of such conserved sites, a single Asp residue appears to be replaced by a Asp-Asp dimer upon transition from primitive organisms to Chordates (Shalaeva et al., 2015).

In case of Apaf-1, it was speculated that an Asp-Asp dimer could provide stronger hydrogen bonding with Lys residues of cytochrome c than a single Asp residue (Shalaeva et al., 2015). By analogy, in case of the tau protein, it is tempting to speculate that several bystanding phosphate residues in higher vertebrates could sustain stronger bonding with the physiological partners—Arg or Lys residues—than a single phosphate group. It was shown that the strength of a bidentate bonding of an Arg residue even with a single phosphate group is compatible with that of a covalent bond (Woods and Ferré, 2005). A bifurcated or bidentate binding between clustered phosphate groups of tau and Arg/Lys residues of its physiological partner(s) could yield an even more tight interaction and, in addition, provide more control possibilities by constraining the mobility of residues involved.

Taken together our data provide evidence that novel, non-MT related tau interactions developed during evolution, which are mediated by tau's N-terminal projection region (NTR and PRR). These evolutionary novel interactions relate to regulation of localization to membranes and regulation of apoptosis, i.e., biological processes, which may be of pathological relevance with respect to tau localization and cell survival. Furthermore, the data indicate that the number of predicted phosphorylation sites in the PRR showed a strong increase with divergence time and show that novel clusters of phosphorylatable residues developed during evolution in the PRR and in an alternatively spliced exon in the NTR. Thus, the data suggest that the propensity of regulation of tau function by phosphorylation (and potential miss-regulation during disease) developed during evolution and may point to isoform-specific regulatory mechanisms of tau isoforms containing N-terminal inserts. In view of the "antagonistic pleiotropy hypothesis," an increase in phosphorylatable residues in the PRR during evolution could be beneficial for the organism's fitness by providing increased ability for regulated interactions, while it would be detrimental at higher age due to increased propensity for miss-regulation and aggregation.

AUTHOR CONTRIBUTIONS

NT, AM and RB designed the research. NT performed the research. NT, LB, AM and RB analyzed, interpreted the data and wrote the article.

ACKNOWLEDGMENTS

We thank Fred Sündermann for providing annotated tau sequences.

SUPPLEMENTARY MATERIAL

FIGURE S1 | Disorder prediction from different algorithms. The average of slope values from all selected algorithms for full-length tau and all selected regions (NTR, PRR, MBR and CTR) are shown. Regions are color-coded as shown in **Figure 2**. Note, that NTR and PRR mainly show an increase in disorder, while the disorder of the CTR decreased.

FIGURE S2 | Comparison of average predicted disorder of tau sequences and its parts for the most represented taxons (i.e., bony fish, birds and mammals, color-coded from yellow to orange). **(A)** Boxplots for all selected disorder prediction algorithms are shown. The background color corresponds to regions of tau as shown in **Figure 2**. Statistical significance was derived from Mann–Whitney test. $^*p < 0.05$, $^{**}p < 0.01$, $^{***}p < 0.001$. **(B)** Numbers of differentially changed disorder for tau sequences divided into regions in selected taxons is shown. Here, table for one level of significance is shown, p-value < 0.05. Note that MBR shows a continuous increase in disorder (MBR), NTR and full-length tau mostly show increase from fish to birds and from fish to mammals, however, in some cases a decrease in disorder from birds to mammals was prominent and finally, CTR shows a continuous decrease in predicted disorder.

FIGURE S3 | Comparison of numbers of predicted phosphorylation sites of tau and its regions for most represented taxons (i.e., bony fish, birds and mammals; color-coded from yellow to orange). **(A)** Boxplots for phosphorylation of tau and its regions are shown. The background colors and filling colors of boxplot correspond to the residue that was predicted to be phosphorylated (all sites—light gray, serine residues—turquoise, threonine residues—dark yellow and tyrosine residues—magenta). Statistical significance was derived from Mann–Whitney U test. $^*p < 0.05$, $^{**}p < 0.01$, $^{***}p < 0.001$. **(B)** Comparison of numbers of predicted phosphorylation sites of tau sequences and its parts for most represented taxons (i.e., bony fish, birds and mammals). Numbers of differentially changed disorder for tau sequences divided into regions in selected taxons is shown. Here, table for one level of significance is shown, p-value < 0.05.

REFERENCES

Aboelnour, A., Van der Spuy, J., Powner, M., and Jeffery, G. (2017). Primate retinal cones express phosphorylated tau associated with neuronal degeneration yet survive in old age. *Exp. Eye Res.* 165, 105–108. doi: 10.1016/j.exer.2017.09.013

Amadoro, G., Serafino, A. L., Barbato, C., Ciotti, M. T., Sacco, A., Calissano, P., et al. (2004). Role of N-terminal tau domain integrity on the survival of cerebellar granule neurons. *Cell Death Differ.* 11, 217–230. doi: 10.1038/sj.cdd.4401314

Andreadis, A., Brown, W. M., and Kosik, K. S. (1992). Structure and novel exons of the human tau gene. *Biochemistry* 31, 10626–10633. doi: 10.1021/bi00158a027

Arendt, T., Stieler, J. T., and Holzer, M. (2016). Tau and tauopathies. *Brain Res. Bull.* 126, 238–292. doi: 10.1016/j.brainresbull.2016.08.018

Atkins, J. D., Boateng, S. Y., Sorensen, T., and McGuffin, L. J. (2015). Disorder prediction methods, their applicability to different protein targets and their usefulness for guiding experimental studies. *Int. J. Mol.sciences* 16, 19040–19054. doi: 10.3390/ijms160819040

Babu, M. M., van der Lee, R., de Groot, N. S., and Gsponer, J. (2011). Intrinsically disordered proteins: regulation and disease. *Curr. Opin. Struct. Biol.* 21, 432–440. doi: 10.1016/j.sbi.2011.03.011

Bah, A., and Forman-Kay, J. D. (2016). Modulation of intrinsically disordered protein function by post-translational modifications. *J. Biol. Chem.* 291, 6696–6705. doi: 10.1074/jbc.r115.695056

Bakota, L., and Brandt, R. (2016). Tau biology and tau-directed therapies for Alzheimer's disease. *Drugs* 76, 301–313. doi: 10.1007/s40265-015-0529-0

Bakota, L., Ussif, A., Jeserich, G., and Brandt, R. (2017). Systemic and network functions of the microtubule-associated protein tau: implications for tau-based therapies. *Mol. Cell. Neurosci.* 84, 132–141. doi: 10.1016/j.mcn.2017.03.003

Barbato, C., Canu, N., Zambrano, N., Serafino, A., Minopoli, G., Ciotti, M. T., et al. (2005). Interaction of Tau with Fe65 links tau to APP. *Neurobiol. Dis.* 18, 399–408. doi: 10.1016/j.nbd.2004.10.011

Barbato, C., Corbi, N., Canu, N., Fanciulli, M., Serafino, A., Ciotti, M., et al. (2003). Rb binding protein Che-1 interacts with Tau in cerebellar granule neurons. Modulation during neuronal apoptosis. *Mol. Cell. Neurosci.* 24, 1038–1050. doi: 10.1016/j.mcn.2003.08.002

Baudier, J., and Cole, R. D. (1988). Interactions between the microtubule-associated tau proteins and S100b regulate tau phosphorylation by the Ca2+/calmodulin-dependent protein kinase II. *J. Biol. Chem.* 263, 5876–5883.

Bindea, G., Mlecnik, B., Hackl, H., Charoentong, P., Tosolini, M., Kirilovsky, A., et al. (2009). ClueGO: a Cytoscape plug-in to decipher functionally grouped gene ontology and pathway annotation networks. *Bioinformatics* 25, 1091–1093. doi: 10.1093/bioinformatics/btp101

Blom, N., Gammeltoft, S., and Brunak, S. (1999). Sequence and structure-based prediction of eukaryotic protein phosphorylation sites. *J. Mol. Biol.* 294, 1351–1362. doi: 10.1006/jmbi.1999.3310

Brandt, R., Léger, J., and Lee, G. (1995). Interaction of tau with the neural plasma membrane mediated by tau's amino-terminal projection domain. *J. Cell Biol.* 131, 1327–1340. doi: 10.1083/jcb.131.5.1327

Brandt, R., and Leschik, J. (2004). Functional interactions of tau and their relevance for Alzheimer's disease. *Curr. Alzheimer Res.* 1, 255–269. doi: 10.2174/1567205043332054

Butner, K. A., and Kirschner, M. W. (1991). Tau protein binds to microtubules through a flexible array of distributed weak sites. *J. Cell Biol.* 115, 717–730. doi: 10.1083/jcb.115.3.717

Caffrey, T. M., Joachim, C., and Wade-Martins, R. (2008). Haplotype-specific expression of the N-terminal exons 2 and 3 at the human MAPT locus. *Neurobiol. Aging* 29, 1923–1929. doi: 10.1016/j.neurobiolaging.2007.05.002

Cao, L., Chen, F., Yang, X., Xu, W., Xie, J., and Yu, L. (2014). Phylogenetic analysis of CDK and cyclin proteins in premetazoan lineages. *BMC Evol. Biol.* 14:10. doi: 10.1186/1471-2148-14-10

Carlier, M. F., Simon, C., Cassoly, R., and Pradel, L. A. (1984). Interaction between microtubule-associated protein tau and spectrin. *Biochimie* 66, 305–311. doi: 10.1016/0300-9084(84)90007-5

Chauderlier, A., Gilles, M., Spolcova, A., Caillierez, R., Chwastyniak, M., Kress, M., et al. (2018). Tau/DDX6 interaction increases microRNA activity. *Biochim. Biophys. Acta Gene Regul. Mech.* 1861, 762–772. doi: 10.1016/j.bbagrm.2018.06.006

Correas, I., Padilla, R., and Avila, J. (1990). The tubulin-binding sequence of brain microtubule-associated proteins, tau and MAP-2, is also involved in actin binding. *Biochem. J.* 269, 61–64. doi: 10.1042/bj2690061

Crowther, R. A. (1991). Straight and paired helical filaments in Alzheimer disease have a common structural unit. *Proc. Natl. Acad. Sci. U S A* 88, 2288–2292. doi: 10.1073/pnas.88.6.2288

Darling, A. L., and Uversky, V. N. (2018). Intrinsic disorder and posttranslational modifications: the darker side of the biological dark matter. *Front. Genet.* 9:158. doi: 10.3389/fgene.2018.00158

Dehmelt, L., and Halpain, S. (2005). The MAP2/Tau family of microtubule-associated proteins. *Genome Biol.* 6:204. doi: 10.1186/gb-2004-6-1-204

Ding, H., Dolan, P. J., and Johnson, G. V. (2008). Histone deacetylase 6 interacts with the microtubule-associated protein tau. *J. Neurochem.* 106, 2119–2130. doi: 10.1111/j.1471-4159.2008.05564.x

Dosztányi, Z., Csizmók, V., Tompa, P., and Simon, I. (2005). The pairwise energy content estimated from amino acid composition discriminates between folded and intrinsically unstructured proteins. *J. Mol. Biol.* 347, 827–839. doi: 10.1016/j.jmb.2005.01.071

Dunker, A. K., Lawson, J. D., Brown, C. J., Williams, R. M., Romero, P., Oh, J. S., et al. (2001). Intrinsically disordered protein. *J. Mol. Graph. Model.* 19, 26–59. doi: 10.1016/S1093-3263(00)00138-8

Dyson, H. J., and Wright, P. E. (2005). Intrinsically unstructured proteins and their functions. *Nat. Rev. Mol. Cell Biol.* 6, 197–208. doi: 10.1038/nrm1589

Eidenmuller, J., Fath, T., Hellwig, A., Reed, J., Sontag, E., and Brandt, R. (2000). Structural and functional implications of tau hyperphosphorylation: information from phosphorylation-mimicking mutated tau proteins. *Biochemistry* 39, 13166–13175. doi: 10.1021/bi001290z

Esposito, A., Dohm, C. P., Kermer, P., Bähr, M., and Wouters, F. S. (2007). α-Synuclein and its disease-related mutants interact differentially with the microtubule protein tau and associate with the actin cytoskeleton. *Neurobiol. Dis.* 26, 521–531. doi: 10.1016/j.nbd.2007.01.014

Farah, C. A., Perreault, S., Liazoghli, D., Desjardins, M., Anton, A., Lauzon, M., et al. (2006). Tau interacts with Golgi membranes and mediates their association with microtubules. *Cell Motil. Cytoskeleton* 63, 710–724. doi: 10.1002/cm.20157

Fath, T., Eidenmüller, J., and Brandt, R. (2002). Tau-mediated cytotoxicity in a pseudohyperphosphorylation model of Alzheimer's disease. *J. Neurosci.* 22, 9733–9741. doi: 10.1523/JNEUROSCI.22-22-09733.2002

Fleming, L. M., Weisgraber, K. H., Strittmatter, W. J., Troncoso, J. C., and Johnson, G. V. (1996). Differential binding of apolipoprotein E isoforms to tau and other cytoskeletal proteins. *Exp. Neurol.* 138, 252–260. doi: 10.1006/exnr.1996.0064

Freilich, R., Betegon, M., Tse, E., Mok, S. A., Julien, O., Agard, D. A., et al. (2018). Competing protein-protein interactions regulate binding of Hsp27 to its client protein tau. *Nat. Commun.* 9:4563. doi: 10.1038/s41467-018-07012-4

Gauthier-Kemper, A., Suárez Alonso, M., Sündermann, F., Niewidok, B., Fernandez, M.-P., Bakota, L., et al. (2018). Annexins A2 and A6 interact with the extreme N-terminus of tau and thereby contribute to tau's axonal localization. *J. Biol. Chem.* 293, 8065–8076. doi: 10.1074/jbc.ra117.000490

Goedert, M., Crowther, R. A., and Spillantini, M. G. (1998). Tau mutations cause frontotemporal dementias. *Neuron* 21, 955–958. doi: 10.1016/s0896-6273(00)80615-7

Goedert, M., Spillantini, M. G., and Crowther, R. A. (1992). Cloning of a big tau microtubule-associated protein characteristic of the peripheral nervous system. *Proc. Natl. Acad. Sci. U S A* 89, 1983–1987. doi: 10.1073/pnas.89.5.1983

Guo, T., Noble, W., and Hanger, D. P. (2017). Roles of tau protein in health and disease. *Acta Neuropathol.* 133, 665–704. doi: 10.1007/s00401-017-1707-9

Gustke, N., Steiner, B., Mandelkow, E. M., Biernat, J., Meyer, H. E., Goedert, M., et al. (1992). The Alzheimer-like phosphorylation of tau protein reduces microtubule binding and involves Ser-Pro and Thr-Pro motifs. *FEBS Lett.* 307, 199–205. doi: 10.1016/0014-5793(92)80767-b

Hanger, D. P., Byers, H. L., Wray, S., Leung, K. Y., Saxton, M. J., Seereeram, A., et al. (2007). Novel phosphorylation sites in tau from Alzheimer brain support a role for casein kinase 1 in disease pathogenesis. *J. Biol. Chem.* 282, 23645–23654. doi: 10.1074/jbc.m703269200

Heinisch, J. J., and Brandt, R. (2016). Signaling pathways and posttranslational modifications of tau in Alzheimer's disease: the humanization of yeast cells. *Microb. Cell* 3, 135–146. doi: 10.15698/mic2016.04.489

Hoenicka, J., Arrasate, M., de Yebenes, J. G., and Avila, J. (2002). A two-hybrid screening of human Tau protein: interactions with Alu-derived domain. *Neuroreport* 13, 343–349. doi: 10.1097/00001756-200203040-00019

Hornbeck, P. V., Zhang, B., Murray, B., Kornhauser, J. M., Latham, V., and Skrzypek, E. (2015). PhosphoSitePlus, 2014: mutations, PTMs and recalibrations. *Nucleic Acids Res.* 43, D512–D520. doi: 10.1093/nar/gku1267

Ittner, A., Chua, S. W., Bertz, J., Volkerling, A., van der Hoven, J., Gladbach, A., et al. (2016). Site-specific phosphorylation of tau inhibits amyloid-β toxicity in Alzheimer's mice. *Science* 354, 904–908. doi: 10.1126/science.aah6205

Ittner, L. M., Ke, Y. D., and Götz, J. (2009). Phosphorylated Tau interacts with c-Jun N-terminal kinase-interacting protein 1 (JIP1) in Alzheimer disease. *J. Biol. Chem.* 284, 20909–20916. doi: 10.1074/jbc.m109.014472

Ivashko-Pachima, Y., Maor-Nof, M., and Gozes, I. (2019). NAP (davunetide) preferential interaction with dynamic 3-repeat Tau explains differential protection in selected tauopathies. *PLoS One* 14:e0213666. doi: 10.1371/journal.pone.0213666

Jahshan, A., Esteves-Villanueva, J. O., and Martic-Milne, S. (2016). Evaluation of ferritin and transferrin binding to tau protein. *J. Inorg. Biochem.* 162, 127–134. doi: 10.1016/j.jinorgbio.2016.06.022

Jha, A. K., Colubri, A., Freed, K. F., and Sosnick, T. R. (2005). Statistical coil model of the unfolded state: resolving the reconciliation problem. *Proc. Natl. Acad. Sci. U S A* 102, 13099–13104. doi: 10.1073/pnas.0506078102

Joo, Y., Schumacher, B., Landrieu, I., Bartel, M., Smet-Nocca, C., Jang, A., et al. (2015). Involvement of 14-3-3 in tubulin instability and impaired axon development is mediated by Tau. *FASEB J.* 29, 4133–4144. doi: 10.1096/fj.14-265009

Kadavath, H., Hofele, R. V., Biernat, J., Kumar, S., Tepper, K., Urlaub, H., et al. (2015). Tau stabilizes microtubules by binding at the interface between tubulin heterodimers. *Proc. Natl. Acad. Sci. U S A* 112, 7501–7516. doi: 10.1073/pnas.1504081112

Kamah, A., Cantrelle, F. X., Huvent, I., Giustiniani, J., Guillemeau, K., Byrne, C., et al. (2016). Isomerization and oligomerization of truncated and mutated tau forms by FKBP52 are independent processes. *J. Mol. Biol.* 428, 1080–1090. doi: 10.1016/j.jmb.2016.02.015

Kang, J. H., Korecka, M., Toledo, J. B., Trojanowski, J. Q., and Shaw, L. M. (2013). Clinical utility and analytical challenges in measurement of cerebrospinal fluid amyloid-$\beta_{(1-42)}$ and tau proteins as Alzheimer disease biomarkers. *Clin. Chem.* 59, 903–916. doi: 10.1373/clinchem.2013.202937

Kellogg, E. H., Hejab, N. M. A., Poepsel, S., Downing, K. H., Dimaio, F., and Nogales, E. (2018). Near-atomic model of microtubule-tau interactions. *Science* 360, 1242–1246. doi: 10.1126/science.aat1780

Kempf, M., Clement, A., Faissner, A., Lee, G., and Brandt, R. (1996). Tau binds to the distal axon early in development of polarity in a microtubule- and microfilament-dependent manner. *J. Neurosci.* 16, 5583–5592. doi: 10.1523/JNEUROSCI.16-18-05583.1996

Krivov, G. G., Shapovalov, M. V., and Dunbrack, R. L. Jr. (2009). Improved prediction of protein side-chain conformations with SCWRL4. *Proteins* 77, 778–795. doi: 10.1002/prot.22488

Kumar, S., Stecher, G., Suleski, M., and Hedges, S. B. (2017). TimeTree: a resource for timelines, timetrees and divergence times. *Mol. Biol. Evol.* 34, 1812–1819. doi: 10.1093/molbev/msx116

Künze, G., Barré, P., Scheidt, H. A., Thomas, L., Eliezer, D., and Huster, D. (2012). Binding of the three-repeat domain of tau to phospholipid membranes induces an aggregated-like state of the protein. *Biochim. Biophys. Acta* 1818, 2302–2313. doi: 10.1016/j.bbamem.2012.03.019

Kuraku, S., and Kuratani, S. (2006). Time scale for cyclostome evolution inferred with a phylogenetic diagnosis of hagfish and lamprey cDNA sequences. *Zoolog. Sci.* 23, 1053–1064. doi: 10.2108/zsj.23.1053

Langridge, T. D., Tarver, M. J., and Whitten, S. T. (2014). Temperature effects on the hydrodynamic radius of the intrinsically disordered N-terminal region of the p53 protein. *Proteins* 82, 668–678. doi: 10.1002/prot.24449

Lee, G., Neve, R. L., and Kosik, K. S. (1989). The microtubule binding domain of tau protein. *Neuron* 2, 1615–1624. doi: 10.1016/0896-6273(89)90050-0

Lee, G., Newman, S. T., Gard, D. L., Band, H., and Panchamoorthy, G. (1998). Tau interacts with src-family non-receptor tyrosine kinases. *J. Cell Sci.* 111, 3167–3177.

Li, H.-L., Wang, H.-H., Liu, S.-J., Deng, Y.-Q., Zhang, Y.-J., Tian, Q., et al. (2007). Phosphorylation of tau antagonizes apoptosis by stabilizing β-catenin, a mechanism involved in Alzheimer's neurodegeneration. *Proc. Natl. Acad. Sci. U S A* 104, 3591–3596. doi: 10.1073/pnas.0609303104

Liu, F., Liang, Z., Shi, J., Yin, D., El-Akkad, E., Grundke-Iqbal, I., et al. (2006). PKA modulates GSK-3β- and cdk5-catalyzed phosphorylation of tau in site- and kinase-specific manners. *FEBS Lett.* 580, 6269–6274. doi: 10.1016/j.febslet.2006.10.033

Lopes, S., Vaz-Silva, J., Pinto, V., Dalla, C., Kokras, N., Bedenk, B., et al. (2016). Tau protein is essential for stress-induced brain pathology. *Proc. Natl. Acad. Sci. U S A* 113, E3755–E3763. doi: 10.1073/pnas.1600953113

Maas, T., Eidenmüller, J., and Brandt, R. (2000). Interaction of tau with the neural membrane cortex is regulated by phosphorylation at sites that are modified in paired helical filaments. *J. Biol. Chem.* 275, 15733–15740. doi: 10.1074/jbc.m000389200

Magnani, E., Fan, J., Gasparini, L., Golding, M., Williams, M., Schiavo, G., et al. (2007). Interaction of tau protein with the dynactin complex. *EMBO J.* 26, 4546–4554. doi: 10.1038/sj.emboj.7601878

Magri, A., and Messina, A. (2017). Interactions of VDAC with proteins involved in neurodegenerative aggregation: an opportunity for advancement on therapeutic molecules. *Curr. Med. Chem.* 24, 4470–4487. doi: 10.2174/0929867324666170601073920

Malia, T. J., Teplyakov, A., Ernst, R., Wu, S. J., Lacy, E. R., Liu, X., et al. (2016). Epitope mapping and structural basis for the recognition of phosphorylated tau by the anti-tau antibody AT8. *Proteins* 84, 427–434. doi: 10.1002/prot.24988

Malki, I., Cantrelle, F. X., Sottejeau, Y., Lippens, G., Lambert, J. C., and Landrieu, I. (2017). Regulation of the interaction between the neuronal BIN1 isoform 1 and Tau proteins—role of the SH3 domain. *FEBS J.* 284, 3218–3229. doi: 10.1111/febs.14185

Manczak, M., and Reddy, P. H. (2012). Abnormal interaction between the mitochondrial fission protein Drp1 and hyperphosphorylated tau in Alzheimer's disease neurons: implications for mitochondrial dysfunction and neuronal damage. *Hum. Mol. Genet.* 21, 2538–2547. doi: 10.1093/hmg/dds072

Manczak, M., and Reddy, P. H. (2013). RNA silencing of genes involved in Alzheimer's disease enhances mitochondrial function and synaptic activity. *Biochim. Biophys. Acta* 1832, 2368–2378. doi: 10.1016/j.bbadis.2013.09.008

Maurage, C. A., Sergeant, N., Ruchoux, M. M., Hauw, J. J., and Delacourte, A. (2001). Paradoxical phosphorylation of the serine 199 on tau proteins from young individuals. *Neuroreport* 12, 3177–3181. doi: 10.1097/00001756-200110290-00007

Mondragón-Rodríguez, S., Trillaud-Doppia, E., Dudilot, A., Bourgeois, C., Lauzon, M., Leclerc, N., et al. (2012). Interaction of endogenous tau protein with synaptic proteins is regulated by N-methyl-D-aspartate receptor-dependent tau phosphorylation. *J. Biol. Chem.* 287, 32040–32053. doi: 10.1074/jbc.m112.401240

Moraga, D. M., Nuñez, P., Garrido, J., and Maccioni, R. B. (1993). A tau fragment containing a repetitive sequence induces bundling of actin filaments. *J. Neurochem.* 61, 979–986. doi: 10.1111/j.1471-4159.1993.tb03611.x

Morishima-Kawashima, M., Hasegawa, M., Takio, K., Suzuki, M., Yoshida, H., Titani, K., et al. (1995). Proline-directed and non-proline-directed phosphorylation of PHF-tau. *J. Biol. Chem.* 270, 823–829. doi: 10.1074/jbc.270.2.823

Nelson, P. T., Alafuzoff, I., Bigio, E. H., Bouras, C., Braak, H., Cairns, N. J., et al. (2012). Correlation of Alzheimer disease neuropathologic changes with cognitive status: a review of the literature. *J. Neuropathol. Exp. Neurol.* 71, 362–381. doi: 10.1097/NEN.0b013e31825018f7

Niewidok, B., Igaev, M., Sündermann, F., Janning, D., Bakota, L., and Brandt, R. (2016). Presence of a carboxy-terminal pseudorepeat and disease-like pseudohyperphosphorylation critically influence tau's interaction with microtubules in axon-like processes. *Mol. Biol. Cell* 27, 3537–3549. doi: 10.1091/mbc.e16-06-0402

Noble, W., Olm, V., Takata, K., Casey, E., Mary, O., Meyerson, J., et al. (2003). Cdk5 is a key factor in tau aggregation and tangle formation *in vivo*. *Neuron* 38, 555–565. doi: 10.1016/s0896-6273(03)00259-9

Notredame, C., Higgins, D. G., and Heringa, J. (2000). T-Coffee: a novel method for fast and accurate multiple sequence alignment. *J. Mol. Biol.* 302, 205–217. doi: 10.1006/jmbi.2000.4042

Padilla, R., Maccioni, R. B., and Avila, J. (1990). Calmodulin binds to a tubulin binding site of the microtubule-associated protein tau. *Mol. Cell. Biochem.* 97, 35–41. doi: 10.1007/bf00231699

Pei, L., Wang, S., Jin, H., Bi, L., Wei, N., Yan, H., et al. (2015). A novel mechanism of spine damages in stroke *via* DAPK1 and tau. *Cereb. Cortex* 25, 4559–4571. doi: 10.1093/cercor/bhv096

Peng, Z., Mizianty, M. J., and Kurgan, L. (2014). Genome-scale prediction of proteins with long intrinsically disordered regions. *Proteins* 82, 145–158. doi: 10.1002/prot.24348

Peng, K., Radivojac, P., Vucetic, S., Dunker, A. K., and Obradovic, Z. (2006). Length-dependent prediction of protein intrinsic disorder. *BMC Bioinformatics* 7:208. doi: 10.1186/1471-2105-7-208

Pérez, M., Cuadros, R., Benítez, M. J., and Jiménez, J. S. (2004). Interaction of Alzheimer's disease amyloid β peptide fragment 25–35 with tau protein and with a tau peptide containing the microtubule binding domain. *J. Alzheimers Dis.* 6, 461–467. doi: 10.3233/jad-2004-6501

Pérez, M., Valpuesta, J. M., Medina, M., Montejo De Garcini, E., and Avila, J. (1996). Polymerization of tau into filaments in the presence of heparin:

the minimal sequence required for tau-tau interaction. *J. Neurochem.* 67, 1183–1190. doi: 10.1046/j.1471-4159.1996.67031183.x

Porzig, R., Singer, D., and Hoffmann, R. (2007). Epitope mapping of mAbs AT8 and Tau5 directed against hyperphosphorylated regions of the human tau protein. *Biochem. Biophys. Res. Commun.* 358, 644–649. doi: 10.1016/j.bbrc. 2007.04.187

Prinzinger, R., Preßmar, A., and Schleucher, E. (1991). Body temperature in birds. *Comp. Biochem. Physiol. A Physiol.* 99, 499–506. doi: 10.1016/0300-9629(91)90122-S

Qi, H., Cantrelle, F. X., Benhelli-Mokrani, H., Smet-Nocca, C., Buée, L., Lippens, G., et al. (2015). Nuclear magnetic resonance spectroscopy characterization of interaction of Tau with DNA and its regulation by phosphorylation. *Biochemistry* 54, 1525–1533. doi: 10.1021/bi5014613

Qureshi, H. Y., Li, T., MacDonald, R., Cho, C. M., Leclerc, N., and Paudel, H. K. (2013). Interaction of 14-3-3ζ with microtubule-associated protein tau within Alzheimer's disease neurofibrillary tangles. *Biochemistry* 52, 6445–6455. doi: 10.1021/bi400442d

Radli, M., and Rüdiger, S. G. D. (2018). Dancing with the diva: Hsp90-client interactions. *J. Mol. Biol.* 430, 3029–3040. doi: 10.1016/j.jmb.2018.05.026

Ramirez-Rios, S., Denarier, E., Prezel, E., Vinit, A., Stoppin-Mellet, V., Devred, F., et al. (2016). Tau antagonizes end-binding protein tracking at microtubule ends through a phosphorylation-dependent mechanism. *Mol. Biol. Cell* 27, 2924–2934. doi: 10.1091/mbc.e16-01-0029

Richey, P. L., Siedlak, S. L., Smith, M. A., and Perry, G. (1995). Apolipoprotein E interaction with the neurofibrillary tangles and senile plaques in Alzheimer disease: implications for disease pathogenesis. *Biochem. Biophys. Res. Commun.* 208, 657–663. doi: 10.1006/bbrc.1995.1389

Riederer, B. M., Mourton-Gilles, C., Frey, P., Delacourte, A., and Probst, A. (2001). Differential phosphorylation of tau proteins during kitten brain development and Alzheimer's disease. *J. Neurocytol.* 30, 145–158. doi: 10.1023/A:1011991207942

Roberson, E. D., Scearce-Levie, K., Palop, J. J., Yan, F., Cheng, I. H., Wu, T., et al. (2007). Reducing endogenous tau ameliorates amyloid β-induced deficits in an Alzheimer's disease mouse model. *Science* 316, 750–754. doi: 10.1126/science. 1141736

Romero, P., Obradovic, Z., Li, X., Garner, E. C., Brown, C. J., and Dunker, A. K. (2001). Sequence complexity of disordered protein. *Proteins* 42, 38–48. doi: 10.1002/1097-0134(20010101)42:1<38::aid-prot50>3.0.co;2-3

Rowland, M. A., Harrison, B., and Deeds, E. J. (2015). Phosphatase specificity and pathway insulation in signaling networks. *Biophys J.* 108, 986–996. doi: 10.1016/j.bpj.2014.12.011

Russell, C. L., Mitra, V., Hansson, K., Blennow, K., Gobom, J., Zetterberg, H., et al. (2017). Comprehensive quantitative profiling of tau and phosphorylated tau peptides in cerebrospinal fluid by mass spectrometry provides new biomarker candidates. *J. Alzheimers Dis.* 55, 303–313. doi: 10.3233/JAD-160633

Sarkar, M., Kuret, J., and Lee, G. (2008). Two motifs within the tau microtubule-binding domain mediate its association with the hsc70 molecular chaperone. *J. Neurosci. Res.* 86, 2763–2773. doi: 10.1002/jnr.21721

Sayas, C. L., Medina, M., Cuadros, R., Ollá, I., García, E., Pérez, M., et al. (2019). Role of tau N-terminal motif in the secretion of human tau by End Binding proteins. *PLoS One* 14:e0210864. doi: 10.1371/journal.pone. 0210864

Schoch, K. M., DeVos, S. L., Miller, R. L., Chun, S. J., Norrbom, M., Wozniak, D. F., et al. (2016). Increased 4R-tau induces pathological changes in a human-tau mouse model. *Neuron* 90, 941–947. doi: 10.1016/j.neuron.2016.04.042

Selden, S. C., and Pollard, T. D. (1986). Interaction of actin filaments with microtubules is mediated by microtubule-associated proteins and regulated by phosphorylation. *Ann. NY Acad. Sci.* 466, 803–812. doi: 10.1111/j.1749-6632. 1986.tb38464.x

Shalaeva, D. N., Dibrova, D. V., Galperin, M. Y., and Mulkidjanian, A. Y. (2015). Modeling of interaction between cytochrome c and the WD domains of Apaf-1: bifurcated salt bridges underlying apoptosome assembly. *Biol. Direct* 10:29. doi: 10.1186/s13062-015-0059-4

Shanley, M. R., Hawley, D., Leung, S., Zaidi, N. F., Dave, R., Schlosser, K. A., et al. (2015). LRRK2 facilitates tau phosphorylation through strong interaction with tau and cdk5. *Biochemistry* 54, 5198–5208. doi: 10.1021/acs.biochem.5b00326

Shannon, P., Markiel, A., Ozier, O., Baliga, N. S., Wang, J. T., Ramage, D., et al. (2003). Cytoscape: a software environment for integrated models of biomolecular interaction networks. *Genome Res.* 13, 2498–2504. doi: 10.1101/gr.1239303

Sibille, N., Sillen, A., Leroy, A., Wieruszeski, J. M., Mulloy, B., Landrieu, I., et al. (2006). Structural impact of heparin binding to full-length Tau as studied by NMR spectroscopy. *Biochemistry* 45, 12560–12572. doi: 10.1021/bi0 60964o

Sluchanko, N. N., Seit-Nebi, A. S., and Gusev, N. B. (2009). Phosphorylation of more than one site is required for tight interaction of human tau protein with 14-3-3ζ. *FEBS Lett.* 583, 2739–2742. doi: 10.1016/j.febslet.2009. 07.043

Sluchanko, N. N., Sudnitsyna, M. V., Seit-Nebi, A. S., Antson, A. A., and Gusev, N. B. (2011). Properties of the monomeric form of human 14-3-3ζ protein and its interaction with tau and HspB6. *Biochemistry* 50, 9797–9808. doi: 10.1021/bi201374s

Smet, C., Sambo, A. V., Wieruszeski, J. M., Leroy, A., Landrieu, I., Buee, L., et al. (2004). The peptidyl prolyl cis/trans-isomerase Pin1 recognizes the phospho-Thr212-Pro213 site on Tau. *Biochemistry* 43, 2032–2040. doi: 10.1021/bi035479x

Søberg, K., Jahnsen, T., Rognes, T., Skålhegg, B. S., and Laerdahl, J. K. (2013). Evolutionary paths of the cAMP-dependent protein kinase (PKA) catalytic subunits. *PLoS One* 8:e60935. doi: 10.1371/journal.pone. 0060935

Sobue, K., Agarwal-Mawal, A., Li, W., Sun, W., Miura, Y., and Paudel, H. K. (2000). Interaction of neuronal Cdc2-like protein kinase with microtubule-associated protein tau. *J. Biol. Chem.* 275, 16673–16680. doi: 10.1074/jbc.m0007 84200

Sontag, E., Nunbhakdi-Craig, V., Lee, G., Brandt, R., Kamibayashi, C., Kuret, J., et al. (1999). Molecular interactions among protein phosphatase 2A, tau and microtubules: implications for the regulation of tau phosphorylation and the development of tauopathies. *J. Biol. Chem.* 274, 25490–25498. doi: 10.1074/jbc. 274.36.25490

Sontag, J. M., Nunbhakdi-Craig, V., White, C. L. III., Halpain, S., and Sontag, E. (2012). The protein phosphatase PP2A/Bα binds to the microtubule-associated proteins Tau and MAP2 at a motif also recognized by the kinase Fyn: implications for tauopathies. *J. Biol. Chem.* 287, 14984–14993. doi: 10.1074/jbc. m111.338681

Sottejeau, Y., Bretteville, A., Cantrelle, F.-X., Malmanche, N., Demiaute, F., Mendes, T., et al. (2015). Tau phosphorylation regulates the interaction between BIN1's SH3 domain and Tau's proline-rich domain. *Acta Neuropathol. Commun.* 3:58. doi: 10.1186/s40478-015-0237-8

Spillantini, M. G., Murrell, J. R., Goedert, M., Farlow, M. R., Klug, A., and Ghetti, B. (1998). Mutation in the tau gene in familial multiple system tauopathy with presenile dementia. *Proc. Natl. Acad. Sci. U S A* 95, 7737–7741. doi: 10.1073/pnas.95.13.7737

Stefanoska, K., Volkerling, A., Bertz, J., Poljak, A., Ke, Y. D., Ittner, L. M., et al. (2018). An N-terminal motif unique to primate tau enables differential protein-protein interactions. *J. Biol. Chem.* 293, 3710–3719. doi: 10.1074/jbc.ra118. 001784

Stieler, J. T., Bullmann, T., Kohl, F., Toien, O., Bruckner, M. K., Hartig, W., et al. (2011). The physiological link between metabolic rate depression and tau phosphorylation in mammalian hibernation. *PLoS One* 6:e14530. doi: 10.1371/journal.pone.0014530

Sun, W., Qureshi, H. Y., Cafferty, P. W., Sobue, K., Agarwal-Mawal, A., Neufield, K. D., et al. (2002). Glycogen synthase kinase-3β is complexed with tau protein in brain microtubules. *J. Biol. Chem.* 277, 11933–11940. doi: 10.1074/jbc.M107182200

Sündermann, F., Fernandez, M. P., and Morgan, R. O. (2016). An evolutionary roadmap to the microtubule-associated protein MAP Tau. *BMC Genomics* 17:264. doi: 10.1186/s12864-016-2590-9

Surridge, C. D., and Burns, R. G. (1994). The difference in the binding of phosphatidylinositol distinguishes MAP2 from MAP2C and Tau. *Biochemistry* 33, 8051–8057. doi: 10.1021/bi00192a009

Takashima, A., Murayama, M., Murayama, O., Kohno, T., Honda, T., Yasutake, K., et al. (1998). Presenilin 1 associates with glycogen synthase kinase-3β and its substrate tau. *Proc. Natl. Acad. Sci. U S A* 95, 9637–9641. doi: 10.1073/pnas.95. 16.9637

Taylor, I. R., Ahmad, A., Wu, T., Nordhues, B. A., Bhullar, A., Gestwicki, J. E., et al. (2018). The disorderly conduct of Hsc70 and its interaction with the Alzheimer's-related Tau protein. *J. Biol. Chem.* 293, 10796–10809. doi: 10.1074/jbc.RA118.002234

Taylor, S. S., Meharena, H. S., and Kornev, A. P. (2019). Evolution of a dynamic molecular switch. *IUBMB Life* 71, 672–684. doi: 10.1002/iub.2059

Tortosa, E., Adolfs, Y., Fukata, M., Pasterkamp, R. J., Kapitein, L. C., and Hoogenraad, C. C. (2017). Dynamic palmitoylation targets MAP6 to the axon to promote microtubule stabilization during neuronal polarization. *Neuron* 94, 809.e7–825.e7. doi: 10.1016/j.neuron.2017.04.042

Trushina, N. I., Mulkidjanian, A. Y., and Brandt, R. (2019). The microtubule skeleton and the evolution of neuronal complexity in vertebrates. *Biol. Chem.* 400, 1163–1179. doi: 10.1515/hsz-2019-0149

Tugaeva, K. V., Tsvetkov, P. O., and Sluchanko, N. N. (2017). Bacterial co-expression of human Tau protein with protein kinase A and 14-3-3 for studies of 14-3-3/phospho-Tau interaction. *PLoS One* 12:e0178933. doi: 10.1371/journal.pone.0178933

Usardi, A., Pooler, A. M., Seereeram, A., Reynolds, C. H., Derkinderen, P., Anderton, B., et al. (2011). Tyrosine phosphorylation of tau regulates its interactions with Fyn SH2 domains, but not SH3 domains, altering the cellular localization of tau. *FEBS J.* 278, 2927–2937. doi: 10.1111/j.1742-4658.2011.08218.x

Uversky, V. N. (2009). Intrinsically disordered proteins and their environment: effects of strong denaturants, temperature, pH, counter ions, membranes, binding partners, osmolytes and macromolecular crowding. *Protein J.* 28, 305–325. doi: 10.1007/s10930-009-9201-4

Uversky, V. N. (2015). Intrinsically disordered proteins and their (disordered) proteomes in neurodegenerative disorders. *Front. Aging Neurosci.* 7:18. doi: 10.3389/fnagi.2015.00018

Vanderweyde, T., Apicco, D. J., Youmans-Kidder, K., Ash, P. E. A., Cook, C., Lummertz Da Rocha, E., et al. (2016). Interaction of tau with the RNA-binding protein TIA1 regulates tau pathophysiology and toxicity. *Cell Rep.* 15, 1455–1466. doi: 10.1016/j.celrep.2016.04.045

Vanmechelen, E., Vanderstichele, H., Davidsson, P., Van Kerschaver, E., Van Der Perre, B., Sjogren, M., et al. (2000). Quantification of tau phosphorylated at threonine 181 in human cerebrospinal fluid: a sandwich ELISA with a synthetic phosphopeptide for standardization. *Neurosci. Lett.* 285, 49–52. doi: 10.1016/s0304-3940(00)01036-3

Walsh, I., Martin, A. J., Di Domenico, T., and Tosatto, S. C. (2012). ESpritz: accurate and fast prediction of protein disorder. *Bioinformatics* 28, 503–509. doi: 10.1093/bioinformatics/btr682

Wang, X. F., Dong, C. F., Zhang, J., Wan, Y. Z., Li, F., Huang, Y. X., et al. (2008). Human tau protein forms complex with PrP and some GSS- and fCJD-related PrP mutants possess stronger binding activities with tau *in vitro*. *Mol. Cell. Biochem.* 310, 49–55. doi: 10.1007/s11010-007-9664-6

Wang, Z. F., Yin, J., Zhang, Y., Zhu, L. Q., Tian, Q., Wang, X. C., et al. (2010). Overexpression of tau proteins antagonizes amyloid-β-potentiated apoptosis through mitochondria-caspase-3 pathway in N2a cells. *J. Alzheimers Dis.* 20, 145–157. doi: 10.3233/jad-2010-1351

Weissmann, C., Reyher, H. J., Gauthier, A., Steinhoff, H. J., Junge, W., and Brandt, R. (2009). Microtubule binding and trapping at the tip of neurites regulate tau motion in living neurons. *Traffic* 10, 1655–1668. doi: 10.1111/j.1600-0854.2009.00977.x

Williams, G. C. (1957). Pleiotropy, natural selection, and the evolution of senescence. *Evolution* 11, 398–411. doi: 10.2307/2406060

Woods, A. S., and Ferré, S. (2005). Amazing stability of the arginine-phosphate electrostatic interaction. *J. Proteome Res.* 4, 1397–1402. doi: 10.1021/pr050077s

Xu, L. R., Liu, X. L., Chen, J., and Liang, Y. (2013). Protein disulfide isomerase interacts with tau protein and inhibits its fibrillization. *PLoS One* 8:e76657. doi: 10.1371/journal.pone.0076657

Yan, X., Uronen, R. L., and Huttunen, H. J. (2018). The interaction of α-synuclein and Tau: a molecular conspiracy in neurodegeneration? *Semin. Cell Dev. Biol.* doi: 10.1016/j.semcdb.2018.05.005 [Epub ahead of print].

Youssef, S. A., Capucchio, M. T., Rofina, J. E., Chambers, J. K., Uchida, K., Nakayama, H., et al. (2016). Pathology of the aging brain in domestic and laboratory animals and animal models of human neurodegenerative diseases. *Vet. Pathol.* 53, 327–348. doi: 10.1177/0300985815623997

Yu, W. H., and Fraser, P. E. (2001). S100β interaction with tau is promoted by zinc and inhibited by hyperphosphorylation in Alzheimer's disease. *J. Neurosci.* 21, 2240–2246. doi: 10.1523/jneurosci.21-07-02240.2001

Zhong, Q., Congdon, E. E., Nagaraja, H. N., and Kuret, J. (2012). Tau isoform composition influences rate and extent of filament formation. *J. Biol. Chem.* 287, 20711–20719. doi: 10.1074/jbc.m112.364067

Zhou, Y., Hayashi, I., Wong, J., Tugusheva, K., Renger, J. J., and Zerbinatti, C. (2014). Intracellular clusterin interacts with brain isoforms of the bridging integrator 1 and with the microtubule-associated protein Tau in Alzheimer's disease. *PLoS One* 9:e103187. doi: 10.1371/journal.pone.0103187

Zhou, M., Li, Y., Hu, Q., Bai, X. C., Huang, W., Yan, C., et al. (2015). Atomic structure of the apoptosome: mechanism of cytochrome c- and dATP-mediated activation of Apaf-1. *Genes Dev.* 29, 2349–2361. doi: 10.1101/gad.272278.115

Zhou, L., Mcinnes, J., Wierda, K., Holt, M., Herrmann, A. G., Jackson, R. J., et al. (2017). Tau association with synaptic vesicles causes presynaptic dysfunction. *Nat. Commun.* 8:15295. doi: 10.1038/ncomms15295

Zhu, H. L., Fernandez, C., Fan, J. B., Shewmaker, F., Chen, J., Minton, A. P., et al. (2010). Quantitative characterization of heparin binding to Tau protein: implication for inducer-mediated Tau filament formation. *J. Biol. Chem.* 285, 3592–3599. doi: 10.1074/jbc.m109.035691

15

Astroglia and Tau: New Perspectives

Gabor G. Kovacs[1,2,3]*

[1]Tanz Centre for Research in Neurodegenerative Disease, University of Toronto, Toronto, ON, Canada, [2]Department of Laboratory Medicine and Pathobiology, University of Toronto, Toronto, ON, Canada, [3]Laboratory Medicine Program, University Health Network, Toronto, ON, Canada

***Correspondence:**
Gabor G. Kovacs
gabor.kovacs@uhnresearch.ca;
gabor.kovacs@utoronto.ca

Astrocytes contribute to the pathogenesis of neurodegenerative proteinopathies as influencing neuronal degeneration or neuroprotection, and also act as potential mediators of the propagation or elimination of disease-associated proteins. Protein astrogliopathies can be observed in different forms of neurodegenerative conditions. Morphological characterization of astrogliopathy is used only for the classification of tauopathies. Currently, at least six types of astrocytic tau pathologies are distinguished. Astrocytic plaques (AP), tufted astrocytes (TAs), ramified astrocytes (RA), and globular astroglial inclusions are seen predominantly in primary tauopathies, while thorn-shaped astrocytes (TSA) and granular/fuzzy astrocytes (GFA) are evaluated in aging-related tau astrogliopathy (ARTAG). ARTAG can be seen in the white and gray matter and subpial, subependymal, and perivascular locations. Some of these overlap with the features of tau pathology seen in Chronic traumatic encephalopathy (CTE). Furthermore, gray matter ARTAG shares features with primary tauopathy-related astrocytic tau pathology. Sequential distribution patterns have been described for tau astrogliopathies. Importantly, astrocytic tau pathology in primary tauopathies can be observed in brain areas without neuronal tau deposition. The various morphologies of tau astrogliopathy might reflect a role in the propagation of pathological tau protein, an early response to a yet unidentified neurodegeneration-inducing event, or, particularly for ARTAG, a response to a repeated or prolonged pathogenic process such as blood-brain barrier dysfunction or local mechanical impact. The concept of tau astrogliopathies and ARTAG facilitated communication among research disciplines and triggered the investigation of the significance of astrocytic lesions in neurodegenerative conditions.

Keywords: ARTAG, astroglia, astrogliopathy, neurodegeneration, proteinopathy, propagation, tau

INTRODUCTION: CONCEPTS OF NEURODEGENERATIVE DISEASES

Neurodegenerative diseases (NDDs) are characterized by progressive dysfunction of neuronal networks. Recent studies have emphasized the role of the supporting tissue, which in the central nervous system comprises astroglia, microglia, and oligodendroglia. Glial responses characterize neuroinflammatory processes and have consequences in the maintenance of the functionality and ion-homeostasis of neurons, and conduction of nerve impulses (Heneka et al., 2014; Ettle et al., 2016; Ferrer, 2017; Verkhratsky et al., 2017). A central aspect of NDDs is the deposition of physicochemically altered variants of physiological proteins in the nervous system (Kovacs, 2019a). Molecular biological, biochemical, genetic and morphological studies identified a spectrum of immunohistochemically and biochemically detectable proteins, which serve as a basis for protein-based disease classification (Kovacs, 2016). Importantly, these pathological proteins accumulate in neurons, astrocytes, and oligodendrocytes (Kovacs et al., 2017a). The microtubule-associated protein tau is one of many proteins that accumulate in pathological forms in NDDs. Additional abnormally deposited proteins include Amyloid-β (Aβ), which is cleaved from the transmembrane amyloid precursor protein (APP), α-Synuclein, Prion protein, Transactive response (TAR) DNA-binding protein 43 (TDP-43), and FET proteins, comprising the fused in sarcoma (FUS), Ewing's sarcoma RNA-binding protein 1 (EWSR1), and TATA-binding protein-associated factor 15 (TAF15). Other proteins are associated with hereditary disorders encoded by genes linked to neurological trinucleotide repeat disorders, neuroserpin, ferritin-related NDDs, and familial cerebral amyloidoses (Kovacs, 2016). Importantly, in addition to the hallmark pathological lesions of NDDs, combinations of pathological alterations can be observed in the same brain, described as concomitant proteinopathies (comorbidities) with or without additional non-neurodegenerative conditions (i.e., metabolic or vascular), designated as multimorbidities (Kovacs et al., 2008; Rahimi and Kovacs, 2014; Kovacs, 2019b). Therefore, analyses of glial responses should be considered in the context of comorbidities and multimorbidities.

Due to their crucial neuron-supporter role, astroglia reacts to the classical pathogenic events associated with NDDs, such as metabolic changes, molecular damage, and dysregulation of energetic and ion homeostasis (von Bernhardi and Eugenin, 2012). Since protein accumulation is a central event for NDDs, the relationship of astroglia and protein processing systems including the ubiquitin-proteasome system and the autophagy-lysosome pathway (Nijholt et al., 2011) and the unfolded protein response (Cornejo and Hetz, 2013) is important in disease mechanisms. Indeed, the novel concept, referred to as prion-like spreading, suggesting that the proteins associated with NDDs propagate in the nervous system (Brettschneider et al., 2015), have turned scientific interest to the role of glia in the propagation of pathological proteins. The prion-like concept stems from prion disease research, which proposes a template-directed protein misfolding of pathological proteins (Brettschneider et al., 2015). A critical aspect when discussing the role of glia in the processing of pathological proteins is that most of the NDD-related proteins are not expressed by glia in their physiological form. The cell-to-cell propagation theory and the recognition of sequential involvement of anatomical regions led to the description of stages and phases of pathological protein deposits (Kovacs, 2019a). Currently, however, these staging schemes have primarily focused on neuronal (e.g., α-synuclein in Lewy body disorders or tau for neurofibrillary tangle (NFT) formation in Alzheimer's disease, AD) or extracellular protein deposits (e.g., Aβ in AD), without consideration of glial involvement (Liddelow and Sofroniew, 2019).

To understand the complex interaction of the tau protein and astroglia in NDDs the following points require consideration: (1) alterations of tau protein in disease; (2) which cell types accumulate pathological tau in different disorders; (3) how pathological tau is distributed in the human brain; (4) whether astroglia contributes to the propagation of pathological tau; and finally (5) whether the accumulation of tau in astroglia influence the degeneration of neurons or cause alterations in the physiological neuron-supporting roles of the astroglia.

FUNDAMENTALS OF TAUOPATHIES WITH RELEVANCE TO ASTROGLIA

Tauopathies are biochemically, morphologically, and genetically heterogenous NDDs characterized by the accumulation of pathological forms of tau protein in diverse anatomical distribution patterns. Conditions where tau pathology is the driving force in the pathogenesis are called primary tauopathies. They are grouped based on the ratio of 3repeat (R)- and 4R-tau isoforms and two or three major bands (60, 64, and 68 kDa) in the Western blot of sarkosyl-insoluble fractions, the distinct involvement of anatomical areas and cell types affected, and ultrastructural features of tau filaments (Kovacs, 2017; Forrest et al., 2019b). Mutations in the microtubule-associated tau (MAPT) gene are associated with various tau pathologies, which recapitulate features of sporadic tauopathies in the majority of cases (Ghetti et al., 2015; Forrest et al., 2018).

Biochemical Aspects

Tau protein undergoes several post-translational modifications such as oxidation, glycation, deamination, isomerization, or enzymatically through phosphorylation, methylation, acetylation, O-GlcNAcylation, nitration, proteolytic cleavage (truncation), sumoylation, and ubiquitination (Spillantini and Goedert, 2013; Rösler et al., 2019). These modifications are major driving forces for neurodegeneration, however, tau hyperphosphorylation is thought to be the most important. This potentially leads to altered binding affinity and then to microtubular malfunction with a loss of function mechanism.

Importantly, post-translational modifications of tau are examined in human brains by preparing homogenates of brain tissue that contain different cell types. To evaluate cell-specific modifications, however, mostly immunohistochemical methods are applied. According to a comprehensive study on glial tau pathologies, tau in astrocytes is hyperphosphorylated at different sites including Thr181, Ser199, Ser202-Thr205, Thr212/Ser214, Thr231, Ser262, Ser396-Ser404, and Ser422 (Ferrer et al., 2014). Antibodies Alz50 (amino acids 5–15) and MC-1 (amino acids 312–322) tau revealed an altered conformation of tau in astroglia in tauopathies, but most of the phosphorylated-tau-positive astrocytes are not stained with the antibody tau-C3, which recognizes tau truncated at aspartic acid 421 (Ferrer et al., 2014). Application of antibodies against the carboxy-terminal, middle segment, and amino-terminal of tau show important differences between astroglial tau pathologies [i.e., astrocytic plaques (AP), tufted and ramified astrocytes (RA)] suggesting different truncation patterns (Ferrer et al., 2014, 2018; Ferrer, 2018). Interestingly, astrocytes accumulate predominantly the 4R tau isoform and 3R immunoreactivity is rarely observed (Ferrer et al., 2014). In summary, for an understanding of the role of astroglia in pathological processes involving tau, the application of different tau-antibodies in scientific reports must be carefully considered as this may lead to distinct interpretations.

Neuropathological Phenotypes

Currently, the nomenclature of primary tauopathies overlaps with that of frontotemporal lobar degeneration (FTLD), and are referred to FTLD-tau (Forrest et al., 2019b). The terminology of clinicopathological phenotypes refers to clinical symptoms, such as progressive supranuclear palsy (PSP), to anatomical distribution of neuronal degeneration, such as corticobasal degeneration (CBD); to morphological features, such as argyrophilic grain disease (AGD) and globular glial tauopathies (GGT); to both clinical and morphological features, such as NFT predominant dementia, which is now included in the spectrum of primary age-related tauopathy (PART); and to a physician referred to as Pick's disease (PiD). Except for PART, all primary tauopathies accumulate pathological tau in astrocytes. However, in the diagnostic neuropathological practice, astrocytic tau pathology is considered for the distinction of PSP and CBD, and GGT.

Neuropathological definitions of primary tauopathies can be summarized as follows (Kovacs, 2017): (1) Neuronal cytoplasmic spherical Pick bodies that are 3R-tau immunoreactive characterize PiD; (2) PSP is a 4R tauopathy with NFTs in hallmark subcortical structures including the subthalamic nucleus, basal ganglia and brainstem, and additionally tufted astrocytes (TAs), oligodendroglial coiled bodies, and threads; (3) CBD is a 4R tauopathy with diffuse neuronal cytoplasmic immunoreactivity and spherical neuronal inclusions, threads in the white and gray matter, coiled bodies and astrocytic plaques (AP); (4) Neuropathology of AGD include argyrophilic and 4R-tau immunoreactive grains in medial temporal lobe structures that are variably associated with pretangles, oligodendroglial coiled bodies, and astrocytic tau immunoreactivity; (5) Argyrophilic (Gallyas) and 4R-tau immunoreactive globular oligodendroglial and non-argyrophilic (Gallyas), 4R-tau immunoreactive globular astroglial inclusions (GOI and GAI, respectively) characterize three types of GGTs; and (6) Histopathological features of the combined 3R and 4R tauopathy, PART, include NFTs restricted to the hippocampus and medial temporal lobe. Tau morphologies in PART are similar to those observed in AD except for the absence or infrequent Aβ plaques (Crary et al., 2014).

Further peculiar tau pathology in the aging brain is aging-related tau astrogliopathy (ARTAG), which describes tau-positive astroglia accumulating 4R isoform of tau in subpial, subependymal, and perivascular locations, and the white and gray matter (Kovacs et al., 2016). Chronic traumatic encephalopathy (CTE) is the neuropathological term describing mixed 3R- and 4R-tau pathology primarily in neurons with additional astroglial tau morphologies following mild repetitive head injury (McKee et al., 2016). Mostly neuronal 3R- and 4R-tau pathology is associated with an autoimmune process anti-IgLON5 (IgLON family member 5)-related encephalopathy that predominantly affects subcortical structures (Gelpi et al., 2016). Several conditions, including post-infectious, metabolic, and non-*MAPT* gene-related hereditary disorders are associated with tau pathologies primarily affecting neurons (Kovacs, 2017).

Highlights of Pathogenesis

As a microtubule-associated protein, tau functions in promoting the polymerization and assembly of microtubules (Weingarten et al., 1975). Although tau isoforms with 3R and 4R are equally expressed in the adult human brain (Sergeant et al., 1997), neuronal populations show variability in the expression of 3R- and 4R-tau isoforms (Goedert et al., 1989; Buée et al., 2000). Full-length tau protein is primarily located in axons (Trojanowski et al., 1989; Lee et al., 2001) and is also present in nuclear or somatodendritic compartments of neurons (Tashiro et al., 1997). Further studies suggest that oligodendrocytes (Klein et al., 2002) also express tau and that tau can be detected in interstitial fluid (Yamada et al., 2011). Stimulation of neuronal activity induces tau release from healthy, mature cortical neurons and the phosphorylation of extracellular tau appears reduced in comparison with intracellular tau (Pooler et al., 2013). Tau may also play a role in cell signaling (or act as a buffer for cell signaling), and binds to nucleic acids, and may be involved in chromatin remodeling (for review, see Jadhav et al., 2019). In disease conditions, secreted tau is thought to be crucial in the propagation of tau pathology. It has been suggested that tau is secreted within extracellular vesicles as exosomes (Wang et al., 2017) and ectosomes, which are plasma membrane-originating vesicles, and when it accumulates, the exosomal pathway is activated (Dujardin et al., 2014).

Prion-like cell-to-cell spreading is considered in the propagation of protein (including tau) pathology in a range of NDDs (Brettschneider et al., 2015). This implies that the release of pathological tau is followed by uptake in related neurons leading to the formation of aggregates inside the recipient cells following a seeding process (Goedert et al., 2017b; Mudher et al., 2017; Goedert, 2018). Mice transgenic for wild-type human tau inoculated with homogenates from human primary tauopathy brain extracts recapitulate the hallmark lesions of the original inoculated tauopathies, including astroglial tau pathology (Clavaguera et al., 2009). A recent study also described the rapid and distinct cell-type-specific spread of pathological tau following intracerebral injections of CBD brain extracts into young human mutant P301S tau transgenic mice (Boluda et al., 2015). These studies support the concept of tau strains. This terminology has been used in prion disease research to describe the event that disease-associated proteins maintain unique conformations and associate with similar patterns of pathology. Indeed, a study using a cell system to isolate tau strains from five different tauopathies described different sets of strains related to tau diseases (Sanders et al., 2014). Furthermore, a recent study identified distinct tau strain potency between tauopathies in non-transgenic mice (Narasimhan et al., 2017). Studies supporting the concept of strains have been recently complemented by research investigating the structure of tau filaments in diverse conditions with tau pathology, including AD, PiD and CTE (Falcon et al., 2018a,b; Falcon et al., 2019).

Whether astroglial disease-associated tau itself is capable of seeding is difficult to address in human studies since brain homogenates contain a mixture of neuronal and glial (astroglia and oligodendroglia) pathological tau in primary tauopathies. However, recent reports used brain homogenates derived from brain regions showing ARTAG pathology. Accordingly, it was shown that seeding is produced in neurons of the hippocampal complex, astrocytes, oligodendroglia and along fibers of the corpus callosum, fimbria and fornix following inoculation into the hippocampus of wild type using brain homogenates of ARTAG pathology (Ferrer et al., 2018). Thus, the host tau is also relevant for the seeding and spreading of tau pathology (Ferrer et al., 2020b).

In summary, regarding these pathogenic aspects, the question remains how astrocytes come into contact with modifications of tau proteins and whether astrocytes are major players or bystanders in tau-induced neurodegeneration and propagation of tau pathology.

THE MORPHOLOGICAL SPECTRUM OF ASTROCYTES ACCUMULATING TAU

For many decades silver stains were the gold standard in neuropathological diagnostic practice. These were used to recognize unusual structures, such as NFTs and inclusion-bodies in degenerating neurons. Although later pathological phenomena have been identified in astrocytes using silver stains (in particular Gallyas staining), their widespread involvement in the pathological process of tauopathies was discovered with the application of immunostaining for phosphorylated tau. Astroglial tau pathologies were described originally as glial fibrillary tangles, by analogy to neuronal NFTs. Later, however, it was recognized that tauopathies associate with dramatically different morphologies. Unfortunately, many studies used different descriptions and terminology when reporting these pathologies, complicating the comparison of studies. However, interpretations still vary between experts calling for consensus studies (Kovacs et al., 2017d). A study aiming to describe aging-related astroglial tau pathologies recommended the distinction of six major morphologies, such as AP, TAs, RA, GAIs, which are seen mostly in primary tauopathies, and thorn-shaped astrocytes (TSA) and granular/fuzzy astrocytes (GFA) observed in ARTAG (Kovacs et al., 2016; **Figure 1**). It must be emphasized that these are predominating astrocytic inclusions, which distinguish the different tauopathies. However, a variety of additional astroglial morphologies of tau accumulation can be detected in these disorders that do not have, and for the current diagnostic practice not require specific designations. These various morphologies yet to be defined might reflect the different phases of tau aggregation and accumulation in astrocytes whereas the six main morphological types depict the mature and characteristic morphologies.

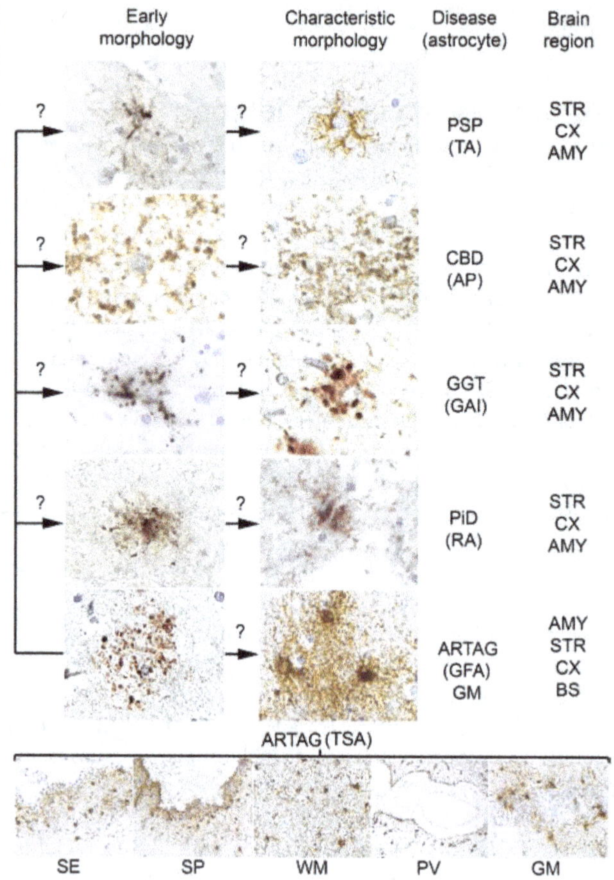

FIGURE 1 | Conceptual summary of astrocytic tau pathologies. Fine granular tau deposition is seen in all primary tauopathies and in gray matter aging-related tau astrogliopathy (ARTAG), which might be interpreted as preceding forms of early morphologies (left column of the upper panel) of disease characteristic morphologies (right column of the upper panel) such as TAs in progressive supranuclear palsy (PSP), astrocytic plaques (AP) in corticobasal degeneration (CBD), globular astroglial inclusions (GAI) in globular glial tauopathies (GGT), ramified astrocytes (RA) in Pick's disease (PiD) and granular fuzzy astrocytes (GFA) of gray matter ARTAG. Thorn-shaped astrocytes (TSA) are different morphologies detected in subependymal (SE), subpial (SP), white matter (WM), perivascular (PV) location, and rarely in gray matter (GM, here exemplified by the dentate gyrus of the hippocampal formation). Question marks indicate that these aspects are hypothetical. The predominantly affected regions are listed on the right, which does not exclude that other regions show these morphologies. AMY, amygdala; STR, striatum; CX, cortex; BS, brainstem.

A further concept that an early event in the development of astrocytic pathology might be the fine granular accumulation of tau in astrocytic processes (Kovacs et al., 2017a,c), which is similar to early pretangle formation in AD, which precedes NFT development (Bancher et al., 1989). This concept suggests that first tau becomes hyperphosphorylated, then misfolds and aggregates, and then forms fibrillar structures. During this process, fine tau deposits are then redistributed to proximal (TAs) or distal (AP) segments of the astrocytic processes, aggregate and become detectable in some silver-stains (Ikeda et al., 2016; Kovacs et al., 2017c; **Figure 1**).

Tufted Astrocytes

TAs are hallmark lesions of PSP. Although in 1988, Probst et al. (1988) described stellate neurons showing Gallyas positive material, which could be interpreted today as TAs. The term tufts of abnormal fibers were used first by Hauw et al. (1990) in PSP cases using the Bodian silver method and tau IHC. This was then confirmed to be related to astrocytes (Yamada et al., 1992, 1993). Currently, TAs are defined as astrocytes showing phosphorylated-tau immunoreactivity in the proximal segments of astrocytic processes (Kovacs et al., 2016). TAs are detected in Gallyas and modified Bielschowsky silver staining. Ultrastructural observations describe tubular profiles in these (Nishimura et al., 1992; Arima, 2006). Interestingly, TAs of PSP and AP of CBD seem to accumulate close to blood vessels (Shibuya et al., 2011).

PSP pathology associates with different clinical presentations (Dickson et al., 2010), therefore, the amount and distribution of astrocytic pathology might vary between these forms. Although descriptions of astrocytic tau pathologies vary considerably, rare tuft-shaped astrocytes in the cortex have been reported in cases with a mutation in *MAPT*. These include mutations on exon 1 R5H (Hayashi et al., 2002), TAs in exon 1 R5L mutation (Poorkaj et al., 2002), in intron 9 and 10 *MAPT* mutations (Malkani et al., 2006; Ghetti et al., 2011), and wide range of astrocytic tau morphologies, referred to as tufted forms, have been linked to the deln296 *MAPT* mutation (Ferrer et al., 2003). TAs and AP have also been described in the P301L, P301t, and P301S *MAPT* mutations (Ghetti et al., 2011). Glial tangles and TAs (Stanford et al., 2000) and AP (Halliday et al., 2006) have been described in the S305S mutation.

Astrocytic Plaques

AP are hallmark lesions of CBD. The observation of tau positive pathology in CBD resembling neuritic plaques without Aβ cores (Mattiace et al., 1991), mainly in the distal parts of astrocytic processes (Feany and Dickson, 1995), opened new avenues for the research on CBD. AP show densely tau-immunoreactive stubby dilatations of distal processes of astrocytes giving a plaque-like appearance (Kovacs et al., 2016), which are argyrophilic on Gallyas silver. Ultrastructurally, AP are characterized by randomly arranged bundles of twisted and straight tubules with diameters of 15–20 nm (Yoshida, 2014). TAs in PSP and AP in CBD are immunoreactive for antibodies detecting the carboxyl-terminal and middle region of tau but do not show immunoreactivity to antibodies detecting the amino-terminal region of tau, suggesting that the latter is reduced or lacking in astrocytic tau pathologies (Ferrer, 2018).

Incidental CBD cases have been reported with astroglial tau pathology in the cortex in the absence of neuronal tau. These findings suggest that tau accumulation in astroglia might represent one of the initial pathological steps in the onset of CBD (Ling et al., 2016). Indeed, CBD pathology can exist in individuals without overt clinical symptoms suggesting that AP are not the major substrates for clinical symptomatology in CBD (Milenkovic and Kovacs, 2013; Martínez-Maldonado et al., 2016), supporting the notion that the regional distribution of neuronal degeneration and tau pathology underlies more the clinical phenotype. In contrast to the predominance of AP in preclinical asymptomatic CBD, neuronal tau aggregates predominated in rapidly progressive fulminant forms of CBD (Ling et al., 2020). In addition to the mutations in *MAPT* associated with TAs in PSP (above), several mutations in *MAPT* are also associated with AP in CBD including the S305S, IVS10+16 and R406W mutations (Forrest et al., 2018).

Ramified Astrocytes

RA are the characteristic astrocytic lesion in PiD. However, compared to neuronal tau pathology in PiD, the reported density and distribution of RA varies between cases and studies. This is likely attributed to the variability of definitions of PiD before the application of isoform-specific antibodies (Dickson, 1998; Kovacs et al., 2013b). Feany et al. (1996) precisely described that these astrocytic inclusions in PiD "tended to occupy more of the cell body and to ramify into the astrocytic cell processes," and that they were "often localized to one side of the cell soma." RA may show 3R-tau immunoreactivity (Kovacs et al., 2013b; Ferrer et al., 2014).

Globular Astroglial Inclusions

Globular astroglial inclusions are seen in GGT in the gray matter and are defined as tau-immunoreactive globules (1–5 μm) and dots (1–2 μm) in the proximal parts of astrocytic processes and perikarya (Kovacs et al., 2016). These can be reminiscent of TAs in morphology and distribution, but they are non-argyrophilic on Gallyas and Bielschowsky silver stains (Ahmed et al., 2013; Kovacs, 2015). GGT types (I–III) are distinguished based on the anatomical involvement and the predominance of oligodendroglial or astroglial inclusions (Ahmed et al., 2013). Globular astroglial inclusions have been associated with mutations in *MAPT* including IVS10+16, P301L, K317N, and K317M (Zarranz et al., 2005; Tacik et al., 2015, 2017; Forrest et al., 2018, 2019a). Altered expression of several functional markers of astroglia (and oligodendroglia) in GGT supports the notion that these are primary astrogliopathies (and oligodendrogliopathies; Ferrer et al., 2020a) opening new avenues to understand NDDs.

Thorn-Shaped Astrocytes

Currently, TSAs are discussed in the frame of ARTAG (Kovacs et al., 2016). They are defined as tau-immunoreactivity in astrocytic perikarya with extension into the proximal astrocytic processes, as well as tau-immunopositive inclusions in the astrocytic endfeet at the glia limitans at the pial surface and around blood vessels (Kovacs et al., 2016). TSAs are argyrophilic on Gallyas silver. Nishimura et al. (1992) reported argyrophilic masses with flame- or thorn-like shape in addition to TAs in PSP, which is likely to represent an early description of TSAs. TSAs were also reported in the aging brain in the subpial and subependymal regions, and frequently in the depths of gyri, and the basal forebrain and brainstem (Ikeda et al., 1995, 1998; Ikeda, 1996). Schultz et al. (2000, 2004) reported a high prevalence of TSAs at the level of the amygdala, furthermore, they observed similar astroglial tau pathology in aged baboons. TSAs are immunoreactive for antibodies detecting the carboxyl- and amino-terminals and middle region of tau, show 4Rtau phosphorylation at several specific sites and abnormal tau conformation, but they lack ubiquitin and show increased superoxide dismutase

2 (SOD2) immunoreactivity (Ferrer et al., 2018). Moreover, phosphoproteomics of dissected vulnerable regions identifies an increase of phosphorylation marks in a large number of proteins such as GFAP, aquaporin 4, several serine-threonine kinases, microtubule-associated proteins and other neuronal proteins (Ferrer et al., 2018).

Granular-Fuzzy Astrocytes

GFA is the second type of astrocytic inclusions associated with ARTAG. GFAs are characterized by fine granular tau-immunoreactivity in processes of gray matter astrocytes with dense tau-immunoreactivity in the perinuclear soma also observed in most astrocytic inclusions (Kovacs et al., 2016). GFAs are largely non-argyrophilic on Gallyas silver-staining, except some of the dense perikaryal accumulations.

In addition to the characteristic tau-immunopositive grains, tau-immunopositive astrocytes have been described in AGD. These are referred to as bush-like astrocytes and have a similar anatomical distribution to GFAs in ARTAG (Botez et al., 1999). Due to the morphological similarities and anatomical overlap of astrocytic inclusions in AGD and ARTAG, the bush-like astrocytes in AGD are better interpreted as GFAs (Kovacs et al., 2016). A study on PSP and AGD indicated that some GFA-like morphologies (termed tufted astrocyte (TA)-like astrocytic lesions in that study) can potentially evolve into Gallyas-positive TAs in AGD brains (Ikeda et al., 2016). GFAs can be seen in a wide range of neurodegenerative conditions, including frontotemporal tauopathies, AD, prion disease and Huntington's disease, and neurologically normal controls (Kovacs et al., 2017b,c; Baskota et al., 2019).

Other Morphologies and Combinations

Additional tau-immunoreactive astrocytes are also described in cases with mutations in *MAPT*. However, meticulous descriptions of the morphological and anatomical distributions of tau inclusions in astrocytes are often missing in publications and the lack of concise consensus nomenclature on astroglial tau pathologies does not facilitate clear comparison of these publications. Usually, mutations in *MAPT* on exons 1, 10, 11, and 12, as well as introns following exons 9 and 10, show astroglial inclusions (Ghetti et al., 2011). A peculiar type of astrocytic tau pathology has been described in a familial behavioral variant frontotemporal dementia disorder where no known mutations in *APP, PSEN1, PSEN2, MAPT, GRN, TARDBP*, and *FUS* and no pathological expansion in *C9ORF72* have been found (Ferrer et al., 2018). The morphology of astrocytic inclusions were similar to reactive astrocytes. In addition to the cytoplasm, perivascular foot processes around cortical blood vessels, furthermore cerebellar Bergmann glia were also immunostained with the AT8 antibody (double-phosphorylation sites Ser202-Thr205; Ferrer et al., 2015). Widespread TSAs and GFAs have also been described in a novel *GRN* nonsense mutation (c.5G>A: p.Trp2*; Gómez-Tortosa et al., 2019); a mixture of bushy and TAs in *TARDBP* mutation p.Ile383Val (Gelpi et al., 2014); and AP and ARTAG in 17q21.31 duplication (Alexander et al., 2016; Le Guennec et al., 2017).

WHAT IS THE RELEVANCE OF ARTAG?

Types of ARTAG

ARTAG is an umbrella term that includes a spectrum of astrocytic tau morphologies mainly in the aging brain (Kovacs et al., 2016). ARTAG includes morphologies described as TSA and GFA, which can be present in the same brains and anatomical regions together (Kovacs et al., 2016). The two types of tau immunoreactivities are present in different locations defined as types of ARTAG. TSAs are seen mostly in subpial, subependymal, or perivascular areas, as well as in the white matter (WM). TSAs are less frequently observed in the gray matter. In contrast, GFAs are observed only in the gray matter. Accordingly, ARTAG is classified as subependymal, subpial, perivascular, white or gray matter ARTAG. Clustering of TSAs and GFAs can be observed in both the white and gray matter.

Distribution Patterns of ARTAG

Using conditional probability and logistic regression to model the sequential distribution of ARTAG across different brain regions, a recent study evaluated the frequencies and hierarchical clustering of anatomical involvement of astrocytic inclusions (Kovacs et al., 2018a). Overlapping sequential distribution patterns have been recognized for the different types of ARTAG.

In the aging brain subpial ARTAG shows two distinct patterns (**Figures 2A,B**; Kovacs et al., 2018a). Pattern 1 is characterized by the involvement of basal forebrain regions first (stage 1). This is followed by a sequence either rostral (lobar, stage 2a) or caudal (brainstem, stage 2b), which regions are then affected together (stage 3). Pattern 2 starts in lobar regions (stage 1a) or the brainstem (stage 1b), followed by the involvement of both (stage 2) and preceding basal forebrain regions (stage 3). Importantly, subpial astrocytic tau accumulation is prominent in CBD, which must be distinguished from subpial TSAs in aging and other conditions on a morphological level and the distinct distribution pattern (Kovacs et al., 2018a).

Pattern 1 described above for subpial ARTAG is also recognized for WM ARTAG. In the second pattern of WM ARTAG, lobar involvement (stage 1) is followed by basal forebrain regions (stage 2a) or the brainstem (stage 2b), finally evolving into the involvement of all regions (stage 3; Kovacs et al., 2018a).

Gray matter ARTAG (GFA morphology) seems to follow two distinct patterns (**Figures 2C–E**). One involves the striatal pathway, which is reminiscent of the pattern seen in PSP but lacking further morphological characteristics of PSP (i.e., subcortical NFTs and accumulation of typical TAs). Accordingly, from the striatum (stage 1) astroglial tau in the form of GFAs proceeds to the amygdala (stage 2a), cortex (stage 2b) or rarely to the brainstem (stage 2c). Following stage 3a (striatum and amygdala and cortex), or stage 3b (striatum and amygdala and brainstem), all regions are affected (stage 4; Kovacs et al., 2018a). The constellation of striatum and cortical and brainstem GFA involvement has not been observed, hence the absence of a stage 3c. The second pattern of gray matter ARTAG is referred to as the "amygdala first" pattern where involvement of the amygdala (stage 1)

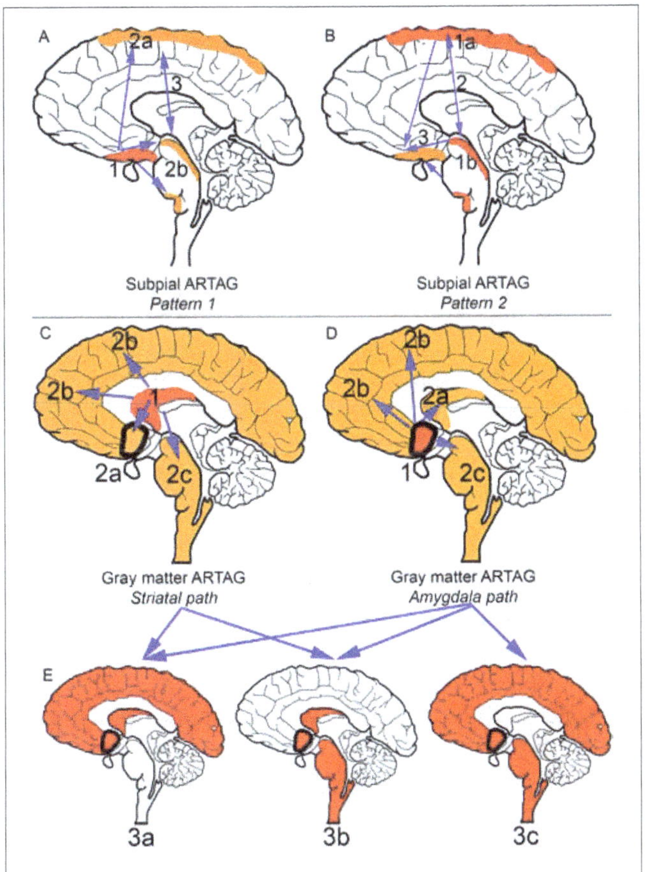

FIGURE 2 | Distribution patterns of subpial and gray matter ARTAG. In all panels, brain regions colored red represent initial or combined regions of astrocytic involvement and brain regions colored orange represent subsequent brain regions involved. Brain regions outlined in a thick black line represent the amygdala. **(A)** Subpial ARTAG, pattern 1. Basal brain regions show subpial ARTAG first (stage 1), which is followed by a bidirectional sequence to rostral (lobar, stage 2a) or caudal (brainstem, stage 2b) regions. Both brain regions are usually affected together (stage 3, indicated by double-headed arrow). **(B)** Subpial ARTAG, pattern 2. Lobar (stage 1a) or brainstem (1b) involvement is followed by the involvement of both brain regions (stage 2), followed by the involvement of basal brain regions (stage 3, indicated by double-headed arrow). **(C)** Gray matter ARTAG, striatal pathway. From the striatum (stage 1), astrocytic tau accumulation proceeds towards the amygdala (stage 2a, blue arrow), or cortex (stage 2b, blue arrow), or rarely to the brainstem (stage 2c, blue arrow). **(D)** Gray matter ARTAG, amygdala pathway. The amygdala (stage 1) precedes the involvement of the striatum (stage 2a, blue arrow), the cortex (stage 2b, blue arrow) or the brainstem (stage 2c, blue arrow). **(E)** Both striatal and amygdala pathway includes stage 3a (striatum + amygdala + cortex), or stage 3b (striatum + amygdala + brainstem), and only the amygdala pathway stage 3c (amygdala +cortex + brainstem), which then eventually involve all regions (stage 4, not indicated).

precedes the striatum (stage 2a), the cortex (stage 2b) or the brainstem (stage 2c). This evolves into three combinations of stage 3 (a: amygdala and striatum and cortex; b: amygdala and striatum and brainstem; c: amygdala and cortex and brainstem) and finally all regions are involved (stage 4; Kovacs et al., 2018a).

The sequential pattern of GFA involvement in the gray matter could represent the involvement of astroglia in the propagation of pathological tau. However, for subpial, WM, perivascular, and subependymal, ARTAG, it might reflect the consequences of a repeated or permanent pathogenic process, such as one associated with the blood-brain barrier. This is supported by the observation of increased connexin-43 (gap junction protein in astrocytes) and aquaporin-4 (a marker of astrocytes associated with water transfer) in these astrocytes (Kovacs et al., 2018b). Subpial ARTAG initiated in basal regions (i.e., pattern 1) proceeding towards the convexity of the brain could suggest a disease mechanism related to the circulation of the cerebrospinal fluid (Kovacs et al., 2018a). In contrast, ARTAG initiated in the dorsolateral lobar areas (i.e., pattern 2) and dorsolateral parts of the brainstem suggest a local inducing factor (i.e., mechanical), including in some cases mild traumatic brain injury (Kovacs et al., 2018a).

Clinical Relevance of ARTAG

Following the examination of patients with a non-fluent variant of primary progressive aphasia associated with AD pathology (logopenic variant of primary progressive aphasia), Munoz et al. (2007) was the first group to discuss the possibility that TSAs may have clinical significance. The authors referred to these astrocytic inclusions as "argyrophilic thorny astrocyte clusters (ATACs)" and described them in the frontal, temporal, and parietal cortices and in the subcortical WM (Munoz et al., 2007). Other studies, however, did not found a clear association between ATACs and focal syndromes (Mesulam et al., 2008; Bigio et al., 2010). Recent studies have shown that lobar WM ARTAG is frequent in AD-related pathology (Kovacs et al., 2017c). A recent study confirmed this and further demonstrated that lobar ARTAG correlates with older age and higher Braak stage. However, ARTAG pathology was found equally prevalent in AD cases with typical and atypical clinical presentations (Nolan et al., 2019). A further interesting aspect of WM ARTAG in AD has been recently highlighted. Accordingly, irrespective of the regional NFT burden worsening language and visuospatial functions were correlated with higher TSA density in language-related and visuospatial-related regions, respectively (Resende et al., 2020).

Widespread distribution of gray matter GFAs has also been reported in elderly patients with cognitive decline with or without parkinsonism (Kovacs et al., 2011). In a subsequent study in an aging cohort, four different patterns of ARTAG were described based on the anatomical distribution of the tau astrogliopathy and its combination with neuronal tau pathology (Kovacs et al., 2013a). These include: (1) medial temporal lobe type; (2) amygdala type; (3) limbic-basal ganglia-nigral type with neuronal tauopathy; and (4) hippocampus-dentate gyrus-amygdala type with neuronal tauopathy (Kovacs et al., 2013a). These different ARTAG patterns overlap with the sequential distribution patterns described above for gray matter ARTAG (Kovacs et al., 2018a). However, TSAs in the dentate gyrus of the hippocampus seems to be an unusual feature, which was recognized by other groups as well (Lace et al., 2012). Indeed, mathematical modeling of hippocampal tau immunolabeling patterns suggested tau astrogliopathy in the elderly involve hippocampal subregions in a different pattern from that observed in primary tauopathies (Milenkovic et al., 2014). The remarkable involvement of the dentate gyrus suggests a distinct pathogenesis, particularly that this subregion might eventually show alterations related to (preclinical?) epileptic mechanisms. A further study involving individuals aged 90 years or older with cognitive decline found an association with cortical ARTAG independent of AD pathology (Robinson et al., 2018).

In summary, depending on the type (e.g., gray matter) and location (e.g., limbic system or WM adjacent to regions related to focal cortical symptoms) of ARTAG pathology it might be a pathological indicator of a reduced threshold, which might lead to decompensation of cognitive functions. Moreover, in combination with other pathologies, even with a different pathogenesis, an additive effect of ARTAG to reach the individual threshold for cognitive decompensation might be seen.

The Peculiar Relation of ARTAG and CTE

The current neuropathological consensus definition of CTE emphasizes the occurrence of neuronal and astrocytic tau "around small vessels in an irregular pattern at the depths of the cortical sulci" (McKee et al., 2016). However, this definition has been used with various interpretations, which makes many studies difficult to reconcile. Some studies interpret subpial TSAs in the depth of cortical sulci as CTE whereas other studies interpret the definition verbatim, and without neuronal tau did not use the term CTE. Examples of overlapping aspects of astrocytic tau accumulation in brains with CTE and that seen in ARTAG in aging cohorts include accumulation of astrocytes in basal brain regions and dorsolateral lobar areas in subpial, perivascular and gray matter locations, association with ventricular enlargement, or overrepresentation of males (McKee et al., 2013, 2015, 2016; Liu et al., 2016; Kovacs et al., 2017c). Forrest et al. (2019c) assessed the brain regions involved in early CTE stages (i.e., frontal, temporal and parietal cortices) in 310 aged participants in a European community-based population for the presence of CTE and ARTAG. This study found that no cases satisfied current diagnostic criteria for CTE although 117 displayed cortical ARTAG. Isolated phosphorylated-tau pathologies occurring at the depths of cortical sulci were found in 25 individuals (8%; 7 Forrest et al., 2019c), but due to the lack of neuronal tau accumulation in a pathognomonic location (McKee et al., 2016), these isolated features did not warrant the diagnosis of CTE. These observations supported the notion that ARTAG is a common age-related pathology in community populations and CTE is absent or rarely observed (Forrest et al., 2019c). Together, with an additional study, these observations corroborate that isolated phosphorylated-tau immunoreactivities in the correct context could be interpreted only as a possible feature (Bieniek et al., 2020) or component (Forrest et al., 2019c), but in isolation not diagnostic, of CTE pathology.

Today, it is difficult to prove or exclude the possibility that some kinds of traumatic brain injuries (which might be different than those associated with currently defined CTE-related pathology) induce astrocytic tau pathologies in isolation or that astrocytic tau pathologies are the first in some cases of whatever type of trauma. There is a lack of standardized questionnaires on mild and repeated head injuries in population-based studies that have evaluated astrocytic tau pathology systematically, which makes the interpretation of results difficult. Current knowledge suggests that the neuronal tau pathology component is required to diagnose CTE. The generation of a CTE-specific tau antibody could help to reconcile this question. Alternatively, in well-documented cohorts of mild traumatic brain injury, the "components" (Forrest et al., 2019c) or "features" (Bieniek et al., 2020) of CTE pathology could be evaluated in isolation and together. Theoretically, in the same brain, there are likely regions with neuronal tau in the "correct location" for CTE while other regions will show astrocytic pathology in isolation.

The Relation of ARTAG and Primary Tauopathy-Related Astrogliopathies

TSAs and GFAs are commonly observed in primary tauopathies, although they are not the distinguishing astrocytic inclusions. The concept of the maturation of tau deposition in astrocytes can lead to the appearance of GFA-like morphologies in PSP, CBD, PiD and GGT (Kovacs et al., 2017a,c). The distribution of the striatal type pattern of gray matter ARTAG in the ageing brain is reminiscent of the distribution of astrocytic tau pathology in PSP. Indeed, in PSP striatum (stage 1) is followed by cortical (frontal-parietal to temporal to occipital) involvement (stage 2a and b, respectively) proceeding then to the amygdala (stage 3) and the brainstem (stage 4; Kovacs et al., 2018a). In contrast, for CBD first involves the frontal (including premotor) and parietal cortices (stage 1) proceeding to the temporal and occipital cortices (stage 2). Subsequently and parallelly subcortical areas, including either, or both, the striatum and the amygdala (stage 3) are involved, followed by the brainstem (stage 4) including the midbrain followed rarely by the pons and medulla oblongata.

Moreover, in CBD a distinct morphology, characterized by tau immunoreactivity of subpial astrocytic end-feet, has been recognized. This is the predominant subpial astrocytic tau pathology in CBD independently of subpial ARTAG in basal brain regions (together representing stage 1). This is followed by the involvement of the brainstem, representing stage 2. This was termed a "masked" bidirectional sequence (Kovacs et al., 2018a). This means that pattern 1 described above for subpial ARTAG in non-CBD cases starting at basal areas and proceeding towards lobar subpial location is masked by the predominant end-feet tau immunoreactivity in subpial locations of lobar areas in CBD (Kovacs et al., 2018a). This concept exemplifies that classical ARTAG and its sequential distribution patterns can be present as "comorbid tauopathy" in primary tauopathies characterized by prominent and distinctive astroglial tau pathologies such as TAs or AP. Thus, these overlaps and combinations of astroglial pathologies might influence interpretations of tau immunoreactivities.

SYNTHESIS: THE PATHOGENIC RELATION OF TAU AND ASTROGLIA

The factor or event that triggers tau aggregation in diverse conditions is yet to be identified. The pathological process of tau aggregation is thought to lead to a *gain of toxic function* paralleled by a loss of physiological functions of tau which alter synaptic functions (Goedert et al., 2017a). Overexpression of mutant human tau leads to filament formation and recapitulates features of human tauopathies (Goedert, 2016). However, overexpression of wild-type human tau in mouse brain does not result in the accumulation of filamentous inclusions in astroglia (Götz et al., 1995), which might question the early role of astroglia in the aggregation process of tau. On the other hand, astroglial activation and reaction seems to precede neuronal loss in PiD (and other FTLD proteinopathies; Kersaitis et al., 2004), supporting an early role of astroglia in the pathogenesis of neurodegeneration itself, eventually before protein aggregation takes place.

Interestingly, divergent patterns of transcriptional associations for neuronal and astroglial tau lesions have been described in PSP (Allen et al., 2018). While neuronal tau pathology is positively associated with a brain co-expression network enriched for synaptic and PSP candidate risk genes, astroglial tau pathology is positively associated with a microglial gene-enriched immune network (Allen et al., 2018). This observation can facilitate the understanding of why there is a difference between brain regions and whether different brain regions preferentially accumulate more neuronal or astroglial tau.

To interpret astrocytic tau accumulation the following theoretical possibilities can be considered (**Figure 3**). First, that astroglia does express subtle (or with current methods is undetectable) levels of tau, which is upregulated and then hyperphosphorylated as a response to an unidentified neurodegeneration-inducing event. There are only scarce studies, which claim that tau might be expressed in astrocytes. For example, positive immunostaining for tau in the normal human brain and astrocytic tumors (Shin et al., 1991; Miyazono et al., 1993) and mRNA expression of tau in astrocytic tumors (Miyazono et al., 1993) have been reported, and the authors considered that astrocytes have a potential to express tau through neoplastic transformation and reactive processes (Miyazono et al., 1993). These observations need to be replicated using current methods, since this would widen the pathophysiological interpretation of astrocytic tau accumulation in NDDs and normal brain aging. However, it is currently more favoured that astrocytes do not contain endogenous tau. Indeed, the pioneering study on tau mRNA expression examining samples of the hippocampus and cerebral cortex evaluated dark-field photomicrographs following hybridization with different probes and found expression only in neurons and not glia (Goedert et al., 1989). In this respect, it is still a puzzle why phosphorylated-tau positive astrocytes are observed in ARTAG without neuronal tau accumulation. This could support the concept of low amounts of tau expression astroglia and

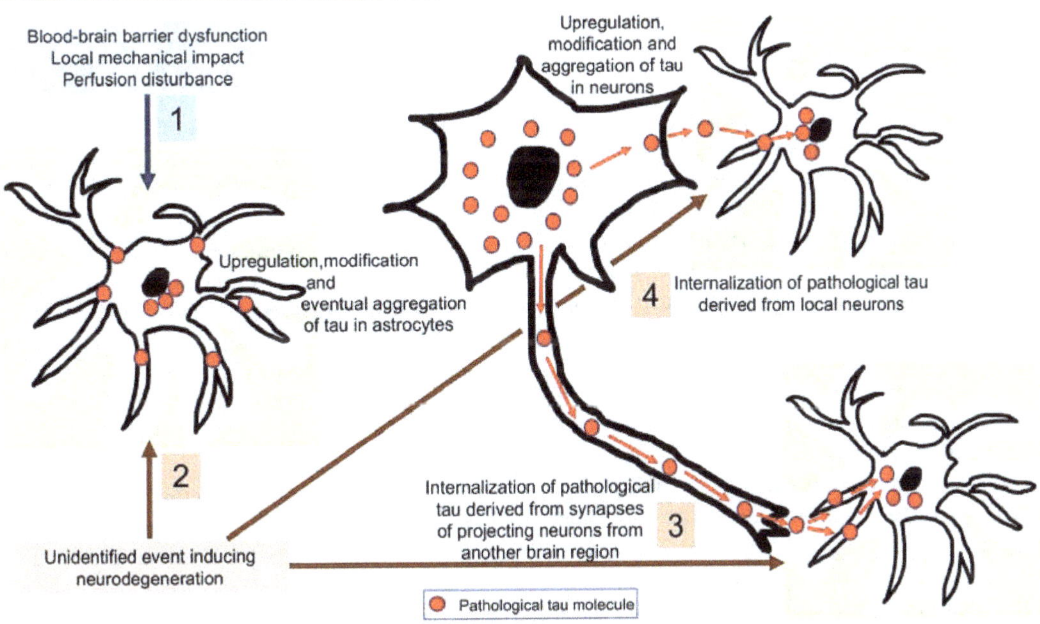

FIGURE 3 | Interpretation of astrocytic tau accumulation. 1: Astroglia expresses subtle levels of tau, which is upregulated and then hyperphosphorylated as a response to a yet unidentified neurodegeneration-inducing event. 2: Tau-overexpression and hyperphosphorylation occurs in astrocytes as a response to a non-neurodegenerative event such as blood-brain barrier dysfunction, perfusion disturbance or a local mechanical impact. 3: Internalization of pathological tau derived from synapses of projecting neurons from another brain region. 4: Internalization of pathological tau derived from local neurons.

suggest that accumulation of tau in astrocytes does happen independently from neuronal tau, but does not necessarily represent a neurodegenerative cause. As exemplified by ARTAG, tau accumulation in astrocytes might reflect the various impacts that individuals can be affected by during life including mechanical impact, perfusion disturbance, or barrier dysfunction.

The most universal view is that astrocytic tau can only be explained by its internalization from the extracellular milieu since astrocytes have been found to express phagocytic receptors such as those phagocytizing synapses (Chung et al., 2013) or axonal mitochondria (Davis et al., 2014) in the brain. Although heparan sulfate proteoglycans have been proposed to be responsible for fibrillary tau uptake in various cell types, astrocytic uptake of tau uptake was found to be an independent process (Perea et al., 2019). Since some brain regions accumulate pathological tau in astroglia before neurons (Ling et al., 2016; Kovacs et al., 2018a), it can be also proposed that these tau-positive astrocytes might phagocytize pathological tau derived from projecting neurons. Another possibility is that astrocytes take up tau secreted from the cytoplasm of local neurons. For these scenarios, presynaptic vesicular secretion, direct translocation from the neuronal cytoplasm across the plasma membrane, release *via* secretory lysosomes, microvesicle shedding, or exosome release could be the source of pathological tau (Sebastián-Serrano et al., 2018) for uptake by astroglia. The observation of an inverse correlation between astroglial and neuronal tau pathology in experimental models was interpreted as support for the transmission of pathological tau from neurons to neighboring astrocytes, or as inter-astrocytic transfer of tau (Narasimhan et al., 2017). Accumulation of tau in astroglia might clear tau from the extracellular space and buffer the neurotoxicity of pathological tau until astrocytes become overloaded. Even without accumulating tau, astroglia in a brain affected by tauopathy might show dysfunction. This is exemplified by an observation indicating that astrocyte transplantation may be neuroprotective in a mouse line transgenic for human P301S tau (Hampton et al., 2010). On the other hand, astroglial tau could be detrimental to neurons. Indeed, neuronal degeneration can be detected in the absence of neuronal tau inclusions but associated with astroglial tau pathology (Forman et al., 2005). Further studies speculated that oxidative damage leads to GFAP fragmentation, indicating dysfunction of pathological tau-harboring protoplasmic astrocytes in PSP, associated with neuronal dysfunction (Santpere and Ferrer, 2009; Song et al., 2009). Studies in cultured hippocampal neurons suggest that extracellular tau oligomers accumulate in astrocytes followed by disrupted intracellular Ca^{2+} signaling and Ca^{2+}-dependent release of gliotransmitters altogether contributing to synaptic dysfunction (Piacentini et al., 2017). In summary, the neuroprotective function of astroglia, in particular the proper protection of neurons from glutamate neurotoxicity, may be impaired early in tauopathies and/or astroglia may gain novel neurotoxic properties (Sidoryk-Wegrzynowicz and Struzyńska, 2019). The latter might be linked to neuroinflammatory responses also, in particular that astroglia may upregulate genes encoding pro-inflammatory mediators and that microglial activation may induce the formation of a subtype of astrocytes (A1; Liddelow et al., 2017) with potential detrimental effects on neurons (Sidoryk-Wegrzynowicz and Struzyńska, 2019).

In AD, evaluation of the astroglial response is complicated by the fact that in addition to tau, Aβ is also present and this might lead to different reactions as in primary tauopathies or ARTAG. Indeed, astrocytes may directly participate in APP metabolism and Aβ clearance (Ries and Sastre, 2016) but they seem to be implicated in neurofibrillary degeneration of AD where the number of activated astrocytes correlates not only with the burden of tangles (Serrano-Pozo et al., 2011) but with the stage of tangle formation (i.e., pretangles to ghost tangles) formation (Sheng et al., 1997). Ultrastructural examination of ghost tangles revealed the presence of astrocytic processes with paired-helical filaments suggesting their incorporation by astrocytes (Ikeda et al., 1992). On the other hand, a population-based study suggested that classical Alzheimer-type pathology is a poor explanatory variable for the astrocyte response seen in the aging brain and rather that astrocytes may respond to other age-associated events (Simpson et al., 2010). Thus, the astroglial response in the neurodegenerating or aging brain might not exactly reflect the pathogenesis of primary tauopathy-related astroglia response where tau protein itself accumulates in these cells.

QUESTIONS TO BE ANSWERED

Astroglia accumulate pathological tau in various disease conditions and normal brain aging. The question remains whether astrocytic tau accumulation uniformly precedes, parallels, or follows neuronal tau in all situations. It also remains unknown whether and how astroglial tau accumulation can develop independently from neuronal tau (see for example subpial TSAs). There is a paucity of data on whether different populations of astrocytes are vulnerable in different disorders accumulating tau in astrocytes and where astrocytic tau originates from, including the mechanism of secretion of tau taken up potentially by astrocytes. There is currently a lack of data on whether astrocytes have a peculiar biochemical tau signatures that differs from neurons. Finally, it remains to be determined whether tau neuroimaging or bodily fluid tau-biomarkers represent astroglial tau accumulation or purely neuronal tau accumulation. Thus, the role of astroglia in tau-associated diseases has still unexplored fields that require communication between glia researchers and tau experts.

AUTHOR CONTRIBUTIONS

GK wrote the article.

REFERENCES

Ahmed, Z., Bigio, E. H., Budka, H., Dickson, D. W., Ferrer, I., Ghetti, B., et al. (2013). Globular glial tauopathies (GGT): consensus recommendations. *Acta Neuropathol.* 126, 537–544. doi: 10.1007/s00401-013-1171-0

Alexander, J., Kalev, O., Mehrabian, S., Traykov, L., Raycheva, M., Kanakis, D., et al. (2016). Familial early-onset dementia with complex neuropathologic phenotype and genomic background. *Neurobiol. Aging* 42, 199–204. doi: 10.1016/j.neurobiolaging.2016.03.012

Allen, M., Wang, X., Serie, D. J., Strickland, S. L., Burgess, J. D., Koga, S., et al. (2018). Divergent brain gene expression patterns associate with distinct cell-specific tau neuropathology traits in progressive supranuclear palsy. *Acta Neuropathol.* 136, 709–727. doi: 10.1007/s00401-018-1900-5

Arima, K. (2006). Utrastructural characteristics of tau filaments in tauopathies: immuno-electron microscopic demonstration of tau filaments in tauopathies. *Neuropathology* 26, 475–483. doi: 10.1111/j.1440-1789.2006.00669.x

Bancher, C., Brunner, C., Lassmann, H., Budka, H., Jellinger, K., Seitelberger, F., et al. (1989). Tau and ubiquitin immunoreactivity at different stages of formation of Alzheimer neurofibrillary tangles. *Prog Clin Biol Res* 317, 837–848. doi: 10.1097/00002093-198802030-00051

Baskota, S. U., Lopez, O. L., Greenamyre, J. T., and Kofler, J. (2019). Spectrum of tau pathologies in Huntington's disease. *Lab. Invest.* 99, 1068–1077. doi: 10.1038/s41374-018-0166-9

Bieniek, K. F., Blessing, M. M., Heckman, M. G., Diehl, N. N., Serie, A. M., Paolini, M. A. II., et al. (2020). Association between contact sports participation and chronic traumatic encephalopathy: a retrospective cohort study. *Brain Pathol.* 30, 63–74. doi: 10.1111/bpa.12757

Bigio, E. H., Mishra, M., Hatanpaa, K. J., White, C. L. III., Johnson, N., Rademaker, A., et al. (2010). TDP-43 pathology in primary progressive aphasia and frontotemporal dementia with pathologic Alzheimer disease. *Acta Neuropathol.* 120, 43–54. doi: 10.1007/s00401-010-0681-2

Boluda, S., Iba, M., Zhang, B., Raible, K. M., Lee, V. M., and Trojanowski, J. Q. (2015). Differential induction and spread of tau pathology in young PS19 tau transgenic mice following intracerebral injections of pathological tau from Alzheimer's disease or corticobasal degeneration brains. *Acta Neuropathol.* 129, 221–237. doi: 10.1007/s00401-014-1373-0

Botez, G., Probst, A., Ipsen, S., and Tolnay, M. (1999). Astrocytes expressing hyperphosphorylated tau protein without glial fibrillary tangles in argyrophilic grain disease. *Acta Neuropathol.* 98, 251–256. doi: 10.1007/s004010051077

Brettschneider, J., Del Tredici, K., Lee, V. M., and Trojanowski, J. Q. (2015). Spreading of pathology in neurodegenerative diseases: a focus on human studies. *Nat. Rev. Neurosci.* 16, 109–120. doi: 10.1038/nrn3887

Buée, L., Bussière, T., Buée-Scherrer, V., Delacourte, A., and Hof, P. R. (2000). Tau protein isoforms, phosphorylation, and role in neurodegenerative disorders. *Brain Res. Rev.* 33, 95–130. doi: 10.1016/s0165-0173(00)00019-9

Chung, W. S., Clarke, L. E., Wang, G. X., Stafford, B. K., Sher, A., Chakraborty, C., et al. (2013). Astrocytes mediate synapse elimination through MEGF10 and MERTK pathways. *Nature* 504, 394–400. doi: 10.1038/nature12776

Clavaguera, F., Bolmont, T., Crowther, R. A., Abramowski, D., Frank, S., Probst, A., et al. (2009). Transmission and spreading of tauopathy in transgenic mouse brain. *Nat. Cell Biol.* 11, 909–913. doi: 10.1038/ncb1901

Cornejo, V. H., and Hetz, C. (2013). The unfolded protein response in Alzheimer's disease. *Semin. Immunopathol.* 35, 277–292. doi: 10.1007/s00281-013-0373-9

Crary, J. F., Trojanowski, J. Q., Schneider, J. A., Abisambra, J. F., Abner, E. L., Alafuzoff, I., et al. (2014). Primary age-related tauopathy (PART): a common pathology associated with human aging. *Acta Neuropathol.* 128, 755–766. doi: 10.1007/s00401-014-1349-0

Davis, C. H., Kim, K. Y., Bushong, E. A., Mills, E. A., Boassa, D., Shih, T., et al. (2014). Transcellular degradation of axonal mitochondria. *Proc. Natl. Acad. Sci. U S A* 111, 9633–9638. doi: 10.1073/pnas.1404651111

Dickson, D. W. (1998). Pick's disease: a modern approach. *Brain Pathol.* 8, 339–354. doi: 10.1111/j.1750-3639.1998.tb00158.x

Dickson, D. W., Ahmed, Z., Algom, A. A., Tsuboi, Y., and Josephs, K. A. (2010). Neuropathology of variants of progressive supranuclear palsy. *Curr. Opin. Neurol.* 23, 394–400. doi: 10.1097/WCO.0b013e32833be924

Dujardin, S., Bégard, S., Caillierez, R., Lachaud, C., Delattre, L., Carrier, S., et al. (2014). Ectosomes: a new mechanism for non-exosomal secretion of tau protein. *PLoS One* 9:e100760. doi: 10.1371/journal.pone.0100760

Ettle, B., Schlachetzki, J. C. M., and Winkler, J. (2016). Oligodendroglia and myelin in neurodegenerative diseases: more than just bystanders? *Mol. Neurobiol.* 53, 3046–3062. doi: 10.1007/s12035-015-9205-3

Falcon, B., Zhang, W., Murzin, A. G., Murshudov, G., Garringer, H. J., Vidal, R., et al. (2018a). Structures of filaments from Pick's disease reveal a novel tau protein fold. *Nature* 561, 137–140. doi: 10.1038/s41586-018-0454-y

Falcon, B., Zhang, W., Schweighauser, M., Murzin, A. G., Vidal, R., Garringer, H. J., et al. (2018b). Tau filaments from multiple cases of sporadic and inherited Alzheimer's disease adopt a common fold. *Acta Neuropathol.* 136, 699–708. doi: 10.1007/s00401-018-1914-z

Falcon, B., Zivanov, J., Zhang, W., Murzin, A. G., Garringer, H. J., Vidal, R., et al. (2019). Novel tau filament fold in chronic traumatic encephalopathy encloses hydrophobic molecules. *Nature* 568, 420–423. doi: 10.1038/s41586-019-1026-5

Feany, M. B., and Dickson, D. W. (1995). Widespread cytoskeletal pathology characterizes corticobasal degeneration. *Am. J. Pathol.* 146, 1388–1396.

Feany, M. B., Mattiace, L. A., and Dickson, D. W. (1996). Neuropathologic overlap of progressive supranuclear palsy, Pick's disease and corticobasal degeneration. *J. Neuropathol. Exp. Neurol.* 55, 53–67. doi: 10.1097/00005072-199601000-00006

Ferrer, I. (2017). Diversity of astroglial responses across human neurodegenerative disorders and brain aging. *Brain Pathol.* 27, 645–674. doi: 10.1111/bpa.12538

Ferrer, I. (2018). Astrogliopathy in tauopathies. *Neuroglia* 1, 126–150. doi: 10.3390/neuroglia1010010

Ferrer, I., Andrés-Benito, P., Zelaya, M. V., Aguirre, M. E. E., Carmona, M., Ausin, K., et al. (2020a). Familial globular glial tauopathy linked to MAPT mutations: molecular neuropathology and seeding capacity of a prototypical mixed neuronal and glial tauopathy. *Acta Neuropathol.* 139, 735–771. doi: 10.1007/s00401-019-02122-9

Ferrer, I., Zelaya, M. V., Aguiló Garcia, M., Carmona, M., López-González, I., Andrés-Benito, P., et al. (2020b). Relevance of host tau in tau seeding and spreading in tauopathies. *Brain Pathol.* 30, 298–318. doi: 10.1111/bpa.12778

Ferrer, I., García, M. A., González, I. L., Lucena, D. D., Villalonga, A. R., Tech, M. C., et al. (2018). Aging-related tau astrogliopathy (ARTAG): not only tau phosphorylation in astrocytes. *Brain Pathol.* 28, 965–985. doi: 10.1111/bpa.12593

Ferrer, I., Legati, A., García-Monco, J. C., Gomez-Beldarrain, M., Carmona, M., Blanco, R., et al. (2015). Familial behavioral variant frontotemporal dementia associated with astrocyte-predominant tauopathy. *J. Neuropathol. Exp. Neurol.* 74, 370–379. doi: 10.1097/nen.0000000000000180

Ferrer, I., López-González, I., Carmona, M., Arregui, L., Dalfó, E., Torrejón-Escribano, B., et al. (2014). Glial and neuronal tau pathology in tauopathies: characterization of disease-specific phenotypes and tau pathology progression. *J. Neuropathol. Exp. Neurol.* 73, 81–97. doi: 10.1097/nen.0000000000000030

Ferrer, I., Pastor, P., Rey, M. J., Muñoz, E., Puig, B., Pastor, E., et al. (2003). Tau phosphorylation and kinase activation in familial tauopathy linked to deln296 mutation. *Neuropathol. Appl. Neurobiol.* 29, 23–34. doi: 10.1046/j.1365-2990.2003.00435.x

Forman, M. S., Lal, D., Zhang, B., Dabir, D. V., Swanson, E., Lee, V. M., et al. (2005). Transgenic mouse model of tau pathology in astrocytes leading to nervous system degeneration. *J. Neurosci.* 25, 3539–3550. doi: 10.1523/JNEUROSCI.0081-05.2005

Forrest, S. L., Halliday, G. M., Shepherd, C. E., Kwok, J. B., Hallupp, M., and Kril, J. J. (2019a). Are mutations in MAPT associated with GGT type III? *Neuropathol. Appl. Neurobiol.* doi: 10.1111/nan.12583 [Epub ahead of print].

Forrest, S. L., Kril, J. J., and Halliday, G. M. (2019b). Cellular and regional vulnerability in frontotemporal tauopathies. *Acta Neuropathol.* 138, 705–727. doi: 10.1007/s00401-019-02035-7

Forrest, S. L., Kril, J. J., Wagner, S., Hönigschnabl, S., Reiner, A., Fischer, P., et al. (2019c). Chronic traumatic encephalopathy (CTE) is absent from a european community-based aging cohort while cortical aging-related tau astrogliopathy (ARTAG) is highly prevalent. *J. Neuropathol. Exp. Neurol.* 78, 398–405. doi: 10.1093/jnen/nlz017

Forrest, S. L., Kril, J. J., Stevens, C. H., Kwok, J. B., Hallupp, M., Kim, W. S., et al. (2018). Retiring the term FTDP-17 as MAPT mutations are genetic forms of sporadic frontotemporal tauopathies. *Brain* 141, 521–534. doi: 10.1093/brain/awx328

Gelpi, E., Höftberger, R., Graus, F., Ling, H., Holton, J. L., Dawson, T., et al. (2016). Neuropathological criteria of anti-IgLON5-related tauopathy. *Acta Neuropathol.* 132, 531–543. doi: 10.1007/s00401-016-1591-8

Gelpi, E., van der Zee, J., Turon Estrada, A., Van Broeckhoven, C., and Sanchez-Valle, R. (2014). TARDBP mutation p.Ile383Val associated with semantic dementia and complex proteinopathy. *Neuropathol. Appl. Neurobiol.* 40, 225–230. doi: 10.1111/nan.12063

Ghetti, B., Oblak, A. L., Boeve, B. F., Johnson, K. A., Dickerson, B. C., and Goedert, M. (2015). Invited review: frontotemporal dementia caused by microtubule-associated protein tau gene (MAPT) mutations: a chameleon for neuropathology and neuroimaging. *Neuropathol. Appl. Neurobiol.* 41, 24–46. doi: 10.1111/nan.12213

Ghetti, B., Wszolek, Z., Boeve, B., Spina, S., and Goedert, M. (2011). "Frontotemporal dementia and parkinsonism linked to chromosome 17," in *Neurodegeneration: The Molecular Pathology of Dementia and Movement Disorders*, eds D. W. Dickson and R. O. Weller (Chichester, UK: Blackwell Publishing Ltd.), 110–134.

Goedert, M. (2016). The ordered assembly of tau is the gain-of-toxic function that causes human tauopathies. *Alzheimers Dement.* 12, 1040–1050. doi: 10.1016/j.jalz.2016.09.001

Goedert, M. (2018). Tau filaments in neurodegenerative diseases. *FEBS Lett.* 592, 2383–2391. doi: 10.1002/1873-3468.13108

Goedert, M., Eisenberg, D. S., and Crowther, R. A. (2017a). Propagation of tau aggregates and neurodegeneration. *Annu. Rev. Neurosci.* 40, 189–210. doi: 10.1146/annurev-neuro-072116-031153

Goedert, M., Masuda-Suzukake, M., and Falcon, B. (2017b). Like prions: the propagation of aggregated tau and α-synuclein in neurodegeneration. *Brain* 140, 266–278. doi: 10.1093/brain/aww230

Goedert, M., Spillantini, M. G., Potier, M. C., Ulrich, J., and Crowther, R. A. (1989). Cloning and sequencing of the cDNA encoding an isoform of microtubule-associated protein tau containing four tandem repeats: differential expression of tau protein mRNAs in human brain. *EMBO J.* 8, 393–399. doi: 10.1002/j.1460-2075.1989.tb03390.x

Gómez-Tortosa, E., Baradaran-Heravi, Y., González Alvarez, V., Sainz, M. J., Prieto-Jurczynska, C., Guerrero-López, R., et al. (2019). Presence of tau astrogliopathy in frontotemporal dementia caused by a novel Grn nonsense (Trp2*) mutation. *Neurobiol. Aging* 76, 214.e211–214.e215. doi: 10.1016/j.neurobiolaging.2018.11.010

Götz, J., Probst, A., Spillantini, M. G., Schäfer, T., Jakes, R., Bürki, K., et al. (1995). Somatodendritic localization and hyperphosphorylation of tau protein in transgenic mice expressing the longest human brain tau isoform. *EMBO J.* 14, 1304–1313. doi: 10.1002/j.1460-2075.1995.tb07116.x

Halliday, G. M., Song, Y. J., Creasey, H., Morris, J. G., Brooks, W. S., and Kril, J. J. (2006). Neuropathology in the S305S tau gene mutation. *Brain* 129:E40. doi: 10.1093/brain/awh720

Hampton, D. W., Webber, D. J., Bilican, B., Goedert, M., Spillantini, M. G., and Chandran, S. (2010). Cell-mediated neuroprotection in a mouse model of human tauopathy. *J. Neurosci.* 30, 9973–9983. doi: 10.1523/JNEUROSCI.0834-10.2010

Hauw, J. J., Verny, M., Delaere, P., Cervera, P., He, Y., and Duyckaerts, C. (1990). Constant neurofibrillary changes in the neocortex in progressive supranuclear palsy. Basic differences with Alzheimer's disease and aging. *Neurosci. Lett.* 119, 182–186. doi: 10.1016/0304-3940(90)90829-x

Hayashi, S., Toyoshima, Y., Hasegawa, M., Umeda, Y., Wakabayashi, K., Tokiguchi, S., et al. (2002). Late-onset frontotemporal dementia with a novel exon 1 (Arg5His) tau gene mutation. *Ann. Neurol.* 51, 525–530. doi: 10.1002/ana.10163

Heneka, M. T., Kummer, M. P., and Latz, E. (2014). Innate immune activation in neurodegenerative disease. *Nat. Rev. Immunol.* 14, 463–477. doi: 10.1038/nri3705

Ikeda, K. (1996). Glial fibrillary tangles and argyrophilic threads: classification and disease specificity. *Neuropathology* 16, 71–77. doi: 10.1111/j.1440-1789.1996.tb00158.x

Ikeda, K., Akiyama, H., Arai, T., and Nishimura, T. (1998). Glial tau pathology in neurodegenerative diseases: their nature and comparison with neuronal tangles. *Neurobiol. Aging* 19, S85–S91. doi: 10.1016/s0197-4580(98)00034-7

Ikeda, K., Akiyama, H., Kondo, H., Haga, C., Tanno, E., Tokuda, T., et al. (1995). Thorn-shaped astrocytes: possibly secondarily induced tau-positive glial fibrillary tangles. *Acta Neuropathol.* 90, 620–625. doi: 10.1007/bf00318575

Ikeda, K., Haga, C., Akiyama, H., Kase, K., and Iritani, S. (1992). Coexistence of paired helical filaments and glial filaments in astrocytic processes within ghost tangles. *Neurosci. Lett.* 148, 126–128. doi: 10.1016/0304-3940(92)90820-w

Ikeda, C., Yokota, O., Nagao, S., Ishizu, H., Oshima, E., Hasegawa, M., et al. (2016). The relationship between development of neuronal and astrocytic tau pathologies in subcortical nuclei and progression of argyrophilic grain disease. *Brain Pathol.* 26, 488–505. doi: 10.1111/bpa.12319

Jadhav, S., Avila, J., Scholl, M., Kovacs, G. G., Kövari, E., Skrabana, R., et al. (2019). A walk through tau therapeutic strategies. *Acta Neuropathol. Commun.* 7:22. doi: 10.1186/s40478-019-0664-z

Kersaitis, C., Halliday, G. M., and Kril, J. J. (2004). Regional and cellular pathology in frontotemporal dementia: relationship to stage of disease in cases with and without Pick bodies. *Acta Neuropathol.* 108, 515–523. doi: 10.1007/s00401-004-0917-0

Klein, C., Kramer, E. M., Cardine, A. M., Schraven, B., Brandt, R., and Trotter, J. (2002). Process outgrowth of oligodendrocytes is promoted by interaction of fyn kinase with the cytoskeletal protein tau. *J. Neurosci.* 22, 698–707. doi: 10.1523/JNEUROSCI.22-03-00698.2002

Kovacs, G. G. (2015). Invited review: neuropathology of tauopathies: principles and practice. *Neuropathol. Appl. Neurobiol.* 41, 3–23. doi: 10.1111/nan.12208

Kovacs, G. G. (2016). Molecular pathological classification of neurodegenerative diseases: turning towards precision medicine. *Int. J. Mol. Sci.* 17:E189. doi: 10.3390/ijms17020189

Kovacs, G. G. (2017). Tauopathies. *Handb. Clin. Neurol.* 145, 355–368. doi: 10.1016/B978-0-12-802395-2.00025-0

Kovacs, G. G. (2019a). Molecular pathology of neurodegenerative diseases: principles and practice. *J. Clin. Pathol.* 72, 725–735. doi: 10.1136/jclinpath-2019-205952

Kovacs, G. G. (2019b). Are comorbidities compatible with a molecular pathological classification of neurodegenerative diseases? *Curr. Opin. Neurol.* 32, 279–291. doi: 10.1097/WCO.0000000000000664

Kovacs, G. G., Alafuzoff, I., Al-Sarraj, S., Arzberger, T., Bogdanovic, N., Capellari, S., et al. (2008). Mixed brain pathologies in dementia: the BrainNet Europe consortium experience. *Dement. Geriatr. Cogn. Disord.* 26, 343–350. doi: 10.1159/000161560

Kovacs, G. G., Ferrer, I., Grinberg, L. T., Alafuzoff, I., Attems, J., Budka, H., et al. (2016). Aging-related tau astrogliopathy (ARTAG): harmonized evaluation strategy. *Acta Neuropathol.* 131, 87–102. doi: 10.1007/s00401-015-1509-x

Kovacs, G. G., Lee, V. M., and Trojanowski, J. Q. (2017a). Protein astrogliopathies in human neurodegenerative diseases and aging. *Brain Pathol.* 27, 675–690. doi: 10.1111/bpa.12536

Kovacs, G. G., Rahimi, J., Ströbel, T., Lutz, M. I., Regelsberger, G., Streichenberger, N., et al. (2017b). Tau pathology in Creutzfeldt-Jakob disease revisited. *Brain Pathol.* 27, 332–344. doi: 10.1111/bpa.12411

Kovacs, G. G., Robinson, J. L., Xie, S. X., Lee, E. B., Grossman, M., Wolk, D. A., et al. (2017c). Evaluating the patterns of aging-related tau astrogliopathy unravels novel insights into brain aging and neurodegenerative diseases. *J. Neuropathol. Exp. Neurol.* 76, 270–288. doi: 10.1093/jnen/nlx007

Kovacs, G. G., Xie, S. X., Lee, E. B., Robinson, J. L., Caswell, C., Irwin, D. J., et al. (2017d). Multisite assessment of aging-related tau astrogliopathy (ARTAG). *J. Neuropathol. Exp. Neurol.* 76, 605–619. doi: 10.1093/jnen/nlx041

Kovacs, G. G., Milenkovic, I., Wohrer, A., Hoftberger, R., Gelpi, E., Haberler, C., et al. (2013a). Non-Alzheimer neurodegenerative pathologies and their combinations are more frequent than commonly believed in the elderly brain: a community-based autopsy series. *Acta Neuropathol.* 126, 365–384. doi: 10.1007/s00401-013-1157-y

Kovacs, G. G., Rozemuller, A. J., Van Swieten, J. C., Gelpi, E., Majtenyi, K., Al-Sarraj, S., et al. (2013b). Neuropathology of the hippocampus in FTLD-Tau with Pick bodies: a study of the BrainNet Europe Consortium. *Neuropathol. Appl. Neurobiol.* 39, 166–178. doi: 10.1111/j.1365-2990.2012.01272.x

Kovacs, G. G., Molnar, K., Laszlo, L., Strobel, T., Botond, G., Honigschnabl, S., et al. (2011). A peculiar constellation of tau pathology defines a subset of dementia in the elderly. *Acta Neuropathol.* 122, 205–222. doi: 10.1007/s00401-011-0819-x

Kovacs, G. G., Xie, S. X., Robinson, J. L., Lee, E. B., Smith, D. H., Schuck, T., et al. (2018a). Sequential stages and distribution patterns of aging-related tau astrogliopathy (ARTAG) in the human brain. *Acta Neuropathol. Commun.* 6:50. doi: 10.1186/s40478-018-0552-y

Kovacs, G. G., Yousef, A., Kaindl, S., Lee, V. M., and Trojanowski, J. Q. (2018b). Connexin-43 and aquaporin-4 are markers of ageing-related tau astrogliopathy (ARTAG)-related astroglial response. *Neuropathol. Appl. Neurobiol.* 44, 491–505. doi: 10.1111/nan.12427

Lace, G., Ince, P. G., Brayne, C., Savva, G. M., Matthews, F. E., De Silva, R., et al. (2012). Mesial temporal astrocyte tau pathology in the MRC-CFAS ageing brain cohort. *Dement. Geriatr. Cogn. Disord.* 34, 15–24. doi: 10.1159/000341581

Lee, V. M., Goedert, M., and Trojanowski, J. Q. (2001). Neurodegenerative tauopathies. *Annu. Rev. Neurosci.* 24, 1121–1159. doi: 10.1146/annurev.neuro.24.1.1121

Le Guennec, K., Quenez, O., Nicolas, G., Wallon, D., Rousseau, S., Richard, A. C., et al. (2017). 17q21.31 duplication causes prominent tau-related dementia with increased MAPT expression. *Mol. Psychiatry* 22, 1119–1125. doi: 10.1038/mp.2016.226

Liddelow, S. A., Guttenplan, K. A., Clarke, L. E., Bennett, F. C., Bohlen, C. J., Schirmer, L., et al. (2017). Neurotoxic reactive astrocytes are induced by activated microglia. *Nature* 541, 481–487. doi: 10.1038/nature21029

Liddelow, S. A., and Sofroniew, M. V. (2019). Astrocytes usurp neurons as a disease focus. *Nat. Neurosci.* 22, 512–513. doi: 10.1038/s41593-019-0367-6

Ling, H., Gelpi, E., Davey, K., Jaunmuktane, Z., Mok, K. Y., Jabbari, E., et al. (2020). Fulminant corticobasal degeneration: a distinct variant with predominant neuronal tau aggregates. *Acta Neuropathol.* 139, 717–734. doi: 10.1007/s00401-019-02119-4

Ling, H., Kovacs, G. G., Vonsattel, J. P., Davey, K., Mok, K. Y., Hardy, J., et al. (2016). Astrogliopathy predominates the earliest stage of corticobasal degeneration pathology. *Brain* 139, 3237–3252. doi: 10.1093/brain/aww256

Liu, A. K., Goldfinger, M. H., Questari, H. E., Pearce, R. K., and Gentleman, S. M. (2016). ARTAG in the basal forebrain: widening the constellation of astrocytic tau pathology. *Acta Neuropathol. Commun.* 4:59. doi: 10.1186/s40478-016-0330-7

Malkani, R., D'Souza, I., Gwinn-Hardy, K., Schellenberg, G. D., Hardy, J., and Momeni, P. (2006). A MAPT mutation in a regulatory element upstream of exon 10 causes frontotemporal dementia. *Neurobiol. Dis.* 22, 401–403. doi: 10.1016/j.nbd.2005.12.001

Martínez-Maldonado, A., Luna-Muñoz, J., and Ferrer, I. (2016). Incidental corticobasal degeneration. *Neuropathol. Appl. Neurobiol.* 42, 659–663. doi: 10.1111/nan.12339

Mattiace, L. A., Wu, E., Aronson, M., and Dickson, D. W. (1991). A new type of neuritic plaque without amyloid in corticonigral degeneration without achromasia. *J. Neuropathol. Exp. Neurol.* 50:310.

McKee, A. C., Cairns, N. J., Dickson, D. W., Folkerth, R. D., Keene, C. D., Litvan, I., et al. (2016). The first NINDS/NIBIB consensus meeting to define neuropathological criteria for the diagnosis of chronic traumatic encephalopathy. *Acta Neuropathol.* 131, 75–86. doi: 10.1007/s00401-015-1515-z

McKee, A. C., Stein, T. D., Kiernan, P. T., and Alvarez, V. E. (2015). The neuropathology of chronic traumatic encephalopathy. *Brain Pathol.* 25, 350–364. doi: 10.1111/bpa.12248

McKee, A. C., Stern, R. A., Nowinski, C. J., Stein, T. D., Alvarez, V. E., Daneshvar, D. H., et al. (2013). The spectrum of disease in chronic traumatic encephalopathy. *Brain* 136, 43–64. doi: 10.1093/brain/aws307

Mesulam, M., Wicklund, A., Johnson, N., Rogalski, E., Leger, G. C., Rademaker, A., et al. (2008). Alzheimer and frontotemporal pathology in subsets of primary progressive aphasia. *Ann. Neurol.* 63, 709–719. doi: 10.1002/ana.21388

Milenkovic, I., and Kovacs, G. G. (2013). Incidental corticobasal degeneration in a 76-year-old woman. *Clin. Neuropathol.* 32, 69–72. doi: 10.5414/np300515

Milenkovic, I., Petrov, T., and Kovacs, G. G. (2014). Patterns of hippocampal tau pathology differentiate neurodegenerative dementias. *Dement. Geriatr. Cogn. Disord.* 38, 375–388. doi: 10.1159/000365548

Miyazono, M., Iwaki, T., Kitamoto, T., Shin, R. W., Fukui, M., and Tateishi, J. (1993). Widespread distribution of tau in the astrocytic elements of glial tumors. *Acta Neuropathol.* 86, 236–241. doi: 10.1007/bf00304137

Mudher, A., Colin, M., Dujardin, S., Medina, M., Dewachter, I., Alavi Naini, S. M., et al. (2017). What is the evidence that tau pathology spreads through prion-like propagation? *Acta Neuropathol. Commun.* 5:99. doi: 10.1186/s40478-017-0488-7

Munoz, D. G., Woulfe, J., and Kertesz, A. (2007). Argyrophilic thorny astrocyte clusters in association with Alzheimer's disease pathology in possible primary progressive aphasia. *Acta Neuropathol.* 114, 347–357. doi: 10.1007/s00401-007-0266-x

Narasimhan, S., Guo, J. L., Changolkar, L., Stieber, A., Mcbride, J. D., Silva, L. V., et al. (2017). Pathological tau strains from human brains recapitulate the diversity of tauopathies in nontransgenic mouse brain. *J. Neurosci.* 37, 11406–11423. doi: 10.1523/jneurosci.1230-17.2017

Nijholt, D. A., De Kimpe, L., Elfrink, H. L., Hoozemans, J. J., and Scheper, W. (2011). Removing protein aggregates: the role of proteolysis in neurodegeneration. *Curr. Med. Chem.* 18, 2459–2476. doi: 10.2174/092986711795843236

Nishimura, M., Namba, Y., Ikeda, K., and Oda, M. (1992). Glial fibrillary tangles with straight tubules in the brains of patients with progressive supranuclear palsy. *Neurosci. Lett.* 143, 35–38. doi: 10.1016/0304-3940(92)90227-x

Nolan, A., De Paula Franca Resende, E., Petersen, C., Neylan, K., Spina, S., Huang, E., et al. (2019). Astrocytic tau deposition is frequent in typical and atypical Alzheimer disease presentations. *J. Neuropathol. Exp. Neurol.* 78, 1112–1123. doi: 10.1093/jnen/nlz094

Perea, J. R., Lopez, E., Diez-Ballesteros, J. C., Avila, J., Hernandez, F., and Bolos, M. (2019). Extracellular monomeric tau is internalized by astrocytes. *Front. Neurosci.* 13:442. doi: 10.3389/fnins.2019.00442

Piacentini, R., Li Puma, D. D., Mainardi, M., Lazzarino, G., Tavazzi, B., Arancio, O., et al. (2017). Reduced gliotransmitter release from astrocytes mediates tau-induced synaptic dysfunction in cultured hippocampal neurons. *Glia* 65, 1302–1316. doi: 10.1002/glia.23163

Pooler, A. M., Phillips, E. C., Lau, D. H., Noble, W., and Hanger, D. P. (2013). Physiological release of endogenous tau is stimulated by neuronal activity. *EMBO Rep.* 14, 389–394. doi: 10.1038/embor.2013.15

Poorkaj, P., Muma, N. A., Zhukareva, V., Cochran, E. J., Shannon, K. M., Hurtig, H., et al. (2002). An R5L tau mutation in a subject with a progressive supranuclear palsy phenotype. *Ann. Neurol.* 52, 511–516. doi: 10.1002/ana.10340

Probst, A., Langui, D., Lautenschlager, C., Ulrich, J., Brion, J. P., and Anderton, B. H. (1988). Progressive supranuclear palsy: extensive neuropil threads in addition to neurofibrillary tangles. Very similar antigenicity of subcortical neuronal pathology in progressive supranuclear palsy and Alzheimer's disease. *Acta Neuropathol.* 77, 61–68. doi: 10.1007/bf00688244

Rahimi, J., and Kovacs, G. G. (2014). Prevalence of mixed pathologies in the aging brain. *Alzheimers Res. Ther.* 6:82. doi: 10.1186/s13195-014-0082-1

Resende, E. P. F., Nolan, A. L., Petersen, C., Ehrenberg, A. J., Spina, S., Allen, I. E., et al. (2020). Language and spatial dysfunction in Alzheimer disease with white matter thorn-shaped astrocytes: astrocytic tau, cognitive function, and Alzheimer disease. *Neurology* doi: 10.1212/wnl.0000000000008937 [Epub ahead of print].

Ries, M., and Sastre, M. (2016). Mechanisms of Aβ clearance and degradation by glial cells. *Front Aging Neurosci* 8:160. doi: 10.3389/fnagi.2016.00160

Robinson, J. L., Corrada, M. M., Kovacs, G. G., Dominique, M., Caswell, C., Xie, S. X., et al. (2018). Non-Alzheimer's contributions to dementia and cognitive resilience in The 90+ Study. *Acta Neuropathol.* 136, 377–388. doi: 10.1007/s00401-018-1872-5

Rösler, T. W., Tayaranian Marvian, A., Brendel, M., Nykänen, N. P., Höllerhage, M., Schwarz, S. C., et al. (2019). Four-repeat tauopathies. *Prog. Neurobiol.* 180:101644. doi: 10.1016/j.pneurobio.2019.101644

Sanders, D. W., Kaufman, S. K., Devos, S. L., Sharma, A. M., Mirbaha, H., Li, A., et al. (2014). Distinct tau prion strains propagate in cells and mice and define different tauopathies. *Neuron* 82, 1271–1288. doi: 10.1016/j.neuron.2014.04.047

Santpere, G., and Ferrer, I. (2009). Delineation of early changes in cases with progressive supranuclear palsy-like pathology. Astrocytes in striatum are primary targets of tau phosphorylation and GFAP oxidation. *Brain Pathol.* 19, 177–187. doi: 10.1111/j.1750-3639.2008.00173.x

Schultz, C., Dehghani, F., Hubbard, G. B., Thal, D. R., Struckhoff, G., Braak, E., et al. (2000). Filamentous tau pathology in nerve cells, astrocytes, and oligodendrocytes of aged baboons. *J. Neuropathol. Exp. Neurol.* 59, 39–52. doi: 10.1093/jnen/59.1.39

Schultz, C., Ghebremedhin, E., Del Tredici, K., Rub, U., and Braak, H. (2004). High prevalence of thorn-shaped astrocytes in the aged human medial temporal lobe. *Neurobiol. Aging* 25, 397–405. doi: 10.1016/s0197-4580(03)00113-1

Sebastián-Serrano, Á., de Diego-García, L., and Díaz-Hernández, M. (2018). The neurotoxic role of extracellular tau protein. *Int. J. Mol. Sci.* 19:E998. doi: 10.3390/ijms19040998

Sergeant, N., David, J. P., Goedert, M., Jakes, R., Vermersch, P., Buee, L., et al. (1997). Two-dimensional characterization of paired helical filament-tau from Alzheimer's disease: demonstration of an additional 74-kDa component and age-related biochemical modifications. *J. Neurochem.* 69, 834–844. doi: 10.1046/j.1471-4159.1997.69020834.x

Serrano-Pozo, A., Mielke, M. L., Gomez-Isla, T., Betensky, R. A., Growdon, J. H., Frosch, M. P., et al. (2011). Reactive glia not only associates with plaques but also parallels tangles in Alzheimer's disease. *Am. J. Pathol.* 179, 1373–1384. doi: 10.1016/j.ajpath.2011.05.047

Sheng, J. G., Mrak, R. E., and Griffin, W. S. (1997). Glial-neuronal interactions in Alzheimer disease: progressive association of IL-1α^+ microglia and S100β^+ astrocytes with neurofibrillary tangle stages. *J. Neuropathol. Exp. Neurol.* 56, 285–290. doi: 10.1097/00005072-199703000-00007

Shibuya, K., Yagishita, S., Nakamura, A., and Uchihara, T. (2011). Perivascular orientation of astrocytic plaques and tuft-shaped astrocytes. *Brain Res.* 1404, 50–54. doi: 10.1016/j.brainres.2011.06.014

Shin, R. W., Iwaki, T., Kitamoto, T., and Tateishi, J. (1991). Hydrated autoclave pretreatment enhances tau immunoreactivity in formalin-fixed normal and Alzheimer's disease brain tissues. *Lab. Invest.* 64, 693–702.

Sidoryk-Wegrzynowicz, M., and Strużyńska, L. (2019). Astroglial contribution to tau-dependent neurodegeneration. *Biochem. J.* 476, 3493–3504. doi: 10.1042/bcj20190506

Simpson, J. E., Ince, P. G., Lace, G., Forster, G., Shaw, P. J., Matthews, F., et al. (2010). Astrocyte phenotype in relation to Alzheimer-type pathology in the ageing brain. *Neurobiol. Aging* 31, 578–590. doi: 10.1016/j.neurobiolaging.2008.05.015

Song, Y. J., Halliday, G. M., Holton, J. L., Lashley, T., O'Sullivan, S. S., Mccann, H., et al. (2009). Degeneration in different parkinsonian syndromes relates to astrocyte type and astrocyte protein expression. *J. Neuropathol. Exp. Neurol.* 68, 1073–1083. doi: 10.1097/nen.0b013e3181b66f1b

Spillantini, M. G., and Goedert, M. (2013). Tau pathology and neurodegeneration. *Lancet Neurol.* 12, 609–622. doi: 10.1016/S1474-4422(13)70090-5

Stanford, P. M., Halliday, G. M., Brooks, W. S., Kwok, J. B., Storey, C. E., Creasey, H., et al. (2000). Progressive supranuclear palsy pathology caused by a novel silent mutation in exon 10 of the tau gene: expansion of the disease phenotype caused by tau gene mutations. *Brain* 123, 880–893. doi: 10.1093/brain/123.5.880

Tacik, P., Deture, M., Lin, W. L., Sanchez Contreras, M., Wojtas, A., Hinkle, K. M., et al. (2015). A novel tau mutation, p.K317N, causes globular glial tauopathy. *Acta Neuropathol.* 130, 199–214. doi: 10.1007/s00401-015-1425-0

Tacik, P., Sanchez-Contreras, M., Deture, M., Murray, M. E., Rademakers, R., Ross, O. A., et al. (2017). Clinicopathologic heterogeneity in frontotemporal dementia and parkinsonism linked to chromosome 17 (FTDP-17) due to microtubule-associated protein tau (MAPT) p.P301L mutation, including a patient with globular glial tauopathy. *Neuropathol. Appl. Neurobiol.* 43, 200–214. doi: 10.1111/nan.12367

Tashiro, K., Hasegawa, M., Ihara, Y., and Iwatsubo, T. (1997). Somatodendritic localization of phosphorylated tau in neonatal and adult rat cerebral cortex. *Neuroreport* 8, 2797–2801. doi: 10.1097/00001756-199708180-00029

Trojanowski, J. Q., Schuck, T., Schmidt, M. L., and Lee, V. M. (1989). Distribution of tau proteins in the normal human central and peripheral nervous system. *J. Histochem. Cytochem.* 37, 209–215. doi: 10.1177/37.2.2492045

Verkhratsky, A., Zorec, R., and Parpura, V. (2017). Stratification of astrocytes in healthy and diseased brain. *Brain Pathol.* 27, 629–644. doi: 10.1111/bpa.12537

von Bernhardi, R., and Eugenin, J. (2012). Alzheimer's disease: redox dysregulation as a common denominator for diverse pathogenic mechanisms. *Antioxid. Redox Signal.* 16, 974–1031. doi: 10.1089/ars.2011.4082

Wang, Y., Balaji, V., Kaniyappan, S., Kruger, L., Irsen, S., Tepper, K., et al. (2017). The release and trans-synaptic transmission of Tau *via* exosomes. *Mol. Neurodegener.* 12:5. doi: 10.1186/s13024-016-0143-y

Weingarten, M. D., Lockwood, A. H., Hwo, S. Y., and Kirschner, M. W. (1975). A protein factor essential for microtubule assembly. *Proc. Natl. Acad. Sci. U S A* 72, 1858–1862. doi: 10.1073/pnas.72.5.1858

Yamada, T., Calne, D. B., Akiyama, H., Mcgeer, E. G., and Mcgeer, P. L. (1993). Further observations on Tau-positive glia in the brains with progressive supranuclear palsy. *Acta Neuropathol.* 85, 308–315. doi: 10.1007/bf00227727

Yamada, K., Cirrito, J. R., Stewart, F. R., Jiang, H., Finn, M. B., Holmes, B. B., et al. (2011). *In vivo* microdialysis reveals age-dependent decrease of brain interstitial fluid tau levels in P301S human tau transgenic mice. *J. Neurosci.* 31, 13110–13117. doi: 10.1523/jneurosci.2569-11.2011

Yamada, T., McGeer, P. L., and McGeer, E. G. (1992). Appearance of paired nucleated, Tau-positive glia in patients with progressive supranuclear palsy brain tissue. *Neurosci. Lett.* 135, 99–102. doi: 10.1016/0304-3940(92)90145-w

Yoshida, M. (2014). Astrocytic inclusions in progressive supranuclear palsy and corticobasal degeneration. *Neuropathology* 34, 555–570. doi: 10.1111/neup.12143

Zarranz, J. J., Ferrer, I., Lezcano, E., Forcadas, M. I., Eizaguirre, B., Atares, B., et al. (2005). A novel mutation (K317M) in the MAPT gene causes FTDP and motor neuron disease. *Neurology* 64, 1578–1585. doi: 10.1212/01.wnl.0000160116.65034.12

16

Role of Microglial Cells in Alzheimer's Disease Tau Propagation

Ena Španić [1†], Lea Langer Horvat [1†], Patrick R. Hof [2] and Goran Šimić [1]*

[1] *Laboratory for Developmental Neuropathology, Department of Neuroscience, Croatian Institute for Brain Research, University of Zagreb School of Medicine, Zagreb, Croatia,* [2] *Nash Family Department of Neuroscience, Ronald M. Loeb Center for Alzheimer's Disease, Friedman Brain Institute, Icahn School of Medicine at Mount Sinai, New York, NY, United States*

***Correspondence:**
Goran Šimić
gsimic@hiim.hr

† These authors have contributed equally to this work

Uncontrolled immune response in the brain contributes to the progression of all neurodegenerative disease, including Alzheimer's disease (AD). Recent investigations have documented the prion-like features of tau protein and the involvement of microglial changes with tau pathology. While it is still unclear what sequence of events is causal, it is likely that tau seeding potential and microglial contribution to tau propagation act together, and are essential for the development and progression of degenerative changes. Based on available evidence, targeting tau seeds and controlling some signaling pathways in a complex inflammation process could represent a possible new therapeutic approach for treating neurodegenerative diseases. Recent findings propose novel diagnostic assays and markers that may be used together with standard methods to complete and improve the diagnosis and classification of these diseases. In conclusion, a novel perspective on microglia-tau relations reveals new issues to investigate and imposes different approaches for developing therapeutic strategies for AD.

Keywords: Alzheimer's disease, blood-brain barrier, inflammation, microglia, neurodegeneration, tau protein propagation

INTRODUCTION

The most common cause of dementia is Alzheimer's disease (AD), a progressive neurodegenerative disease that affects nearly 50 million people in the world. Histopathological features of AD are extracellular amyloid-β (Aβ) plaques and intracellular aggregation of hyperphosphorylated tau protein in a form of neurofibrillary tangles (NFTs; Braak and Braak, 1991a). The disease is also characterized by loss of neurons and synapses and elevated levels of inflammatory factors (Kinney et al., 2018). Many studies have shown the harmful effect of tau protein oligomers and its potential to propagate through synaptically connected regions (Kfoury et al., 2012; Liu et al., 2012; Plouffe et al., 2012; Smolek et al., 2019). Tau protein aggregation and neurofibrillary lesions also show the highest correlation with the clinical symptoms of the disease (Arriagada et al., 1992; Bierer et al., 1995). As such, tau protein aggregation, neurofibrillary lesions, and cytoskeletal abnormalities are considered to be a central pathogenetic mechanism of AD (Šimić et al., 1998) important for its progressive nature (Clavaguera et al., 2009; Šimić et al., 2017). Inflammation is another crucial factor that can contribute to disease progression. Neuroinflammation occurs in many neurodegenerative diseases, including AD. Several studies confirmed elevated levels of pro-inflammatory cytokines and stronger microglial activation during disease progression (Griffin et al., 1989; Lanzrein et al., 1998; Minghetti, 2005). For example, we observed Iba1-expressing microglia to be present in various stages of activation

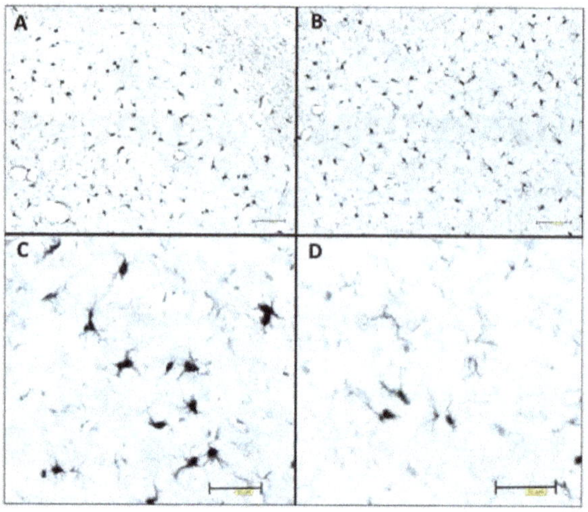

FIGURE 1 | Immunocytochemical expression of the Iba1 marker visualizes the morphology of microglia. Illustrative examples of Iba1-expressing microglia in various stages of activation in the adult Wistar rat brain 3 days after inoculation of 4 μg of preformed synthetic tau fibrils (gift of Dr. Rakez Kayed, Galveston, TX, USA) into the entorhinal cortex. **(A)** Hippocampus (CA1), **(B)** entorhinal cortex, **(C)** activated microglia, **(D)** resting microglia. Scale bars **(A,B)** 100 μm, **(C,D)** 50 μm.

in the rat brain after inoculation of synthetic tau fibrils (**Figure 1**). Activated microglia have been found near NFT-bearing neurons (Sheffield et al., 2000). There is also a better correlation between numbers of activated microglia and NFT than between microglial cells' activation and amyloid plaques distribution (Serrano-Pozo et al., 2011). Several lines of evidence suggest that inflammation may even precede the development of tau pathology (Yoshiyama et al., 2007; Denver and McClean, 2018). Therefore, controlling the components in a complex inflammatory process represents a new possible therapeutic approach for neurodegenerative diseases (for review see Šimić et al., 2019).

MICROGLIAL CELLS

Microglial cells are a population of brain myeloid cells that represent a part of the innate immunity system. Myeloid cells arise from the yolk sac and colonize the central nervous system (CNS) during early embryonic development. Their appropriate response is crucial for maintaining homeostasis and to carry out the immune response in the CNS (Ginhoux et al., 2013). Innate and adaptive immunity are the two main components of the immune response in the human body. Innate immunity is a general response, recognizing pathogen-associated molecular patterns (PAMPs) and damage-associated molecular patterns (DAMPs) through pattern recognition receptors (PRRs). In contrast, the adaptive immune response is based on the recognition of specific antigen components and acts against a specific pathogen. Adaptive immunity includes the formation of specific antibodies and involves memory cells to eliminate pathogens more efficiently upon recurrence after first exposure (Medzhitov, 2007). Based on specific gene expression microglial cells can be divided into three groups, early, pre-microglia, and adult microglia (Matcovitch-Natan et al., 2016). Microglial cells have different functions depending on their micro- and macro-environment or their developmental stage (Lavin et al., 2014; Matcovitch-Natan et al., 2016). Although, their role as immune agents during pathological conditions is still a matter of debate, microglial cells also play a key role during brain development. Through their phagocytic activity, they control the formation and depletion of the synapses, which is crucial for normal brain development. It has been suggested that synaptic pruning can be regulated by the chemokine receptor fractalkine (CX3CR1) expressed on microglia. In mouse model lacking CX3CR1, synaptic pruning was reduced, which led to the formation of immature brain and synapses (Paolicelli et al., 2011; Hoshiko et al., 2012). Furthermore, it appears that the CX3CR1/CX3CL1 complex has also a neuroprotective effect while lacking either fractalkine (CX3CL1) or its receptor leads to neurodegeneration. Elevated microglia cell activation and neuronal loss have been also noticed in SOD1G93A/CX3CR1$^{-/-}$ mice (Liu et al., 2019). One study showed that microglia can regulate the number of neural precursor cells in the developing brain. These authors suggested that the number or activation state of microglia affect the precursor cells number and concluded that any factor that can change the number or activation state of microglia can affect neural development as well as behavioral outcomes (Cunningham et al., 2013). Depletion of the synapses is complement-dependent and it is mediated by complement receptor 3 (CR3) together with neuronal activity (Schafer et al., 2012). By releasing specific mediators that promote cell genesis, health, and dendritic growth, microglia has additional beneficial roles too (Lenz and Nelson, 2018).

In the mature brain, microglia play an important role as the main immune agents. Under physiological conditions, microglial cells are in the resting state, but they actively survey the brain parenchyma with motile processes (Nimmerjahn et al., 2005). In this state, microglia are sensitive to a wide range of stimuli like injury, toxins, pathogens, misfolded proteins, and damaged neurons (von Bernhardi et al., 2015). Similar to the polarization of macrophages in peripheral organs, it was proposed that microglia differentiate into two different phenotypes depending on their extracellular environment (Michelucci et al., 2009). The M1 or pro-inflammatory phenotype releases inflammatory mediators such as interleukin 1-β (IL-1β), tumor necrosis factor-α (TNF-α), nitric oxide (NO), reactive oxygen species (ROS), proteases, and many others in order to eliminate the potential pathogens. In contrast, the M2 phenotype is considered neuroprotective due to its phagocytic activity and anti-inflammatory effect. M2 microglia support tissue repair, reconstruction of extracellular matrix, and releases anti-inflammatory cytokines, which together promote a homeostatic environment (von Bernhardi et al., 2015; Tang and Le, 2016). Although the M1/M2 model is widely adopted, a recent study proposed a different perspective relating to the microglia disease phenotype (Keren-Shaul et al., 2017). Single-cell RNA sequencing of microglia cells from human AD brain and 5xFAD mice identified a unique subtype of microglia, called disease-associated microglia (DAM) that is characterized by a specific gene expression profile. These authors found elevated expression of some AD-related genes but decreased expression of some genes normally expressed in homeostatic microglia. Two stages in DAM activation were suggested, a triggering receptor expressed on myeloid cells 2 (TREM2) independent stage followed by TREM2-dependent activation (Keren-Shaul et al., 2017). Similar to the M1/M2, another study proposed the existence of pro-inflammatory and anti-inflammatory DAM phenotypes and the potential benefits of suppressing pro-inflammatory DAM (Rangaraju et al., 2018).

INFLAMMATION IN AD

Neuroinflammation occurs in most neurodegenerative diseases (for review see Stephenson et al., 2018). Even though activation of microglial cells should be protective in the short-term, under altered conditions microglia sometimes promote continuous inflammation and oxidative stress which defeats homeostasis (Minghetti, 2005; Sardi et al., 2011; von Bernhardi et al., 2015; Jiang et al., 2019). In AD, microglia are supposed to be in an continuously activated state due to Aβ or some other extra- or intracellular product(s) of APP metabolism as well as due to neurofibrillary changes (Bellucci et al., 2004; Sasaki et al., 2008; Serrano-Pozo et al., 2011; Appel et al., 2014; Kametani and Hasegawa, 2018). A consequence of severe and constant microglial activation is the excessive production of pro-inflammatory mediators that creates a cytotoxic environment. Overactive microglia are associated with neuronal loss and decline of cognitive functions (Cagnin et al., 2001; Qin et al., 2002). It seems that the overproduction of ROS contributes the most to the deleterious effects of inflammation. Oxidative stress further induces production of pro-inflammatory cytokines consequently creating a vicious cycle that results in neurodegeneration (Wu et al., 2016). One study showed that microglia activation by Aβ could suppress cell proliferation and promote apoptosis of neural stem cells due to oxidative stress (Jiang et al., 2016a). In another study the same group demonstrated that activated microglia could release NO and pro-inflammatory cytokines that increased ROS levels and induced oxidative stress injury in dopaminergic neurons (Jiang et al., 2019), suggesting that harmful effects of inflammation cannot be ignored when considering potential therapeutic approaches for neurodegenerative diseases. Peripheral immune cells infiltrate the brain during neurodegeneration (Zilka et al., 2009; Sardi et al., 2011). The detrimental effect of inflammation contributes to the disruption of the blood-brain barrier in AD (Sardi et al., 2011). Therefore, a greater influx of the peripheral immune cells can occur. Although what the effects of these peripheral immune cells might be is not completely clear, it has been proposed that these cells further exacerbate inflammation (Sardi et al., 2011), while others have argued that there may be beneficial effects of the peripheral cells influx (Dionisio-Santos et al., 2019). In this context, it is interesting to note that the beneficial effect of non-steroidal anti-inflammatory drugs (NSAID) on AD incidence has been noted early in in t' Veld et al. (2001) and Zandi et al. (2002). Apart from human studies in animal models, it has been documented that neurotrophin treatment caused a decrease in pro-inflammatory cytokines IL-1β IL-6 (TNF-α), elevation of brain-derived neurotrophic factor (BDNF), and less cognitive impairment, Aβ deposition, and microglial activation (Fang et al., 2019). Interferon-β1a (IFNβ1a) is largely used to attenuate the progression of multiple sclerosis and its anti-inflammatory effect could be beneficial also for AD patients. In an AD rat model, treatment with IFNβ1a improved memory impairment and decreased inflammation and ROS production (Mudò et al., 2019). Such possible interventions have not yet been tested in AD patients.

PROPAGATION OF TAU PROTEIN

Tau protein is mainly expressed in neurons and is essential for microtubule assembly and stabilization of the cytoskeleton (Weingarten et al., 1975). Tau is encoded by the *MAPT* gene and different RNA splicing can produce six tau isoforms in the human brain. Isoforms of tau have either three or four microtubule-binding repeats (Neve et al., 1986; Goedert et al., 1989). Phosphorylation is one of the main posttranslational changes of tau and is crucial for the regulation of tau functions as it can reduce its ability to bind to microtubules (Lindwall and Cole, 1984). Therefore, only the correct pattern of tau phosphorylation can be effective. It was proposed that hyperphosphorylation can cause abnormal folding of tau. This is also supported by *in vitro* findings, where we showed that exhaustive tau phosphorylation is either not essential for the stability of the putative tau oligomer once it is formed, or is necessary for initial oligomer formation (Boban et al., 2019). Once formed, tau oligomers can be stable even upon dephosphorylation (Boban et al., 2019), but misfolded tau is not able to stabilize microtubules properly, consequently causing its degradation and intracellular self-aggregation. Thus, the accumulation of abnormally phosphorylated tau is one of the earliest changes in the process of NFT formation (Bancher et al., 1989; Braak et al., 1994; Šimić et al., 2016). Because of the positive correlation between NFT formation and loss of cognitive function (Arriagada et al., 1992; Bierer et al., 1995) and the specific patterns of disease progression, the disease is usually described in terms of the Braak and Braak stages. This topographic progression of the disease is classified into six stages. The first two stages are called transentorhinal because of the progression from the entorhinal region to the hippocampal formation. Further, in stages III and IV, the disease spreads to the temporal, frontal and parietal neocortex and finally, in late stages V and VI, sensory and motor areas of the neocortex are affected (Braak and Braak, 1991b). The pathogenic spread hypothesis can explain the characteristic spread of tau, but alternative mechanisms about selective vulnerability should also be considered (Walsh and Selkoe, 2016). Both mechanisms may be acting together and contribute to spatial distribution of protein aggregates. The concept of selective neuronal vulnerability refers to a situation where certain neurons are more vulnerable than others to pathogenic processes that cause the misfolding and aggregation of tau proteins. This is perhaps determined by biochemical, genomic, connectomic, electrophysiological, and morphological properties of vulnerable neurons (Šimić et al., 2017, 2019) and region-specific microenvironments (Jackson, 2014). There are other possible reasons for vulnerability due to differential protein expression: for example, in regions that are always affected by tau pathology, elevated expression of some proteins that co-aggregate with tau and Aβ, with lower expression of proteins that can prevent aggregation of tau and Aβ has been observed, when compared to regions less susceptible to the disease (Freer et al., 2016). Recent evidence suggests that abnormal forms of tau proteins appear in a small number of neurons and propagate to other regions inducing disease progression in a prion-like manner (Clavaguera et al., 2009; Hall and Patuto, 2012; Walker and Jucker, 2015). Prions, or proteinaceous infectious particles, represent the misfolded prion protein that causes several neurological diseases known as transmissible spongiform encephalopathies (Prusiner, 1982, 2013). Prions are considered infectious due to their potential to induce misfolding of normally folded PrP molecules in neighboring cells. It is likely that prions are transmitted between cells through synaptic or vesicular transport (Aguzzi and Rajendran, 2009). Until recently, it was believed that only cell-autonomous mechanisms are responsible for sporadic neurodegenerative disease development. Cell-autonomous mechanisms imply that protein aggregation emerges independently in several cells. It has however been shown that first local inclusion propagates towards healthy cells *via* non-cell-autonomous mechanisms, which leads to degeneration (Goedert et al., 2017). For pathogenic spread of tau proteins there are few initial steps that have to occur. It has been proposed that initially a tau-competent monomer is formed. This means that such specific conformation of monomer is competent to assemble into nuclei, a supposedly rate-limiting stage for the rapid growth of tau fibrils. Elongation of the tau-competent conformers or fragmentation of tau aggregates/fibrils may produce short fragments ("seeds"), which are able to act as templates and thus recruit native tau monomers to rapid growth of tau aggregates (**Figure 2A**), thus skipping a long early, rate-limiting, stage (Nizynski et al., 2017). There are many experimental animal and *in vitro* studies that describe the trans-synaptic spread of tau along anatomically connected brain regions. One study demonstrated this kind of propagation in transgenic mice that differentially express pathological human tau in the entorhinal cortex (Liu et al., 2012). Furthermore, injection of insoluble tau isolated from human AD brain induces neurofibrillary pathology in rats expressing non-mutated truncated tau (Smolek et al., 2019), as well as in several non-transgenic mouse models (Clavaguera et al., 2013; Boluda et al., 2015; Guo et al., 2016; Gibbons et al., 2017; Narasimhan et al., 2017). When protein aggregates were injected into specific mouse brain region pathology progressed only into brain regions synaptically connected to the injected site, leaving the closer but unconnected neurons unaffected (Clavaguera et al., 2013). *In vitro* studies also support the prion-like feature of tau (Kfoury et al., 2012; Plouffe et al., 2012). Using an ultrasensitive FRET-based flow cytometry biosensor assay, tau seeding was detected 4 weeks earlier than other pathological tau species, marked with common histological markers in P301S mouse (Holmes et al., 2014). The same technology detected tau seeding activity in some regions that usually lack pathological tau detected with histological markers in human postmortem AD brains. The majority of Braak stage 1 samples had seeding activity in the hippocampus and some of them in some neocortical regions although histological markers of tau pathology are limited to the entorhinal cortex in stage 1. Tau seeding was found frequently in frontal and parietal lobes of stage 2 cases, where tau pathology is generally restricted to the limbic system. Some stage 3 samples exhibited tau seeding even in the cerebellum which is not typically affected by tau pathology. This suggests that seeding activity precedes other histological markers of pathological tau and could be the earliest indication of tau pathology. This assay may thus be used together with standard neuropathological methods to refine the classification of tauopathies (Furman et al., 2017). To test whether there is a direct trans-synaptic spread of protein aggregates we need to restrict aggregated protein expression to one regional population of neurons and demonstrate conversion of natively folded tau protein in synaptically connected neurons. Hyperphosphorylation and misfolding of tau can enhance neuronal tau uptake (Takeda et al., 2015; Šimić et al., 2016). Takeda et al. (2015) detected soluble phosphorylated high-molecular-weight (HMW) tau species as tau with the greatest ability to propagate in a prion-like manner. Using differential centrifugation and size-exclusion chromatography they isolated propagating tau and then assessed its uptake. Tau uptake was present only in neurons treated with extracts that contained HMW tau. Further characterization revealed small amounts of HMW tau in those extracts and only small globular tau aggregates in HMW tau fraction (Takeda et al., 2015). Tau from brain intestinal fluid (ISF) and cerebrospinal fluid (CSF) of mouse model applied on the cell culture is taken up by neurons where it can promote the formation of intracellular aggregates. As the CSF from AD patients also contains HMW tau, these results provide evidence that extracellular tau from the diseased brain can be bioactive and that HMW tau has a major seeding potential because even small amounts of bioactive HMW tau can promote its further propagation (Takeda et al., 2015, 2016). Can be taken up by neurons in culture.

TAU RELEASE *VIA* EXOSOMES

The prion-like hypothesis of tau transmission proposes that misfolded tau acts as a seed causing further misfolding of proteins inside healthy cells, implying that tau needs to be released outside of the cells. Tau released in the ISF can induce stronger microglial activation which in turn may promote the propagation of tau pathology. It is well known that the CSF levels of tau are elevated in AD patients (Zetterberg and Blennow, 2013; Babic et al., 2014; Blennow et al., 2015; Babic Leko et al., 2018), and this was also confirmed in tau transgenic mice model (Barten et al., 2011). One study detected tau in the ISF of wild-type mice, suggesting that tau is released into the ISF under normal conditions (Yamada et al., 2011). These investigators also tested tau levels in P301S transgenic mice. Tau levels were approximately 5-fold higher in P301S brain than in wild-type and similar differences were observed in ISF tau levels. This results

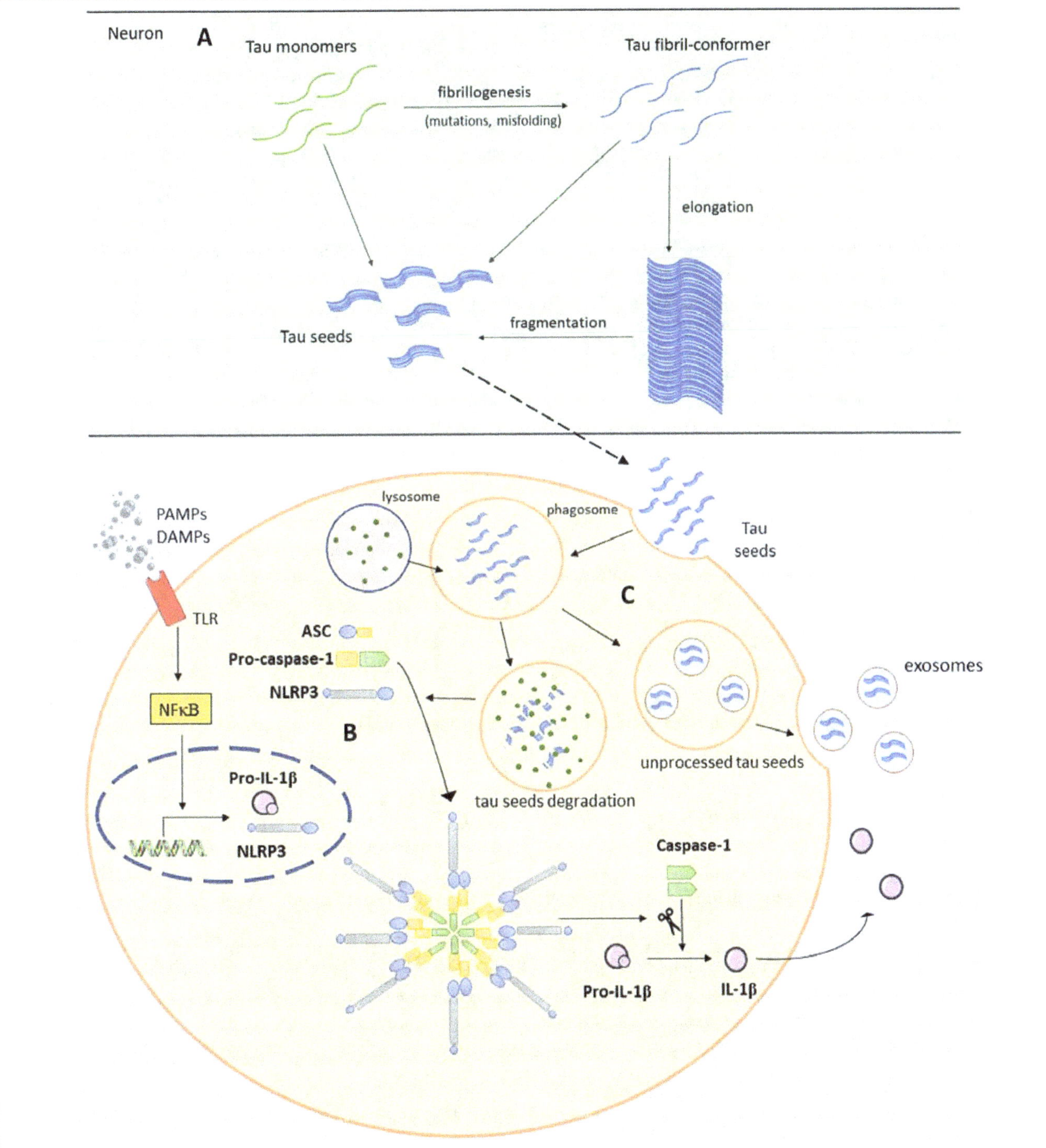

FIGURE 2 | Schematic representation of Panel **(A)**. Tau seeds formation (based on Nizynski et al., 2017). **(B)** NLRP3 inflammasome activation (based on data by Stancu et al., 2019), and **(C)** microglia releasing tau seeds in exosomes (based on Hopp et al., 2018). Aβ, amyloid β; ASC, apoptosis-associated speck-like protein containing a C-terminal caspase recruitment domain (CARD); DAMPs, damage-associated molecular patterns; mtROS, mitochondrial reactive oxygen species (ROS); NLRP3, NACHT, LRR and PYD domains-containing protein 3; PAMPs, pathogen-associated molecular patterns; TLR, toll-like receptor. See text for details.

proved that intracellular and extracellular tau levels are related (Yamada et al., 2011) and even though tau is predominantly a cytosolic protein, it can be actively secreted outside of the cell. Tau does not have a signal peptide for the secretory pathway, which means it cannot be released through the endoplasmic reticulum (ER)-Golgi secretory pathway. Several studies have proposed possible mechanisms of tau release and uptake. Some mentioned tau can be secreted *via* unconventional secretory pathways like other proteins lacking signal peptides (Rabouille et al., 2012; Katsinelos et al., 2018). One of the mechanisms described is tau secretion *via* exosomes. This mechanism was demonstrated in cell cultures *in vitro* such as M1C (Saman et al., 2012), N2a, and also in primary neurons (Wang et al., 2017). Exosome release is regulated by cell activity and depolarization of neurons promotes the release of tau-containing exosomes. Also, another study showed that synaptic connection is crucial for tau transmission *via* exosomes (Wang et al., 2017) which supports the possibility that synaptic connections are the main factor that influences the specific way of tau spreading and disease progression across brain regions. Exosomes isolated from the CSF of AD patients and control subjects contain tau (Saman et al., 2012; Wang et al., 2017). It is interesting that exosomes from AD and control CSF can promote aggregation of tau protein in cultured cells. Exosomes from AD patients induces slightly higher, yet statistically not significant, aggregation (Wang et al., 2017). Based on exosomes-associated tau presence in the CSF it is of interest to examine the diagnostic potential of CSF exosomes. Levels of blood exosomal tau are higher in AD patients than in control subjects (Fiandaca et al., 2015). Higher sensitivity and therefore better diagnostic potential of exosomal tau was reported compared to statistically significant tau levels evaluated only from fluid-phase. More importantly, elevated exosomal levels of tau, together with $A\beta_{1-42}$ levels were detected up to 10 years prior to clinical diagnosis (Fiandaca et al., 2015). Exosomes and other extracellular vesicles, therefore, represent potential new biomarkers for AD and could help predict the course of the disease (Fiandaca et al., 2015). As it stands, we are still lacking standardized protocols for isolation or characterization of extracellular vesicles for clinical purpose (Gámez-Valero et al., 2019).

MICROGLIA-TAU RELATIONSHIPS

It is well known that tau can mediate an inflammatory response in neurodegenerative disease. Many studies show microglial activation upon tau pathology (Bellucci et al., 2004; Sasaki et al., 2008; Zilka et al., 2009, 2012). Activated microglia were found near NFT-bearing neurons (Sheffield et al., 2000). Also, there is a better correlation between the number of activated microglia and NFT than between glial activation and plaques distribution (Serrano-Pozo et al., 2011). In a transgenic rat model, reactive microglia were associated with neurofibrillary changes and was absent within regions with smaller neurofibrillary degeneration (Zilka et al., 2009). It was recently hypothesized that inflammation even precedes the development of tau pathology (Sheffield et al., 2000; Yoshiyama et al., 2007; Ghosh et al., 2013). In a mouse model of tauopathy, microglial activation and synaptic pathology were identified as the earliest manifestations of neurodegeneration. These authors suggested that activated microglia exacerbate tau pathology by damaging dendrites and axons. This study also provided evidence that inhibition of the inflammatory response may ameliorate consequences of tau pathology (Yoshiyama et al., 2007). Experiments in various transgenic mice models demonstrated the importance of proper microglial response in maintaining healthy brain environment. High levels of pro-inflammatory cytokine IL-1 exacerbate tau phosphorylation (Li et al., 2003; Ghosh et al., 2013). Elevated tau phosphorylation and aggregation were noticed in the absence of TREM2 or fractalkine receptor (Bhaskar et al., 2010; Maphis et al., 2015; Bemiller et al., 2017). Tau binding to CX3CR1 initiate its uptake and absence of CX3CR1 resulted in altered uptake and degradation of tau by microglia. It is proposed that tau competes with CX3CL1 to bind to this receptor (Bolós et al., 2017). Overexpression of TREM2 improves cognitive impairments, attenuates synapse loss and tau hyperphosphorylation (Jiang et al., 2016b). Another interesting study shows the different effect of partial and complete depletion of TREM2 on the progression of tau pathology, pointing out worse outcome in the case of partial TREM2 depletion (Sayed et al., 2018). These studies emphasize the importance of TREM2 and CX3CR1 signaling pathways in regulating microglial response and tau pathology. Controlling those signaling pathways outlines possible future therapeutic strategies. Furthermore, inflammatory factors from microglia cells cause upregulation of tau protein *in vitro*. Interestingly, microglia pretreated with NSAID attenuated tau overexpression (Lee et al., 2015). Microglia can actively phagocytize tau (Asai et al., 2015; Bolós et al., 2015; Luo et al., 2015; Hopp et al., 2018). Depending on tau isoform or microglial response, internalized tau can be processed in different ways. Microglia-mediated degradation of tau can be enhanced by an anti-tau monoclonal antibody (Luo et al., 2015). Moreover, if microglia fail to process tau completely into a non-toxic form, tau seeds can be released within exosomes making microglia competent to promote tau seeding in adjacent cells (**Figure 2C**; Hopp et al., 2018). Asai et al. (2015) tested the role of microglia in tau propagation *in vitro* and *in vivo*. AT8 and PHF1 tau colocalized within hippocampal Iba1-expressing microglia, which convincingly demonstrate microglial uptake of tau (Asai et al., 2015). *In vitro* test supported this conclusion, showing more efficient phagocytic activity by microglia when compared to neurons and astroglia (Asai et al., 2015). Activation of microglia also induced tau ubiquitination (modification important for exosomal incorporation of tau) and secretion of exosomal tau. An exosomal fraction from microglia applied on pyramidal neurons in culture or injected in the mouse brain caused neuronal uptake of exosome derived tau. Finally, it has been demonstrated that depletion of microglia and inhibition of exosome synthesis reduce tau propagation *in vitro* and *in vivo* (Asai et al., 2015).

TAU SEEDS INDUCE INFLAMMASOME ACTIVATION

A recent study revealed one possible molecular mechanism that can explain noticed microglial changes in response to tau pathology and microglial contribution to tau propagation (**Figure 2B**; Stancu et al., 2019). Aggregated tau acting as prion-like seeds activate NLRP3-ASC inflammasome. Nod-like receptors (NLR) are one of the sensors important for activation of innate immune response. Molecular binding to NLRP3 induces the formation of ASC heteromer which further causes microglial activation and elevation of pro-inflammatory cytokine production. Stancu et al. (2019) propose that activation of NLRP3-ASC inflammasome follows microglial uptake of tau, therefore in such way inflammasome activation can promote further exogenously and non-exogenously tau seeded pathology. In ASC deficient microglia, tau-induced IL-1β secretion was blocked and in mice lacking ASC, tau pathology was significantly reduced compared with mice expressing ASC. Using NLRP3 inhibitor MCC950, they also confirmed ASC formation is dependent on NLRP3 activation (Stancu et al., 2019). Prior research by Franklin et al. (2014) revealed that ASC accumulates outside of the cells consequently inducing further IL-1β elevation. In addition, microglial uptake of ASC causes its activation, but it also can promote damage inside the cells. Based on these observations, it appears that the inflammasome can be activated in neighboring cells not just because of the tau seeds but also because of extracellular ASC heteromer uptake which creates a vicious cycle promoting constant microglial activation and severe inflammation that spreads within affected areas (Franklin et al., 2014; Stancu et al., 2019).

CONCLUSIONS

The harmful effect of tau protein oligomers and its potential to propagate through synaptically connected regions has been well established by recent evidence, along with microglial changes in close vicinity of tau pathology. Uncontrolled microglial response in the brain contributes to the progression of many neurodegenerative diseases and several lines of evidence suggest that inflammation may even precede the development of tau pathology in AD. Exosomes could be an important link between tau propagation and microglial activation. Reduction of microglial cells number and exosome synthesis inhibition reduces tau propagation (Asai et al., 2015). Further, phagocytosed tau seeds induce inflammasome activation inside microglia causing overactive microglia state. That could be one of the mechanisms that promote the constant inflammatory response in AD. Based on the recent results presented in this mini-review, we concluded that seeding potential of tau protein and microglial activation are probably acting together and contribute to tau propagation, which could be crucial for the development and progression of degenerative changes. In conclusion, a novel perspective on microglia-tau relations reveals new issues to investigate and imposes different approaches for developing therapeutic and preventative strategies.

ETHICS STATEMENT

All animal experiments were conducted according to the Principles of Laboratory Animal Care and ARRIVE guidelines[1], with the approval of the Ethical Committee of the University of Zagreb Faculty of Science (EP 02/2015 from 15th August 2015) and in accordance with relevant laws (Animal Welfare Law 135/06 and 37/13) and regulations of the The Ministry of Agriculture of The Republic of Croatia (approval no. NP-999/15-01/15) from 12th October 2015).

AUTHOR CONTRIBUTIONS

GŠ conceived the manuscript. All authors edited the drafts of the manuscript.

REFERENCES

Aguzzi, A., and Rajendran, L. (2009). The transcellular spread of cytosolic amyloids, prions and prionoids. *Neuron* 64, 783–790. doi: 10.1016/j.neuron.2009.12.016

Appel, S., Beers, D., and Zhao, W. (2014). Role of inflammation in neurodegenerative diseases. *Neurobiol. Brain Dis.* 380–395. doi: 10.1016/B978-0-12-398270-4.00025-2

Arriagada, P. V., Growdon, J. H., Hedley-Whyte, E. T., and Hyman, B. T. (1992). Neurofibrillary tangles but not senile plaques parallel duration and severity of Alzheimer's disease. *Neurology* 42, 631–639. doi: 10.1212/wnl.42.3.631

Asai, H., Ikezu, S., Tsunoda, S., Medalla, M., Luebke, J., Haydar, T., et al. (2015). Depletion of microglia and inhibition of exosome synthesis halt tau propagation. *Nat. Neurosci.* 18, 1584–1593. doi: 10.1038/nn.4132

Babić, M., Švob Štrac, D., Mück-Šeler, D., Pivac, N., Stanić, G., Hof, P. R., et al. (2014). Update on the core and developing cerebrospinal fluid biomarkers for Alzheimer's disease. *Croat. Med. J.* 55, 347–365. doi: 10.3325/cmj.2014.55.347

Babić Leko, M., Willumsen, N., Nikolac Perković, M., Klepac, N., Borovečki, F., Hof, P. R., et al. (2018). Association of MAPT haplotype-tagging polymorphisms with cerebrospinal fluid biomarkers of Alzheimer's disease: a preliminary study in a Croatian cohort. *Brain Behav.* 8:e01128. doi: 10.1002/brb3.1128

Bancher, C., Brunner, C., Lassmann, H., Budka, H., Jellinger, K., Wiche, G., et al. (1989). Accumulation of abnormally phosphorylated tau precedes the formation of neurofibrillary tangles in Alzheimer's disease. *Brain Res.* 477, 90–99. doi: 10.1016/0006-8993(89)91396-6

Barten, D. M., Cadelina, G. W., Hoque, N., DeCarr, L. B., Guss, V. L., Yang, L., et al. (2011). Tau transgenic mice as models for cerebrospinal fluid tau biomarkers. *J Alzheimers Dis.* 24, 127–141. doi: 10.3233/JAD-2011-110161

Bellucci, A., Westwood, A. J., Ingram, E., Casamenti, F., Goedert, M., and Spillantini, M. G. (2004). Induction of inflammatory mediators and microglial activation in mice transgenic for mutant human P301S tau protein. *Am. J. Pathol.* 165, 1643–1652. doi: 10.1016/s0002-9440(10)63421-9

Bemiller, S. M., McCray, T. J., Allan, K., Formica, S. V., Xu, G., Wilson, G., et al. (2017). TREM2 deficiency exacerbates tau pathology through dysregulated kinase signaling in a mouse model of tauopathy. *Mol. Neurodegener.* 12:74. doi: 10.1186/s13024-017-0216-6

Bhaskar, K., Konerth, M., Kokiko-Cochran, O. N., Cardona, A., Ransohoff, R. M., and Lamb, B. T. (2010). Regulation of tau pathology by the microglial fractalkine receptor. *Neuron* 68, 19–31. doi: 10.1016/j.neuron.2010.08.023

Bierer, L. M., Patrick, R., Schmeidler, J., Perl, D. P., and Carlin, L. (1995). Neocortical neurofibrillary tangles correlate with dementia severity in Alzheimer's disease. *Arch. Neurol.* 52, 81–88. doi: 10.1001/archneur.1995.00540250089017

Blennow, K., Dubois, B., Fagan, A. M., Lewczuk, P., de Leon, M. J., and Hampel, H. (2015). Clinical utility of cerebrospinal fluid biomarkers in the diagnosis of early Alzheimer's disease. *Alzheimers Dement.* 11, 58–69. doi: 10.1016/j.jalz.2014.02.004

Boban, M., Babić Leko, M., Miškić, T., Hof, P. R., and Šimić, G. (2019). Human neuroblastoma SH-SY5Y cells treated with okadaic acid express phosphorylated high molecular weight tau-immunoreactive protein species. *J. Neurosci. Methods* 319, 60–68. doi: 10.1016/j.jneumeth.2018.09.030

Bolós, M., Llorens-Martín, M., Jurado-Arjona, J., Hernández, F., Rábano, A., and Avila, J. (2015). Direct evidence of internalization of tau by microglia *in vitro* and *in vivo*. *J. Alzheimers Dis.* 50, 77–87. doi: 10.3233/JAD-150704

Bolós, M., Llorens-Martín, M., Perea, J. R., Jurado-Arjona, J., Rábano, A., Hernández, F., et al. (2017). Absence of CX3CR1 impairs the internalization of tau by microglia. *Mol. Neurodegener.* 12:59. doi: 10.1186/s13024-017-0200-1

Boluda, S., Iba, M., Zhang, B., Raible, K. M., Lee, V. M.-Y., and Trojanowski, J. Q. (2015). Differential induction and spread of tau pathology in young PS19 tau transgenic mice following intracerebral injections of pathological tau from Alzheimer's disease or corticobasal degeneration brains. *Acta Neuropathol.* 129, 221–237. doi: 10.1007/s00401-014-1373-0

Braak, H., and Braak, E. (1991a). Demonstration of amyloid deposits and neurofibrillary changes in whole brain sections. *Brain Pathol.* 1, 213–216. doi: 10.1111/j.1750-3639.1991.tb00661.x

Braak, H., and Braak, E. (1991b). Neuropathological stageing of Alzheimer-related changes. *Acta Neuropathol.* 82, 239–259. doi: 10.1007/bf00308809

Braak, E., Braak, H., and Mandelkow, E. (1994). A sequence of cytoskeleton changes related to the formation of neurofibrillary tangles and neuropil threads. *Acta Neuropathol.* 87, 554–567. doi: 10.1007/bf00293315

Cagnin, A., Brooks, D. J., Kennedy, A. M., Gunn, R. N., Myers, R., Turkheimer, F. E., et al. (2001). *in vivo* measurement of activated microglia in dementia. *Lancet* 358, 461–467. doi: 10.1016/S0140-6736(01)05625-2

Clavaguera, F., Akatsu, H., Fraser, G., Crowther, R. A., Frank, S., Hench, J., et al. (2013). Brain homogenates from human tauopathies induce tau inclusions in mouse brain. *Proc. Natl. Acad. Sci. U S A* 110, 9535–9540. doi: 10.1073/pnas.1301175110

Clavaguera, F., Bolmont, T., Crowther, R. A., Abramowski, D., Frank, S., Probst, A., et al. (2009). Transmission and spreading of tauopathy in transgenic mouse brain. *Nat. Cell Biol.* 11, 909–913. doi: 10.1038/ncb1901

Cunningham, C. L., Martínez-Cerdeño, V., and Noctor, S. C. (2013). Microglia regulate the number of neural precursor cells in the developing cerebral cortex. *J. Neurosci.* 33, 4216–4233. doi: 10.1523/JNEUROSCI.3441-12.2013

Denver, P., and McClean, P. L. (2018). Distinguishing normal brain aging from the development of Alzheimer's disease: inflammation, insulin signaling and cognition. *Neural Regen. Res.* 13, 1719–1730. doi: 10.4103/1673-5374.238608

Dionisio-Santos, D. A., Olschowka, J. A., and O'Banion, M. K. (2019). Exploiting microglial and peripheral immune cell crosstalk to treat Alzheimer's disease. *J. Neuroinflammation* 16:74. doi: 10.1186/s12974-019-1453-0

Fang, W., Liao, W., Zheng, Y., Huang, X., Weng, X., Fan, S., et al. (2019). Neurotropin reduces memory impairment and neuroinflammation via BDNF/NF-κB in a transgenic mouse model of Alzheimer's disease. *Am. J. Transl. Res.* 11, 1541–1554. doi: 10.1093/cercor/bhy039

Fiandaca, M. S., Kapogiannis, D., Mapstone, M., Boxer, A., Eitan, E., Schwartz, J. B., et al. (2015). Identification of preclinical Alzheimer's disease by a profile of pathogenic proteins in neurally derived blood exosomes: a case-control study. *Alzheimers Dement.* 11, 600.e1–607.e1. doi: 10.1016/j.jalz.2014.06.008

Franklin, B. S., Bossaller, L., De Nardo, D., Ratter, J. M., Stutz, A., Engels, G., et al. (2014). The adaptor ASC has extracellular and "prionoid" activities that propagate inflammation. *Nat. Immunol.* 15, 727–737. doi: 10.1038/ni.2913

Freer, R., Sormanni, P., Vecchi, G., Ciryam, P., Dobson, C. M., and Vendruscolo, M. (2016). A protein homeostasis signature in healthy brains recapitulates tissue vulnerability to Alzheimer's disease. *Sci. Adv.* 2:e1600947. doi: 10.1126/sciadv.1600947

Furman, J. L., Vaquer-Alicea, J., White, C. L., Cairns, N. J., Nelson, P. T., Diamond, M. I., et al. (2017). Widespread tau seeding activity at early Braak stages. *Acta Neuropathol.* 133, 91–100. doi: 10.1007/s00401-016-1644-z

Gámez-Valero, A., Beyer, K., and Borràs, F. E. (2019). Extracellular vesicles, new actors in the search for biomarkers of dementias. *Neurobiol. Aging* 74, 15–20. doi: 10.1016/j.neurobiolaging.2018.10.006

Ghosh, S., Wu, M. D., Shaftel, S. S., Kyrkanides, S., LaFerla, F. M., Olschowka, J. A., et al. (2013). Sustained interleukin-1β overexpression exacerbates tau pathology despite reduced amyloid burden in an Alzheimer's mouse model. *J. Neurosci.* 33, 5053–5064. doi: 10.1523/JNEUROSCI.4361-12.2013

Gibbons, G. S., Banks, R. A., Kim, B., Xu, H., Changolkar, L., Leight, S. N., et al. (2017). GFP-mutant human tau transgenic mice develop tauopathy following CNS injections of Alzheimer's brain-derived pathological tau or synthetic mutant human tau fibrils. *J. Neurosci.* 37, 11485–11494. doi: 10.1523/JNEUROSCI.2393-17.2017

Ginhoux, F., Lim, S., Hoeffel, G., Low, D., Huber, T., and Cuadros, M. A. (2013). Origin and differentiation of microglia. *Front. Cell. Neurosci.* 7:45. doi: 10.3389/fncel.2013.00045

Goedert, M., Eisenberg, D. S., and Crowther, R. A. (2017). Propagation of tau aggregates and neurodegeneration. *Annu. Rev. Neurosci.* 40, 189–210. doi: 10.1146/annurev-neuro-072116-031153

Goedert, M., Spillantini, M. G., Jakes, R., Rutherford, D., and Crowther, R. A. (1989). Multiple isoforms of human microtubule-associated protein tau: sequences and localization in neurofibrillary tangles of Alzheimer's disease. *Neuron* 3, 519–526. doi: 10.1016/0896-6273(89)90210-9

Griffin, W. S., Stanley, L. C., Ling, C., White, L., MacLeod, V., Perrot, L. J., et al. (1989). Brain interleukin 1 and S-100 immunoreactivity are elevated in down syndrome and Alzheimer disease. *Proc. Natl. Acad. Sci. U S A* 86, 7611–7615. doi: 10.1073/pnas.86.19.7611

Guo, J. L., Narasimhan, S., Changolkar, L., He, Z., Stieber, A., Zhang, B., et al. (2016). Unique pathological tau conformers from Alzheimer's brains transmit tau pathology in nontransgenic mice. *J. Exp. Med.* 213, 2635–2654. doi: 10.1084/jem.20160833

Hall, G. F., and Patuto, B. A. (2012). Is tau ready for admission to the prion club? *Prion* 6, 223–233. doi: 10.4161/pri.19912

Holmes, B. B., Furman, J. L., Mahan, T. E., Yamasaki, T. R., Mirbaha, H., Eades, W. C., et al. (2014). Proteopathic tau seeding predicts tauopathy *in vivo*. *Proc. Natl. Acad. Sci. U S A* 111, E4376–4385. doi: 10.1073/pnas.1411649111

Hopp, S. C., Lin, Y., Oakley, D., Roe, A. D., DeVos, S. L., Hanlon, D., et al. (2018). The role of microglia in processing and spreading of bioactive tau seeds in Alzheimer's disease. *J. Neuroinflammation* 15:269. doi: 10.1186/s12974-018-1309-z

Hoshiko, M., Arnoux, I., Avignone, E., Yamamoto, N., and Audinat, E. (2012). Deficiency of the microglial receptor CX3CR1 impairs postnatal functional development of thalamocortical synapses in the barrel cortex. *J. Neurosci.* 32, 15106–15111. doi: 10.1523/JNEUROSCI.1167-12.2012

in t' Veld, B. A., Ruitenberg, A., Hofman, A., Launer, L. J., van Dujin, C. M., Stijnen, T., et al. (2001). Nonsteroidal antiinflammatory drugs and the risk of Alzheimer's disease. *N. Engl. J. Med.* 345, 1515–1521. doi: 10.1056/NEJMoa010178

Jackson, W. S. (2014). Selective vulnerability to neurodegenerative disease: the curious case of prion protein. *Dis. Model Mech.* 7, 21–29. doi: 10.1242/dmm.012146

Jiang, D.-Q., Ma, Y.-J., Wang, Y., Lu, H.-X., Mao, S.-H., and Zhao, S.-H. (2019). Microglia activation induces oxidative injury and decreases SIRT3 expression in dopaminergic neuronal cells. *J. Neural Transm.* 126, 559–568. doi: 10.1007/s00702-019-02005-z

Jiang, D.-Q., Wei, M.-D., Wang, K.-W., Lan, Y.-X., Zhu, N., and Wang, Y. (2016a). Nicotine contributes to the neural stem cells fate against toxicity of microglial-derived factors induced by Aβ via the Wnt/β-catenin pathway. *Int. J. Neurosci.* 126, 257–268. doi: 10.3109/00207454.2015.1008696

Jiang, T., Zhang, Y.-D., Chen, Q., Gao, Q., Zhu, X.-C., Zhou, J.-S., et al. (2016b). TREM2 modifies microglial phenotype and provides neuroprotection in P301S tau transgenic mice. *Neuropharmacology* 105, 196–206. doi: 10.1016/j.neuropharm.2016.01.028

Kametani, F., and Hasegawa, M. (2018). Reconsideration of amyloid hypothesis and tau hypothesis in Alzheimer's disease. *Front. Neurosci.* 12:25. doi: 10.3389/fnins.2018.00025

Katsinelos, T., Zeitler, M., Dimou, E., Karakatsani, A., Müller, H.-M., Nachman, E., et al. (2018). Unconventional secretion mediates the trans-cellular spreading of tau. *Cell Rep.* 23, 2039–2055. doi: 10.1016/j.celrep.2018.04.056

Keren-Shaul, H., Spinrad, A., Weiner, A., Matcovitch-Natan, O., Dvir-Szternfeld, R., Ulland, T. K., et al. (2017). A unique microglia type associated with restricting development of Alzheimer's disease. *Cell* 169, 1276.e17–1290.e17. doi: 10.1016/j.cell.2017.05.018

Kfoury, N., Holmes, B. B., Jiang, H., Holtzman, D. M., and Diamond, M. I. (2012). Trans-cellular propagation of tau aggregation by fibrillar species. *J. Biol. Chem.* 287, 19440–19451. doi: 10.1074/jbc.M112.346072

Kinney, J. W., Bemiller, S. M., Murtishaw, A. S., Leisgang, A. M., Salazar, A. M., and Lamb, B. T. (2018). Inflammation as a central mechanism in Alzheimer's disease. *Alzheimers Dement.* 4, 575–590. doi: 10.1016/j.trci.2018.06.014

Lanzrein, A.-S., Johnston, C. M., Perry, V. H., Jobst, K. A., King, E. M., and Smith, A. D. (1998). Longitudinal study of inflammatory factors in serum, cerebrospinal fluid and brain tissue in Alzheimer disease. *Alzheimer Dis. Assoc. Disord.* 12, 215–227. doi: 10.1097/00002093-199809000-00016

Lavin, Y., Winter, D., Blecher-Gonen, R., David, E., Keren-Shaul, H., Merad, M., et al. (2014). Tissue-resident macrophage enhancer landscapes are shaped by the local microenvironment. *Cell* 159, 1312–1326. doi: 10.1016/j.cell.2014.11.018

Lee, M., McGeer, E., and McGeer, P. L. (2015). Activated human microglia stimulate neuroblastoma cells to upregulate production of beta amyloid protein and tau: implications for Alzheimer's disease pathogenesis. *Neurobiol. Aging* 36, 42–52. doi: 10.1016/j.neurobiolaging.2014.07.024

Lenz, K. M., and Nelson, L. H. (2018). Microglia and beyond: innate immune cells as regulators of brain development and behavioral function. *Front. Immunol.* 9:698. doi: 10.3389/fimmu.2018.00698

Li, Y., Liu, L., Barger, S. W., and Griffin, W. S. T. (2003). Interleukin-1 mediates pathological effects of microglia on tau phosphorylation and on synaptophysin synthesis in cortical neurons through a p38-MAPK pathway. *J. Neurosci.* 23, 1605–1611. doi: 10.1523/jneurosci.23-05-01605.2003

Lindwall, G., and Cole, R. D. (1984). Phosphorylation affects the ability of tau protein to promote microtubule assembly. *J. Biol. Chem.* 259, 5301–5305.

Liu, L., Drouet, V., Wu, J. W., Witter, M. P., Small, S. A., Clelland, C., et al. (2012). Trans-synaptic spread of tau pathology *in vivo*. *PLoS One* 7:e31302. doi: 10.1371/journal.pone.0031302

Liu, C., Hong, K., Chen, H., Niu, Y., Duan, W., Liu, Y., et al. (2019). Evidence for a protective role of the CX3CL1/CX3CR1 axis in a model of amyotrophic lateral sclerosis. *Biol. Chem.* 400, 651–661. doi: 10.1515/hsz-2018-0204

Luo, W., Liu, W., Hu, X., Hanna, M., Caravaca, A., and Paul, S. M. (2015). Microglial internalization and degradation of pathological tau is enhanced by an anti-tau monoclonal antibody. *Sci. Rep.* 5:11161. doi: 10.1038/srep11161

Maphis, N., Xu, G., Kokiko-Cochran, O. N., Jiang, S., Cardona, A., Ransohoff, R. M., et al. (2015). Reactive microglia drive tau pathology and contribute to the spreading of pathological tau in the brain. *Brain* 138, 1738–1755. doi: 10.1093/brain/awv081

Matcovitch-Natan, O., Winter, D. R., Giladi, A., Vargas Aguilar, S., Spinrad, A., Sarrazin, S., et al. (2016). Microglia development follows a stepwise program to regulate brain homeostasis. *Science* 353:aad8670. doi: 10.1126/science.aad8670

Medzhitov, R. (2007). Recognition of microorganisms and activation of the immune response. *Nature* 449, 819–826. doi: 10.1038/nature06246

Michelucci, A., Heurtaux, T., Grandbarbe, L., Morga, E., and Heuschling, P. (2009). Characterization of the microglial phenotype under specific pro-inflammatory and anti-inflammatory conditions: effects of oligomeric and fibrillar amyloid-β. *J. Neuroimmunol.* 210, 3–12. doi: 10.1016/j.jneuroim.2009.02.003

Minghetti, L. (2005). Role of inflammation in neurodegenerative diseases. *Curr. Opin. Neurol.* 18, 315–321. doi: 10.1097/01.wco.0000169752.54191.97

Mudò, G., Frinchi, M., Nuzzo, D., Scaduto, P., Plescia, F., Massenti, M. F., et al. (2019). Anti-inflammatory and cognitive effects of interferon-β1a (IFNβ1a) in a rat model of Alzheimer's disease. *J. Neuroinflammation* 16:44. doi: 10.1186/s12974-019-1417-4

Narasimhan, S., Guo, J. L., Changolkar, L., Stieber, A., McBride, J. D., Silva, L. V., et al. (2017). Pathological tau strains from human brains recapitulate the diversity of tauopathies in nontransgenic mouse brain. *J. Neurosci.* 37, 11406–11423. doi: 10.1523/JNEUROSCI.1230-17.2017

Neve, R. L., Harris, P., Kosik, K. S., Kurnit, D. M., and Donlon, T. A. (1986). Identification of cDNA clones for the human microtubule-associated protein tau and chromosomal localization of the genes for tau and microtubule-associated protein 2. *Brain Res.* 387, 271–280. doi: 10.1016/0169-328x(86)90033-1

Nimmerjahn, A., Kirchhoff, F., and Helmchen, F. (2005). Resting microglial cells are highly dynamic surveillants of brain parenchyma *in vivo*. *Science* 308, 1314–1318. doi: 10.1126/science.1110647

Nizynski, B., Dzwolak, W., and Nieznanski, K. (2017). Amyloidogenesis of tau protein. *Proten Sci.* 26, 2126–2150. doi: 10.1002/pro.3275

Paolicelli, R. C., Bolasco, G., Pagani, F., Maggi, L., Scianni, M., Panzanelli, P., et al. (2011). Synaptic pruning by microglia is necessary for normal brain development. *Science* 333, 1456–1458. doi: 10.1126/science.1202529

Plouffe, V., Mohamed, N.-V., Rivest-McGraw, J., Bertrand, J., Lauzon, M., and Leclerc, N. (2012). Hyperphosphorylation and cleavage at D421 enhance tau secretion. *PLoS One* 7:e36873. doi: 10.1371/journal.pone.0036873

Prusiner, S. B. (1982). Novel proteinaceous infectious particles cause scrapie. *Science* 216, 136–144. doi: 10.1126/science.6801762

Prusiner, S. B. (2013). Biology and genetics of prions causing neurodegeneration. *Annu. Rev. Genet.* 47, 601–623. doi: 10.1146/annurev-genet-110711-155524

Qin, L., Liu, Y., Cooper, C., Liu, B., Wilson, B., and Hong, J.-S. (2002). Microglia enhance beta-amyloid peptide-induced toxicity in cortical and mesencephalic neurons by producing reactive oxygen species. *J. Neurochem.* 83, 973–983. doi: 10.1046/j.1471-4159.2002.01210.x

Rabouille, C., Malhotra, V., and Nickel, W. (2012). Diversity in unconventional protein secretion. *J. Cell Sci.* 125, 5251–5255. doi: 10.1242/jcs.103630

Rangaraju, S., Dammer, E. B., Raza, S. A., Rathakrishnan, P., Xiao, H., Gao, T., et al. (2018). Identification and therapeutic modulation of a pro-inflammatory subset of disease-associated-microglia in Alzheimer's disease. *Mol. Neurodegener.* 13:24. doi: 10.1186/s13024-018-0254-8

Saman, S., Kim, W., Raya, M., Visnick, Y., Miro, S., Saman, S., et al. (2012). Exosome-associated tau is secreted in tauopathy models and is selectively phosphorylated in cerebrospinal fluid in early Alzheimer disease. *J. Biol. Chem.* 287, 3842–3849. doi: 10.1074/jbc.M111.277061

Sardi, F., Fassina, L., Venturini, L., Inguscio, M., Guerriero, F., Rolfo, E., et al. (2011). Autoimmunity reviews Alzheimer's disease, autoimmunity and inflammation. The good, the bad and the ugly. *Autoimmun. Rev.* 11, 149–153. doi: 10.1016/j.autrev.2011.09.005

Sasaki, A., Kawarabayashi, T., Murakami, T., Matsubara, E., Ikeda, M., Hagiwara, H., et al. (2008). Microglial activation in brain lesions with tau deposits: comparison of human tauopathies and tau transgenic mice TgTauP301L. *Brain Res.* 1214, 159–168. doi: 10.1016/j.brainres.2008.02.084

Sayed, F. A., Telpoukhovskaia, M., Kodama, L., Li, Y., Zhou, Y., Le, D., et al. (2018). Differential effects of partial and complete loss of TREM2 on microglial injury response and tauopathy. *Proc. Natl. Acad. Sci. U S A* 115, 10172–10177. doi: 10.1073/pnas.1811411115

Schafer, D. P., Lehrman, E. K., Kautzman, A. G., Koyama, R., Mardinly, A. R., Yamasaki, R., et al. (2012). Microglia sculpt postnatal neural circuits in an activity and complement-dependent manner. *Neuron* 74, 691–705. doi: 10.1016/j.neuron.2012.03.026

Serrano-Pozo, A., Mielke, M. L., Gómez-Isla, T., Betensky, R. A., Growdon, J. H., Frosch, M. P., et al. (2011). Reactive glia not only associates with plaques but also parallels tangles in Alzheimer's disease. *Am. J. Pathol.* 179, 1373–1384. doi: 10.1016/j.ajpath.2011.05.047

Sheffield, L. G., Marquis, J. G., and Berman, N. E. (2000). Regional distribution of cortical microglia parallels that of neurofibrillary tangles in Alzheimer's disease. *Neurosci. Lett.* 285, 165–168. doi: 10.1016/s0304-3940(00)01037-5

Šimić, G., Babić Leko, M., Wray, S., Harrington, C., Delalle, I., Jovanov-Milošević, N., et al. (2016). Tau protein hyperphosphorylation and aggregation in Alzheimer's disease and other tauopathies and possible neuroprotective stragegies. *Biomolecules* 6:6. doi: 10.3390/biom6010006

Šimić, G., Babić Leko, M., Wray, S., Harrington, C. R., Delalle, I., Jovanov-Milošević, N., et al. (2017). Monoaminergic neuropathology in Alzheimer's disease. *Prog. Neurobiol.* 151, 101–138. doi: 10.1016/j.pneurobio.2016.04.001

Šimić, G., Gnjidić, M., and Kostović, I. (1998). Cytoskeletal changes as an alternative view on pathogenesis of Alzheimer's disease. *Period Biol.* 100, 165–173.

Šimić, G., Španić, E., Langer Horvat, L., and Hof, P. R. (2019). Blood-brain barrier and innate immunity in the pathogenesis of Alzheimer's disease. *Prog. Mol. Biol. Transl. Sci.* 168:47. doi: 10.1016/bs.pmbts.2019.06.003

Smolek, T., Jadhav, S., Brezovakova, V., Cubinkova, V., Valachova, B., Novak, P., et al. (2019). First-in-rat study of human Alzheimer's disease tau propagation. *Mol. Neurobiol.* 56, 621–631. doi: 10.1007/s12035-018-1102-0

Stancu, I.-C., Cremers, N., Vanrusselt, H., Couturier, J., Vanoosthuyse, A., Kessels, S., et al. (2019). Aggregated tau activates NLRP3-ASC inflammasome exacerbating exogenously seeded and non-exogenously seeded tau pathology *in vivo*. *Acta Neuropathol.* 137, 599–617. doi: 10.1007/s00401-018-01957-y

Stephenson, J., Nutma, E., van der Valk, P., and Amor, S. (2018). Inflammation in CNS neurodegenerative diseases. *Immunology* 154, 204–219. doi: 10.1111/imm.12922

Takeda, S., Commins, C., DeVos, S. L., Nobuhara, C. K., Wegmann, S., Roe, A. D., et al. (2016). Seed-competent high-molecular-weight tau species accumulates in the cerebrospinal fluid of Alzheimer's disease mouse model and human patients. *Ann. Neurol.* 80, 355–367. doi: 10.1002/ana.24716

Takeda, S., Wegmann, S., Cho, H., DeVos, S. L., Commins, C., Roe, A. D., et al. (2015). Neuronal uptake and propagation of a rare phosphorylated high-molecular-weight tau derived from Alzheimer's disease brain. *Nat. Commun.* 6:8490. doi: 10.1038/ncomms9490

Tang, Y., and Le, W. (2016). Differential roles of M1 and M2 microglia in neurodegenerative diseases. *Mol. Neurobiol.* 53, 1181–1194. doi: 10.1007/s12035-014-9070-5

von Bernhardi, R., Eugenín-von Bernhardi, L., and Eugenín, J. (2015). Microglial cell dysregulation in brain aging and neurodegeneration. *Front. Aging Neurosci.* 7:124. doi: 10.3389/fnagi.2015.00124

Walker, L. C., and Jucker, M. (2015). Neurodegenerative diseases: expanding the prion concept. *Annu. Rev. Neurosci.* 38, 87–103. doi: 10.1146/annurev-neuro-071714-033828

Walsh, D. M., and Selkoe, D. J. (2016). A critical appraisal of the pathogenic protein spread hypothesis of neurodegeneration. *Nat. Rev. Neurosci.* 17, 251–260. doi: 10.1038/nrn.2016.13

Wang, Y., Balaji, V., Kaniyappan, S., Krüger, L., Irsen, S., Tepper, K., et al. (2017). The release and trans-synaptic transmission of tau via exosomes. *Mol. Neurodegener.* 12:5. doi: 10.1186/s13024-016-0143-y

Weingarten, M. D., Lockwood, A. H., Hwo, S. Y., and Kirschner, M. W. (1975). A protein factor essential for microtubule assembly. *Proc. Natl. Acad. Sci. U S A* 72, 1858–1862. doi: 10.1073/pnas.72.5.1858

Wu, Z., Yu, J., Zhu, A., and Nakanishi, H. (2016). Nutrients, microglia aging and brain aging. *Oxid. Med. Cell. Longev.* 2016:7498528. doi: 10.1155/2016/7498528

Yamada, K., Cirrito, J. R., Stewart, F. R., Jiang, H., Finn, M. B., Holmes, B. B., et al. (2011). *in vivo* microdialysis reveals age-dependent decrease of brain interstitial fluid tau levels in P301S human tau transgenic mice. *J. Neurosci.* 31, 13110–13117. doi: 10.1523/JNEUROSCI.2569-11.2011

Yoshiyama, Y., Higuchi, M., Zhang, B., Huang, S.-M., Iwata, N., Saido, T. C., et al. (2007). Synapse loss and microglial activation precede tangles in a P301S tauopathy mouse model. *Neuron* 53, 337–351. doi: 10.1016/j.neuron.2007.01.010

Zandi, P. P., Anthony, J. C., Hayden, K. M., Mehta, K., Mayer, L., and Breitner, J. C. S. (2002). Reduced incidence of AD with NSAID but not H2 receptor antagonists: the cache county study. *Neurology* 59, 880–886. doi: 10.1212/wnl.59.6.880

Zetterberg, H., and Blennow, K. (2013). Cerebrospinal fluid biomarkers for Alzheimer's disease: more to come? *J. Alzheimers Dis.* 33, S361–S369. doi: 10.3233/JAD-2012-129035

Zilka, N., Kazmerova, Z., Jadhav, S., Neradil, P., Madari, A., Obetkova, D., et al. (2012). Who fans the flames of Alzheimer's disease brains? Misfolded tau on the crossroad of neurodegenerative and inflammatory pathways. *J. Neuroinflammation* 9:47. doi: 10.1186/1742-2094-9-47

Zilka, N., Stozicka, Z., Kovac, A., Pilipcinec, E., Bugos, O., and Novak, M. (2009). Human misfolded truncated tau protein promotes activation of microglia and leukocyte infiltration in the transgenic rat model of tauopathy. *J. Neuroimmunol.* 209, 16–25. doi: 10.1016/j.jneuroim.2009.01.013

17

Involvement of Oligodendrocytes in Tau Seeding and Spreading in Tauopathies

Isidro Ferrer[1,2,3,4*], *Meritxell Aguiló García*[1], *Margarita Carmona*[1,3], *Pol Andrés-Benito*[1,3], *Benjamin Torrejón-Escribano*[5], *Paula Garcia-Esparcia*[1,3] and *José Antonio del Rio*[3,4,6,7]

[1] *Department of Pathology and Experimental Therapeutics, University of Barcelona, Barcelona, Spain,* [2] *Senior Consultant, Bellvitge University Hospital, IDIBELL (Bellvitge Biomedical Research Centre), Barcelona, Spain,* [3] *CIBERNED (Network Centre of Biomedical Research of Neurodegenerative Diseases), Institute of Health Carlos III, Ministry of Economy and Competitiveness, Madrid, Spain,* [4] *Institute of Neurosciences, University of Barcelona, Barcelona, Spain,* [5] *Biology Unit, Scientific and Technical Services, Hospitalet de Llobregat, University of Barcelona, Barcelona, Spain,* [6] *Molecular and Cellular Neurobiotechnology, Institute of Bioengineering of Catalonia (IBEC), Barcelona Institute for Science and Technology, Parc Científic de Barcelona, Barcelona, Spain,* [7] *Department of Cell Biology, Physiology and Immunology, Faculty of Biology, University of Barcelona, Barcelona, Spain*

Correspondence:
Isidro Ferrer
8082ifa@gmail.com

Introduction: Human tau seeding and spreading occur following intracerebral inoculation into different gray matter regions of brain homogenates obtained from tauopathies in transgenic mice expressing wild or mutant tau, and in wild-type (WT) mice. However, little is known about tau propagation following inoculation in the white matter.

Objectives: The present study is geared to learning about the patterns of tau seeding and cells involved following unilateral inoculation in the corpus callosum of homogenates from sporadic Alzheimer's disease (AD), primary age-related tauopathy (PART: neuronal 4Rtau and 3Rtau), pure aging-related tau astrogliopathy (ARTAG: astroglial 4Rtau with thorn-shaped astrocytes TSAs), globular glial tauopathy (GGT: 4Rtau with neuronal tau and specific tau inclusions in astrocytes and oligodendrocytes, GAIs and GOIs, respectively), progressive supranuclear palsy (PSP: 4Rtau with neuronal inclusions, tufted astrocytes and coiled bodies), Pick's disease (PiD: 3Rtau with characteristic Pick bodies in neurons and tau containing fibrillar astrocytes), and frontotemporal lobar degeneration linked to P301L mutation (FTLD-P301L: 4Rtau familial tauopathy).

Methods: Adult WT mice were inoculated unilaterally in the lateral corpus callosum with sarkosyl-insoluble fractions or with sarkosyl-soluble fractions from the mentioned tauopathies; mice were killed from 4 to 7 months after inoculation. Brains were fixed in paraformaldehyde, embedded in paraffin and processed for immunohistochemistry.

Results: Tau seeding occurred in the ipsilateral corpus callosum and was also detected in the contralateral corpus callosum. Phospho-tau deposits were found in oligodendrocytes similar to coiled bodies and in threads. Moreover, tau deposits co-localized with active (phosphorylated) tau kinases p38 and ERK 1/2, suggesting active tau phosphorylation of murine tau. TSAs, GAIs, GOIs, tufted astrocytes, and tau-containing fibrillar astrocytes were not seen in any case. Tau deposits were often associated with slight myelin disruption and the presence of small PLP1-immunoreactive globules and dots in the ipsilateral corpus callosum 6 months after inoculation of sarkosyl-insoluble fractions from every tauopathy.

Conclusions: Seeding and spreading of human tau in the corpus callosum of WT mice occurs in oligodendrocytes, thereby supporting the idea of a role of oligodendrogliopathy in tau seeding and spreading in the white matter in tauopathies. Slight differences in the predominance of threads or oligodendroglial deposits suggest disease differences in the capacity of tau seeding and spreading among tauopathies.

Keywords: tau, tauopathies, seeding and spreading, AD, ARTAG, GGT, PiD

INTRODUCTION

Tauopathies are progressive neurodegenerative diseases characterized by the accumulation of abnormal hyper-phosphorylated tau deposits in neurons and glial cells. These diseases are classified according to the clinical symptoms and neuropathological features, including particular regional and cellular vulnerability, together with biochemical and genetic determinants (Kovacs, 2015a,b). Biochemical factors are mainly defined by the accumulation of particular tau isoforms; protein tau in human brain (encoded by *MAPT* gene) is expressed in six isoforms arising from alternative splicing of exons 2 and 3 which encode N-terminal sequences, and exon 10 which encodes a microtubule-binding repeat domain; isoforms with 352 (3R/0N), 381 (3R/1N), and 410 (3R/2N) amino acids are 3Rtau; and isoforms with 383 (4R/0N), 412 (4R/1N), and 441 (4R/2N) amino acids are 4Rtau (Goedert et al., 1989, 1992; Spillantini and Goedert, 1998). Genetic factors largely depend on the mutation of *MAPT* which leads to familial frontotemporal lobar degeneration with tau deposits (fFTLD-tau).

The main sporadic tauopathies are Alzheimer's disease (AD), which is a 4Rtau+3Rtau plus β-amyloidopathy characterized by the combined accumulation of abnormal tau and β-amyloid in β-amyloid plaques and cerebral blood vessels in β-amyloid angiopathy (Duyckaerts and Dickson, 2011; Lowe and Kalaria, 2015); primary age related tauopathy (PART), a pure neuronal 3Rtau+4Rtau tauopathy; aging-related tau astrogliopathy (ARTAG), a pure 4Rtau astroglial tauopathy characterized by thorn-shaped astrocytes (TSAs) and granular/fuzzy astrocytes; globular glial tauopathy (GGT), a 4Rtau neuronal and glial tauopathy with distinctive globular astroglial and oligodendroglial inclusions (GAIs and GOIs, respectively); Pick's disease (PiD), a 3Rtau mainly neuronal tauopathy with some tau deposits in fibrillar astrocytes; progressive supranuclear palsy (PSP), a 4Rtau neuronal and glial tauopathy with characteristic tufted astrocytes (TAs) and coiled bodies; corticobasal degeneration (CBD), a 4Rtau neuronal and glial tauopathy with characteristic astrocytic plaques and coiled bodies; and argyrophilic grain disease (AGD), a 4Rtau neuronal and glial tauopathy with neuronal pre-tangles, grains in the neuropil, TSAs, and coiled bodies (Tolnay et al., 1997; Jellinger, 1998; Bigio et al., 2001; Ferrer et al., 2003, 2008, 2013; Powers et al., 2003; Piao et al., 2005; Josephs et al., 2006; Giaccone et al., 2008; Kovacs et al., 2008, 2016, 2017; Fu et al., 2010; Ahmed et al., 2011, 2013; Dickson et al., 2011; Muñoz et al., 2011; Tolnay and Braak, 2011; Crary et al., 2014; Duyckaerts et al., 2015; Jellinger et al., 2015; Ferrer, 2018a; Kovacs, 2018).

The main familial tauopathies are familial AD (fAD), linked to mutations in the genes encoding β-amyloid precursor protein (*APP*); presenilin 1 (*PSEN1*) and presenilin 2 (*PSEN2*), with biochemical characteristics similar to those in sporadic AD (sAD) (Bertram and Tanzi, 2011); and familial frontotemporal lobar degeneration linked to tau mutations (fFTLD-tau), in which the clinical features, neuropathology, and biochemical attributes largely depend on the localization of the mutation in *MAPT* together with individual variations (Spillantini et al., 1997; Iseki et al., 2001; Muñoz and Ferrer, 2008; Spina et al., 2008; Ghetti et al., 2011; Tacik et al., 2016, 2017; Borrego-Écija et al., 2017).

One of the mechanisms involved in the progression of tauopathies is inter-cellular and trans-regional propagation of the altered protein tau (de Calignon et al., 2012; Liu et al., 2012; Iba et al., 2013; Dujardin et al., 2014; Peeraer et al., 2015; Stancu et al., 2015; Lewis and Dickson, 2016; Goedert and Spillantini, 2017; Mudher et al., 2017). Studies analyzing tau seeding and propagation *in vivo* have been performed following inoculation of human homogenates in mice expressing human tau (Clavaguera et al., 2009, 2013a,b, 2015; Ahmed et al., 2014; Boluda et al., 2015) or in WT mice (Audouard et al., 2016; Guo et al., 2016; Narasimhan et al., 2017). Homogenates are obtained from transgenic mice expressing human tau or, more commonly, from human neuronal or mixed neuronal and glial tauopathies; these studies are focused on neurons as main targets of tau propagation although glial cells are also involved (Clavaguera et al., 2009, 2013a,b, 2015; Ahmed et al., 2014; Boluda et al., 2015; Audouard et al., 2016; Guo et al., 2016; Narasimhan et al., 2017). However, tau seeding and spreading occurs in neurons, astrocytes, and oligodendrocytes following intrahippocampal inoculation of homogenates from pure ARTAG in WT mice (Ferrer et al., 2018), raising the important question of the relevance of astrocytes in the pathogenesis and progression of at least certain tauopathies. On the other hand, tau homogenates have been inoculated into different gray matter regions including cerebral cortex, hippocampus, striatum and locus ceruleus, among other gray matter centers. Little attention has been paid regarding direct and selective tau inoculation into the white matter.

In this line of thinking, and considering that (1) the white matter is involved, often severely, in the majority of tauopathies; and (2) the majority of cells in the white matter are oligodendrocytes, the present study has been designed to learn about the capacity of seeding and spreading of abnormal tau and the involvement of oligodendrocytes in the process, following unilateral inoculation of sarkosyl-insoluble and sarkosyl-soluble fractions from distinct human tauopathies, including AD, PART, ARTAG, GGT, PiD, PSP, and fFTLD-tau linked to P301L mutation (fFTLD-P301L or P301L), into the lateral corpus callosum of WT mice.

MATERIALS AND METHODS

Human Cases

Brain tissue was obtained from the Institute of Neuropathology HUB-ICO-IDIBELL Biobank following the guidelines of Spanish legislation on this matter (Real Decreto de Biobancos 1716/2011) and approval of the local ethics committee. One hemisphere was immediately cut in coronal sections, 1 cm thick, and selected areas of the encephalon were rapidly dissected, frozen on metal plates over dry ice, placed in individual air-tight plastic bags, and stored at −80°C until use for biochemical studies. The other hemisphere was fixed by immersion in 4% buffered formalin for 3 weeks for morphological studies and neuropathological diagnoses.

Cases were categorized and selected following well-established neuropathological criteria (Braak et al., 2006; Dickson et al., 2011; Muñoz et al., 2011; Ahmed et al., 2013; Crary et al., 2014; Kovacs et al., 2016; Borrego-Écija et al., 2017) excluding cases with combined pathologies (excepting discrete small blood vessel disease related to age, and atherosclerosis), systemic diseases, and prolonged terminal hypoxia. It is worth stressing that ARTAG cases were pure forms without additional tau pathology excepting PART stage I-II (without involvement of the hippocampus). The cause of death was variable and included bronchopneumonia, rupture of aortic aneurysm, respiratory failure, cardiac arrest, kidney failure, pulmonary thromboembolism, and metastatic carcinoma. Post-mortem delay from death to tissue processing was between 4 h and 18 h. The final selection of inocula was based on the optimal profile of the western blot bands of sarkosyl-insoluble fractions visualized with anti-P-tauSer422 antibodies (see below). Selected samples were from sporadic AD (Braak stage VI/C: one man and one woman aged 82 and 76 years, respectively); PART (Braak stage IV: one man and one woman aged 68 and 72, respectively); pure ARTAG (two women aged 68 and 72, and one man 68 years old); GGT (one man and one woman aged 49 and 43 years, respectively); PiD (a 67-year-old man); PSP (one woman aged 72 years old); fFTLD-P301L (one man 53 years old); and one control (one man 61 years old).

Sarkosyl-Insoluble and Sarkosyl-Soluble Fractions Used for Inoculations

Human brain samples used for brain inoculation in mice were obtained from the hippocampus in cases of AD, PART, PiD, fFTLD-P301L, and control; temporal white matter in cases of ARTAG; striatum in PSP; and prefrontal cortex area 8 in GGT cases.

Frozen samples of about 1 g were lysed in 10 volumes (w/v) with cold suspension buffer (10 mM Tris-HCl, pH 7.4, 0.8 M NaCl, 1 mM EGTA) supplemented with 10% sucrose, protease, and phosphatase inhibitors (Roche, GE). The homogenates were first centrifuged at 20,000×g for 20 min (Ultracentrifuge Beckman with 70Ti rotor), and the supernatant (S1) was saved. The pellet was re-homogenized in 5 volumes of homogenization buffer and re-centrifuged at 20,000×g for 20 min (Ultracentrifuge Beckman with 70Ti rotor). The two supernatants (S1 + S2) were then mixed and incubated with 0.1% N-lauroylsarkosynate (sarkosyl) for 1 h at room temperature while being shaken. Samples were then centrifuged at 100,000×g for 1 h (Ultracentrifuge Beckman with 70Ti rotor). Sarkosyl-insoluble pellets (P3) were re-suspended (0.2 ml/g) in 50 mM Tris–HCl (pH 7.4). Protein concentrations were quantified with the bicinchoninic acid assay (BCA) assay (Pierce, Waltham, MA). Sarkosyl-insoluble and sarkosyl-soluble fractions were frozen at −80°C until use.

Western Blotting of Sarkosyl-Insoluble Fractions

Samples were mixed with loading sample buffer and heated at 95°C for 5 min. Sixty microgram of protein was separated by electrophoresis in SDS-PAGE gels and transferred to nitrocellulose membranes (200 mA per membrane, 90 min). The membranes were blocked for 1 h at room temperature with 5% non-fat milk in TBS containing 0.2% tween and were then incubated with the primary antibody, anti-tau Ser422 (diluted 1:1,000; Thermo Fisher (Waltham, MA, USA). After washing with TBS-T, blots were incubated with the appropriate secondary antibody (anti-rabbit IgG conjugated with horseradish peroxidase diluted at 1:2,000, DAKO, DE) for 45 min at room temperature. Immune complexes were revealed by incubating the membranes with chemiluminescence reagent (Amersham, GE Healthcare, Buckinghamshire, UK) (Ferrer et al., 2018).

Animals and Tissue Processing

Wild-type C57BL/6 mice from our colony were used. All animal procedures were carried out following the guidelines of the European Communities Council Directive 2010/63/EU and with the approval of the local ethical committee (University of Barcelona, Spain). The age and number of animals, and the survival times, are listed in **Table 1**.

Inoculation Into the Lateral Corpus Callosum

Mice were inoculated unilaterally with sarkosyl-insoluble fractions or with sarkosyl-soluble fractions from the above-mentioned tauopathies. In parallel, other mice were injected with 50 mM Tris-HCl (pH 7.4) as vehicle (negative) controls. Mice were deeply anesthetized by intra-peritoneal ketamin/xylazine/buprenorphine cocktail injection and placed in a stereotaxic frame after assuring lack of reflexes. Injections were done using a Hamilton syringe; the coordinates for lateral

TABLE 1 | Mice used in the study of unilateral inoculation in the lateral corpus callosum, age of inoculation, age of killing, survival, and type of inoculum; AD, Alzheimer's disease stage VI; PART, primary age-related tauopathy; ARTAG, aging related tau astrogliopathy; GGT, globular glial tauopathy; PSP, progressive supranuclear palsy; PiD, Pick's disease; and fFTLD-P301L, familial frontotemporal lobar degeneration linked to P301L mutation in *MAPT*.

Age inoculation month	Age killed month	Survival months	Inoculum	Tau-positive oligodendrocytes in ipsilateral/contralateral corpus callosum	Tau-positive threads/dots in ipsilateral/contralateral corpus callosum	PLP1-immunoreactive globules and balls in ipsilateral/contralateral corpus callosum
7	11	4	Control	–/–	–/–	–/–
			Control	–/–	–/–	–/–
			AD	++/–	ϕϕ/–	+/–
			ADs	–/–	–/–	–/–
			GGT	±	ϕ/–	–/–
			GGT	±	ϕ/–	–/–
			GGT	±	ϕ/–	–/–
			GGT	±	ϕ/–	–/–
			GGTs	–/–	–/–	–/–
			GGTs	–/–	–/–	–/–
			GGTs	–/–	–/–	–/–
12	18–19	6–7	AD	+ + +/+ + +	ϕϕ/ϕϕ	±
			AD	+ + +/+ + +	ϕϕ/ϕϕ	±
			PART	+ + +/+ + +	ϕϕ/ϕϕ	±
			PART	+ + +/+ + +	ϕϕ/ϕϕ	±
			PART	+ + +/++	ϕϕ/ϕ	±
			PART	+ + +/++	ϕ/ϕ	±
			ARTAG	+ + +/+	ϕϕ/ϕ	±
			ARTAG	+ + +/+ + +	ϕ/ϕ	±
			ARTAG	+ + +/++	ϕϕ/ϕ	±
			GGT	++/+	ϕϕ/ϕ	±
			GGT	++/++	ϕϕ/ϕϕ	±
			GGT	+/+	ϕϕ/ϕ	–/–
			GGT	–/–	–/–	–/–
			control	–/–	–/–	–/–
			control	–/–	–/–	–/–
			ARTAGs	–/–	–/–	–/–
			ARTAGs	–/–	–/–	–/–
10-12	16-18	6	PSP	++/+	ϕ/ϕ	±
			PSP	++/+	ϕ/ϕ	–/–
			PSP	+ + +/++	ϕ/ϕ	±
			PiD	+/+	ϕϕ/ϕ	–/–
			PiD	+/+	ϕϕ/ϕ	–/–
			PiD	+/+	ϕϕ/ϕ	±
			PiD	–/–	–/–	–/–
			fFTLD-P301L	+/+	ϕϕ/ϕ	±
			fFTLD-P301L	±	ϕϕ/ϕ	–/–
			fFTLD-P301L	+/+	ϕϕ/ϕ	–/–

The column on the right is a summary of the efficiency of the injection referred to the presence of deposits in oligodendrocytes (percentage of tau-containing oligodendrocytes of the total number of oligodendrocytes per section) in the ipsilateral and contralateral corpus callosum in each mouse. Inoculum refers to sarkosyl-insoluble fractions of the corresponding human tauopathies with the exception of ADs, GGTs, and ARTAGs, which indicate sarkosyl-soluble fractions of AD, GGT, and ARTAG, respectively. Signs of the semiquantitative study: –, indicate no tau-positive oligodendrocytes; +, 5–9% tau-positive oligodendrocytes; ++, 10–39%, and + + +, 40–65% tau-positive oligodendrocytes of the total number of oligodendrocytres per section as revealed with double-labeling immunofluorescence with Olig2 and AT8 antibodies and visualization with confocal microscopy. Tau-containing threads and dots along the corpus callosum were evaluated as: –, no deposits; ϕ, a few per section; ϕϕ, some per section; and ϕϕϕ, many per section. Regarding myelin alterations in PLP1-immunostained sections: –, no alterations; +, present.

corpus callosum inoculations were: −1.9 AP; ± 1.4 ML relative to Bregma and −1.0 DV from the dural surface. A volume of 1.2 μl was injected at a rate of 0.1 μl/min. The syringe was retired slowly over a period of 10 min to avoid leakage of the inoculum. Each mouse was injected with inoculum from a single human case. Following surgery, mice were kept in a warm blanket and monitored until they recovered from the anesthesia. Carprofen analgesia was administered immediately after surgery and once a day during the following 2 days. Animals were housed individually with full access to food and water.

Inoculation Into the Hippocampus of AD Homogenates

For comparative purposes two mice aged 10 months were inoculated with sarkosyl-insoluble fractions and two mice of similar age with sarkosyl-soluble fractions of AD cases into the hippocampus and killed at the age of 16 months following the same protocol. The coordinates for hippocampal injections were −1.9 AP; ± 1.4 ML relative to Bregma and −1.5 DV from the dural surface. A volume of 1.5 μl was injected at a rate of 0.05 μl/min in the hippocampus.

Tissue Processing

Animals were killed under anesthesia and the brains were rapidly fixed with paraformaldehyde in phosphate buffer, and then embedded in paraffin. Consecutive serial sections, 4 μm thick, were obtained with a sliding microtome. De-waxed sections were stained with haematoxylin and eosin or processed for immunohistochemistry using the antibodies AT8 (directed against P-tau at Ser202/Thr205), PLP1 (directed against proteolipid protein 1) and RT97 (directed against neurofilaments of 200 kDa) Following incubation with the primary antibody, the sections were incubated with EnVision + system peroxidase for 30 min at room temperature. The peroxidase reaction was visualized with diaminobenzidine and H_2O_2. Control of the immunostaining included omission of the primary antibody; no signal was obtained following incubation with only the secondary antibody.

Double-labeling immunofluorescence was carried out on the de-waxed sections, 4μm thick, which were stained with a saturated solution of Sudan black B (Merck, DE) for 15 min to block autofluorescence of lipofuscin granules present in cell bodies, and then rinsed in 70% ethanol and washed in distilled water. The sections were boiled in citrate buffer to enhance antigenicity and blocked for 30 min at room temperature with 10% fetal bovine serum diluted in PBS. Then the sections were incubated at 4°C overnight with combinations of AT8 and one of the following primary antibodies: glial fibrillary acidic protein (GFAP), Iba-1, Olig2, and phospho-p38: p38-P (Thr180-Tyr182). Other sections were immunostained with anti-phospho-tauThr181 and anti-phospho ERK 1/2 (Thr202/Tyr204) (see **Table 2** for the characteristics of the antibodies). After washing, the sections were incubated with Alexa488 or Alexa546 fluorescence secondary antibodies against the corresponding host species. Nuclei were stained with DRAQ5^{TM}.

The characteristics of the antibodies are listed in **Table 2**. Then the sections were mounted in Immuno-Fluore mounting medium, sealed, and dried overnight. Sections were examined with a Leica TCS-SL confocal microscope.

Semi-quantitative studies were carried in the ipsilateral corpus callosum and contralateral corpus callosum in three non-consecutive sections per case. Data were expressed as the percentage of oligodendrocytes (as revealed with the Olig2 antibody) with tau deposits (as seen with the antibody AT8) compared with the total number of oligodendrocytes in the same field following double-labeling immunofluorescence and examination with the confocal microcopy. Signs: −, indicates no tau deposits in oligodendrocytes; +, 5–9% tau-positive oligodendrocytes; ++, 10–39%, and + + +, 40–65% oligodendrocytes containing tau deposits from the total number of oligodendrocytes in the same field. Regarding the number of oligodendrocytes co-expressing phospho-tau and phospho-p38, data were expressed as the percentage of tau-positive oligodendrocytes containing active p38 from the total number of tau-containing oligodendrocytes in three non-consecutive sections in every case. Tau-containing threads and dots along the corpus callosum were evaluated as: −, no deposits; ϕ, a few per section; ϕϕ, some per section; and ϕϕϕ, many per section. Regarding myelin alterations in PLP1-immunostained sections: −, no alterations; +, present.

RESULTS

Biochemical Characterization of Tau Inocula

Western blots of sarkosyl-insoluble fractions incubated with anti P-tau Ser422 antibodies showed the expected phospho-tau band pattern for each tauopathy. AD and PART were characterized by bands of 68, 64, and 60 kDa indicative of 3Rtau + 4Rtau tauopathies; longer exposure showed bands of 50 kDa and about 30–37 kDa, and lower bands of about 20 kDa. ARTAG, GGT, PSP, and fFTLD-P301L revealed two bands of 68 and 64 kDa specific to 4Rtau tauopathies. GGT also showed several bands of about 50 and 55 kDa, and lower bands of truncated tau of about 20 kDa. In contrast, PiD showed two bands of 64 and 60 kDa, distinctive of 3Rtau tauopathies, in addition to some smears of ∼35 kDa (**Figure 1**).

Tau Seeding and Spreading in Mice Inoculated in the Hippocampus and Lateral Corpus Callosum With Sarkosyl-Insoluble Fractions From AD

This set of experiments was used to show different regional vulnerability of the same type of homogenates when injected in the hippocampus with large numbers of neurons, and the corpus callosum with a major predominance of oligodendrocytes.

Two mice unilaterally injected in the hippocampus with sarkosyl-insoluble fractions of AD at the age of 10 months and killed at the age of 16 months showed tau deposition in neurons and rare glial cells of the hippocampus (dentate gyrus and CA1 region), in glial cells in the fimbria (**Figures 2A–C**), and in some fibers and neurons in septal nuclei and periventricular hypothalamus (data not shown). One mouse unilaterally injected in the corpus callosum with sarkosyl-insoluble fractions from AD at the age of 7 months and killed at the age of 11 months showed phospho-tau deposits in the ipsilateral corpus callosum in threads and glial cells, and rarely extending to the middle corpus callosum

TABLE 2 | : Characteristics of the antibodies used.

Antibody	Mono-/polyclonal	Dilution	Supplier	Country
Iba1	Rabbit polyclonal	1:1000	Wako	Richmond, VA, USA
phospho-tau Thr181	Rabbit polyclonal	1:50	Cell Signaling	Danvers, MA,USA
phospho-tau Ser422	Rabbit polyclonal	1:1000	Thermo Fisher	Waltham, MA, USA
AT8 (Ser202/Thr205)	Monoclonal	1:50	Innogenetics	Ghent, BE
glial fibrillary acidic protein (GFAP)	Rabbit polyclonal	1:500	Dako	Glostrup, DK
P38-P (Thr180-Tyr182)	Rabbit polyclonal	1:100	Cell Signaling	Danvers, MA, USA
ERK 1/2-P (Thr202/Tyr204)	Monoclonal	1:50	Merck-Millipore	Billerica, MA, USA
Olig2	Rabbit polyclonal	1:500	Abcam	Cambridge, UK
PLP1	Monoclonal	1:100	Lifespan Biosci	Seattle, WA, USA
RT97	Monoclonal	1:50	Novocastra, Leica Biosyst	Barcelona, Spain

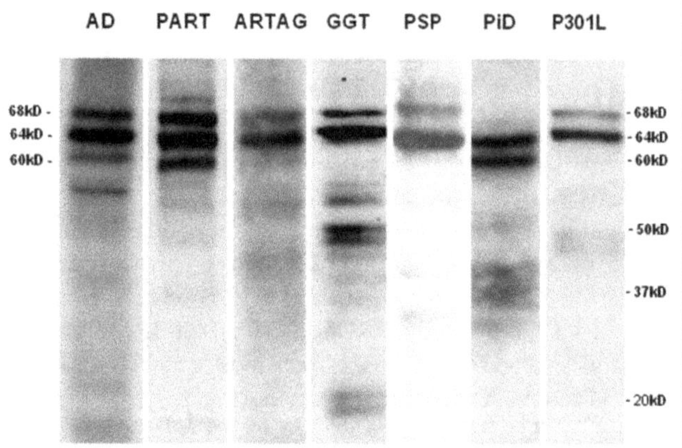

FIGURE 1 | Sarkosyl-insoluble fractions of brain homogenates blotted with anti-tauSer422 in AD, PART, ARTAG, GGT, PSP, PiD, and fFTLD-P301L cases. The band pattern of AD and PART is characterized by three bands of 68, 64, and 60 kDa. AD shows, in addition, bands of low molecular weight some of them of about 20kDa and lower. The ARTAG case is characterized by two bands of 68 and 64 kDa. GGT shows bands of 68 and 64 kDa, bands between 50 and 37 kDa, and bands of truncated tau of about 20 kDa. PSP is characterized by two bands of 68 and 64 kDa whereas PiD is characterized by two bands of 64 and 60 kDa. Finally, fFTLD-P301L (P301L) shows two bands of 68 and 64 kDa.

(data not shown). Two mice unilaterally injected into the corpus callosum with sarkosyl-insoluble fractions of AD at the age of 12 months and killed at the age of 18 months showed tau deposition only in glial cells and threads of the ipsilateral (D), middle region (E) and contralateral (F) corpus (**Figures 2D–F**). Double-labeling immunofluorescence in the corpus callosum showed almost absent co-localization of GFAP and AT8 (**Figure 2G**), but numerous oligodendroglial cells with phospho-tau deposits (**Figure 2H**) (**Table 1**). No tau-positive deposits co-localized with the microglial marker Iba1 (not shown).

One mouse aged 7 months and two mice aged 10 months were inoculated with sarkosyl-soluble fractions from AD (ADs). No tau deposits were seen 4 months and 6 months, respectively, after the inoculation (**Table 1**).

Tau Seeding and Spreading in Mice Inoculated in the Lateral Corpus Callosum With Sarkosyl-Insoluble and Sarkosyl-Soluble Fractions From Pure Tauopathies

Inoculation of sarkosyl-insoluble fractions obtained from pure tauopathies PART, ARTAG, GGT, PSP, PiD, and fFTLD-P301L was very effective as seen in **Table 1**. Of the 25 inoculated animals in the corpus callosum, only two (one inoculated with GGT and another with PiD) did not show phospho-tau deposits. Control cases (two mice inoculated at the age of 7 months and killed at the age 11 months, and two mice inoculated at the age 12 months and killed at the age of 18–19 months) were negative, as expected (**Table 1**).

Mice inoculated with sarkosyl-soluble fractions from GGT and ARTAG cases (GGTs and ARTAGs) did not show tau deposits at 4 months and 6 months, respectively, after unilateral inoculation into the corpus callosum (**Table 1**).

Mice injected with sarkosyl-insoluble fractions from GGT at the age of 7 months and killed 4 months later showed phospho-tau deposits in the ipsilateral corpus callosum in threads and glial cells, rarely extending to the middle corpus callosum. Mice inoculated at the age of 10–12 months and surviving 6 to 7 months showed phospho-tau deposition in threads and glial cells in the ipsilateral corpus callosum, middle region and throughout the contralateral corpus callosum. The pattern was similar using PART, ARTAG, GGT, PSP, PiD, and fFTLD-P301L sarkosyl-insoluble fractions of brain homogenates, although with disease differences regarding tau immunostaining. PART and ARTAG homogenates showed the most dramatic capacity for phospho-tau labeling of oligodendrocytes followed by PSP. Phospho-tau in oligodendrocytes was less marked in GGT, PiD and fFTLD-P301L when compared with the other tauopathies (**Figures 3, 4; Table 1**). The morphology of tau deposits in glial cells was perinuclear, with certain coma-like enlargements in some cells, mimicking coiled bodies in human tauopathies; labeled cells were commonly arranged as oligodendrocyte rows. Glial cells with the

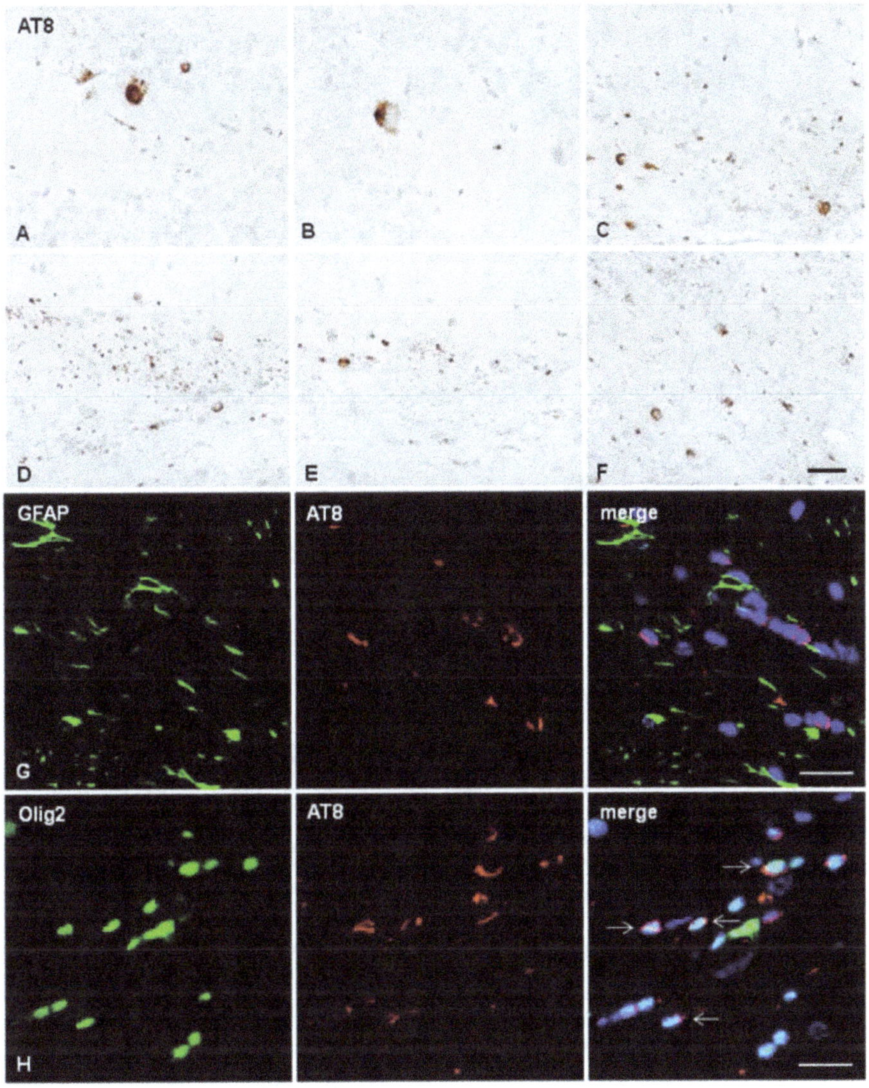

FIGURE 2 | Hyper-phosphorylated tau containing cells and fibers following unilateral intra-hippocampal injection **(A–C)** and unilateral inoculation into the corpus callosum **(D–H)** of sarkosyl-insoluble fractions from AD cases into WT mice at the age of 10 and 12 months, respectively, and killed 6 months later. **(A,B)** tau-containing neurons and rare glial cells in the hippocampus; **(C)** tau-containing glial cells and threads in the fimbria. Tau- containing glial cells and threads in the ipsilateral **(D)**, middle region **(E)** and contralateral corpus callosum **(F)**. Paraffin sections immunostained with AT8 antibody and slightly counterstained with hematoxylin; **(A–F)**, bar = 25 μm. **(G,H)** Double-labeling immunofluorescence to GFAP (green) and AT8 (red) **(G)**, and to Olig2 (green) and AT8 (red) in the corpus callosum of WT mice inoculated with sarkosyl-insoluble fractions from AD at the age of 12 months and killed at the age of 18 months after unilateral inoculation in the corpus callosum. No tau deposits are seen in astrocytes **(G)**, but phospho-tau is present in oligodendrocytes (arrows). Paraffin sections, nuclei stained with DRAQ5™ (blue); bar = 20 μm.

morphology of thorn-shaped astrocytes (TSAs), globular astrocytic inclusions (GAIs), tufted astrocytes (TAs), and fibrillary astrocytes were not visualized in any cases. Importantly, globular oligodendroglial inclusions (GOIs) were not observed following inoculation of sarkosyl-insoluble fractions from GGT homogenates.

In addition to glial cells, tau-immunoreactive threads and dots along nerve fibers were observed in every positive case. However, threads were more common in GGT, PiD, and fFTLD-P301L when compared with the other tauopathies (**Table 1**).

Tau deposits were restricted to the corpus callosum, no neurons and other cells were stained in the contralateral cortex or in any other region at 6–7 months after inoculation into the corpus callosum.

Identification of Hyper-Phosphorylated Tau-Containing Cells Using Double-Labeling Immunofluorescence and Confocal Microscopy

Double-labeling immunofluorescence was carried out using monoclonal anti-phospho-tau (clone AT8) and rabbit

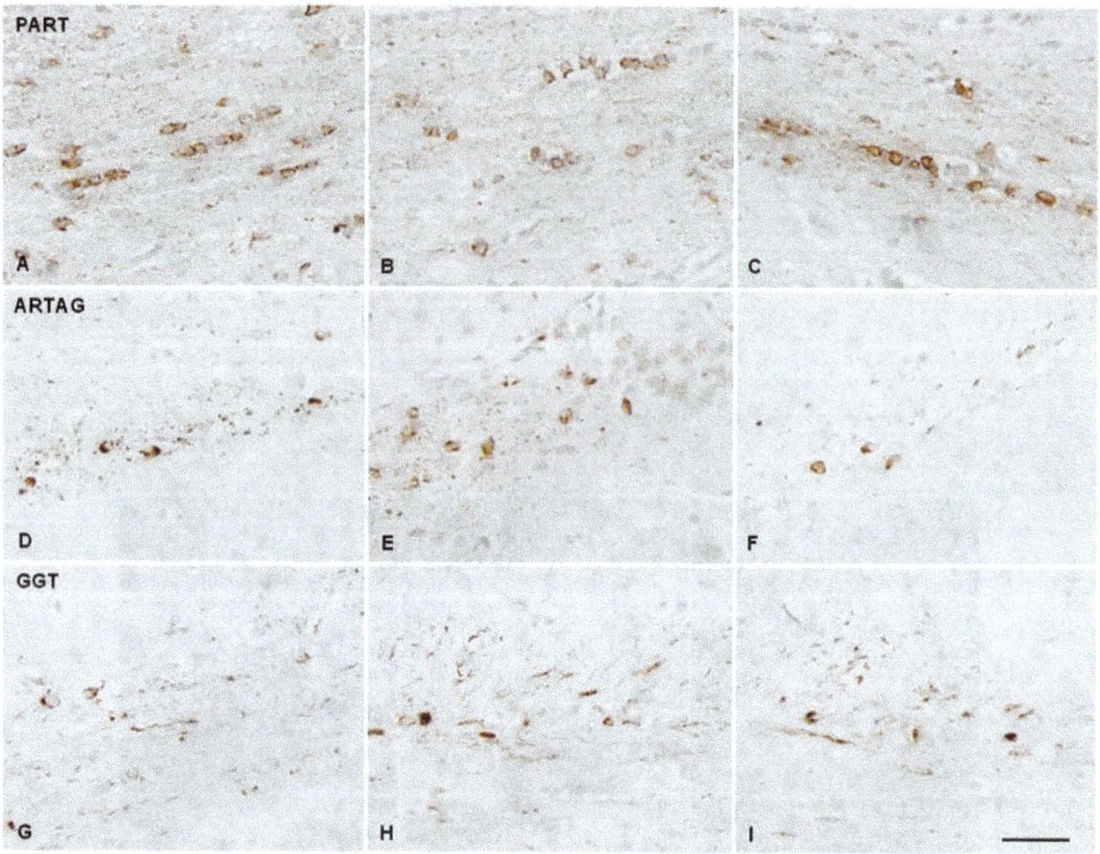

FIGURE 3 | Hyper-phosphorylated tau-containing cells and threads following unilateral inoculation of sarkosyl-insoluble fractions into the lateral corpus callosum from PART, ARTAG, and GGT cases in WT mice at the age of 12 months and killed 6–7 months later; **(A,D,G)** correspond to the injected corpus callosum; **(B,E,H)** to the middle region of the corpus callosum; and **(C,F,I)** to the contralateral corpus callosum. Paraffin sections immunostained with antibodies AT8 slightly counterstained with hematoxylin; bar = 25 μm.

polyclonal antibodies to microglia (Iba1), astrocytes (GFAP), and oligodendroglia (Olig2).

As in the case of inoculation of AD sarkosyl-insoluble fractions, no tau deposits were seen in microglia at any age (mice with short survival: 4 months; and mice with long survival: 6–7 months). Phospho-tau deposits in astrocytes were rarely seen only in ARTAG, as detailed in a previous work (Ferrer et al., 2018). The vast majority of tau-containing cells in the corpus callosum were oligodendrocytes, independently of the tauopathy (**Figure 5**). The morphology of tau deposits was similar in all the tauopathies: PART, ARTAG, GGT, PSP, PiD, and fFTLD-P301L. The distribution of tau was perinuclear, forming caps or coma-like deposits, the latter resembling coiled bodies (**Figure 5**). Phospho-tau-labeled oligodendrocytes were found in the ipsilateral corpus callosum, middle region and contralateral corpus callosum (**Figure 6**). Semi-quantitative studies were carried out in double-immunolabeled sections using Olig2 and AT8 antibodies in three non-consecutive sections per case. Data were expressed as the percentage of oligodendroglia with tau deposits compared with the total number of oligodendrocytes in the same field. As summarized in **Table 1**, the percentage of labeled oligodendrocytes in the ipsilateral and contralateral hippocampus was higher in AD, PART and ARTAG than in GGT, and lower in PiD- and P301L-inoculated mice.

Tau in Oligodendrocytes Is Associated With Activation of Tau-kinases in Tau-Positive Cells

Double-labeling immunofluorescence with anti-phospho-tau antibodies (AT8) and antibodies directed to phosphorylated p38 kinase (p38-P Thr180-Tyr182), examined with confocal microscopy, identified co-localization of tau and active p38 (p38-P) in oligodendrocytes in mice inoculated with sarkosyl-insoluble fractions from tauopathies. Co-localization occurred in oligodendrocytes in the ipsilateral corpus callosum, middle region and contralateral corpus callosum (**Figures 7A–C**). Semiquantitative studies showed that between 20 and 30% of tau-containing oligodendrocytes co-localized phosphorylated p38 kinase.

Similarly, double-labeling immunofluorescence with anti-phospho-tauThr181 and phospho-ERK 1/2 (Thr202/Tyr204) showed co-localization of tau and phospho-ERK 1/2-P in oligodendrocytes in the corpus callosum of mice inoculated

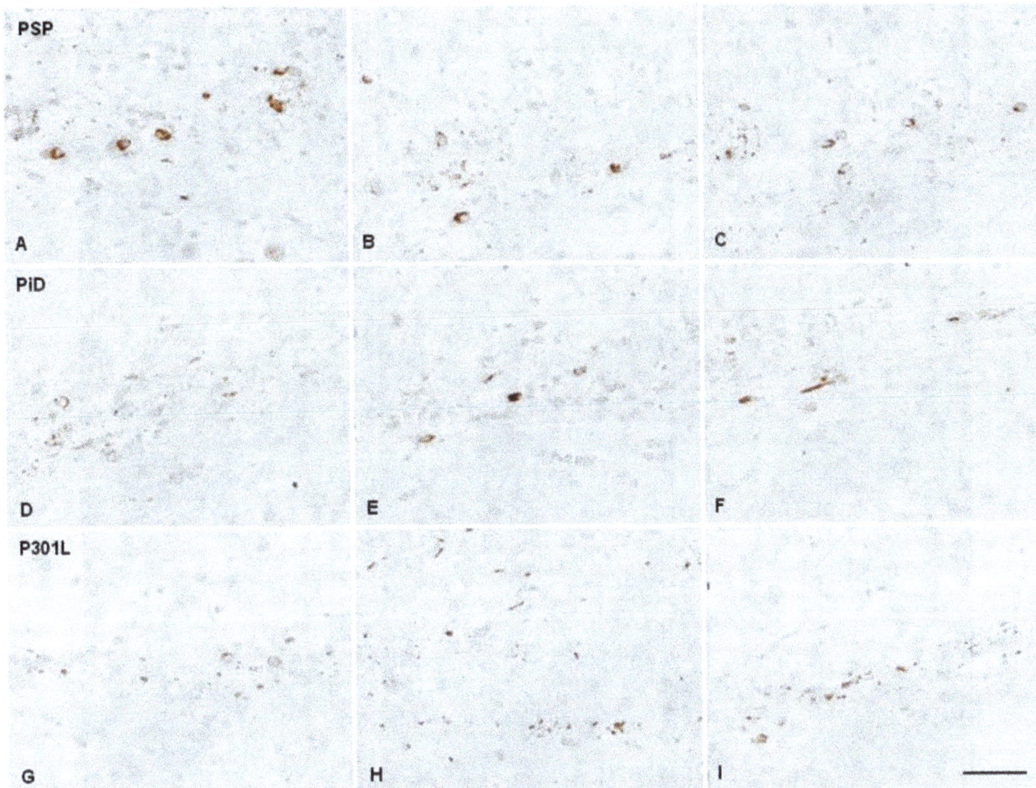

FIGURE 4 | Hyper-phosphorylated tau-containing cells and threads following unilateral inoculation of sarkosyl-insoluble fractions into the lateral corpus callosum from PSP, PiD, and fFTLD-P3101L in WT mice at the age of 10–12 months and killed at the age of 16–18 months; **(A,D,G)** correspond to the injected corpus callosum; **(B,E,H)** to the middle region of the corpus callosum; and **(C,F,I)** to the contralateral corpus callosum. Paraffin sections immunostained with antibodies AT8 slightly counterstained with hematoxylin; bar = 25 μm.

with sarkosyl-insoluble fractions from tauopathies (**Figure 7D**). The number of oligodendrocytes co-localizing phospho-tau and phospho-ERK 1/2 was between 25 and 35% of the total number of tau-containing oligodendrocytes.

The same pattern was seen in the different tauopathies (**Figures 7E–G**).

No expression of phospho-p38 and phospho-ERK 1/2 was observed outside the sites of phospho-tau deposits.

Long-Term Effects on Myelin Linked to Tau Spreading

To learn whether tau deposition in oligodendrocytes and threads had any impact on myelin and nerve fibers, consecutive sections to those used for AT8 immunohistochemistry were immunostained with anti-PLP1 antibody, as a marker of myelin, and with the antibody RT97 as a marker of neurofilaments 200 kDa.

Myelin lesions in the corpus callosum were very rare in inoculated animals killed 4 months after the injection. However, PLP1 immunohistochemistry disclosed slight myelin disruption and the presence of small globules and balls in the ipsilateral corpus callosum 6 months after the inoculation in some cases. These changes were observed in all samples in all tauopathies with tau deposits, although with disease-dependent variability; lesions were more common following inoculation of AD, PART, and ARTAG followed by GGT than following inoculation of homogenates from PSP, PiD, and fFTLD-P301L (**Figure 8**; **Table 1**). No changes were seen in cases inoculated with sarkosyl-soluble fractions and in controls.

In contrast to myelin alterations, no modifications were observed in parallel sections immunostained with the antibody RT97 (data not shown).

DISCUSSION

The present findings are in line with previous observations concerning tau seeding and spreading of abnormal tau derived from human brain homogenates of different tauopathies inoculated into the brain of mice (Clavaguera et al., 2009, 2013a,b, 2015; Ahmed et al., 2014; Boluda et al., 2015; Audouard et al., 2016; Guo et al., 2016; Narasimhan et al., 2017; Ferrer et al., 2018). In all these experimental paradigms, studies are focused on the neuronal involvement following inoculation in different regions of the gray matter including cerebral cortex, hippocampus, striatum and locus ceruleus, among others. However, the effects

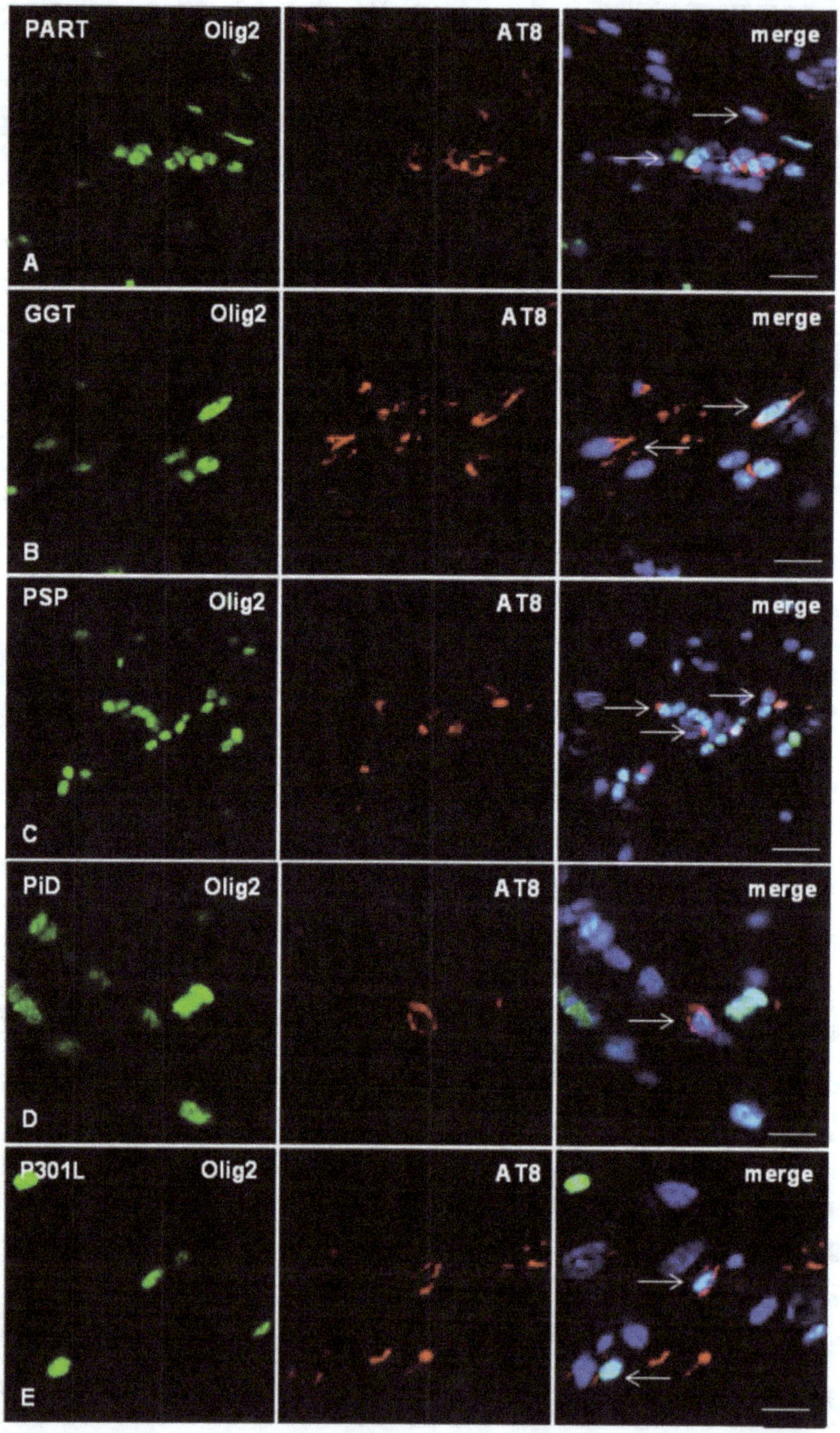

FIGURE 5 | Double-labeling immunofluorescence to Olig2 (green) and AT8 (red) in the corpus callosum of WT mice inoculated with sarkosyl-insoluble fractions from PART, GGT, PSP, PiD, and FTLD-P301L and killed 6–7 months after unilateral inoculation showing phospho-tau deposition in oligodendrocytes (arrows). Paraffin sections, nuclei stained with DRAQ5^{TM} (blue); **(A)** bar = 15 μm; **(B,D,E)**, bar = 10 μm; **(C)** bar = 20 μm.

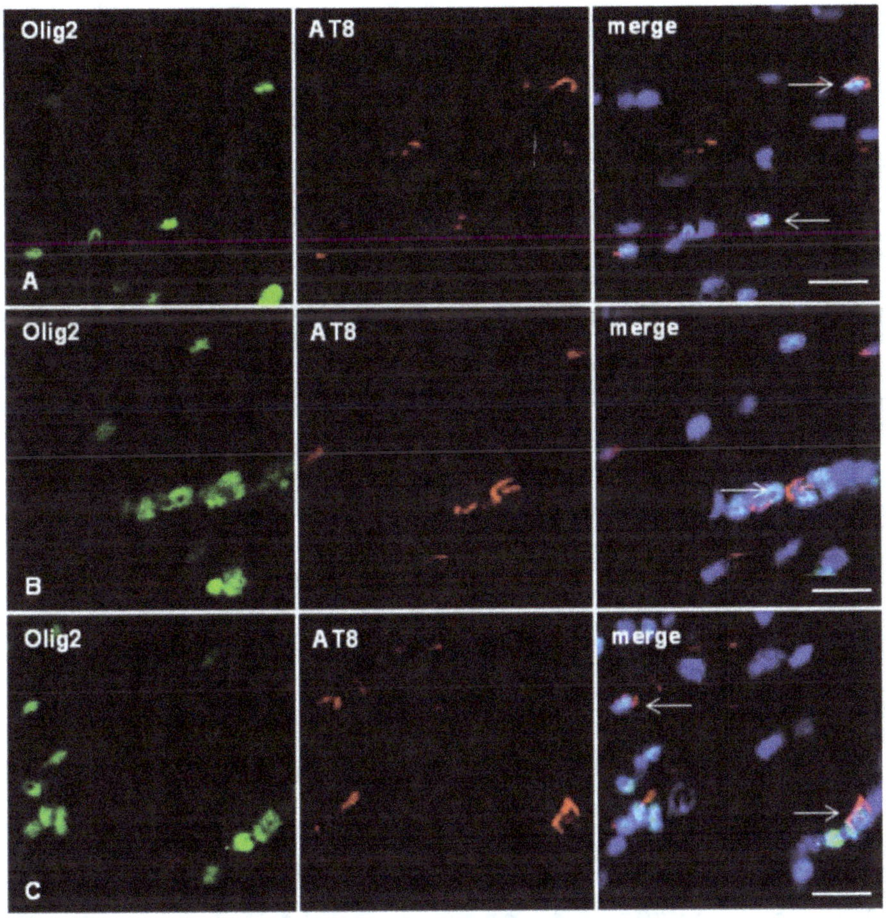

FIGURE 6 | Double-labeling immunofluorescence to Olig2 (green) and AT8 (red) in the corpus callosum of WT mice inoculated with sarkosyl-insoluble fractions from ARTAG at 12 months and killed at 19 months showing oligodendrocytes (arrows) containing hyper-phosphorylated tau in the injected corpus callosum **(A)**, middle region **(B)**, and contralateral corpus callosum **(C)**. Paraffin sections, nuclei stained with DRAQ5^{TM} (blue); bar = 15 μm.

of inoculation of abnormal tau in the white matter have not been examined in detail.

The present observations show tau seeding and spreading in the corpus callosum of WT mice following inoculation of homogenates from AD (4R+3R tauopathy + β-amyloidopathy), and pure neuronal 4R+3R tauopathy (PART), pure astrocyte 4R tauopathy (ARTAG), combined neuronal and glial 4R tauopathy (PSP), neuronal and glial 4R tauopathy with specific globular glial inclusions (GGT), 3R tauopathy (PiD), and familial FTLD-P301L. In all these paradigms, oligodendrocytes, and threads are the main if not the only targets of abnormal tau, albeit with variations in the capacity for seeding and spreading, depending on the tauopathy.

The overwhelming presence of tau in oligodendrocytes in comparison to astrocytes following abnormal tau inoculation into the corpus callosum may be explained because oligodendrocytes represent about 75.4 ± 5.1% of cells in the human corpus callosum, (Yeung et al., 2014), and the great majority of oligodendrocytes in mouse corpus callosum are not replaced during the animal's lifetime (Tripathi et al., 2017). Other targets of tau seeding and spreading, as neurons in gray matter regions, are well documented (Clavaguera et al., 2009, 2013a,b, 2015; Ahmed et al., 2014; Boluda et al., 2015; Audouard et al., 2016; Guo et al., 2016; Narasimhan et al., 2017; Ferrer et al., 2018), and here supported as complementary data using the same homogenates of AD employed for callosal inoculation following injection into the hippocampus; inoculation of homogenates into the hippocampus produced tau deposition in neurons and their projections, in addition to glial cells in the fimbria.

Slight peculiarities in relation with the amount of labeled oligodendrocytes and threads in the analyzed tauopathies are probably related to particular characteristics of tau in the different diseases. This possibility is in agreement with the observation that distinct artificially-generated strains of tau produce different types of neuronal and glial inclusions depending on the strain (Sanders et al., 2014; Kaufman et al., 2016).

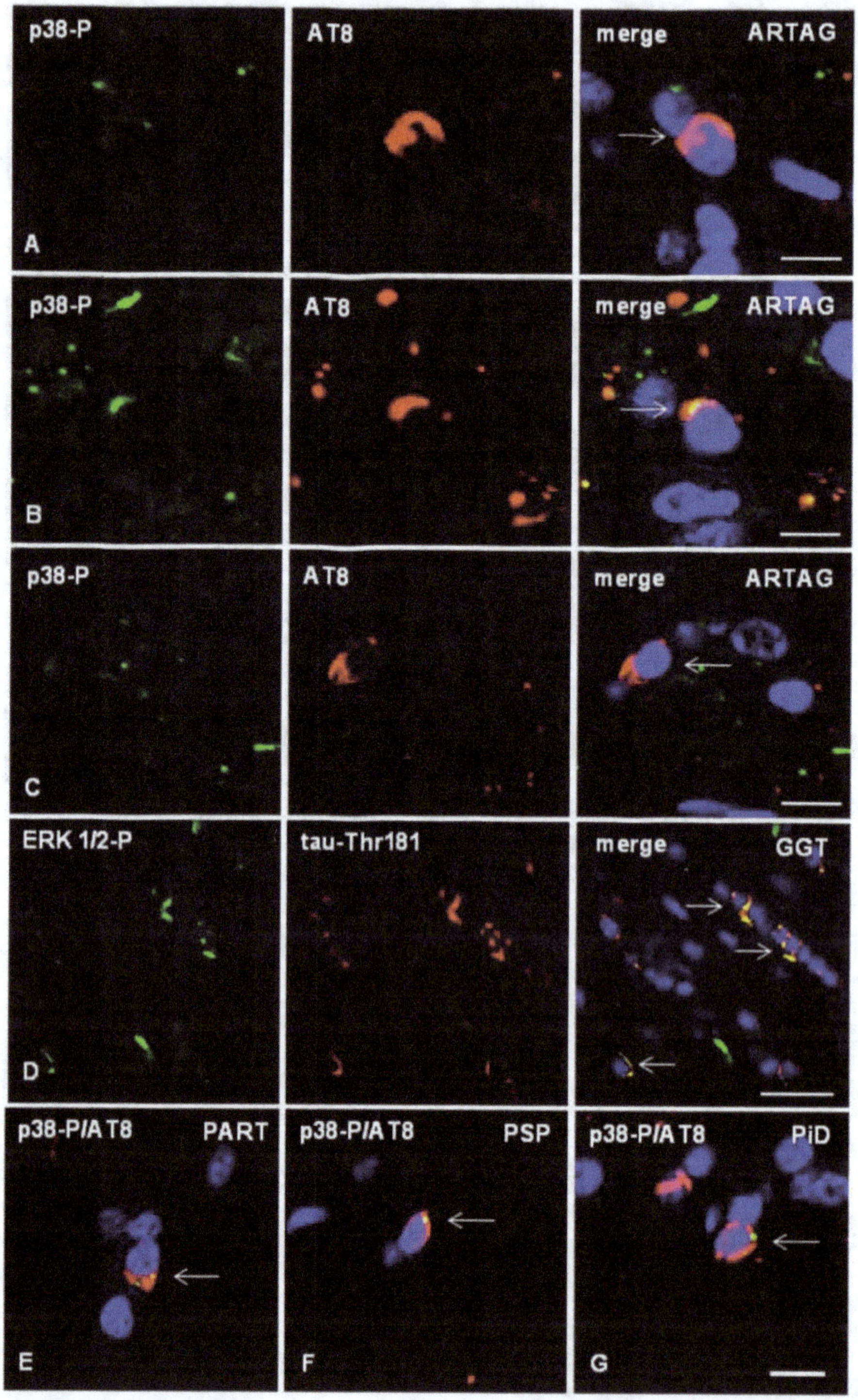

FIGURE 7 | (A–C) Double-labeling immunofluorescence to phosphorylated p38 (p38-P: Thr180-182) (green) and AT8 (red) in the corpus callosum of WT mice inoculated unilaterally with sarkosyl-insoluble fractions from ARTAG at the age of 12 months and killed at the age of 19 months. Phospho-p38 kinase (p38-P) co-localizes with tau deposits (arrows) in oligodendrocytes in the ipsilateral corpus callosum **(A)**, middle region **(B),** and contralateral corpus callosum **(C)**. **(D)** Double-labeling immunofluorescence to phospho-ERK 1/2 (Thr202/Tyr204) (green) and phospho-tau Thr181 (red) in the corpus callosum of WT mice inoculated with sarkosyl-insoluble fractions from GGT at the age of 12 months and killed at the age of 19 months. Phospho-ERK 1/2 co-localizes with tau deposits (arrows) in oligodendrocytes. **(E–G)** Double-labeling immunofluorescence to p38-P and AT8 (merge) in oligodendroglial cells of the corpus callosum of WT mice inoculated unilaterally with sarkosyl-insoluble fractions from PART **(E)**, PSP **(F)**, or PiD **(G)** at the age of 10–12 months and killed 6 months later. Paraffin sections, nuclei stained with DRAQ5™ (blue), **(A,B)**, bar = 5 μm; **(C)** bar = 10 μm; **(D)** bar = 20 μm; **(E–G)**, bar in **(G)** = 10 μm.

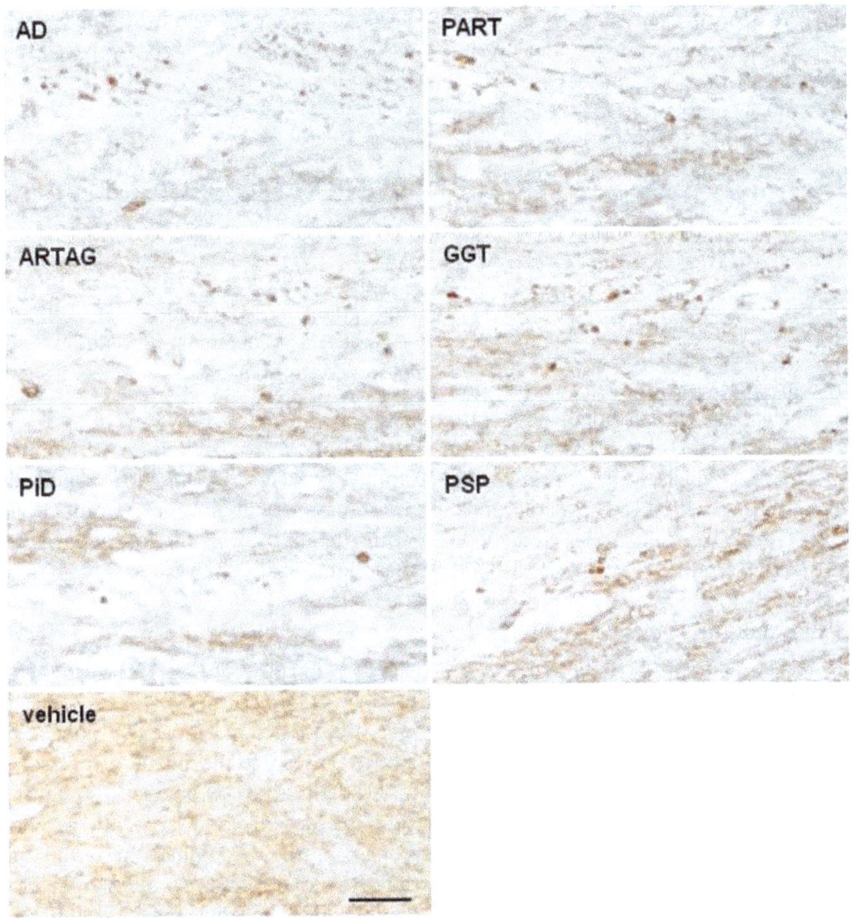

FIGURE 8 | Representative sections of the corpus callosum immunostained with antibodies anti-PLP1 (proteolipid protein 1) in WT mice following inoculation of AD, PART, ARTAG, GGT, PiD, and PSP in the lateral corpus callosum at the age of 10–12 months and killed 6 months later. Disrupted myelin with occasional formation of small PLP1-immunoreactive balls is observed, when compared with mice inoculated with vehicle (control). Paraffin sections immunostained with antibodies PLP1 slightly counterstained with hematoxylin; bar = 50 μm.

Morphological characteristics of tau inclusions in oligodendrocytes in the present experiments are reminiscent to coiled bodies which are the most typical tau oligodendroglial inclusions in the majority of human tauopathies. However, coiled-like bodies are also observed following inoculation of AD and PART sarkosyl-insoluble homogenates thus indicating that pure neuronal tauopathies (AD and PART) have the capacity to induce tau seeding and spreading in oligodendrocytes in WT mice. On the other hand, GOIs, which are typical of GGT, are not seen following inoculation of sarkosyl-insoluble homogenates from GGT cases. Based on these findings, it may be suggested that, in addition to the postulated tau strains, the characteristics of the host tau and the region of inoculation help determine the characteristics of tau seeding and spreading of human tau inoculated into WT mice. Therefore, the present observations show that inoculation of homogenates from specific tauopathies into the corpus callosum does not replicate important aspects of the corresponding human tauopathies. Regarding astrocytes, TSAs typical of ARTAG, GAIs typical of GGT, tau-containing fibrillary astrocytes found in PiD, and TA of PSP are not reproduced in WT following intracallosal inoculation of homogenates from the corresponding tauopathies. This may be due, in part, to the predominance of GAIs and TAs in gray matter regions in human diseases, while TSAs are typically localized in the white matter.

Importantly, sarkosyl-soluble fractions have no capacity of tau seeding in any cases.

It may be suggested that the progressive appearance of threads along the corpus callosum is due to diffusion of the seeds. However, it can be posed that tau seeding and spreading in oligodendrocytes is an active process. On the one hand, inoculated tau has a half-life of a few days (Guo et al., 2016), whereas tau immunostaining in the corpus callosum extends over greater distances with longer survival time. Moreover, abnormal tau deposits in inoculated mice particularly those in oligodendrocytes co-express phospho-kinase p-38 and phospho-ERK-1/2; expression of phospho-kinase p38 and phospho-ERK-1/2 is restricted to the regions with phospho-tau deposits including threads and dots, thus suggesting active phosphorylation of resident murine tau (Ferrer et al., 2001a,b, 2005; Ferrer, 2004; Puig et al., 2004).

Coiled bodies are present in most non-AD tauopathies, and the white matter is affected in the majority of tauopathies. Various transgenic mice expressing tau mutations have oligodendroglial, in addition to neuronal and astroglial inclusions (Götz et al., 2001; Lin et al., 2003, 2005; Ren et al., 2014; Ferrer, 2018b). Moreover, selective over-expression of mutant tau in oligodendrocytes using CNP promoter in mice produces filamentous inclusions in oligodendrocytes and progressive impairment of axonal transport, followed by myelin and axonal disruption (Higuchi et al., 2005). Finally, *in vitro* studies have also shown deleterious effects of abnormal tau expression and deposition in oligodendrocytes which are causative of degeneration in particular settings (Richter-Lansberg, 2008; Richter-Landsberg, 2016). Functional deficiencies linked to phospho-tau deposition in oligodendrocytes and threads is also supported in the present study by the demonstration of slightly disrupted myelin and the occasional presence of PLP1-immunoreactive balls and dots in the ipsilateral corpus callosum following inoculation of sarkosyl-enriched fractions from AD, PART, ARTAG and less commonly with GGT, PSP, PiD, and fFTLD-301L.

Together, the present findings show that the white matter may be involved in tau seeding and spreading in a variety of experimentally-induced tauopathies. This is in accordance with the well-recognized, although often minimized, tau involvement of the white matter in most human tauopathies. Moreover, the present observations point to oligodendrocytes as targets of tau seeding and spreading in the white matter, thus highlighting oligodendrogliopathy (Ferrer, 2018b) as a component in the pathogenesis of tauopathies.

ETHICS STATEMENT

Brain tissue was obtained from the Institute of Neuropathology HUB-ICO-IDIBELL Biobank following the guidelines of Spanish legislation on this matter (Real Decreto de Biobancos 1716/2011) and approval of the local ethics committee.

Wild-type C57BL/6 mice from our colony were used. All animal procedures were carried out following the guidelines of the European Communities Council Directive 2010/63/EU and with the approval of the local ethical committee (University of Barcelona, Spain).

AUTHOR CONTRIBUTIONS

MA and PG-E carried out the inoculations of the animals. PA-B and MC prepared the inocula, processed brain tissue and checked tissue lesions. BT-E obtained confocal microscopy images. IF and JdR designed the experiments and summarized the main conclusions. IF examined the brains of all inoculated animals, interpreted the lesions, and wrote the manuscript which was circulated for approval by all the authors.

REFERENCES

Ahmed, Z., Bigio, E. H., Budka, H., Dickson, D. W., Ferrer, I., Ghetti, B., et al. (2013). Globular glial tauopathies (GGT): consensus recommendations. *Acta Neuropathol.* 126, 537–544. doi: 10.1007/s00401-013-1171-0

Ahmed, Z., Cooper, J., Murray, T. K., Garn, K., McNaughton, E., Clarke, H., et al. (2014). A novel *in vivo* model of tau propagation with rapid and progressive neurofibrillary tangle pathology: the pattern of spread is determined by connectivity, not proximity. *Acta Neuropathol.* 127, 667–683. doi: 10.1007/s00401-014-1254-6

Ahmed, Z., Doherty, K. M., Silveira-Moriyama, L., Bandopadhyay, R., Lashley, T., Mamais, A., et al. (2011). Globular glial tauopathies (GGT) presenting with motor neuron disease or frontotemporal dementia: an emerging group of 4-repeat tauopathies. *Acta Neuropathol.* 122, 415–428. doi: 10.1007/s00401-011-0857-4

Audouard, E., Houben, S., Masaracchia, C., Yilmaz, Z., Suain, V., Authelet, M., et al. (2016). High-molecular weight paired helical filaments from Alzheimer brain induces seeding of wild-type mouse tau into argyrophilic 4Rtau pathology *in vivo*. *Am. J. Pathol.* 186, 2709–2722. doi: 10.1016/j.ajpath.2016.06.008

Bertram, L., and Tanzi, R. E. (2011). "Genetics of Alzheimer's disease," in *Neurodegeneration: The Molecular Pathology of Dementia and Movement Disorders, Second Edition*, eds D. W. Dickson and R. O. Weller (Chichester: Wiley-Blackwell), 151–161. doi: 10.1002/9781444341256.ch9

Bigio, E. H., Lipton, A. M., Yen, S. H., Hutton, M. L., Baker, M., Nacharaju, P., et al. (2001). Frontal lobe dementia with novel tauopathy: sporadic multiple system tauopathy with dementia. *J. Neuropathol. Exp. Neurol.* 60, 328–341. doi: 10.1093/jnen/60.4.328

Boluda, S., Iba, M., Zhang, B., Raible, K. M., Lee, V. M., and Trojanowski, J. Q. (2015). Differential induction and spread of tau pathology in young PS19 tau transgenic mice following intracerebral injections of pathological tau from Alzheimer's disease or corticobasal degeneration brains. *Acta Neuropathol.* 129, 221–237. doi: 10.1007/s00401-014-1373-0

Borrego-Écija, S., Morgado, J., Palencia-Madrid, L., Grau-Rivera, O., Reñé, R., Hernández, I., et al. (2017). Frontotemporal dementia caused by the P301L mutation in the MAPT gene: clinicopathological features of 13 cases from the same geographical origin in Barcelona, Spain. *Dement. Geriatr. Cogn. Disord.* 44, 213–221. doi: 10.1159/000480077

Braak, H., Alafuzoff, I., Arzberger, T., Kretzschmar, H., and del Tredici, K. (2006). Staging of Alzheimer disease-associated neurofibrillary pathology using paraffin sections and immunocytochemistry. *Acta Neuropathol.* 112, 389–404. doi: 10.1007/s00401-006-0127-z

Clavaguera, F., Akatsu, H., Fraser, G., Crowther, R. A., Frank, S., Hench, J., et al. (2013a). Brain homogenates from human tauopathies induce tau inclusions in mouse brain. *Proc. Natl. Acad. Sci. U.S.A.* 110, 9535–9540. doi: 10.1073/pnas.1301175110

Clavaguera, F., Bolmont, T., Crowther, R. A., Abramowski, D., Frank, S., Probst, A., et al. (2009). Transmission and spreading of tauopathy in transgenic mouse brain. *Nat. Cell Biol.* 11, 909–913. doi: 10.1038/ncb1901

Clavaguera, F., Hench, J., Goedert, M., and Tolnay, M. (2015). Invited review: Prion-like transmission and spreading of tau pathology. *Neuropathol. Appl. Neurobiol.* 41, 47–58. doi: 10.1111/nan.12197

Clavaguera, F., Lavenir, I., Falcon, B., Frank, S., Goedert, M., and Tolnay, M. (2013b). "Prion-like" templated misfolding in tauopathies. *Brain Pathol.* 23, 342–349. doi: 10.1111/bpa.12044

Crary, J. F., Trojanowski, J. Q., Schneider, J. A., Abisambra, J. F., Abner, E. L., Alafuzoff, I., et al. (2014). Primary age-related tauopathy (PART): a common pathology associated with human aging. *Acta Neuropathol.* 128, 755–766. doi: 10.1007/s00401-014-1349-0

de Calignon, A., Polydoro, M., Suárez-Calvet, M., William, C., Adamowicz, D. H., Kopeikina, K. J., et al. (2012). Propagation of tau pathology in a model of early Alzheimer's disease. *Neuron* 73, 685–697. doi: 10.1016/j.neuron.2011.11.033

Dickson, D. W., Hauw, J. J., Agid, Y., and Litvan, I. (2011). "Progressive supranuclear palsy and corticobasal degeneration," in *Neurodegeneration: The Molecular Pathology of Dementia and Movement Disorders, Second Edition*, eds D. W. Dickson and R. O. Weller (Chichester: Wiley-Blackwell), 135–155. doi: 10.1002/9781444341256.ch15

Dujardin, S., Lécolle, K., Caillierez, R., Bégard, S., Zommer, N., Lachaud, C., et al. (2014). Neuron to neuron wild-type tau protein transfer through a trans-synaptic mechanism: relevance to sporadic tauopathies. *Acta Neuropathol. Commun.* 2:14. doi: 10.1186/2051-5960-2-14

Duyckaerts, C., Braak, H., Brion, J. P., Buée, L., and Del Tredici, K., Goedert, M., et al. (2015). PART is part of Alzheimer disease. *Acta Neuropathol.* 129, 749–756. doi: 10.1007/s00401-015-1390-7

Duyckaerts, C., and Dickson, D. (2011). "Neuropathology of Alzheimer's disease," in: *Neurodegeneration: The Molecular Pathology of Dementia and Movement Disorders, Second Edition*, eds D. W. Dickson, and R. O. Weller (Chichester: Wiley-Blackwell), 62–96. doi: 10.1002/9781444341256.ch10

Ferrer, I. (2004). Stress kinases involved in tau phosphorylation in Alzheimer's disease, tauopathies and APP transgenic mice. *Neurotox Res.* 6, 469–475. doi: 10.1007/BF03033283

Ferrer, I. (2018a). Astrogliopathy in tauopathies. *Neuroglia* 1, 126–150. doi: 10.3390/neuroglia1010010

Ferrer, I. (2018b). Oligodendrogliopathy in neurodegenerative diseases with abnormal protein aggregates: the forgotten partner. *Prog. Neurobiol.* 169, 24–54. doi: 10.1016/j.pneurobio.2018.07.004

Ferrer, I., Aguiló-García, M., López-González, I., Diaz-Lucena, D., Roig-Villalonga, A., Carmona, M., et al. (2018). Aging-related tau astrogliopathy (ARTAG): Not only tau phosphorylation in astrocytes. *Brain Pathol.* 28, 965–985. doi: 10.1111/bpa.12593

Ferrer, I., Blanco, R., Carmona, M., and Puig, B. (2001a). Phosphorylated mitogen-activated protein kinase (MAPK/ERK-P), protein kinase of 38 kDa (p38-P), stress-activated protein kinase (SAPK/JNK-P), and calcium/calmodulin-dependent kinase II (CaM kinase II) are differentially expressed in tau deposits in neurons and glial cells in tauopathies. *J. Neural. Transm.* 108, 1397–1415. doi: 10.1007/s007020100016

Ferrer, I., Blanco, R., Carmona, M., Ribera, R., Goutan, E., Puig, B., et al. (2001b). Phosphorylated map kinase (ERK1, ERK2) expression is associated with early tau deposition in neurones and glial cells, but not with increased nuclear DNA vulnerability and cell death, in Alzheimer disease, Pick's disease, progressive supranuclear palsy and corticobasal degeneration. *Brain Pathol.* 11, 144–158. doi: 10.1111/j.1750-3639.2001.tb00387.x

Ferrer, I., Gomez-Isla, T., Puig, B., Freixes, M., Ribé, E., Dalfó, E., et al. (2005). Current advances on different kinases involved in tau phosphorylation, and implications in Alzheimer's disease and tauopathies. *Curr. Alzheimer Res.* 2, 3–18. doi: 10.2174/1567205052772713

Ferrer, I., Hernandez, I., Boada, M., Llorente, A., Rey, M. J., Cardozo, A., et al. (2003). Primary progressive aphasia as the initial manifestation of corticobasal degeneration and unusual tauopathies. *Acta Neuropathol.* 106, 419–435. doi: 10.1007/s00401-003-0756-4

Ferrer, I., López-González, I., Carmona, M., Arregui, L., Dalfó, E., Torrejón-Escribano, B., et al. (2013). Glial and neuronal tau pathology in tauopathies: characterization of disease-specific phenotypes and tau pathology progression. *J. Neuropathol. Exp. Neurol.* 73, 81–97. doi: 10.1097/NEN.0000000000000030

Ferrer, I., Santpere, G., and van Leeuwen, F. W. (2008). Argyrophilic grain disease. *Brain* 146, 1640–1651. doi: 10.1093/brain/awm305

Fu, Y. J., Nishihira, Y., Kuroda, S., Toyoshima, Y., Ishihara, T., Shinozaki, M., et al. (2010). Sporadic four-repeat tauopathy with frontotemporal lobar degeneration, Parkinsonism, and motor neuron disease: a distinct clinicopathological and biochemical disease entity. *Acta Neuropathol.* 120, 21–32. doi: 10.1007/s00401-010-0649-2

Ghetti, B., Wszolek, Z. K., Boeve, B. F., Spina, S., and Goedert, M. (2011). "Frontotemporal dementia and parkinsonism linked to chromosome 17," in *Neurodegeneration: The Molecular Pathology of Dementia and Movement Disorders, Second Edition*, eds D. W. Dickson, and R. O. Weller (Chichester: Wiley-Blackwell), 110–134. doi: 10.1002/9781444341256.ch14

Giaccone, G., Marcon, G., Mangieri, M., Morbin, M., Rossi, G., Fetoni, V., et al. (2008). Atypical tauopathy with massive involvement of the white matter. *Neuropathol. Appl. Neurobiol.* 34, 468–472. doi: 10.1111/j.1365-2990.2007.00927.x

Goedert, M., and Spillantini, M. G. (2017). Propagation of tau aggregates. *Mol. Brain* 10:18. doi: 10.1186/s13041-017-0298-7

Goedert, M., Spillantini, M. G., Cairns, N. J., and Crowther, R. A. (1992). Tau proteins of Alzheimer paired helical filaments: abnormal phosphorylation of all six brain isoforms. *Neuron* 8, 159–168. doi: 10.1016/0896-6273(92)90117-V

Goedert, M., Spillantini, M. G., Jakes, R., Rutherford, D., and Crowther, R. A. (1989). Multiple isoforms of human microtubule-associated protein tau: sequences and localization in neurofibrillary tangles of Alzheimer's disease. *Neuron* 3, 519–526. doi: 10.1016/0896-6273(89)90210-9

Götz, J., Tolnay, M., Barmettler, R., Chen, F., Probst, A., and Nitsch, R. M. (2001). Oligodendroglial tau filament formation in transgenic mice expressing G272V tau. *Eur. J. Neurosci.* 13, 2131–2140. doi: 10.1046/j.0953-816x.2001.01604.x

Guo, J. L., Narasimhan, S., Changolkar, L., He, Z., Stieber, A., Zhang, B., et al. (2016). Unique pathological tau conformers from Alzheimer's brains transmit tau pathology in nontransgenic mice. *J. Exp. Med.* 213, 2635–2654. doi: 10.1084/jem.20160833

Higuchi, M., Zhang, B., Forman, M. S., Yoshiyama, Y., Trojanowski, J. Q., and Lee, V. M. (2005). Axonal degeneration induced by targeted expression of mutant human tau in oligodendrocytes of transgenic mice that model glial tauopathies. *J. Neurosci.* 25, 9434–9343. doi: 10.1523/JNEUROSCI.2691-05.2005

Iba, M., Guo, J. L., McBride, J. D., Zhang, B., Trojanowski, J. Q., and Lee, V. M. (2013). Synthetic tau fibrils mediate transmission of neurofibrillary tangles in a transgenic mouse model of Alzheimer's-like tauopathy. *J. Neurosci.* 33, 1024–1037. doi: 10.1523/JNEUROSCI.2642-12.2013

Iseki, E., Matsumura, T., Marui, W., Hino, H., Odawara, T., Sugiyama, N., et al. (2001). Familial frontotemporal dementia and parkinsonism with a novel N296H mutation in exon 10 of the tau gene and a widespread tau accumulation in the glial cells. *Acta Neuropathol.* 102, 285–292.

Jellinger, K. A. (1998). Dementia with grains (argyrophilic grain disease). *Brain Pathol.* 8, 377–386. doi: 10.1111/j.1750-3639.1998.tb00161.x

Jellinger, K. A., Alafuzoff, I., Attems, J., Beach, T. G., and Cairns, N. J., Crary, J. F., et al. (2015). PART, a distinct tauopathy, different from classical sporadic Alzheimer disease. *Acta Neuropathol.* 129, 757–762. doi: 10.1007/s00401-015-1407-2

Josephs, K. A., Katsuse, O., Beccano-Kelly, D. A., Lin, W. L., Uitti, R. J., Fujino, Y., et al. (2006). Atypical progressive supranuclear palsy with corticospinal tract degeneration. *J. Neuropathol. Exp. Neurol.* 65, 396–405. doi: 10.1097/01.jnen.0000218446.38158.61

Kaufman, S. K., Sanders, D. W., Thomas, T. L., Ruchinskas, A. J., Vaquer-Alicea, J., Sharma, A. M., et al. (2016). Tau prion strains dictate patterns of cell pathology, progression rate, and regional vulnerability *in vivo*. *Neuron* 92, 796–812. doi: 10.1016/j.neuron.2016.09.055

Kovacs, G. G. (2015a). Invited review: Neuropathology of tauopathies: principles and practice. *Neuropathol. Appl. Neurobiol.* 41, 3–23. doi: 10.1111/nan.12208

Kovacs, G. G. (2015b). "Tauopathies," in *Neuropathology of Neurodegenerative Diseases: A Practical Guide*, eds G. G. Kovacs (Cambridge: Cambridge University Press), 109–148. doi: 10.1017/CBO9781107588660.008

Kovacs, G. G. (2018). Understanding the relevance of aging-related tau astrogliopathy (ARTAG). *Neuroglia* 1, 339–350. doi: 10.3390/neuroglia1020023

Kovacs, G. G., Ferrer, I., Grinberg, L. T., Alafuzoff, I., Attems, J., Budka, H., et al. (2016). Aging-related tau astrogliopathy (ARTAG): harmonized evaluation strategy. *Acta Neuropathol.* 131, 87–102. doi: 10.1007/s00401-015-1509-x

Kovacs, G. G., Lee, V. M., and Trojanowski, J. Q. (2017). Protein astrogliopathies in human neurodegenerative diseases and aging. *Brain Pathol.* 27, 675–690. doi: 10.1111/bpa.12536

Kovacs, G. G., Majtenyi, K., Spina, S., Murrell, J. R., Gelpi, E., Hoftberger, R., et al. (2008). White matter tauopathy with globular glial inclusions: a distinct sporadic frontotemporal lobar degeneration. *J. Neuropathol. Exp. Neurol.* 67, 963–975. doi: 10.1097/NEN.0b013e318187a80f

Lewis, J., and Dickson, D. W. (2016). Propagation of tau pathology: hypotheses, discoveries, and yet unresolved questions from experimental and human brain studies. *Acta Neuropathol.* 131, 27–48. doi: 10.1007/s00401-015-1507-z

Lin, W. L., Lewis, J., Yen, S. H., Hutton, M., and Dickson, D. W. (2003). Filamentous tau oligodendrocytes and astrocytes of transgenic mice expressing the human tau isoform with the P301L mutation. *Am. J. Pathol.* 162, 213–218. doi: 10.1016/S0002-9440(10)63812-6

Lin, W. L., Zehr, C., Lewis, J., Hutton, M., Yen, S. H., and Dickson, D. W. (2005). Progressive white matter pathology in the spinal cord of transgenic mice expressing mutant (P301L) human tau. *J. Neurocytol.* 34, 397–410. doi: 10.1007/s11068-006-8726-0

Liu, L., Drouet, V., Wu, J. W., Witter, M. P., Small, S. A., Clelland, C., et al. (2012). Trans-synaptic spread of tau pathology *in vivo*. *PLoS ONE* 7:e31302. doi: 10.1371/journal.pone.0031302

Lowe, J., and Kalaria, R. (2015). "Dementia," in *Greenfield's Neuropathology, Ninth Edition*, eds S. Love, H. Budka, J. Ironside, and A. Perry (Boca Raton, FL: CRC Press), 858–973.

Mudher, A., Colin, M., Dujardin, S., Medina, M., Dewachter, I., Naini, S. M. A., et al. (2017). What is the evidence that tau pathology spreads through prion-like propagation? *Acta Neuropathol. Commun.* 5:99. doi: 10.1186/s40478-017-0488-7

Muñoz, D. G., and Ferrer, I. (2008). "Neuropathology of hereditary forms of frontotemporal dementia and parkinsonism," in *Handbook of Clinical Neurology: Dementias*, eds C. Duyckaerts and I. Litvan (Edinburgh; London; New York, NY: Elsevier), 393–414. doi: 10.1016/S0072-9752(07)01237-7

Muñoz, D. G., Morris, H. R., and Rossor, M. (2011). "Pick's disease," in *Neurodegeneration: the Molecular Pathology of Dementia and Movement Disorders, Second Edition*, eds D. W. Dickson and R. O. Weller (Chichester: Wiley-Blackwell), 156–164. doi: 10.1002/9781444341256.ch16

Narasimhan, S., Guo, J. L., Changolkar, L., Stieber, A., McBride, J. D., Silva, L. V., et al. (2017). Pathological tau strains from human brains recapitulate the diversity of tauopathies in non-transgenic mouse brain. *J. Neurosci.* 37, 11406–11423. doi: 10.1523/JNEUROSCI.1230-17.2017

Peeraer, E., Bottelbergs, A., Van Kolen, K., Stancu, I. C., Vasconcelos, B., Mahieu, M., et al. (2015). Intracerebral injection of preformed synthetic tau fibrils initiates widespread tauopathy and neuronal loss in the brains of tau transgenic mice. *Neurobiol. Dis.* 73, 83–95. doi: 10.1016/j.nbd.2014.08.032

Piao, Y. S., Tan, C. F., Iwanaga, K., Kakita, A., Takano, H., Nishizawa, M., et al. (2005). Sporadic four-repeat tauopathy with frontotemporal degeneration, parkinsonism and motor neuron disease. *Acta Neuropathol.* 110, 600–609. doi: 10.1007/s00401-005-1086-5

Powers, J. M., Byrne, N. P., Ito, M., Takao, M., Yankopoulou, D., Spillantini, M. G., et al. (2003). A novel leukoencephalopathy associated with tau deposits primarily in white matter glia. *Acta Neuropathol.* 106, 181–187. doi: 10.1007/s00401-003-0719-9

Puig, B., Vinals, F., and Ferrer, I. (2004). Active stress kinase p38 enhances and perpetuates abnormal tau phosphorylation and deposition in Pick's disease. *Acta Neuropathol.* 107, 185–189. doi: 10.1007/s00401-003-0793-z

Ren, Y., Lin, W. L., Sanchez, L., Ceballos, C., Polydoro, M., Spires-Jones, T. L., et al. (2014). Endogenous tau aggregates in oligodendrocytes of rTg4510 mice induced by human P301L tau. *J. Alzheimers Dis.* 38, 589–600. doi: 10.3233/JAD-130986

Richter-Landsberg, C. (2016). Protein aggregate formation in oligodendrocytes: tau and the cytoskeleton at the intersection of neuroprotection and neurodegeneration. *Biol. Chem.* 397, 185–194. doi: 10.1515/hsz-2015-0157

Richter-Lansberg, C. (2008). The cytoskeleton in oligodendrocytes. Microtubule dynamics in health and disease. *J. Mol. Neurosci.* 35, 55–63. doi: 10.1007/s12031-007-9017-7

Sanders, D. W., Kaufman, S. K., DeVos, S. L., Sharma, A. M., Mirbaha, H., Li, A., et al. (2014). Distinct tau prion strains propagate in cells and mice and define different tauopathies. *Neuron* 82, 1271–1288. doi: 10.1016/j.neuron.2014.04.047

Spillantini, M. G., and Goedert, M. (1998). Tau protein pathology in neurodegenerative diseases. *Trends Neurosci.* 21, 428–433. doi: 10.1016/S0166-2236(98)01337-X

Spillantini, M. G., Goedert, M., Crowther, R. A., Murrell, J. R., Farlow, M. R., and Ghetti, B. (1997). Familial multiple system tauopathy with presenile dementia: a disease with abundant neuronal and glial tau filaments. *Proc. Natl. Acad. Sci. U.S.A.* 94, 4113–4118. doi: 10.1073/pnas.94.8.4113

Spina, S., Farlow, M. R., Unverzagt, F. W., Kareken, D. A., Murrell, J. R., Fraser, G., et al. The tauopathy associated with mutation +3 in intron 10 of Tau characterization of the MSTD family. *Brain* (2008) 131:72–89. doi: 10.1093/brain/awm280

Stancu, I. C., Vasconcelos, B., Ris, L., Wang, P., Villers, A., Peeraer, E., et al. (2015). Templated misfolding of tau by prion-like seeding along neuronal connections impairs neuronal network function and associated behavioral outcomes in tau transgenic mice. *Acta Neuropathol.* 129, 875–894. doi: 10.1007/s00401-015-1413-4

Tacik, P., Sanchez-Contreras, M., DeTure, M., Murray, M. E., Rademakers, R., Ross, O. A., et al. (2017). Clinicopathologic heterogeneity in frontotemporal dementia and parkinsonism linked to chromosome 17 (FTDP-17) due to microtubule-associated protein tau (MAPT) p.P301L mutation, including a patient with globular glial tauopathy. *Neuropathol. Appl. Neurobiol.* 43, 200–214. doi: 10.1111/nan.12367

Tacik, P., Sanchez-Contreras, M., Rademakers, R., Dickson, D. W., and Wszolek, Z. K. (2016). Genetic disorders with tau pathology: a review of the literature and report of two patients with tauopathy and positive family histories. *Neurodegener. Dis.* 16, 12–21. doi: 10.1159/000440840

Tolnay, M., and Braak, H. (2011). "Argyrophilic grain disease," in *Neurodegeneration: The Molecular Pathology of Dementia and Movement Disorders, Second Edition*, eds D. W. Dickson and R. O. Weller (Chichester: Wiley-Blackwell), 165–170. doi: 10.1002/9781444341256.ch17

Tolnay, M., Spillantini, M. G., Goedert, M., Ulrich, J., Langui, D., and Probst, A. (1997). Argyrophilic grain disease: widespread hyperphosphorylation of tau protein in limbic neurons. *Acta Neuropathol.* 93, 477–484. doi: 10.1007/s004010050642

Tripathi, R. B., Jackiewicz, M., McKenzie, I. A., Kougioumtzidou, E., Grist, M., and Richardson, W. D. (2017). Remarkable stability of myelinating oligodendrocytes in mice. *Cell Rep.* 21, 316–323. doi: 10.1016/j.celrep.2017.09.050

Yeung, M. S., Zdunek, S., Bergmann, O., Bernard, S., Salehpour, M., Alkass, K., et al. (2014). Dynamics of oligodendrocyte generation and myelination in the human brain. *Cell* 159, 766–774. doi: 10.1016/j.cell.2014.10.011

18

Tau-Cofactor Complexes as Building Blocks of Tau Fibrils

Yann Fichou[1]*, Zachary R. Oberholtzer*[1]*, Hoang Ngo*[1]*, Chi-Yuan Cheng*[1]*,*
Timothy J. Keller[1]*, Neil A. Eschmann*[1] *and Songi Han*[1,2*]

[1] *Department of Chemistry and Biochemistry, University of California, Santa Barbara, Santa Barbara, CA, United States,*
[2] *Department of Chemical Engineering, University of California, Santa Barbara, Santa Barbara, CA, United States*

***Correspondence:**
Songi Han
songihan@ucsb.edu

The aggregation of the human tau protein into neurofibrillary tangles is directly diagnostic of many neurodegenerative conditions termed tauopathies. The species, factors and events that are responsible for the initiation and propagation of tau aggregation are not clearly established, even in a simplified and artificial *in vitro* system. This motivates the mechanistic study of *in vitro* aggregation of recombinant tau from soluble to fibrillar forms, for which polyanionic cofactors are the most commonly used external inducer. In this study, we performed biophysical characterizations to unravel the mechanisms by which cofactors induce fibrillization. We first reinforce the idea that cofactors are the limiting factor to generate ThT-active tau fibrils, and establish that they act as templating reactant that trigger tau conformational rearrangement. We show that heparin has superior potency for recruiting monomeric tau into aggregation-competent species compared to any constituent intermediate or aggregate "seeds." We show that tau and cofactors form intermediate complexes whose evolution toward ThT-active fibrils is tightly regulated by tau-cofactor interactions. Remarkably, it is possible to find mild cofactors that complex with tau without forming ThT-active species, except when an external catalyst (e.g., a seed) is provided to overcome the energy barrier. In a cellular context, we propose the idea that tau could associate with cofactors to form a metastable complex that remains "inert" and reversible, until encountering a relevant seed that can trigger an irreversible transition to β-sheet containing species.

Keywords: tau protein, protein aggregation, tau oligomers, tauopathies, conformational transformation, aggregation seeding, cofactors

INTRODUCTION

The intrinsically disordered human tau protein has the primary function of stabilizing microtubules in healthy individuals, whereas under pathological conditions, soluble tau dissociates from microtubules and aggregates into distinct fibrillar constructs (Goedert et al., 2006). The formation of neurofibrillary tangles from human tau has been verified to be directly part of the diagnosis of Alzheimer's disease and other neurodegenerative diseases including chronic traumatic encephalopathy (CTE) and corticobasal degeneration (CBD), collectively referred to as tauopathies (Lee et al., 2001). However, viable therapeutic approaches do not currently exist to alter the course of such diseases. Tau is believed to be capable of spreading aggregate pathology through interconnected neuronal pathways *in vivo* in a "prion"-like process (Sanders et al., 2014; Stancu et al., 2015; Kaufman et al., 2016; Woerman et al., 2016), making the elucidation of intermediate aggregation species and seeding mechanisms a top priority in the study of the pathological tau aggregation pathway. At the current state of understanding, it is unclear what the defining molecular-level feature of aggregation-prone and seeding-competent tau is, even in a simplified *in vitro* system. The ultimate question in the prion hypothesis is what factor is responsible for converting normal to pathological tau.

Tau protein is highly charged, overall positively, hydrophilic and therefore very stable in aqueous conditions across a large range of pH, temperatures and concentrations. Tau aggregation *in vitro* is most commonly triggered by external inducers or cofactors, such as heparin (Goedert et al., 1996), RNA (Kampers et al., 1996) or arachidonic acid (Wilson and Binder, 1997). The use of cofactors to make and study tau aggregation *in vitro* has two main origins. First, it represents a convenient, reproducible procedure to form tau fibrils in order to mechanistically study the process of amyloid formation. Second, several cofactors have been colocalized with tau neurofibrillary tangles in brain tissue (Goedert et al., 1996; Ginsberg et al., 1997), providing a biological justification for these cofactors. Recently, tau fibrils induced by addition of heparin, the most commonly used cofactor, were found to be heterogeneous and different from brain-extracted fibril structures (Fichou et al., 2018b; Zhang et al., 2019a), thereby questioning the quality of cofactor-induced fibrils as an aggregate model. However, recent studies demonstrated the biological relevance of cofactors in tau aggregation, by indirectly showing its involvement in seeding and fibril stability (Fichou et al., 2018a) and by showing that a cofactor of unknown identity is part of the fibril core in CTE (Falcon et al., 2019) and CBD (Zhang et al., 2019b). Through the study of cofactor-induced aggregation of recombinant tau *in vitro*, we endeavor to find defining molecular features of aggregation-prone or seeding-competent tau species.

At a mechanistic level, how cofactors interact with tau to trigger aggregation is not well understood. Heparin-induced tau aggregation has been modeled in several quantitative studies (Ramachandran and Udgaonkar, 2011; Shammas et al., 2015; Kjaergaard et al., 2018) and has provided a global picture where heparin interacts with tau to form aggregation competent oligomers that evolve to fibrils. However, even a property as basic as the inclusion of heparin into the mature fibrils is disputed, with multiple conflicting reports saying that heparin is either not part of fibrils (von Bergen et al., 2006; Carlson et al., 2007; Ramachandran and Udgaonkar, 2011) or part of the final aggregate (Sibille et al., 2006; Dinkel et al., 2015; Fichou et al., 2018a). It is perhaps due to these observations that heparin's treatment in literature has largely been that of a useful catalyst rather than a critical reactant. In this study, we used heparin and RNA as cofactors to understand the conformational evolution of tau, the population of intermediate species, as well as the role of the cofactors in assisting the seeding of aggregation to further refine the tau-aggregation model.

A previous study of ours used electron paramagnetic resonance (EPR) spectroscopy to reveal experimentally the existence of disordered intermediate aggregates (termed I) of tau lacking β-sheet structure (Pavlova et al., 2016). Additionally, we have identified aggregation-prone soluble tau species with an extended conformation around PHF6$^{(*)}$ (termed S*), distinct

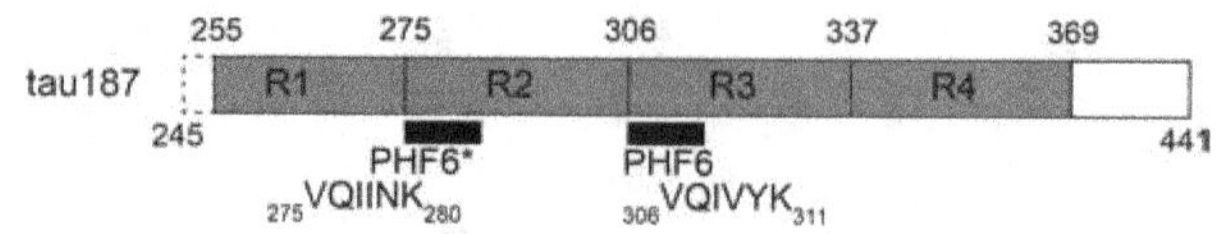

FIGURE 1 | Schematic of tau187. It contains all four repeat domains R1-R4, minus 10 residues of R1, and the C-terminus. The N-terminal end contains a six histidine tag for purification (not shown).

from the pre-heparin-activated tau species which are composed of a more compact conformation around PHF6$^{(*)}$ (termed S) (Eschmann et al., 2017). The key unresolved question is what are the seeding competent species or factors that are responsible for inducing, as well as propagating aggregation? With that in mind, we ask: (1) Do the disordered aggregation intermediates (I) quantitatively convert *on pathway* to mature fibrils? (2) What is the role of heparin in populating the intermediate stages of tau, namely S*, I, and mature fibrils? And (3) should cofactors be considered a constitutive part of tau fibrils?

In order to accomplish these goals, we employed a combination of EPR spectroscopy tools together with multiple biochemical assays which allow for the direct observation and characterization of cofactor-induced aggregation intermediates. We used a truncated version of tau, containing the four repeat regions as well as the C-terminus (residues 255–441 of full length 2N4R), termed tau187 (**Figure 1**). Continuous wave (cw) EPR lineshape analysis was employed to report on spin-label mobility and β-sheet formation as well as to quantify intermediate species, as previously demonstrated (Pavlova et al., 2016). Intra-protein distances and conformational rearrangement around PHF6* (^{275}VQIINK^{280}) were quantified by applying Double Electron-Electron Resonance (DEER) spectroscopy to tau187 doubly labeled with MTSL at sites 272 and 285. We also assessed time-resolved local dehydration around selected tau187 sites by Electron Spin-Echo Envelope Modulation (ESEEM) measurements. This report makes the case that cofactors are active parts of the tau aggregation process and should not be considered as a mere catalyst.

RESULTS

Heparin Stoichiometry Dictates Tau Population Embedded in Fibrils

We first investigated the relation between the quantity of heparin incubated with tau and the fibril quantity formed at equilibrium. Tau187 contains two cysteines, one of which was mutated to serine (C291S) so that only one cysteine (C322) could be spin-labeled for cw-EPR experiments (see subsequent sections). This construct is referred to as tau187 throughout the manuscript. Fluorescence kinetic measurements were carried out using thioflavin T (ThT), a fluorescent dye that has been established to bind specifically to β-sheet structures of amyloid proteins (Nilsson, 2004; Biancalana and Koide, 2010) and thus allowed the determination of the total tau embedded in β-sheet structures. Increase in ThT fluorescence intensity occurs rapidly

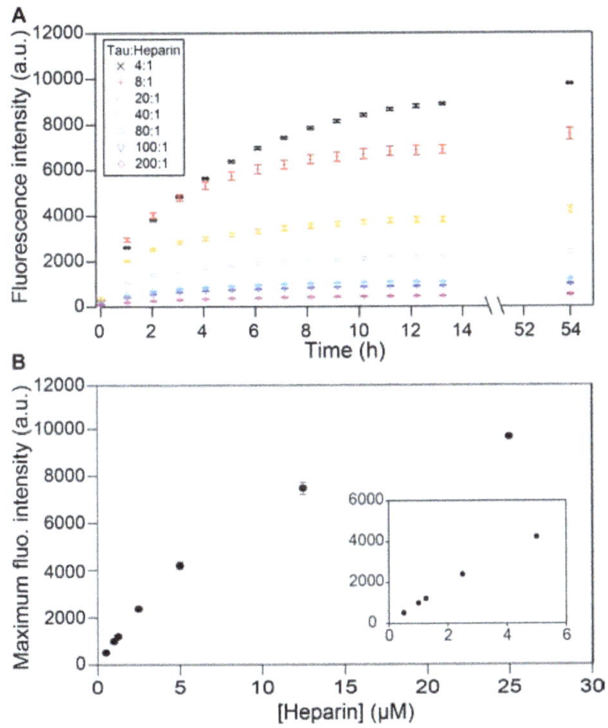

FIGURE 2 | ThT fluorescence measuring β-sheet formation as a function of time and tau:heparin molar ratio. Tau concentration is 100 μM. Kinetic curves **(A)** have plateaued after 53 h and the fluorescence intensities at this time are reported as a function of heparin concentration **(B)**. A zoom at low heparin concentration (**B**, inset) shows a linear behavior. Gaps between 13 and 54 h represent reading interruptions. Error bars represent standard deviation over 3 repeats.

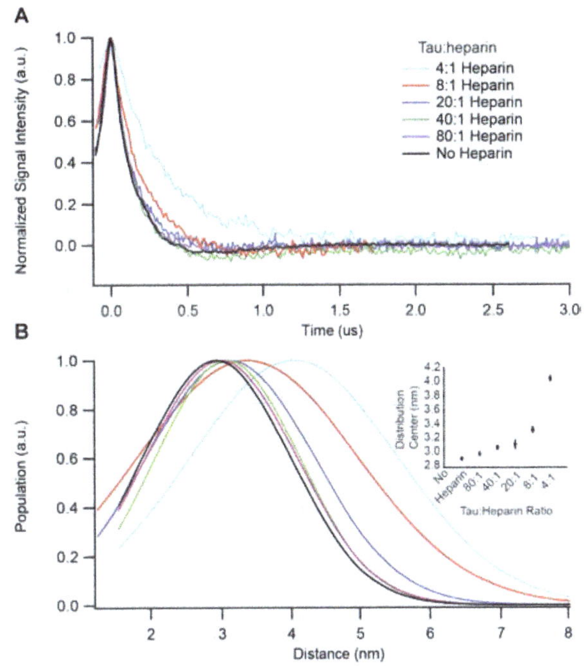

FIGURE 3 | DEER spectroscopy of doubly labeled tau187 at positions 272 and 285. Data points shown are for before (black) and 1 h after addition of the following stoichiometries: 4:1 (cyan), 8:1 (red), 20:1 (blue), 40:1 (green), and 80:1 (purple) tau:heparin molar ratio. **(A)** Background subtracted and normalized DEER time-domain signal. **(B)** Intramolecular distance distribution assuming a Gaussian distribution. The inset shows the Gaussian distribution center as a function of heparin amount. Error bars are estimated from the covariance matrix of the fitting procedure.

after heparin addition to spin-labeled tau187, where no extended lag phase is observed (**Figure 2A**). These measurements were performed with spin-labeled tau187 so that the kinetics could be directly compared with cw-EPR experiments, but the same results were found with unlabeled tau187 (**Supplementary Figure S1**). The ThT fluorescence time course was measured out to 54 h; the results showed that the total β-sheet content does not converge to the same value between samples that contained equal quantities of tau incubated with different quantities of heparin. In fact, the maximum ThT value was found to scale linearly with heparin at low concentrations (**Figure 2B**), but not at higher concentrations, possibly due to the formation of off-pathway oligomers (Ramachandran and Udgaonkar, 2011). In addition, increasing the amount of fibril ends by sonication (**Supplementary Figures S2, S3**) or introduction of intermediates (**Supplementary Figure S4**) did not change the ThT intensity. This result demonstrates that the systematic decrease in β-sheet content seen with decreasing amount of heparin (and unchanged tau content) is not a kinetics driven effect. Rather, the data shows that heparin dictates and limits the quantity of tau transforming into β-sheets at equilibrium, suggesting that heparin is an obligatory reactant of tau187 fibril formation that does not free up even after fibrils are formed.

Heparin Stoichiometry Dictates the Conversion to Aggregation-Prone Conformations

We have identified key structural transformations that tau undergoes during aggregation (Eschmann et al., 2017), however, it is unclear what role heparin plays in these transformation processes. Does heparin facilitate only the formation of aggregation-driving tau species or is it directly involved in each structural transition? We examined the dependence of the S* population, the aggregation-prone conformation of tau that has been identified in an earlier report (Eschmann et al., 2017), on heparin concentration. For that, we used DEER measurements on doubly labeled tau187, at position 272 and 285, to probe the opening of the segments flanking the PHF6* region. In order to ensure that only intra-tau, not inter-tau, distances are measured, spin dilution was employed by mixing MTSL and dMTSL – the diamagnetic analog of MTSL – labeled tau187 at a 1:10 molar ratio (Fichou et al., 2017). At a 4:1 tau:heparin stoichiometry, tau187 is maximally extended at a distance of ~4.1 nm, as shown in **Figure 3**. However, when adding heparin at 5-, 10- or 20-fold dilution (20:1, 40:1, and 80:1 tau:heparin, respectively), we observed no clear conformational extension of the 272–285 tau segment (**Figure 3**) while a twofold dilution (8:1) invoked a small extension around PHF6*. Thus, a fivefold

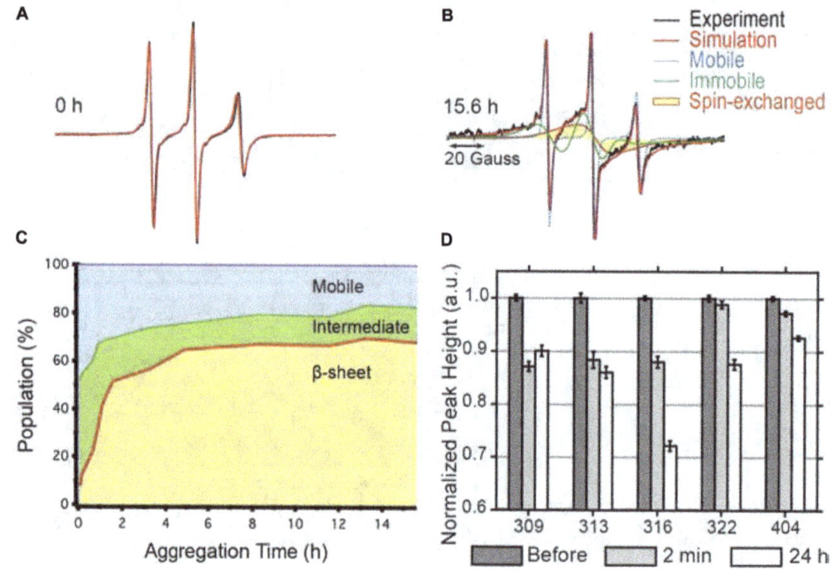

FIGURE 4 | cw-EPR time course of 4:1 tau:heparin molar ratio induced aggregation. **(A)** Before heparin addition, the EPR line shape (black) can be simulated by a single mobile component (red). **(B)** 15.6 h after heparin addition, the spectrum is broadened and the simulation requires the addition of an immobile (green) and spin-exchange (yellow) component in order to obtain a good fit. **(C)** Time evolution of the relative contributions of each component. **(D)** ESEEM relative deuterium peak normalized by the value before heparin addition and plotted versus MTSL-labeled residue. The decrease in peak height, reflecting a local dehydration, at 2 min shows that the arrangement of the intermediates is consistent with the structural features of matures fibrils. Error bars represent the standard deviation of the baseline noise.

reduction in heparin concentration, i.e., the presence of a sub-stoichiometric amount of heparin (tau:heparin 20:1), diminishes the S* population to below our measurement threshold, indicating the direct dependence of the S* population on the tau:heparin stoichiometry. In other words, heparin is necessary to trigger and maintain the conformational rearrangement of S to S* that precedes aggregation. In addition, we spin labeled heparin and measured the cw-EPR lineshape before and after incubation with tau187. The lineshape broadened (most likely due to weak spin exchange or/and lower correlation time) upon addition of tau187 (**Supplementary Figure S5**), revealing a direct and persistent interaction of heparin and tau187. More specifically, the line broadening already occurs within 30 min after incubation, showing that heparin is directly involved in the S to S* transition and intermediate formation measured within 1 h of incubation (**Figure 3**). This result suggests that heparin acts as a templating reactant that triggers the conformational rearrangements necessary for aggregation, in good agreement with a previous report showing that heparin directly participates in the formation of early intermediates (Kjaergaard et al., 2018).

Aggregation Involves the Formation of On-Pathway Oligomers

We sought to gain information on the mechanisms of cofactor-induced aggregation, by measuring the formation of intermediate species along the aggregation pathway. A distinct single line component of the EPR spectra was first recognized and utilized by Margittai and Langen (2004) as a diagnostic tool to characterize parallel β-sheet structures for the study of tau fibrils. Our group has used cw-EPR to quantify the populations of tau molecules that (i) participate in a cross-β sheet arrangement (termed F) giving rise to so-called spin-exchange interaction between the spin labels, (ii) participate in oligomer/aggregate intermediates (termed I) that do not form in-register cross-β sheets but are still characterized by a slow rotational time, and (iii) remains monomeric (termed M) and therefore mobile (Pavlova et al., 2016). Systematically deconvoluting the different contributions to the EPR lineshape allowed for the tracking of the formation and transformation of these tau species as a function of aggregation time.

We tracked the time course of the population and turnover of monomeric (M), intermediate (I) and cross-β-rich (F) species of tau187 (**Figure 4**). Prior to heparin addition, the EPR lineshape is 100% mobile (i.e., population of M is 100%) and displays a narrow nitroxide EPR spectrum (**Figure 4A**). After aggregation, the EPR lineshape is broadened, and contributions from both a slow component (termed immobile) originating from non-amyloid aggregates and a single line spin-exchange component, originating from cross-β structures, are required to simulate the EPR spectra, as shown for the EPR spectra of tau after 15.6 h upon heparin addition (**Figure 4B**). The fit and the raw spectra are overlaid for each time point in **Supplementary Figure S6**. Time evolution of the populations of the different components is summarized in **Figure 4C**. Within 5 min of heparin addition, 44% of the tau population forms I, while the population of tau incorporated in β-sheet F remains small (<10%). As aggregation progresses, the intermediate species that constituted up to ~40% of the total population convert into the F species, which constitute a majority of tau (65%) after 5 h of aggregation. The quantitative conversion of the intermediate population into β-sheet containing species demonstrates that the intermediates are on-pathway to fibrils. The remaining population of the intermediate component after 5 h (less than 15%) might originate from molecules either composing the end of tau fibrils (also previously referred to as interfacial tau; Pavlova et al., 2016) or forming off-pathway intermediates. Interestingly, the ThT-derived measurement of β-sheet structured species (**Figure 2A**, maximum reached after 15 h) systematically lagged behind the populations as quantified by EPR lineshape analysis (**Figure 4C**, maximum reached at about 5 h), i.e., the formation of β-sheet as revealed by EPR occurred more rapidly than captured by ThT fluorescence measurements. The ThT intensity may depend on a threshold aggregate size in contrast to EPR that measures the spin-exchange component as soon as two spin labels come within close proximity.

The dynamic intermediates, I, lack measurable β-sheet structure in the R3 region according to their EPR lineshape (i.e., no spin-exchange), but the question is whether they are deficient of any residual structural features. In other words, does the formation of I occur by structurally directed transitions or by non-specific collapse? We applied ESEEM spectroscopy to measure relative changes in the local water density on the protein surface within a ~3–6 Å shell of a site-specific spin label over the course of aggregation (Volkov et al., 2009). In essence, ESEEM spectroscopy counts the number of deuterated water nuclei around the spin label, where the intensity of the D^2 peak is proportional to the number of these nuclei. We carried out ESEEM spectroscopy with singly MTSL labeled tau187 at several sites within the R3 region (residues 309, 313, 316, 322) and in the C-terminus (residue 404). Decrease in the D^2 peak height, reflecting a decrease in water density, is observed within 2 min after heparin addition for all sites (**Figure 4D**). A gradient of dehydration is observed where sites 309, 313, and 316 exhibit the strongest effect and dehydration becomes progressively less visible for the sites close (322) or in the C-terminal region (404) (**Figure 4D**). After 24 h of aggregation, site 309 experiences a slight recovery in the D^2 density, while the D^2 densities around sites 313, 316, 322, and 404 are systematically decreased. The timing of the initial dehydration (i.e., within 2 min) clearly precedes the development of the amyloid structure seen by EPR lineshape analysis, but it is within the development time scale of the I intermediates (**Figure 4C**). Thus, ESEEM suggests that I species structures are *en route* to aggregates; dehydration is stronger around residues that are expected to be buried in the mature fibrils (Margittai and Langen, 2006; Zhang et al., 2019a).

A Well-Defined Cofactor-Tau Interaction Pattern Is Necessary to Form Fibrils

Aggregation-promoting cofactors, such as heparin or RNA, are usually described as polyanions that somewhat screen the positively charged tau repeat domain (Sibille et al., 2006). We investigated whether this simple charge compensation picture can sufficiently describe cofactor-induced aggregation by varying the nature and length of the cofactors. The heparin typically used in the literature, and elsewhere in this study, is polydisperse as it is directly extracted from porcine intestinal mucosa. Here we used purified monodisperse heparins of various molecular masses to trigger tau aggregation, quantified by ThT fluorescence. For all heparins, a constant tau:heparin mass ratio of 4:1 was used. **Figure 5A** reports the maximum ThT fluorescence reading of fully grown fibrils formed with heparins of different molecular weights. Heparins below 2.3 kDa are incapable of forming tau fibrils. The maximal ThT value increased with heparin's molecular weight until reaching a maximum between 11 and 15 kDa. Addition of higher molecular weight heparin (18 and 22 kDa) decreased the maximum ThT intensity, suggesting an optimal heparin length of 11–15 kDa to promote fibril formation of tau187.

We furthermore looked at the influence of the charges on heparin molecules. Heparin is a highly sulfated glycosaminoglycan that mostly possesses 4 charges per disaccharide (3 sulfate and 1 carboxyl groups). We compared the aggregation triggering propensity of heparin, 2-O desulfated (2OD) and 6-O desulfated (6OD) heparin (**Figure 5B**). Desulfation of either of the two sites resulted in a loss of ThT signal of about one order of magnitude, consistent with the picture that charge interaction is critical for the ability of heparin to trigger aggregation. However, when comparing the aggregation propensity of the two desulfated heparins, we observed that, despite the same charge density, 6OD heparin gives rise to a significantly larger ThT fluorescence signal than 2OD heparin. This modulation of the ThT intensity could originate either from a change in the total amount of fibrils (i.e., 6OD heparin is more potent to induce tau fibrils) or from a change in the fibril structure that would react differently with ThT. Interestingly, this modulation of ThT intensity triggered by the different heparin ($ThT_{heparin} > ThT_{6OD} > ThT_{2OD}$) cannot be explained by a modulation of tau-heparin affinity, as heparin and 2OD heparin have a similar affinity to tau, while 6OD has a drastically lower affinity (Zhao et al., 2017).

In **Figure 5C**, we added excess heparin at a constant tau concentration beyond the 4:1 tau:heparin molar ratio typically used. The data showed that increasing the quantity of heparin, above an optimal ratio of about 1:1 tau:heparin in our conditions, decreased the maximum ThT intensity. This result shows that a defined tau:heparin molar stoichiometry is necessary to trigger optimal aggregation, as previously observed (Carlson et al., 2007; Ramachandran and Udgaonkar, 2011). DEER measurements around PHF6* further confirmed this results by showing the quasi absence of the aggregation-prone open conformation S* at 1:20 tau:heparin (**Figure 5C** inset and **Supplementary Figure S7**).

RNA molecules are other polyanions that have been reported to be capable of triggering tau aggregation (Kampers et al., 1996). Here we tested the efficacy of polyU RNA in aggregating tau187 with and without the disease-associated mutation P301L (**Figure 5D**). In contrast to heparin, polyU does not spontaneously trigger aggregation of tau187 over the time course of 26 h. However, a single-point mutation P301L in tau187, which does not add any charge to tau, led to polyU-induced aggregation, as shown by ThT (**Figure 5D**) and TEM

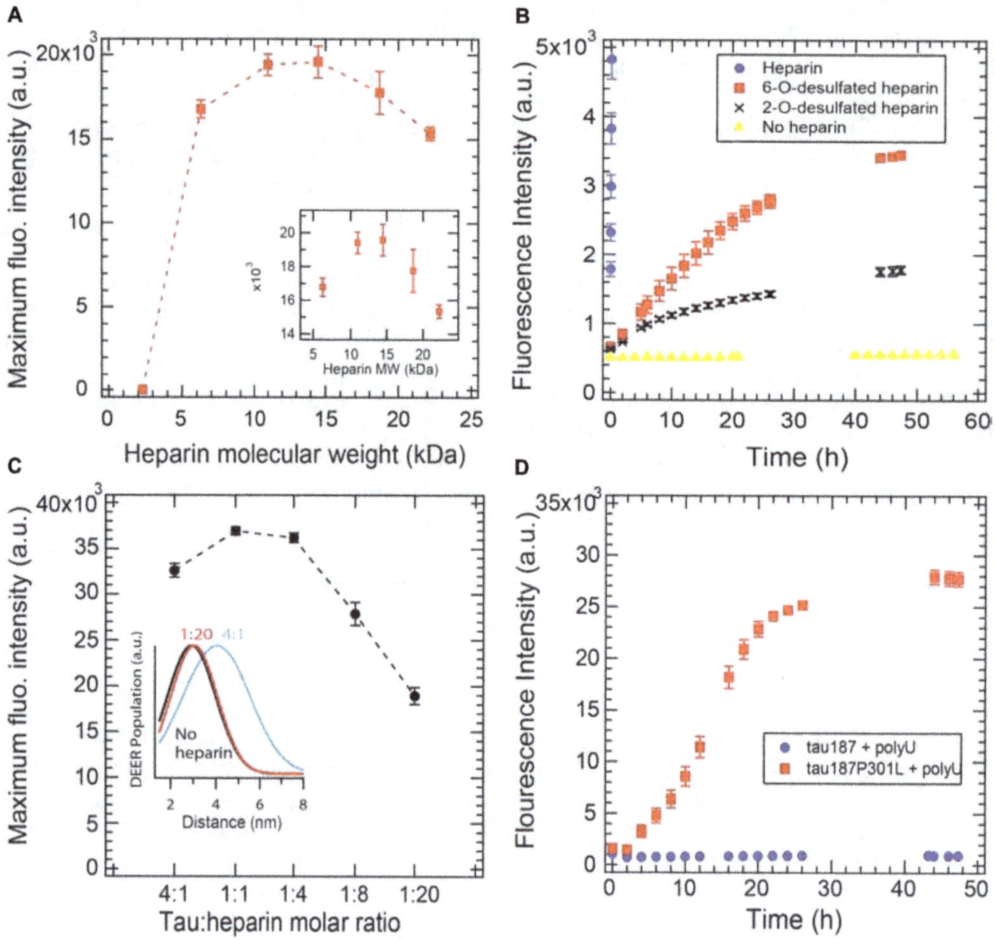

FIGURE 5 | Cofactor length, stoichiometry, charge state and nature modulate tau187 aggregation, as probed by ThT fluorescence. ThT fluorescence was measured over time and the maximum plateau value is plotted for **(A)** different heparin lengths (constant mass ratio) and **(C)** different tau:heparin molar ratios. DEER distance distribution between residues 272 and 285 (inset **C**) shows that S* is not present at 1:20 tau:heparin ratio, **(B)** Tau187 was incubated with fully sulfated (purple circle), 6-O desulfated (red square), 2-O desulfated (black cross) heparin or no heparin (yellow triangle) at 4:1 tau:heparin ratio. The sulfated heparin curve converges to about 3.8×10^4 fluorescence units and was cut to better highlight the difference between 6OD and 2OD. **(D)** PolyU (500 μg/mL) incubated with tau187 and tau187-P301L. The protein concentration was 50 μM in all panels. Gaps in the ThT kinetics **(B,D)** originate from reading interruptions. Error bars represent standard deviation over 3 repeats.

(**Supplementary Figure S8**). Note that the kinetics of polyU-induced tau aggregation is different from heparin-induced aggregation (compare **Figure 5D** with **Figure 2A**), potentially revealing different aggregation pathways. The P301L mutation was recently proposed to promote aggregation by increasing the population of aggregation-prone conformers (Chen et al., 2019). The data here suggests that this conformational rearrangement in combination with the presence of polyU is highly favorable for aggregation. Note that neither tau187 nor tau187-P301L aggregate spontaneously without polyU (**Supplementary Figure S9**).

These results highlight that the simple view of a charge compensation mechanisms, in which the basic tau repeat domains are allowed to self-assemble by adding anions, is not sufficient. Rather, a well-defined pattern of interaction between tau and its cofactor seems to be required, which is influenced by the length, charge state, steric environment, and stoichiometry of the cofactor, as well as the conformational landscape of the protein.

Tau-Cofactor Form a Complex That May Not Spontaneously Evolve to Fibrils

Here we focus on the tau187 + polyU RNA system that evolves into fibrils only in the presence of the P301L mutation (**Figure 5D**). This observation raises the question of how a single-point mutation can completely enable/disable RNA-induced aggregation. We applied multiple techniques to characterize the tau187 + polyU sample, within 20 min after co-incubation, by dynamic light scattering (DLS), cw-EPR lineshape analysis and affinity chromatography. DLS was measured on tau187 alone, polyU alone and a mixture of both (**Figure 6A**). We observed a significant increase of hydrodynamic radius (Rh) when the compounds were mixed together to a value of about 40 nm.

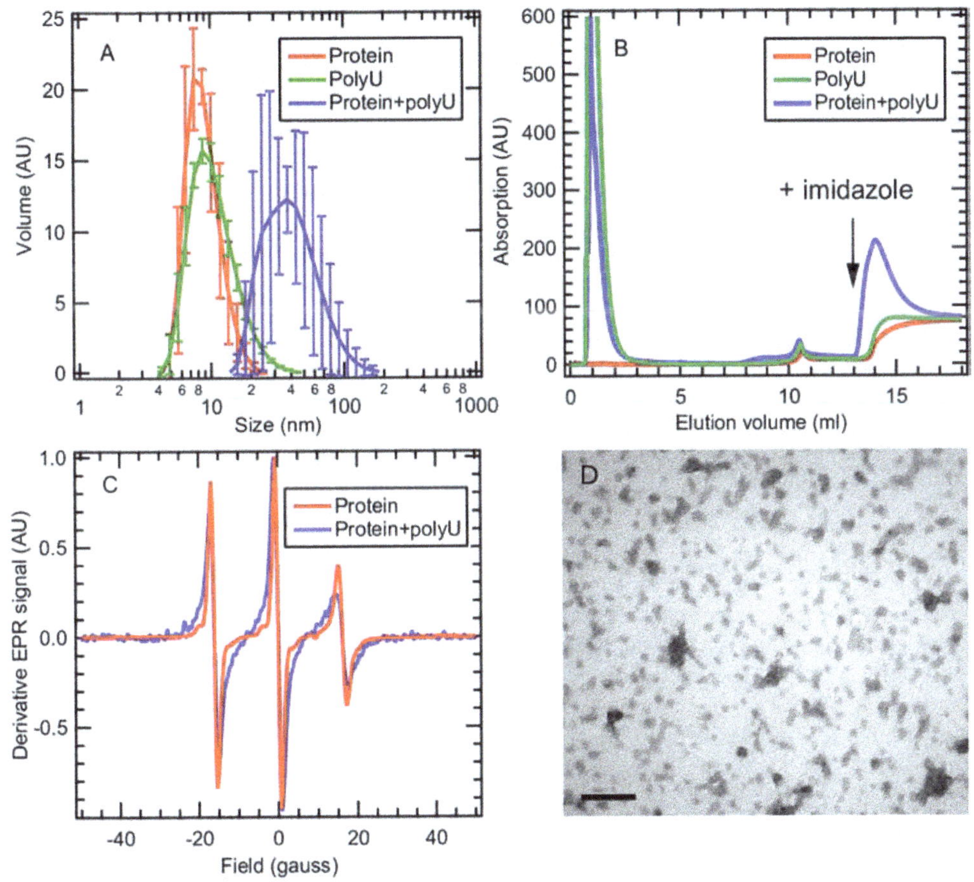

FIGURE 6 | Tau187 and polyU form a complex. **(A)** tau187 (100 µM) incubated with polyU (1 mg/mL) (blue) exhibit a larger hydrodynamic radius than tau187 alone (red) or polyU alone (green), as shown by DLS. Error bars represent standard deviation over 3 independant repeats, each composed of 3 measurements of the same sample. **(B)** tau187, which possesses a histidine tag, can be immobilized onto a Ni-affinity column (mounted on a FPLC system), and eluted by imidazole. The absorption value reports on the presence of polyU, which has an absorption coefficient 100 times larger than that of tau187. The fact that RNA is eluted with imidazole when incubated with tau187 (blue trace) shows that they form a complex that is immobilized in the Ni-column. **(C)** The presence of the complex is further confirmed by cw-EPR applied on tau187 labeled at position 322. The lineshape broadening observed when tau187 is incubated with polyU (blue) reflects a slower correlation time and therefore shows that tau187 is no longer monomeric. **(D)** TEM picture of tau187 incubated with polyU for 10 min. Scale bar is 200 nm.

This Rh is compatible with a small complex containing several molecules, but given the uncertainty on the complex structure, we cannot deduce the exact stoichiometric composition from the Rh. The presence of tau87-polyU complexes was confirmed by electron microscopy (**Figure 6D**) showing oligomers of few tens of nm, in good agreement with DLS data. Interestingly, round-like oligomers of about 30 nm seems to agglomerate in elongated assemblies that might represent prefibrillar assemblies. Note that these oligomers do not originate from liquid-liquid phase separation (LLPS) as they do not appear to merge or be perfectly round. In addition, the tau187:polyU ratio used does not fulfill the charge balance requirement to form LLPS (Lin et al., 2019) (excess of negative charges from RNA). The formation of this complex was further confirmed by cw-EPR that showed a lineshape broadening upon addition of polyU to tau187 (**Figure 6C**). This broadened linshape, which reflects a slowdown of the spin label dynamics, could be fit with a single component (**Supplementary Figure S10**), suggesting that most of the tau molecules are part of a complex. The best fit was obtained utilizing a rotational correlation time of 1.3 ns, which is lower than the one found for the spin labeled part of intermediate species identified in heparin-induced aggregation (~3.4 ns, see **Figure 4** and **Supplementary Table S1**). This difference suggests that the polyU-tau187 complex is smaller than the heparin-induced intermediate species identified in **Figure 4**. Similar lineshape broadening was observed when tau187 was labeled at a different position (residue 272; **Supplementary Figure S11**), suggesting that this decrease in dynamics is not a local effect but reflects the global property of the protein.

We furthermore demonstrated the presence of this complex by affinity chromatography. Tau187 was expressed with a poly-histidine tag that can be immobilized onto a Ni-affinity column. We loaded either tau187 (0.4 mg), tau187 + polyU (0.4 mg + 0.4 mg, respectively) or polyU (0.4 mg) onto the Ni-affinity column connected to a FPLC system and followed the absorption at 280 nm (**Figure 6B**). Note that the absorption at 280 nm is 100-fold lower for tau187 than for polyU (about 0.13 and 11 $mg^{-1}.mL.cm^{-1}$ for tau187 and polyU, respectively), so that it reports on the presence of polyU. The sample was injected at V = 0 mL and the peaks visible at 1–2 mL correspond to the material flowing through the column without interaction. After flowing buffer, imidazole was injected at V = 13 mL to elute the material that was immobilized in the column. Because of the low absorption of tau187, it is essentially invisible from the chromatogram (red trace; the step at 14 mL corresponds to imidazole absorption; **Supplementary Figure S12**). As expected, polyU flows entirely through the column and none of it is eluted with imidazole (green trace). However, when tau187 mixed with polyU are injected, a strong polyU peak is eluted with imidazole. We confirmed that this peak contained both the protein and RNA by running SDS-page gel and acquiring the absorption spectrum (**Supplementary Figure S12**). The elution of polyU from the affinity column (i) demonstrates the existence of a tau187-polyU complex that can be immobilized onto an affinity column via the histidine tag present on the protein and (ii) offers a reliable way to purify this complex by collecting the elution peak. After collection of the elution peak and removal of the imidazole by buffer exchange, we were able to measure the polyU concentration by UV absorption and the protein concentration by spin counting (see section Materials and Methods), which revealed a polyU:tau187 mass ratio of ~2:1. We also showed that this complex could be destabilized either by increasing salt concentration in the buffer (**Supplementary Figure S13**) or by digestion of polyU RNA with RNase A (**Supplementary Figure S14**). These results demonstrate that tau187 mixed with polyU form an electrostatically stabilized complex that does not spontaneously aggregate to fibrils. The existence of this ThT-inactive polyU-tau complex was also shown for other tau187 mutants (with zero and two native cysteines) and for the full length tau 2N4R isoform (**Supplementary Figure S15**), as well as for a different buffer (**Supplementary Figure S16**) and across a wide range of concentration (**Supplementary Figure S17**).

Tau-Cofactor Complex Is Metastable and Form Fibril Building Blocks

We then asked the question whether this complex that appears stable at room temperature could be converted to fibrils. We first mixed tau187 and polyU and purified the complex by affinity chromatography (see previous section). The elution peak was collected and buffer exchanged to remove imidazole. This purified complex was incubated with 5% (protein mass ratio) of mature heparin-induced fibrils as seeds, while monitoring ThT fluorescence (**Figure 7A** and **Supplementary Figure S18**). The ThT intensity significantly increased when seeds were added to the complex, but not when added to the protein alone (i.e., not complexed with polyU), showing that the tau-RNA complex can be efficiently seeded to form ThT-active species. The seed-enabled conversion from oligomer to amyloid fibrils was confirmed by TEM showing that oligomers before seed addition (10 min incubation of polyU + tau187) turned into fibrillary assemblies 24 h after seed addition (**Figure 7B**). Once the ThT signal was maximal and steady (21 h), RNAse A was added to the seeded fibrils, resulting in a significant loss of the ThT signal (**Figure 7A**). This is consistent with previous results (Fichou et al., 2018a) showing that mature cofactor-induced tau fibrils depolymerize upon digestion of the cofactor. The full ThT intensity curves are provided in **Supplementary Figure S18**. These results show that (i) tau187-polyU complex is metastable and can be converted to fibrils given that an appropriate trigger is provided (seed) and (ii) the entire complex (not just tau) is a constituent of the fibrils as removal of the cofactor results in the destabilization of the fibrils.

DISCUSSION

In this report, we first reinforced previous findings showing that (i) the amount of tau aggregates formed by cofactor induction is limited by the stoichiometry of the cofactor relative to tau (Carlson et al., 2007; Ramachandran and Udgaonkar, 2011) and that (ii) tau aggregation to fibril is preceded by the formation of on-pathway intermediates (Ramachandran and Udgaonkar, 2011; Shammas et al., 2015; Kjaergaard et al., 2018). The latter intermediates are directly measured and quantified by EPR lineshape analysis. We furthermore showed that the molar stoichiometry of the cofactor relative to tau dictates the extent of conversion toward aggregation-prone tau conformers (either present as monomers or as part of intermediate species), recalling a chaperone-like activity of the cofactor, but one in which the cofactor remains associated with tau. We highlighted that seemingly relatively small modifications in the polyanionic cofactor, such as changing the charge location, or a single point mutation of tau, can drastically change the aggregation propensity of tau. Remarkably, we found that RNA and tau187 associate to form a soluble complex, apparently stable as it does not spontaneously trigger fibril formation of tau. However, we showed that this complex is metastable and can be converted to fibrils when exposed to a seed.

The importance of the cofactor:tau stoichiometry was studied in great detail by Carlson et al. (2007) as well as Ramachandran and Udgaonkar (2011). Similar to what is reported here, they found the existence of a cofactor-limited regime at low cofactor concentrations, and an inhibitory regime at high cofactor concentration, where addition of cofactor inhibited fibril formation. They postulated that the cofactor converts tau into an aggregation-prone form, acting as an allosteric regulator (Carlson et al., 2007), or into an aggregation-prone intermediate (Ramachandran and Udgaonkar, 2011). However, because they could not detect the cofactors as part of the mature fibrils, the concept of heparin as a catalyst was still compatible with these studies, leaving an unresolved question open as to why the cofactor could not be used multiple times to convert all available tau. The finding here (**Figure 7A**) and elsewhere (Fichou et al., 2018a) that removal of the cofactor by enzymatic digestion destabilizes the mature fibrils uncovers the missing piece of evidence to claim that cofactors are critical reactants of the tau-cofactor aggregation reaction. In other words, we show that the entire tau187-polyU complex (not just tau) is a constituent of the fibrils as removal of the cofactor results in the destabilization of the fibrils. Strikingly, the structure of tau

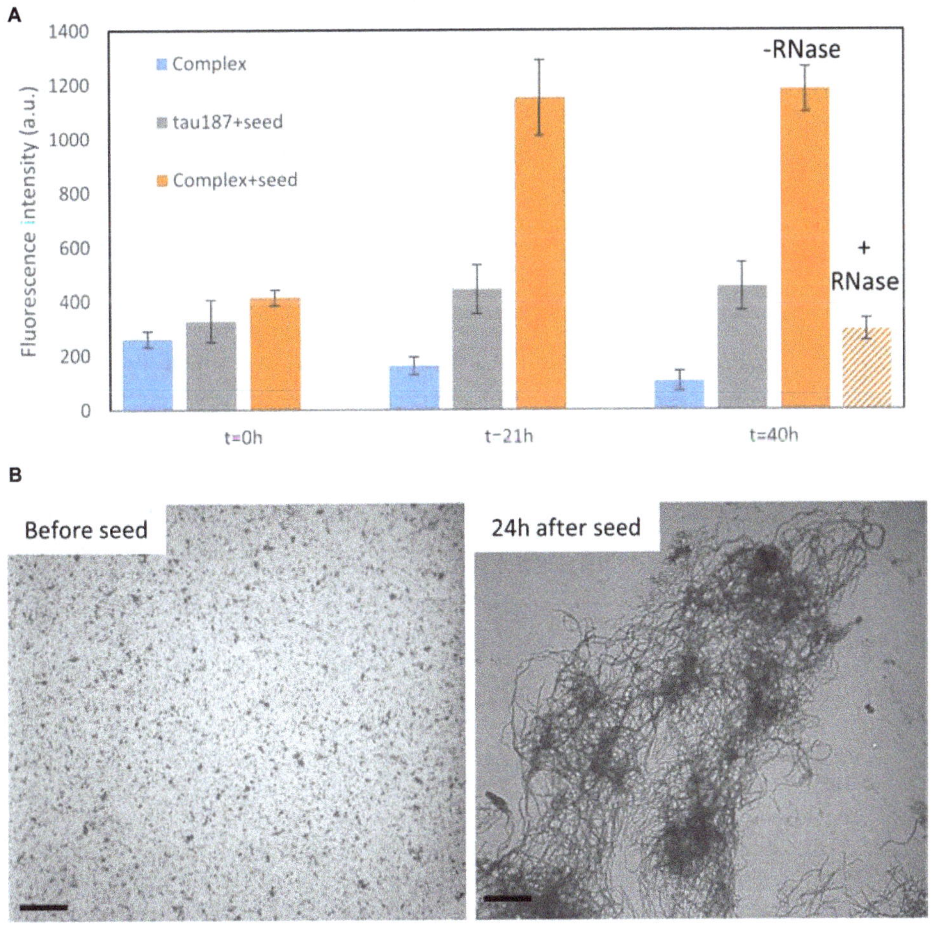

FIGURE 7 | Tau187-polyU complex is stable but can be converted to ThT active species in the presence of a seed. **(A)** ThT intensity of the complex sample eluted from a Ni-affinity column with (orange) or without 5% seed (blue). In comparison, fresh tau187 is incubated with seed (gray). The seed is added at time t = 0 h and the ThT value, reported at 21 h, increased significantly for the seeded complex. RNase is added right after 21 h and significantly reduces the ThT intensity. Full kinetics curves are shown in **Supplementary Figure S18**. **(B)** TEM pictures show tau187-polyU complexes (without Ni-affinity purification) that are converted to fibrillary assemblies 24 h after seed addition. Scale bars are 1 μm.

aggregates present in corticobasal degeneration was solved very recently (Zhang et al., 2019b) and highlighted the incorporation of an unknown polyanionic cofactor in the fibril core. It is important to note that these findings do not exclude the existence of other aggregation pathways that do not involve cofactors. Such pathways could be promoted by specific post-translational modifications (PTMs) (Despres et al., 2017) or fragmentations (Al-Hilaly et al., 2017).

We also found that the population of tau transforming from S (tau adopting a compact conformation around PHF6*) to S* (tau adopting an extended conformation around PHF6*) (**Figure 3**) depends on the heparin concentration, showing that heparin is directly involved in the structural conversion of tau and acts as a templating reactant. Interestingly, when adding an excess amount of heparin (20:1 heparin:tau), this conversion to S* conformations is no longer observed, in good agreement with the low maximum ThT signal (**Figure 5C**). This shows that the stoichiometry between tau and cofactors is critical for the formation of S*. Ramachandran and Udgaonkar (2011) modeled the decrease in ThT signal observed when increasing heparin amount with off-pathway oligomers that have excess of heparin. Our results show that these off-pathway oligomers are lacking the aggregation-prone conformations S*.

We found that, at equal quantity of a heparin cofactor, the length of heparin monomers influences the final population of β-sheet structured species. This finding suggests that heparin templates aggregation via a well-defined structural change that requires an optimal polyanion chain length. Recall that the same tau:heparin mass ratio is compared to ensure the same quantity of saccharide units are present in each experiment. The observation that there is a lower molecular weight cutoff for heparin below which it cannot induce aggregation suggests that a polymer chain of heparin is necessary, not merely the heparin monomers, to trigger aggregation. If we consider the minimum heparin weight to be 2.3 kDa (**Figure 5A**), corresponding to 9 monosaccharides, and if we assume a linear length of 1 nm per disaccharide unit (Carlström, 1957), our results suggest that it is necessary to bridge intraprotein interactions (e.g., to create

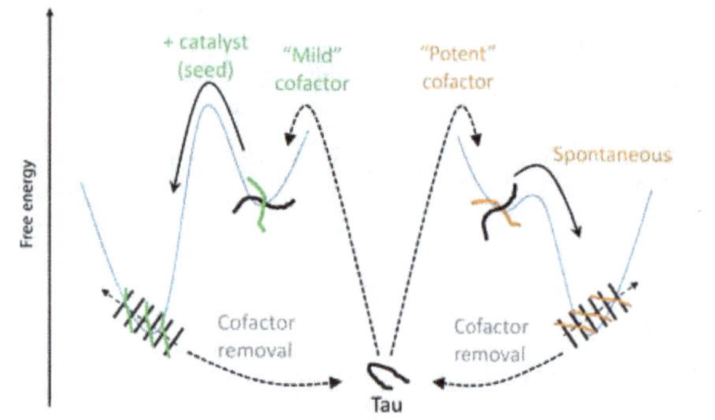

FIGURE 8 | Thermodynamic model of cofactor-induced aggregation and cofactor assisted seeding. Mild cofactors (e.g., polyU) form metastable complexes that do not evolve to β-sheet containing species due to a high energy barrier. This barrier can be overcome by a catalyst such as a seed. In contrast, potent cofactors (e.g., heparin) form intermediate complexes, or oligomers, that spontaneously evolved toward amyloid fibrils. In both cases, removal of the cofactors from the mature fibrils results in their depolymerization, showing that the tau-cofactor complex, and not tau only, is the building block of these fibrils.

the opening from S to S*) or interprotein interactions (e.g., to promote oligomerization; Ramachandran and Udgaonkar, 2011) across at least 4.5 nm distance to generate aggregation-prone species.

We introduce here the idea of "potent" and "mild" cofactors. Potent cofactors create unstable intermediates, such as those identified by EPR (**Figure 4**) and elsewhere in the literature (Shammas et al., 2015; Kjaergaard et al., 2018), which spontaneously convert to fibrils, given a low energy barrier to fibrils (**Figure 8**). The most prominent example of a potent cofactor is heparin that robustly triggers tau aggregation in a broad range of conditions. Mild cofactors create metastable complexes, which in contrast cannot spontaneously transform into fibrils given a considerable energy barrier to fibrils (**Figure 8**). Here we identified polyU RNA as a mild cofactor for tau187, which necessitates either a seed to overcome the energy barrier or an aggregation-prone tau mutant to lower the complex-to-fibril formation barrier. The observation that P301L facilitate the complex-to-fibril transition is in good agreement with early reports that P301L does not significantly increase the β-sheet structure in tau monomers, but rather increase the β-sheet formation upon cofactor addition (von Bergen et al., 2001; Fischer et al., 2007). Because this barrier crossing event is modulated by the nature of both partners, other RNA molecules or experimental conditions might trigger spontaneous aggregation of wild type tau (Kampers et al., 1996). Other mild cofactors are likely numerous under *in vivo* environments, but might have been overlooked because they do not spontaneously respond to commonly used ThT and TEM assays when mixed with tau. This model explains the underlying mechanisms by which RNA has been reported to allow efficient seeding (Meyer et al., 2014; Dinkel et al., 2015; Fichou et al., 2018a); RNA forms a metastable complex with tau that subsequently converts into fibrils in the presence of a seed.

This raises the following important question: in a cofactor-assisted experiment, are the properties of mature fibrils most influenced by the nature of the tau-cofactor complex (and therefore by the cofactor) or by the nature of the seed? This question is essential in the context of prion-like mechanisms (Sanders et al., 2014; Woerman et al., 2016), where one needs to understand the conditions required to ensure the faithful propagation of a given strain. Although cellular work has suggested that strain properties (based on proteolysis patterns and cellular localization of aggregates) can be maintained through seeding (Kaufman et al., 2016), other *in vitro* work suggested that properties of the seeded protein, and not the seed, dictate the structure of the obtained aggregates (Nizynski et al., 2018). Fichou and coworkers (Fichou et al., 2018a) showed that cofactor-assisted seeding achieve a mild degree of structural convergence compared to heterogeneous heparin fibrils, but without deciphering its origin. Recently, the structure of tau fibrils from CTE and CBD revealed the presence of a cofactor, whose identity however remains unknown, that is buried inside the tau aggregates (Falcon et al., 2019; Zhang et al., 2019b). Hence, it is reasonable to postulate that the cofactor-tau interaction would play a significant role in the final tau aggregate structure, in which the protein is "rolled" around the cofactor. In contrast, recently solved high-resolution structures of heparin fibrils (Zhang et al., 2019a) showed that heparin is not part of the core but might be scattered on the outside of the positively charged residues, suggesting that heparin might not be a critical determinant of the fibril morphology. This is consistent with the view that heparin increases the prevalence of aggregation-prone conformers (**Figure 3**) by exposing amyloidogenic segments, but does not specifically dictate the superstructural properties of the fibrils, yielding heterogenous fibrils (Fichou et al., 2018b; Zhang et al., 2019a).

Given the large structural diversity tau aggregates can adopt, we hypothesize that it is the interplay between the properties of (i) tau monomers (fragmentation, post-translational modifications, mutations...), (ii) the seed and (iii) the available cofactor (RNA, sterol, DNA...) that dictates the tau fold and packing that constitutes the structure of the final aggregate. In a cellular context, this hypothesis suggests that a given strain could be created/propagated when tau comes in contact with a specific cofactor [e.g., promoted by tau mislocalization (Thies and Mandelkow, 2007; Hoover et al., 2010) or abnormal homeostasis (Petrov et al., 2017)]. In addition, we highlighted here that tau-cofactor complexes can be isolated *in vitro*, and shown to only convert to fibrils when exposed to a potent seed. This suggests a possible cellular mechanism in which tau could associate with a locally upregulated cofactor, and remain inert until a competent seed is brought to its location, for instance through cell-to-cell propagation (Frost et al., 2009; Wang et al., 2017).

MATERIALS AND METHODS

Protein Expression and Purification

A segment of tau, **Figure 1**, consisting of residues 255-441 was expressed in *E. coli* BL21 (DE3) and purified via nickel affinity chromatography as previously described (Pavlova et al., 2016). The mutation C291S was added by site directed mutagenesis and this construct is referred to as tau187 throughout the manuscript. Briefly, BL21 (DE3) cells transfected with a pET28a vector including the tau187 genes were grown in 1 L cultures of LB broth (Thermo Fisher Scientific) until an optical density of 0.6 A_{600} was achieved. Expression was induced through addition of 1 mM isopropyl β-D-1-thiogalactopyranoside (IPTG, Thermo Fischer Scientific) and incubated for 3 h. Cells were harvested by centrifugation at 6,000 × g (Beckman J-10) for 20 min. Purification was carried out by lysing the cells with 2 mg/ml lysozyme (Sigma-Aldrich) and pelleting cell debris through centrifugation. Subsequently, the supernatant was heated to 65°C for 12 min and unwanted proteins were precipitated and removed by centrifugation. Tau was extracted from the supernatant by binding to nickel affinity resin and subsequently removed by washing with increasing concentration of imidazole buffers. The protein was then buffer exchanged into the desired running buffer (20 mM ammonium acetate with 100 mM NaCl for experiments with heparin and with 0 mM NaCl for experiments with polyU, except when otherwise stated). The pH of the running buffer was 7.4 without protein and shifted to 7.8 with 100 μM tau187, due to poor buffering capacity of ammonium acetate. Several experiments were reproduced in 20 mM HEPES (which maintained pH at 7.4) to verify that the pH drift does not influence the conclusions of the manuscript (**Supplementary Figure S16**).

Fibril Formation Using Heparin

Tau187 was incubated at 37°C with heparin at a tau:heparin molar ratio of 4:1 in 20 mM ammonium acetate and 100 mM NaCl, except when otherwise stated. Polydisperse heparin with an average molecular weight of 11 kDa (Sigma-Aldrich) was used, except when otherwise stated. Monodisperse purified heparin and desulfated heparin were bought from Galen Laboratory Supplies. When length of heparin was varied (**Figure 5A**), a tau:heparin mass ratio of 4:1 was used for each type of heparin. Spin-labeled tau187 was used in **Figures 2** and **4** so that kinetics of ThT reading and EPR experiments could be directly compared. Spin-labeled tau187 was used in **Figure 6B**. Non-spin-labeled tau187 was used elsewhere.

Fibril/Complex Formation Using PolyU

Tau187 was incubated with polyU (Sigma Aldrich, P9528; 10 μg/mL of polyU per 1 μM of tau187) in 20 mM ammonium acetate, except when otherwise stated. For **Figure 6** and **Supplementary Figures S11, S13, S14, S15**, measurements were performed within 20 min after co-incubation of tau187 with polyU.

ThT Fluorescence and Turbidity Measurement

ThT fluorescence intensity was measured with a Tecan M220 Infinite Pro plate reader for data in **Figure 2** and **Supplementary Figures S1, S2, S4, S20** and with a Biotek Synergy II for other data. A 20 μL sample volume was added to a Corning 384 Flat Black low volume well plate and covered with black vinyl electrical tape to prevent evaporation. For the Tecan plate reader, excitation wavelength of 450 nm (9 nm bandwidth) and emission wavelength of 484 nm (20 nm bandwidth) were used. Number of flashes was set to 25 and readings were taken from the bottom. For the Biotek plate reader, an excitation wavelength of 440 nm (30 nm bandwidth) and emission wavelength of 485 nm (20 nm bandwidth) were used. Number of flashes was set to 10 and readings were taken from the bottom. In the tau:heparin ratio study (**Figures 2, 5C** and **Supplementary Figures S1, S3**), the tau187 concentration was fixed to 100. For data in **Figure 5**, the concentrations of tau187 50 μM. For clarity, every 60th time points were shown in the ThT kinetic curves. In parallel of all fluorescence reading, absorption at 500 nm was recorded to verify the absence of liquid droplets (phase separation) in the initial conditions. 20 μM ThT was used for all fluoerescence experiments.

Complex Aggregation Experiments (Figure 7)

After purification of the polyU + tau187 complex from Ni-affinity and subsequent concentration and buffer exchange, the protein concentration was estimated using spin-counting. The complex was diluted to reach 20 μM protein concentration and was mixed with 5% protein mass ratio of seeds. 20 μM ThT was used. The seeds consisted of tau187 mixed with heparin at a 4:1 tau:heparin molar ratio and incubated for 24 h at 37C. At 21 h, 25 μg/mL of RNase A was added in some of wells containing the complex + seed (labeled + RNase) while other wells received the same volume of buffer (labeled–RNase). The data presented in **Figure 7A** represents the ThT intensity measured from the given samples to which was subtracted the average intensity measured in 2 wells containing only buffer and 20 μM ThT. Raw data are presented in **Supplementary Figure S18**. TEM pictures in **Figure 7** are obtained from a preparation of 80 μM tau187 and 0.8 mg/mL polyU after 10 min of incubation ("before seed"). 5% protein mass ratio of seeds was added to this same preparation for 24 h before taking the "24 h after seed" pictures.

Spin Labeling

For experiments showed in **Figures 2–4** and **Supplementary Figure S4**, tau187 was dissolved in 6 M guanidine hydrochloride and labeled by adding a 10-fold molar excess of spin label (1-oxyl-2,2,5,5,-tetramethylpyrroline-3-methyl) methanethiosulfonate (MTSL, Toronto Research Chemicals) or the diamagnetic analog of MTSL (1-Acetoxy-2,2,5,5,-tetramethyl-d-3-pyrroline-3-methyl) methanethiosulfonate (Toronto Research Chemicals), referred as dMTSL. For other experiments. Tau was reduced by addition of TCEP for at least 2 h. After removal of TCEP by PD-10 column, a 10-fold molar excess of MTSL (Toronto Research Chemicals) was added. The excess of spin labels was then removed by standard buffer exchange methods.

Continuous Wave EPR

Continuous wave EPR measurements were acquired using a Bruker EMX X-Band spectrometer and dielectric (ER4123D) cavity. The microwave source applied ~6 mW of power at 9.8 GHz using 0.3 G modulation amplitude and sweep width of 150 G. Samples of 3.5 μL volume were transferred to a 0.6 mm diameter quartz capillary and sealed with wax on both ends. A 2-D EPR spectrum was then acquired stepping through time. The concentration of MTSL labeled tau187 was 100 μM, and aggregation was induced with the appropriate molar ratio (4:1 tau:heparin) of 11 kDa Heparin (Sigma Aldrich) in phosphate final buffer (20 mM Sodium Phosphate, 100 mM Sodium Chloride, 100 μM EDTA, pH 7.0).

Spin Counting

In order to obtain the protein concentration inside the complex, we used cw-EPR to measure the concentration of spin labels and infer the concentration of tau187. We measured the double integral of the acquired derivative spectra, which is proportional to the number of spins in the cavity. A 3rd order polynomial fitted baseline was subtracted to the first integral before applying the second integration. The obtained double integral value was compared to the one from a radical (4-hydroxy-TEMPO) at known concentration to calculate the absolute concentration.

Continuous Wave EPR Lineshape Analysis

EPR lineshape analysis was carried out as previously described (Pavlova et al., 2016) using the MultiComponent software developed by Dr. Christian Altenbach (University of California, Los Angeles), where a microscopic order macroscopic disorder (MOMD) model was used to describe the anisotropic motion of nitroxide radical (Hwang et al., 1975; Budil et al., 1996). The magnetic tensors A and g were fixed to those previously determined for MTSL spin labels attached to proteins (A_{xx} = 6.2 G, A_{yy} = 5.9 G, A_{zz} = 37.0 G, g_{xx} = 2.0078, g_{yy} = 2.0058, and g_{zz} = 2.0022) (Columbus et al., 2001).

In this study, the mobile component of this spin-labeled site was assumed to have isotropic motion with rotational diffusion tensor of $R_x = R_y = R_z$, while the immobile and spin-exchanged components were assumed to have axially symmetric anisotropic motion. The spin-exchange component is subject to an ordering potential described by order parameter, S (Columbus et al., 2001; Pavlova et al., 2016). The number of fit parameters was kept at a minimum, which includes the population for each component (p), rotational diffusion constant (R), and order parameter (S). Rotational correlation time (t_R) was calculated using $t_R = 1/(6R)$.

The single-component fit was carried out from EPR spectra of tau monomer (without heparin addition) assuming the rotational diffusion without a restoring potential. For the three-component fit, in addition to mobile and immobile components, we included Heisenberg exchange frequency ω_{ss} in the third spin-exchanged component. Specifically, in order to fit the single-line, spin-exchanged component in the simulated EPR spectrum, the exchange frequency needs to be greater than the hyperfine interaction, i.e., > 100 MHz. To minimize the number of fitted parameters, we empirically optimized and used a fix value of ω_{ss} = 140 MHz in the simulation. We found that the three-component model using five fit parameters (p_1, p_2, t_{R1}, t_{R2}, S) obtained the best fit for the aggregated tau samples (Pavlova et al., 2016). The fit parameters used in **Figure 2** are summarized in **Supplementary Table S1**.

3-Pulse ESEEM

ESEEM measurements were performed at X-Band on an ELEXSYS E580 spectrometer at 80 K with an Oxford instruments cryostat (CF935P) and temperature controller (ITC503). A Bruker MS3 resonator was maximally overcoupled to a Q-factor of approximately 100 for these measurements. A volume of 20–30 μL of sample was loaded into a 3 mm OD quartz EPR tube and flash frozen in liquid nitrogen before being inserted into the resonator. For each label position, both native cysteines were replaced by a serine while the specified residue number was replaced by a cysteine, which was subsequently labeled, i.e., the following tau187 mutants were measured: C322S/V309C, C322S/V313C, C322S/S316C and C322S/S404C. All experiments were carried out in deuterated phosphate final buffer and 30 wt% sucrose.

The pulse sequence for 3-pulse ESEEM (90°-τ-90°-T-90°-τ) consists of three 90°-pulses which generate a stimulated echo. When the delay between the 2nd and 3rd 90°-pulse is incremented, the amplitude of the stimulated echo is modulated at frequencies which correspond to the nuclear Larmor frequencies of nuclei coupled to the electron spin. The depth of the modulation is related to both the distance and number of nuclei around the electron spin (Erilov et al., 2005; Volkov et al., 2009). For our experiments, we specifically looked at deuterium nuclei in D_2O. By deuterating the solvent water, we can distinguish between solvent nuclei and other nuclei in the sample. This allows us to selectively measure and quantify the water content at specific sites around tau protein.

For 3-pulse ESEEM measurements, the 90°-pulse length was 16 ns, and the delay, τ, between the 1st and 2nd 90°-pulses was set to 204 ns which suppresses ESEEM from proton nuclei. The delay between 2nd and 3rd 90-pulse was set to a starting value of 20 ns and was incremented by steps of 32 ns to a final value of 8160 ns.

The ESEEM data was processed by fitting the background decay to a polynomial (5th degree) and subtracting and dividing by the polynomial fit. The data was subsequently Hamming windowed, zero-filled to twice the original length and Fourier-transformed. The deuterium peak height in frequency domain is proportional to the total number of waters around the electron spin. For our analysis of the ESEEM data, we interpret the relative changes in deuterium peak height as changes in extent of hydration, i.e., large drops in relative peak height correspond to dehydration of the protein surface and indicate less solvent exposure. The raw data are shown in **Supplementary Figures S21, S22.**

DEER

DEER measurement were carried out at Q-band (32 GHz) on an E580 pulsed EPR spectrometer (Bruker) at 50 or 80 K.

Samples were prepared by mixing 50 μM of MTSL doubly labeled tau187 C322S/G272C/S285C at a 1:10 molar ratio with dMTSL labeled tau (500 μM) in 20 mM ammonium acetate buffer (20 mM ammonium acetate, 100 mM NaCl, 100 μM EDTA, pH = 7.0) supplemented with 30% sucrose. The samples were aggregated with appropriate molar ratio of heparin for 1 h at room temperature at which time they were flash frozen in liquid nitrogen. A dead-time free four-pulse DEER sequence was used. The pulse durations for the $(\pi/2)_{obs}$, $(\pi)_{obs}$, and $(\pi)_{pump}$, were 22, 44, and 30 ns, respectively for the before, 4:1, 40:1, and 80:1 samples. The 8:1 and 20:1 samples utilized AWG capability with 32 ns Gaussian pulses. Distance distributions were determined using LongDistances.

DLS

Dynamic light scattering (DLS) was performed on a Malvern Zetasizer Nano ZS. The samples were filtered at 0.22 μM before measurement. 100 μM tau187 and/or 1 mg/mL polyU were used in 20 mM ammonium acetate with 40 mM NaCl. For each sample, three consecutive measurements were acquired. At least three sample preparations were measured for each data set presented in **Figure 6**. Error bars represent the standard deviation among the different sample preparations. The autocorrelation functions were treated with automatic procedures implemented in Zetasizer software 7.10 assuming protein material and using the "general purpose" data analysis mode.

Affinity Chromatography

Tau187 at 80 μM and/or polyU at 800 μg/mL were injected (250 μL injection volume) onto a Bio-Scale Mini Profinity IMAC Cartridge using a Biorad NGC liquid chromatography system. Samples were injected at 0.1 mL/min for 1 mL, before increasing the flow to 1 mL/min. The absorption at 280 nm was measured just after the column.

Absorption Spectroscopy

Absorption spectra (**Supplementary Figure S12**) were acquired in a plate reader Biotek Synergy II. For each sample, 80 μL of sample was placed into a UV transparent plate.

TEM

TEM grids, FORMVAR Carbon film on 300 mesh copper (Electron Microscopy Sciences), were floated on 10 μL of the fixed sample for 1 min and then blotted on filter paper. The grid was touched to 10 μL of deionized water, blotted, touched to 10 μL of the stain solution, 2% Uranyl Acetate (Electron Microscopy Sciences), blotted and then floated on 10 μL of 2% Uranyl Acetate for 1 min before blotting and setting aside to dry for 24 h. Imaging was carried out at room temperature using a JEOL JEM-1230 TEM at the UCSB NRI-MCDB Microscopy facility. Pictures of oligomers were obtained by incubating tau187 with poly U for 10 min at room temperature before preparing the grids.

AUTHOR CONTRIBUTIONS

YF, ZO, and SH prepared the manuscript and coordinated the experiments. C-YC carried out the EPR data acquisition and analysis, and aided in the preparation of figures. TK performed the ESEEM experiments and analysis, and aided in the interpretation and figure preparation. NE coordinated the DEER experiments and carried out the data analysis and figure preparation. ZO, YF, and HN handled the ThT experiments and data. HN and YF carried out the complex characterization by DLS and chromatography. YF, HN, ZO, and NE generated, expressed, and purified the protein mutants. All authors reviewed and approved the final manuscript.

ACKNOWLEDGMENTS

We acknowledge the assistance of Dr. Jennifer Smith, Manager of the Biological Nanostructures Laboratory within the California NanoSystems Institute, supported by the University of California, Santa Barbara and the University of California, Office of the President. We thank Ralph T. Weber and Kalina Ranguelova from Bruker Biospin for their generous assistance in acquiring Q-band DEER data, as well as Enrica Bordignon and Tufa Assafa for assistance with acquiring Q-band DEER data. We thank Yanxian Lin for his contribution in acquiring and analyzing some supplemental data. We acknowledge the use of the NRI-MCDB Microscopy Facility at UC, Santa Barbara. We also acknowledge the use of the MultiComponent software for the analysis of cw-EPR lineshape developed by Dr. Christian Altenbach (University of California, Los Angeles). The program is written in LabVIEW (National Instruments) and can be freely downloaded from the following site: http://www.biochemistry.ucla.edu/Faculty/Hubbell.

REFERENCES

Al-Hilaly, Y. K., Pollack, S. J., Vadukul, D. M., Citossi, F., Rickard, J. E., Simpson, M., et al. (2017). Alzheimer's Disease-like Paired Helical Filament Assembly from Truncated Tau Protein Is Independent of Disulfide Crosslinking. *J. Mol. Biol.* 429, 3650–3665. doi: 10.1016/j.jmb.2017.09.007

Biancalana, M., and Koide, S. (2010). Molecular mechanism of Thioflavin-T binding to amyloid fibrils. *Biochim. Biophys. Acta* 1804, 1405–1412. doi: 10.1016/j.bbapap.2010.04.001

Budil, D. E., Lee, S., Saxena, S., and Freed, J. H. (1996). Nonlinear-Least-Squares Analysis of Slow-Motion EPR Spectra in One and Two Dimensions Using a Modified Levenberg–Marquardt Algorithm. *J. Magn. Reson. A* 120, 155–189. doi: 10.1006/jmra.1996.0113

Carlson, S. W., Branden, M., Voss, K., Sun, Q., Rankin, C. A., and Gamblin, T. C. (2007). A Complex Mechanism for Inducer Mediated Tau Polymerization†. *Biochemistry* 46, 8838–8849. doi: 10.1021/bi700403a

Carlström, D. (1957). The Crystal Structure Of A-Chitin (Poly-N-Acetyl-D-glucosamine). *J. Biophys Biochem. Cytol.* 3, 669–683. doi: 10.1083/jcb.3.5.669

Chen, D., Drombosky, K. W., Hou, Z., Sari, L., Kashmer, O. M., Ryder, B. D., et al. (2019). Tau local structure shields an amyloid-forming motif and controls aggregation propensity. *Nat. Commun.* 10:2493. doi: 10.1038/s41467-019-10355-1

Columbus, L., Kálai, T., Jekö, J., Hideg, K., and Hubbell, W. L. (2001). Molecular Motion of Spin Labeled Side Chains in α-Helices:? Analysis by Variation of Side Chain Structure. *Biochemistry* 40, 3828–3846. doi: 10.1021/bi002645h

Despres, C., Byrne, C., Qi, H., Cantrelle, F.-X., Huvent, I., Chambraud, B., et al. (2017). Identification of the Tau phosphorylation pattern that drives its aggregation. *PNAS* 114, 9080–9085. doi: 10.1073/pnas.1708448114

Dinkel, P. D., Holden, M. R., Matin, N., and Margittai, M. (2015). RNA Binds to Tau Fibrils and Sustains Template-Assisted Growth. *Biochemistry* 54, 4731–4740. doi: 10.1021/acs.biochem.5b00453

Erilov, D. A., Bartucci, R., Guzzi, R., Shubin, A. A., Maryasov, A. G., Marsh, D., et al. (2005). Water concentration profiles in membranes measured by ESEEM of spin-labeled lipids. *J. Phys. Chem. B* 109, 12003–12013. doi: 10.1021/jp050886z

Eschmann, N., Georgieva, E., Ganguly, P., Borbat, P., Rappaport, M., Akdogan, Y., et al. (2017). Signature of an aggregation-prone conformation of tau. *Sci. Rep.* 7:44739. doi: 10.1038/srep44739

Falcon, B., Zivanov, J., Zhang, W., Murzin, A. G., Garringer, H. J., Vidal, R., et al. (2019). Novel tau filament fold in chronic traumatic encephalopathy encloses hydrophobic molecules. *Nature* 568, 420–423. doi: 10.1038/s41586-019-1026-5

Fichou, Y., Eschmann, N. A., Keller, T. J., and Han, S. (2017). Conformation-based assay of tau protein aggregation. *Methods Cell Biol.* 141, 89–112. doi: 10.1016/bs.mcb.2017.06.008

Fichou, Y., Lin, Y., Rauch, J. N., Vigers, M., Zeng, Z., Srivastava, M., et al. (2018a). Cofactors are essential constituents of stable and seeding-active tau fibrils. *PNAS* 115, 13234–13239. doi: 10.1073/pnas.1810058115

Fichou, Y., Vigers, M., Goring, A. K., Eschmann, N. A., and Han, S. (2018b). Heparin-induced tau filaments are structurally heterogeneous and differ from Alzheimer's disease filaments. *Chem. Commun.* 54, 4573–4576. doi: 10.1039/C8CC01355A

Fischer, D., Mukrasch, M. D., von Bergen, M., Klos-Witkowska, A., Biernat, J., Griesinger, C., et al. (2007). Structural and Microtubule Binding Properties of Tau Mutants of Frontotemporal Dementias. *Biochemistry* 46, 2574–2582. doi: 10.1021/bi061318s

Frost, B., Jacks, R. L., and Diamond, M. I. (2009). Propagation of Tau Misfolding from the Outside to the Inside of a Cell. *J. Biol. Chem.* 284, 12845–12852. doi: 10.1074/jbc.M808759200

Ginsberg, S. D., Crino, P. B., Lee, V. M.-Y., Eberwine, J. H., and Trojanowski, J. Q. (1997). Sequestration of RNA in Alzheimer's disease neurofibrillary tangles and senile plaques. *Ann. Neurol.* 41, 200–209. doi: 10.1002/ana.410410211

Goedert, M., Jakes, R., Spillantini, M. G., Hasegawa, M., Smith, M. J., and Crowther, R. A. (1996). Assembly of microtubule-associated protein tau into Alzheimer-like filaments induced by sulphated glycosaminoglycans. *Nature* 383, 550–553. doi: 10.1038/383550a0

Goedert, M., Klug, A., and Crowther, R. A. (2006). Tau protein, the paired helical filament and Alzheimer's disease. *J. Alzheimers Dis.* 9, 195–207.

Hoover, B. R., Reed, M. N., Su, J., Penrod, R. D., Kotilinek, L. A., Grant, M. K., et al. (2010). Tau mislocalization to dendritic spines mediates synaptic dysfunction independently of neurodegeneration. *Neuron* 68, 1067–1081. doi: 10.1016/j.neuron.2010.11.030

Hwang, J. S., Mason, R. P., Hwang, L. P., and Freed, J. H. (1975). Electron spin resonance studies of anisotropic rotational reorientation and slow tumbling in liquid and frozen media. III. Perdeuterated 2,2,6,6-tetramethyl-4-piperidone N-oxide and an analysis of fluctuating torques. *J. Phys. Chem.* 79, 489–511. doi: 10.1021/j100572a017

Kampers, T., Friedhoff, P., Biernat, J., Mandelkow, E. M., and Mandelkow, E. (1996). RNA stimulates aggregation of microtubule-associated protein tau into Alzheimer-like paired helical filaments. *FEBS Lett.* 399, 344–349. doi: 10.1016/s0014-5793(96)01386-5

Kaufman, S. K., Sanders, D. W., Thomas, T. L., Ruchinskas, A. J., Vaquer-Alicea, J., Sharma, A. M., et al. (2016). Tau Prion Strains Dictate Patterns of Cell Pathology, Progression Rate, and Regional Vulnerability In Vivo. *Neuron* 92, 796–812. doi: 10.1016/j.neuron.2016.09.055

Kjaergaard, M., Dear, A. J., Kundel, F., Qamar, S., Meisl, G., Knowles, T. P. J., et al. (2018). Oligomer Diversity during the Aggregation of the Repeat Region of Tau. *ACS Chem. Neurosci.* 9, 3060–3071. doi: 10.1021/acschemneuro.8b00250

Lee, V. M., Goedert, M., and Trojanowski, J. Q. (2001). Neurodegenerative tauopathies. *Annu. Rev. Neurosci.* 24, 1121–1159. doi: 10.1146/annurev.neuro.24.1.1121

Lin, Y., McCarty, J., Rauch, J. N., Delaney, K. T., Kosik, K. S., Fredrickson, G. H., et al. (2019). Narrow equilibrium window for complex coacervation of tau and RNA under cellular conditions. *eLife* 8:e42571. doi: 10.7554/eLife.42571

Margittai, M., and Langen, R. (2004). Template-assisted filament growth by parallel stacking of tau. *Proc. Nat. Acad. Sci. U.S. A.* 101, 10278–10283. doi: 10.1073/pnas.0401911101

Margittai, M., and Langen, R. (2006). Side Chain-dependent Stacking Modulates Tau Filament Structure. *J. Biol. Chem.* 281, 37820–37827. doi: 10.1074/jbc.M605336200

Meyer, V., Dinkel, P. D., Rickman Hager, E., and Margittai, M. (2014). Amplification of Tau Fibrils from Minute Quantities of Seeds. *Biochemistry* 53, 5804–5809. doi: 10.1021/bi501050g

Nilsson, M. R. (2004). Techniques to study amyloid fibril formation in vitro. *Methods* 34, 151–160. doi: 10.1016/j.ymeth.2004.03.012

Nizynski, B., Nieznanska, H., Dec, R., Boyko, S., Dzwolak, W., and Nieznanski, K. (2018). Amyloidogenic cross-seeding of Tau protein: Transient emergence of structural variants of fibrils. *PLoS One* 13:e0201182. doi: 10.1371/journal.pone.0201182

Pavlova, A., Cheng, C.-Y., Kinnebrew, M., Lew, J., Dahlquist, F. W., and Han, S. (2016). Protein structural and surface water rearrangement constitute major events in the earliest aggregation stages of tau. *PNAS* 113, E127–E136. doi: 10.1073/pnas.1504415113

Petrov, A. M., Kasimov, M. R., and Zefirov, A. L. (2017). Cholesterol in the Pathogenesis of Alzheimer's, Parkinson's Diseases and Autism: Link to Synaptic Dysfunction. *Acta Naturae* 9, 26–37. doi: 10.32607/20758251-2017-9-1-26-37

Ramachandran, G., and Udgaonkar, J. B. (2011). Understanding the Kinetic Roles of the Inducer Heparin and of Rod-like Protofibrils during Amyloid Fibril Formation by Tau Protein. *J. Biol. Chem.* 286, 38948–38959. doi: 10.1074/jbc.M111.271874

Sanders, D. W., Kaufman, S. K., DeVos, S. L., Sharma, A. M., Mirbaha, H., Li, A., et al. (2014). Distinct Tau Prion Strains Propagate in Cells and Mice and Define Different Tauopathies. *Neuron* 82, 1271–1288. doi: 10.1016/j.neuron.2014.04.047

Shammas, S. L., Garcia, G. A., Kumar, S., Kjaergaard, M., Horrocks, M. H., Shivji, N., et al. (2015). A mechanistic model of tau amyloid aggregation based on direct observation of oligomers. *Nat. Commun.* 6:7025. doi: 10.1038/ncomms8025

Sibille, N., Sillen, A., Leroy, A., Wieruszeski, J.-M., Mulloy, B., Landrieu, I., et al. (2006). Structural Impact of Heparin Binding to Full-Length Tau As Studied by NMR Spectroscopy†. *Biochemistry* 45, 12560–12572. doi: 10.1021/bi060964o

Stancu, I.-C., Vasconcelos, B., Ris, L., Wang, P., Villers, A., Peeraer, E., et al. (2015). Templated misfolding of Tau by prion-like seeding along neuronal connections impairs neuronal network function and associated behavioral outcomes in Tau transgenic mice. *Acta Neuropathol.* 129, 875–894. doi: 10.1007/s00401-015-1413-1414

Thies, E., and Mandelkow, E.-M. (2007). Missorting of tau in neurons causes degeneration of synapses that can be rescued by the kinase MARK2/Par-1. *J. Neurosci.* 27, 2896–2907. doi: 10.1523/JNEUROSCI.4674-06.2007

Volkov, A., Dockter, C., Bund, T., Paulsen, H., and Jeschke, G. (2009). Pulsed EPR determination of water accessibility to spin-labeled amino acid residues in LHCIIb. *Biophys. J.* 96, 1124–1141. doi: 10.1016/j.bpj.2008.09.047

von Bergen, M., Barghorn, S., Li, L., Marx, A., Biernat, J., Mandelkow, E. M., et al. (2001). Mutations of tau protein in frontotemporal dementia promote aggregation of paired helical filaments by enhancing local beta-structure. *J. Biol. Chem.* 276, 48165–48174. doi: 10.1074/jbc.M105196200

von Bergen, M., Barghorn, S., Müller, S. A., Pickhardt, M., Biernat, J., Mandelkow, E.-M., et al. (2006). The core of tau-paired helical filaments studied by scanning transmission electron microscopy and limited proteolysis†. *Biochemistry* 45, 6446–6457. doi: 10.1021/bi052530j

Wang, Y., Balaji, V., Kaniyappan, S., Krüger, L., Irsen, S., Tepper, K., et al. (2017). The release and trans-synaptic transmission of Tau via exosomes. *Mol. Neurodegener.* 12:5. doi: 10.1186/s13024-016-0143-y

Wilson, D. M., and Binder, L. I. (1997). Free fatty acids stimulate the polymerization of tau and amyloid beta peptides. In vitro evidence for a common effector of pathogenesis in Alzheimer's disease. *Am. J. Pathol.* 150, 2181–2195.

Woerman, A. L., Aoyagi, A., Patel, S., Kazmi, S. A., Lobach, I., Grinberg, L. T., et al. (2016). Tau prions from Alzheimer's disease and chronic traumatic encephalopathy patients propagate in cultured cells. *PNAS* 113, E8187–E8196. doi: 10.1073/pnas.1616344113

Zhang, W., Falcon, B., Murzin, A. G., Fan, J., Crowther, R. A., Goedert, M., et al. (2019a). Heparin-induced tau filaments are polymorphic and differ from those in Alzheimer's and Pick's diseases. *eLife* 8:e43584. doi: 10.7554/eLife.43584

Zhang, W., Tarutani, A., Newell, K. L., Murzin, A. G., Matsubara, T., Falcon, B., et al. (2019b). Novel tau filament fold in corticobasal degeneration, a four-repeat tauopathy. *bioRxvi* [Preprint]. doi: 10.1101/811703

Zhao, J., Huvent, I., Lippens, G., Eliezer, D., Zhang, A., Li, Q., et al. (2017) Glycan Determinants of Heparin-Tau Interaction. *Biophys. J.* 112, 921–932. doi: 10.1016/j.bpj.2017.01.024

19

Novel Functions of the Neurodegenerative-Related Gene Tau in Cancer

Ricardo Gargini[1†], Berta Segura-Collar[2†] and Pilar Sánchez-Gómez[2]*

[1] Centro de Biología Molecular, CSIC, Madrid, Spain, [2] Neurooncology Unit, Instituto de Salud Carlos III-UFIEC, Madrid, Spain

Correspondence:
Pilar Sánchez-Gómez
psanchezg@isciii.es

† These authors have contributed equally to this work

The analysis of global and comparative genomics between different diseases allows us to understand the key biological processes that explain the etiology of these pathologies. We have used this type of approach to evaluate the expression of several neurodegeneration-related genes on the development of tumors, particularly brain tumors of glial origin (gliomas), which are an aggressive and incurable type of cancer. We have observed that genes involved in Amyotrophic lateral sclerosis (ALS), as well as in Alzheimer's and Parkinson's diseases, correlate with better prognosis of gliomas. Within these genes, high *Tau/MAPT* expression shows the strongest correlation with several indicators of prolonged survival on glioma patients. Tau protein regulates microtubule stability and dynamics in neurons, although there have been reports of its expression in glial cells and also in gliomas. However, little is known about the regulation of *Tau/MAPT* transcription in tumors. Moreover, our *in silico* analysis indicates that this gene is also expressed in a variety of tumors, showing a general correlation with survival, although its function in cancer has not yet been addressed. Another remarkable aspect of Tau is its involvement in resistance to taxanes in various tumors types such as breast, ovarian and gastric carcinomas. This is due to the fact that taxanes have the same tubulin-binding site as Tau. In the present work we review the main knowledge about Tau function and expression in tumors, with a special focus on brain cancer. We will also speculate with the therapeutic implications of these findings.

Keywords: Tau/MAPT, gliomas, neurodegenerative diseases, cancer, tumor aggressiveness

INTRODUCTION

Although the incidence of cancer and neurodegenerative diseases increases with age, there are plenty of evidences of an inverse comorbidity of these two conditions. The inverse association with cancer has been observed for Parkinson's disease (PD) (Moller et al., 1995; Inzelberg and Jankovic, 2007), as well as for Hungtington's disease (HD) (Sorensen et al., 1999). Moreover, a decreased risk of tumor incidence has been found after the onset of amyotrophic lateral sclerosis (ALS) (Gibson et al., 2016), although having a cancer diagnosis was not associated with an overall risk of ALS (Fang et al., 2013; Freedman et al., 2014). In the case of Alzheimer's disease (AD), the inverse comorbidity seems to be maintained in both directions, that is, older people with a history of cancer have a reduced risk of AD, and individuals diagnosed with AD have a decreased risk to develop tumors (Roe et al., 2005, 2010; Driver et al., 2012; Musicco et al., 2013; Ou et al., 2013;

Catala-Lopez et al., 2014; Ma et al., 2014). The inverse association between neurodegenerative and oncological diseases appears across many individual types of cancer, even though some studies have reported a positive association of PD with melanoma and prostate cancer (Liu et al., 2011; Kareus et al., 2012). For AD patients there is a more significant decreased risk of lung cancer (Musicco et al., 2013; Ou et al., 2013), and the "protective effect" of previous tumors seems to be greater for smoking related cancers (Driver et al., 2012). Nevertheless, the relationship between smoking and AD is still conflicted. Other question that remains unanswered is what happen with less frequent cancers, like for example brain malignancies, which occur in the same tissue and with the same range of age of the neurodegenerative diseases. The epidemiological evidences in this type of tumors are scarce and sometimes contradictory as they even suggest a direct co-occurrence with AD (Driver et al., 2012). Moreover, a positive correlation has been found between the mortality rate of AD and malignant brain cancer in US (Lehrer, 2010, 2018). Anyhow, these findings support the idea that the two diseases share some environmental and/or genetic risks or that they are governed by similar biological pathways.

Here, we have performed a comprehensive meta-analysis of the genomic and transcriptomic status of genes related to neurodegenerative diseases in brain cancer, particularly in tumors of glial origin (gliomas). Gliomas constitute the most common primary brain tumors and they include astrocytomas, which resemble astrocytes at the histological level, and oligodendrogliomas, with similarities with oligodendrocytes. They are all characterized by their diffuse nature although the WHO (World Health Organization) classify them from the less aggressive grade II, to the grade IV glioblastomas (GBM), whose median overall survival is approximately 15 months (Ceccarelli et al., 2016). Our *in silico* data show a striking inverse correlation between the expression of some of the neurodegenerative genes, especially *Tau/MAPT*, and the clinical progression of gliomas. Here we discuss what could be the implications of these observations and we extend it to the analysis of *Tau/MAPT* in other cancers, where this gene has been associated with resistance to taxanes. The comparative analysis of the biological processes that orchestrate the appearance and the development of gliomas and those that participate in neurodegenerative diseases may potentially lead to a better understanding of both conditions and therefore to the development of more effective therapeutic interventions.

MATERIALS AND METHODS

Analysis of Somatic Mutations and Copy Number Variations

Genetic alterations were analyzed using the TCGA (The Cancer Genome Atlas) data sets. For AD, the genes included were *APP, Tau/MAPT, PSEN1, PSEN2; APOE,* and *GSK3B*; for PD, the genes were *GBA, LRRK2, PARK2 (PRKN), PARK7, PINK1, SNCA,* and *UCHL1*; for *ALS*, the genes were *C9orf72, TARDBP, SOD1, FUS, UBQLN2, and HNRNPA2B1*, which were downloaded from cBioPortal[1] and UCSC cancer browser TCGA databases[2].

Gene Expression Analysis

Information about the progression and the histological types of gliomas was retrieved from the TCGA dataset that includes GBM[3] and LGG (Lower Grade Gliomas)[4]. These parameters were analyzed together with the expression values of *APP, Tau/MAPT, APOE, PARK2, PARK7, PINK1, SNCA, UCHL1, UBQLN2,* and *HNRNPA2B1*[5,6]. The expression of *Tau/MAPT* in different cancers was retrieved from the TCGA PAN-CANCER and GTEx dataset[7,8,9].

In silico Survival Analyses

The expression of *Tau/MAPT* and the follow-up overall survival data from human glioma tumors corresponding to TCGA datasets were downloaded from Xena cancer Browser see text footnote 5 and Gliovis[10], respectively. Kaplan-Meier survival curves were done following patient stratification using *Tau/MAPT* expression values. TCGA-gliomas LGG + GBM patients (n = 690) were stratified in two groups using *Tau/MAPT* median values as thresholds. The significance of the differences in overall survival between groups were calculated using the Log-rank test as Mantel-Cox (Chi square).

Detailed description of how TCGA samples have been processed to generate the dataset of somatic mutations, copy number variations and RNA-seq has been described for LGG dataset [N. Engl. J. Med. 2015 June 25; 372(26):2481–2498] and GBM dataset [Cell. 2013 October 10; 155(2):462–477].

Primary Glioma Cells

The primary glioma cell lines were obtained by dissociation of surgical specimens from "Hospital 12 de Octubre" (Madrid, Spain), after patient's written consent and with the approval of the Ethical Committee (CEI 14/023). They belong to the Biobank of that Hospital. Cells were grown in complete media (CM): Neurobasal supplemented with B27 (1:50) and GlutaMAX (1:100) (Thermo Fisher Scientific); penicillin-streptomycin (1:100) (Lonza); 0.4% heparin (Sigma-Aldrich); and 40 ng/ml EGF and 20 ng/ml bFGF2 (Peprotech).

Mouse Xenograft Assays

Animal care and experimental procedures were performed in accordance to the European Union and National guidelines for the use of animals in research and were reviewed and approved by the Research Ethics and Animal Welfare

[1]http://www.cbioportal.org
[2]https://tcga.xenahubs.net
[3]https://www.cell.com/cell/pdfExtended/S0092-8674(13)01208-7
[4]https://www.nejm.org/doi/full/10.1056/NEJMoa1402121
[5]https://xenabrowser.net
[6]https://www.ncbi.nlm.nih.gov/pubmed/24120142
[7]https://www.ncbi.nlm.nih.gov/pubmed/29022597
[8]https://www.ncbi.nlm.nih.gov/pubmed/25954001
[9]https://www.ncbi.nlm.nih.gov/pubmed/30881377
[10]http://gliovis.bioinfo.cnio.es

Committee at our institution (Instituto de Salud Carlos III, Madrid) (PROEX 244/14). For heterotopic xenografts, 1×10^6 cells were resuspended in culture media with Matrigel (1:10, BD) and then subcutaneously injected into athymic nude Foxn1nu mice (Harlan Iberica). For orthotopic xenografts, stereotactically guided intracranial injections in athymic nude *Foxn1*^{nu} mice were performed by administering 0.5×10^5 cells resuspended in 2 μl of Complete Media. The injections were made into the striatum (coordinates: A-P, −0.5 mm; M-L, +2 mm; D-V, −3 mm; related to Bregma) using a Hamilton syringe. Mice were sacrificed at the onset of symptoms.

Tumor Tissue Analysis

At the endpoint, subcutaneous tumors or brain tumors were dissected and the tissue was fresh frozen for molecular analysis or fixed o/n in 4% paraformaldehyde (Merck) and embedded in paraffin. Paraffin embedded tissue was cut with a microtome (Leica Microsystems) (3 μm sections) and sections were stained with specific antibodies. For that, slides were heated at 60°C for 1 h followed by deparaffinization and hydration, washed with water, placed into antigen retrieval solution (pressure cooking) in 10 mM sodium citrate pH 6.0 for 10 min. Paraffin sections were permeabilized with 1% Triton X-100 (Sigma-Aldrich) in PBS and blocked for 1 h in PBS with 5% BSA (Sigma), 10% FBS (Sigma), and 0,1% Triton X-100 (Sigma). The following primary antibodies (anti-Tau, Dako A0024; anti-Ki67, Dako M7240 and anti-GFAP, M 0761) were incubated O/N at 4°C. The second day, section was washed with PBS three times prior to incubation with the appropriate fluorescent secondary antibody (anti-mouse and anti rabbit Jackson immunoresearch) for 2 h at room temperature. Prior to coverslip application, nuclei were counterstained with DAPI and imaging was done with Leica SP-5 confocal microscope.

Western Blot Analysis

For protein expression analysis, a piece of tissue was processed by mechanical disruption in lysis buffer (Tris–HCl pH 7.6, 1 mM EDTA, 1 mM EGTA, 1% SDS, and 1% Triton X100) followed by heating for 15 min at 96°C. Protein content was quantified using BCA Protein Assay Kit (Thermo Fisher Scientific). Approximately 20 μg of proteins were resolved by 10% or 12% SDS-PAGE and they were then transferred to a nitro cellulose membrane (Hybond-ECL, Amersham Biosciences). The membranes were blocked for 1 h at room temperature in TBS-T [10 mM Tris–HCl (pH 7.5), 100 mM NaCl, and 0.1% Tween-20] with 5% skimmed milk, and then incubated overnight at 4°C with the corresponding primary antibody (anti-Tau Calbiochem, 577801 and anti-Actin Sigma, A2228) diluted in TBS-T. After washing 3 times with TBS-T, the membranes were incubated for 2 h at room temperature with their corresponding secondary antibody (HRP-conjugated anti mouse or anti rabbit, Amersham) diluted in TBS-T. Proteins were visible by enhanced chemiluminiscence with ECL (Pierce) using the Amersham Imager 680.

qRT-PCR Assay

RNA was extracted from the tissue using RNA isolation Kit (Roche). Total RNA (1 μg) was reverse transcribed with PrimeScript RT Reagent Kit (Takara). Quantitative real-time PCR was performed using the Light Cycler 1.5 (Roche) with the SYBR Premix Ex Taq (Takara). The primers used for each reaction were *Tau/MAPT* Fw-GTCGAAGATTGGGTCCCTGG; Rv-GGTCGTAGGGCTGCTGGAA and *HPRT* Fw-TGACACTGG CAAAACAATGCA; Rv- GGTCCTTTTCACCAGCAAGCT. Gene expression was quantified by the delta-delta Ct method.

Statistical Analysis

Quantitative data, represented as mean ± SD, were compared between groups using two-tailed Student's t or multiple ANOVA test. One-way ANOVA analysis was used to establish the differences of gene expression data between three groups and was represented as *F* value (F = the ratio of two mean square values). Differences are presented with statistical significance or *p* value (n.s., not significant). For survival study, patients were grouped into two groups with high and low expression of the gene of interest using median values and were analyzed by Kaplan-Meier method and log-rank tests using GraphPad program.

RESULTS

Genetic Status of Molecules Associated With Neurogedegenerative Diseases in Gliomas

To begin to address if there is a molecular correlation between gliomas and neurodegenerative diseases we analyzed the TCGA merge dataset for LGG and GBM (Ceccarelli et al., 2016) looking for the presence of mutations and copy number alterations in genes associated with AD, PD, and ALS. The genes we chose for AD were *APP* (Amyloid Beta Precursor Protein); *Tau/MAPT*; *PSEN1* (Presenilin 1), *PSEN2* (Presenilin 2), *APOE* (Apolipoprotein E), and *GSK3B* (Glycogen Synthase Kinase 3 Beta). For PD the genes analyzed were *GBA* (Glucosylceramidase Beta), *LRRK2* (Leucine Rich Repeat Kinase 2), *PARK2* (Parkin RBR E3 Ubiquitin Protein Ligase), *PARK7* (Parkinsonism Associated Deglycase), *PINK1* (PTEN Induced Kinase 1), *SNCA* (Synuclein Alpha), and *UCHL1* (Ubiquitin C-Terminal Hydrolase L1). Finally, the genes analyzed for ALS were *C9orf72* (C9orf72-SMCR8 complex subunit); *TARDBP* (TAR DNA Binding Protein), *SOD1* (Superoxide Dismutase 1); *FUS* (FUS RNA Binding Protein), *UBQLN2* (Ubiquilin 2) and *HNRNPA2B1* (Heterogeneous Nuclear Ribonucleoprotein A2/B1). **Figure 1A** shows that there is a very low frequency of somatic mutations or copy number variations (CNV) in glioma samples for all the genes included in the study. The higher percentage of genetic alterations was found in the *C9orf7* gene (3%), mainly associated with deep deletions that, in any case, are not frequently found in ALS patients. Overall, these results suggest that genetic alterations in genes associated with neurodegeneration are not common drivers of gliomas.

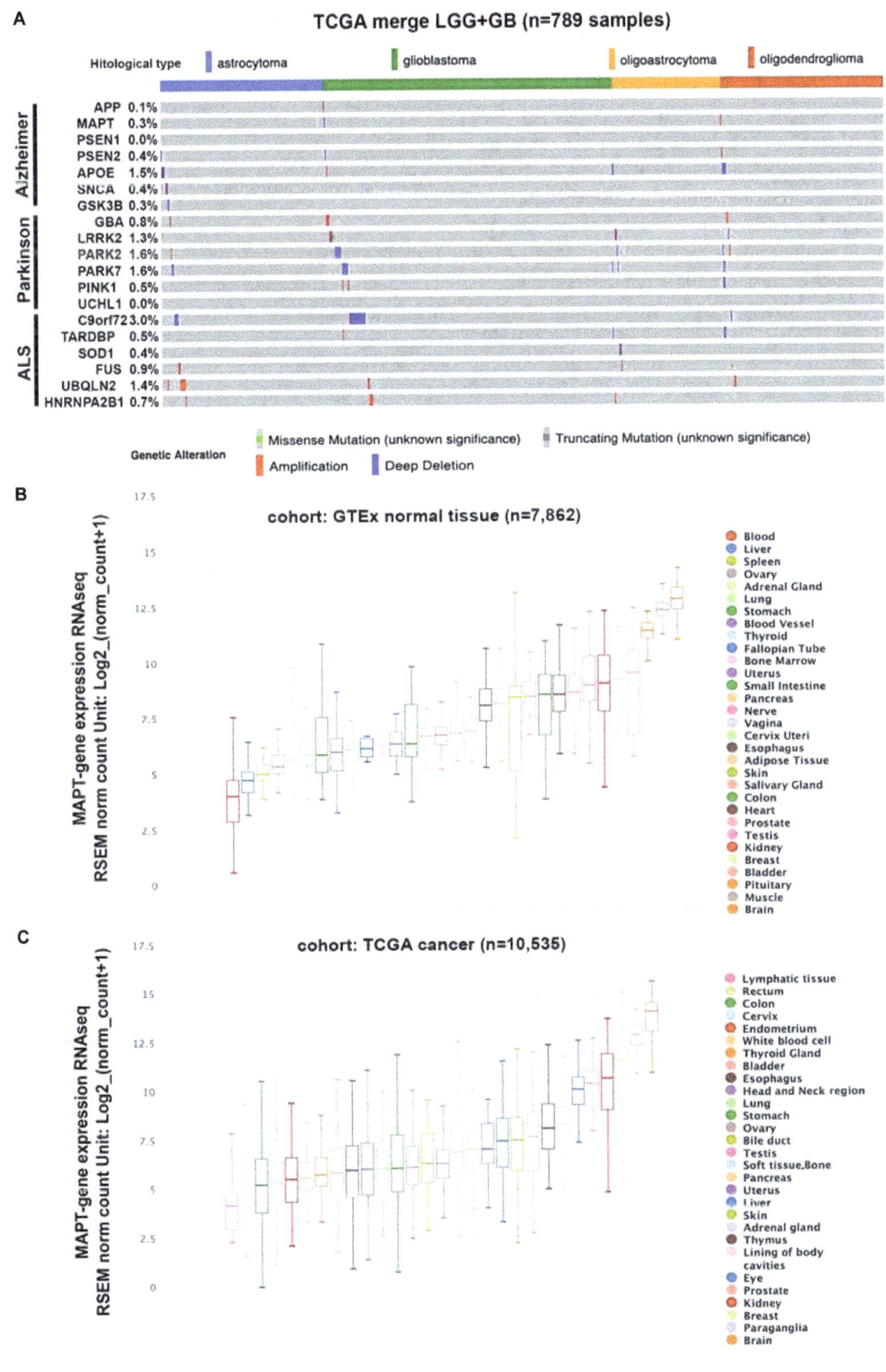

FIGURE 1 | Genetic status and gene expression of neurodegeneration-related genes in cancerous and normal tissues. **(A)** Histogram showing non-silent somatic mutations and copy number variations of genes commonly altered in AD, PD, and ALS on the TCGA cohort of diffuse gliomas (n = 789), grouped according to the WHO classification (histological type). **(B,C)** Box plots showing *Tau/MAPT* relative mRNA levels in different normal tissues **(B)** and tumors **(C)**, extracted from TCGA-TARGET-GTEx cohort, with RNAseq-normalized mRNA expression data.

Expression of Genes Related to Neurodegenerative Diseases in Gliomas

To further assess the involvement of the selected genes in the pathology of gliomas, we analyzed their levels of expression on the same TCGA cohort (Ceccarelli et al., 2016). We summarize in **Table 1** the results obtained for those genes that showed significant changes associated with the disease. It is noteworthy that the expression of most of these candidates appear diminished when we compare primary tumors with normal tissue. Moreover, their levels are even lower after tumor recurrence, suggesting that most of these neurodegeneration-related genes are downregulated as the brain pathology progress. By contrast, the opposite trend was observed for the *HNRNPA2B1* gene, which is highly expressed in recurrent tumors compared to primary gliomas or in the latter vs. normal tissue (**Table 1**).

Following the same type of analysis, we evaluated the expression of the selected genes in relation to the histological grade: from LGG (grade 2 and 3) to the aggressive grade 4 GBMs. In agreement with the previous data, the expression of most of the genes decrease as the tumor grade increases. In the particular case of *HNRNPA2B1*, we did not find a direct correlation with the histological grade as the expression levels were higher in grade 3 than in grade 2 or 4 tumors (**Table 1**).

Finally, we studied what was the implication of the expression of these genes in the survival of glioma patients. Except for *UCHL1* and *HNRNPA2B1*, we found that the high transcriptional levels of the rest of the selected genes are associated significantly with a decrease in tumor burden (**Table 1**). Taken together, these data supports the notion that the expression of many genes associated with neurodegenerative diseases correlate inversely with the progression of the glioma pathology. The strongest correlation was observed for *Tau/MAPT* so we hypothesized that it must play an important role in gliomas, slowing down or preventing the clinical evolution of these tumors. It is worth mentioning that even though the Tau protein is mostly found in neurons, there are few reports of its expression in glial cells and also in brain tumors of glial origin (Miyazono et al., 1993; LoPresti et al., 1995), reinforcing the need for a deep analysis of the function of this protein in gliomas. Besides, we could get some insights on the oncogenic role of Tau by addressing its significance in other cancers.

Expression of Tau/MAPT in Cancer

The primary function of Tau protein is the regulation of the dynamic instability of neuronal microtubules during synaptic transmission (Avila et al., 2016; Wang and Mandelkow, 2016). Moreover, tubulin and microtubules are the key components of the mitotic spindle and therefore they control the cell cycle. Actually, microtubule destabilizing and stabilizing components, which include taxanes, have been widely used as anticancer agents as they induce cell cycle arrest and apoptosis (Loong and Yeo, 2014). Because Tau compete with taxanes for the same tubulin-binding domain, a higher expression of this protein has been linked to resistance to these type of compounds, mainly in non-neuronal cancers (Kar et al., 2003). These observations are related to the fact that Tau expression could be expressed in other tissues outside the brain, as it has been already described (Caillet-Boudin et al., 2015). To corroborate these affirmations, we performed an *in silico* analysis of the levels of *Tau/MAPT* mRNA in normal and cancerous tissues in different organs. As expected, the highest expression of this gene occurs in the normal brain. However, elevated levels were also observed in other tissues like muscle, breast, kidney, and prostate (**Figure 1B**). Remarkably, tumors in those tissues lie among the group of cancers with higher *Tau/MAPT* expression (**Figure 1C**), suggesting that this gene could have other functions beyond chemoresistance and could

TABLE 1 | Correlation of the expression of different neurodegeneration-related genes with the clinical evolution of gliomas.

	Normal brain/Primary tumor/Recurrent		G2/G3/G4 histological grade		Survival test statistics		
	F-value anova	Expression pattern	*F*-value anova	Expression pattern	Media OS (days) high expression	Media OS (days) low expression	Long-rank value
Alzheimer							
APP	7.92	N>P>R	2.3	G2>G3>G4	2660	1209	6 4
MAPT	9.88	N>P>R	241.1	G2>G3>G4	2975	489	148.8
APOE	6.57	N>P>R	42.2	G2>G3>G4	2660	918	44.2
Parkinson							
PARK2	16.27	N>P>R	82.2	G2>G3>G4	2703	880	66.6
PINK1	13.23	N>P>R	77.1	G2>G3>G4	2660	919	45.2
SNCA	15.25	N>P>R	15.1	G2>G3>G4	2235	1137	13.1
UCHL1	10.48	N>P>R	13.9	G2>G3<G4	1233	2000	8.2
ALS							
UBQLN2	7.95	N>P>R	104.4	G2>G3>G4	2875	737	106.5
HNRNPA2B1	4.88	N<P<R	4.4	G2>G3>G4	1120	2000	5.1

Analysis of the expression of genes related to AD, PD, and ALS on the TCGA merged dataset for LGG + GB (Normal brain/Primary tumor/Recurrent tumor, n = 701; G2/G3/G4, n = 702; Overall survival (OS), n = 690 for the merged TCGA dataset (LGG + GB).

be associated with intrinsic properties of the cells in the different organs.

To gain further insight into the relevance of Tau in cancer we analyzed the TCGA cohorts for different cancers and we used the median of *Tau/MAPT* expression to classify tumors into High or Low-Tau. We then studied if there were differences in the overall survival of these two groups. In accordance with our previous data (**Table 1**), gliomas with high levels of *Tau/MAPT* have a much better prognosis (**Table 2**). However, the expression of this gene also correlates with an increase in the overall survival of patients with breast cancer, kidney clear cell carcinoma, lung adenocarcinoma and pheochromocytoma/paraganglioma (**Table 2**). By contrast, we found an inverse correlation between the expression of *Tau/MAPT* and the survival of colon and head and neck cancer (**Table 2**). However, those tumor have one of the lowest transcriptional levels of this gene (**Figure 2**). By contrast, it seems that *Tau/MAPT mRNA* is enriched in those cancers in which it has a significant prognostic value, particularly for breast and kidney tumors (**Table 2**). Collectively, these results suggest that Tau could have an important role in gliomas, but also in other cancers, beyond its competition with microtubule stabilizing agents.

Tau/MAPT Is Expressed on Glioma Cells and Correlates With a Less Aggressive Behavior of These Tumors

The data presented here suggest that *Tau/MAPT* is expressed in certain types of cancers, especially in the brain. Moreover, it allow us to hypothesize that, in some cases, the expression of this gene could be a marker of the less undifferentiated tumors (those that show a better clinical behavior) that get lost during the progression of the disease. In order to gain insight into the possible role of Tau in cancer, particularly in gliomas, we analyzed its expression in a panel of patient-derived-xenografts (PDXs). In these subcutaneous xenografts, in the absence of *Tau/MAPT* positive neurons, we observed that there is a variability in the transcriptional levels of this gene (**Figure 2A**). We then chose 3 of these PDX, with high, intermediate and low expression of *Tau/MAPT*, and we injected the dissociated cells into the

TABLE 2 | Prognostic value of *Tau/MAPT* in different cancers.

	N	Tau(MAPT) exp (Median)	Pro-survival	Median OS (days) high-Tau	Median OS (days) low-Tau	Survival *p* value	Survival log-rank value
Acute myeloid leukemia	132	4.52	n.s				
Adrenocortical cancer	79	6.91	n.s				
Bile duct cancer	**55**	5.65	n.s				
Bladder cancer	429	4.91	n.s				
Breast cancer	**1200**	**10.72**	**Yes**	**3736**	**3472**	**<0.0001**	**21.32**
Cervical cancer	296	4.46	n.s				
Colon cancer	**315**	**6.83**	**No**	**1881**	**3041**	**0.0089**	**6.83**
Endometrioid cancer	188	4.61	n.s				
Esophageal cancer	196	4.74	n.s				
Glioma	**690**	**13.27**	**Yes**	**2875**	**489**	**<0.0001**	**148.8**
Head and neck cancer	**562**	**5.17**	**No**	**1090**	**1732**	**0.0073**	**7.19**
Kidney clear cell carcinoma	**604**	**10.47**	**Yes**	**Undefined**	**2090**	**<0.0001**	**29.67**
Large B-lymphoma	47	3.25	n.s				
Liver cancer	417	6.63	n.s				
Lung adenocarcinoma	**564**	**5.31**	**Yes**	**1632**	**1423**	**0.0334**	**4.52**
Lung cancer	1109	5.14	n.s				
Melanoma	462	6.57	n.s				
Mesothelioma	85	7.48	n.s				
Ovarian cancer	307	5.16	n.s				
Pancreatic cancer	182	6.15	n.s				
Pheochromocytoma/Paraganglioma	**185**	**12.13**	**Yes**	**Undefined**	**Undefined**	**0.0383**	**4.29**
Prostate cancer	549	9.55	n.s				
Rectal cancer	103	3.99	n.s				
Sarcoma	265	6.15	n.s				
Stomach cancer	421	4.92	n.s				
Testicular cancer	139	5.21	n.s				
Thymoma	121	7.23	n.s				
Thyroid cancer	571	4.91	n.s				
Uterine carcinosarcoma	56	6.24	n.s				

Analysis of Tau/MAPT gene expression on the TCGA dataset for the different types of tumors. The median of Tau/MAPT expression was used to separate the high- and low-Tau groups and to calculate the overall survival (OS). Log-rank (Mantel-Cox) analysis was performed to determine the Pro-Survival value of Tau/MAPT expression. Bold words show relevant values for Tau/MAPT. N, number of patients enrolled. n.s., non-significant.

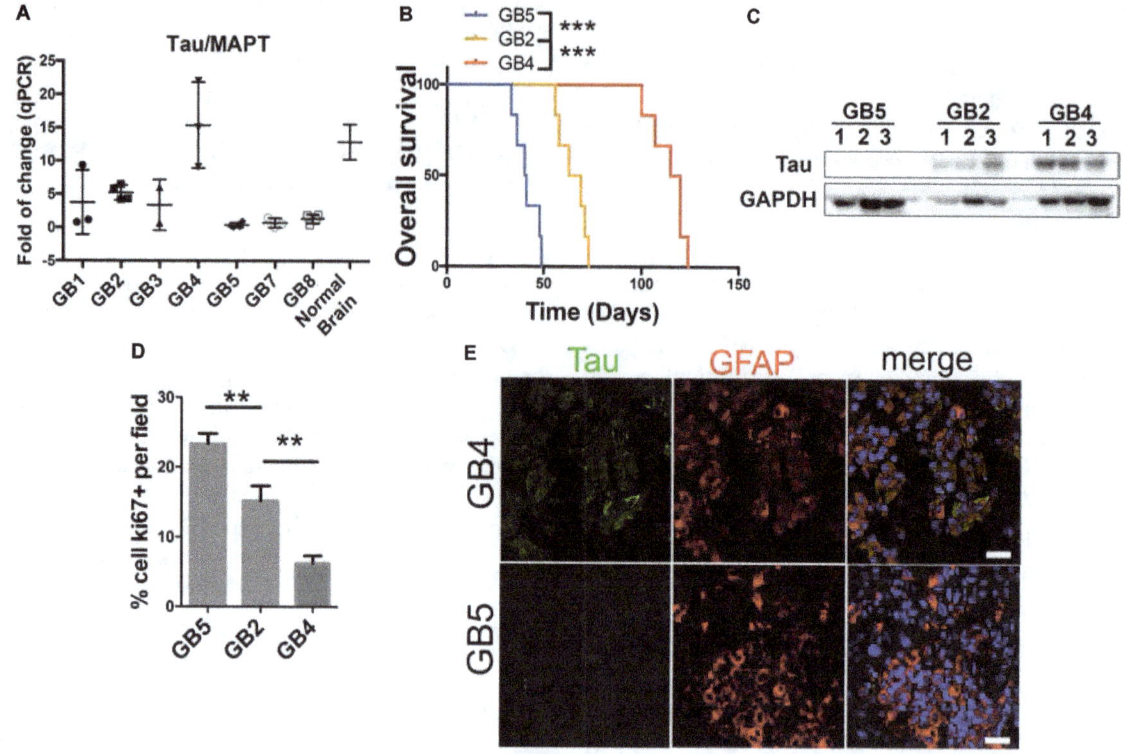

FIGURE 2 | Tau/MAPT expression correlates with less aggressive glioblastomas of PDXs. **(A)** Quantification of Tau/MAPT mRNA expression levels by qPCR in 7 different glioblastomas derived from patients implanted in flanks of nude mice. Normal human brain tissue was used as control. **(B)** Kaplan meier curve of 3 PDXs with different Tau expression levels implanted in the brain of nude mice (n = 6 for each group). **(C)** Tau expression levels analysis by western blot of tissue extracts of the experiment described in B using GAPDH as loading control. **(D)** Quantification of Ki67 cells percentage by immunohistochemistry (IHC) of PDXs tissue of samples described in **(B)**. **(E)** Tau and GFAP expression analysis by IHC in tumor tissue of samples described in **(B)**, showing Tau expression in green and GFAP in red, of the PDXs with high and low expression of Tau. ***p value < 0.0001, **p value < 0.01. Scale bar 25 μm.

brain of immunodeficient mice. We observed a striking inverse correlation between the amount of Tau and the tumor growth (**Figures 2B,C**). In fact, the more aggressive tumors show higher proliferative index (Ki67 staining) (**Figure 2D**). Interestingly, the analysis of the dissected GBM xenografts confirmed that Tau is expressed in a high percentage of tumor cells (co-stained with a GFAP antibody) in the Tau-high PDX, whereas there is very little expression in the Tau-low PDX (**Figure 2E**). Altogether, these results confirm the specific expression of Tau in glioma cells. Moreover, they suggest that the levels of this protein correlate inversely with the progression of this pathology.

DISCUSSION

Epidemiological evidences point toward an inverse comorbidity of neurodegenerative diseases and cancer. This phenomenon could be influenced by environmental factors and drug treatments. However, genetic and molecular pathways should have an important contribution as well. In fact, the two maladies are characterized by opposing cellular behavior in relation to cell growth and survival. In the case of AD, for example, a pathogenesis model has been proposed based on the up-regulation of tumor suppressors (Blalock et al., 2004). In that sense, p53, which promotes apoptosis and protects against cancer, is overexpressed in the central nervous system (CNS) of patients diagnosed with a neurodegenerative disease (Behrens et al., 2009). Others have found that several genes and pathways are upregulated in CNS disorders but downregulated in cancer and the other way round (Ibanez et al., 2014). This particular study has confirmed the dual role for the p53 pathway as well as for two other candidates, the enzyme Pin1 and the Wnt pathway, which are overexpressed or activated in most cancers but downregulated in AD (Behrens et al., 2009). More recently, another functional analysis has suggested that proteosomal, protein folding and mitochondrial processes are regulated oppositely in AD and lung cancer (Sanchez-Valle et al., 2017). The same study found a significant number of immune system and oxidative-phosphorylation-related genes that were deregulated in the same direction in AD and aggressive gliomas. More recently, it has been proposed that GBM-secreted CD44 could induce neuronal degeneration through the activation of Tau pathologies in the brain (Lim et al., 2018). These findings suggest a positive correlation between the last two diseases, something that had already been proposed (Lehrer, 2010, 2018). However, there are no robust epidemiological data on the incidence of gliomas in AD patients or vice versa, probably due to the low frequency of these tumors. Moreover, there are also discrepancies at the molecular level as other authors have found that the ERK/MAPK (associated with cell proliferation and survival) and the Angiopoietin (associated to angiogenesis) signaling pathways are oppositely regulated in the two diseases (Liu et al., 2013). Given this controversy we decided to perform a comprehensive characterization in gliomas of the genetic and transcriptomic status of genes associated with neurodegenerative diseases.

Despite the lack of genetic alterations of our panel of neurodegenerative genes in gliomas, we have observed an important correlation of their transcriptional expression with the clinical behavior of this type of cancer. It is true that almost all the genes tested have a higher expression in normal tissue compared to primary gliomas, nevertheless this could reflect that they are enriched in neurons in comparison to glial cells. However, the most relevant data is that their transcriptional levels diminish in parallel with the clinical evolution of the disease: after recurrence and during the progression of gliomas from low to higher grade tumors. Among the studied genes, we decided to focus on *Tau/MAPT*, as it shows the strongest correlation with the clinical evolution of gliomas. We performed an *in vivo* analysis, with ortho and hetherotopic glioma xenografts, which confirmed that Tau protein is truly expressed in the astrocytic tumor cells. Moreover, we validated the inverse correlation between the Tau and glioma growth. Therefore, our findings suggest that *Tau/MAPT*, and some other genes whose alterations are linked to neurodegenerative diseases, are enriched in the less aggressive gliomas and they probably need to be downregulated for these tumors to progress. This phenomenon could explain their positive correlation with survival in almost all the cases analyzed.

It is worth mentioning that there have been previous reports of deregulations (mutations and copy number losses) observed in *PARK2* in GBM (Veeriah et al., 2010), which argue in favor of a possible tumor suppressor function of this gene in such tumors. Still, our meta-analysis indicates a lower frequency of *PARK2* deletions in the joint cohort of gliomas. However, we only accounted for those CNV that appear in homozygosity, which could explain why we found a reduced percentage of gliomas with these deletions. Nevertheless, our transcriptomic data further supports that this protein could be inhibiting glioma growth as it has been suggested by others (Yeo et al., 2012; Viotti et al., 2014; Gupta et al., 2017). Regarding Tau, it has been recently reported that families affected by genetic tauopathies have a higher risk of developing cancer (Rossi et al., 2018). However, our analysis has found a very small percentage of gliomas (0.3%) with Tau alterations (amplifications and deletions).

Although Tau is highy expressed in neuronal axons, there were evidences of its presence in glial cells (LoPresti et al., 1995) and even in gliomas (Lopes et al., 1992; Miyazono et al., 1993). Moreover, the levels of Tau had been recently associated with LGG survival rates (Zaman et al., 2019), although its role in brain cancer was largely unknown. Our results suggest that gliomas need to lose Tau expression in order to progress into a more aggressive entity. In AD and other tauopathies, it has been postulated that changes in the expression of the different *Tau/MAPT* splicing isoforms might facilitate the neurodegeneration. Besides, Tau becomes increasingly phosphorylated in AD, which is the first step in the formation of toxic aggregates of the protein (gain of toxic function). The phosphorylation and subsequent aggregation of Tau compromises its microtubule-stabilizing functions (loss of physiological function), favoring the evolution of the pathology. In agreement with the loss-of-function model, several groups have reported behavioral changes and neurogenesis in aged Tau knockout mice (Pallas-Bazarra et al., 2016). Therefore, we could postulate that Tau expression and/or function might be lost during the progression of both, gliomas and AD, which might contribute to explain the correlation between the two diseases observed by certain authors. Nevertheless, the mechanism for Tau inhibition could be seemingly different: gene expression regulation in gliomas and posttraductional modifications in AD and other Tauopathies.

In relation to Tau function, our results suggest that the stabilization of the microtubule network might be needed in the earliest stages of gliomas, but it would be lost as the tumors progress. Tau overexpression in immortalized cell lines induces a plethora of changes in the location and trafficking of different organelles, including mitochondria and endosomes. This leads to a decrease in cell proliferation (Ebneth et al., 1998), which could be associated with the reduction in tumor growth that we have observed in the Tau-high gliomas. Moreover, changes in the dynamics of the microtubular cytoskeleton might have important implications in the motility of the tumor cells, affecting their invasive capacity. In adition, the microtubules participate in the process of epithelial-to-mesenchymal transition (EMT), which also occur in gliomas and has been associated with an increase in the aggressivity of these tumors (Bhat et al., 2013). In fact, the higher expression of Tau/MAPT in lower degree gliomas suggest that it could be an accumulation of this protein in the so-called Proneural tumors, which have a better prognosis and tend to suffer a process of mesenchymalization after tumor recurrence (Bhat et al., 2013). Interestingly, we have shown that Proneural gliomas are more prone to invasion whereas mesenchymal tumors are more angiogenic (Garcia-Romero et al., 2016). Therefore, we could speculate that changes in Tau expression could affect at the same time the EMT and the invasion capacity of the glioma cells. In fact, a recent article suggests that Tau downregulation in a glioma cell line leads to a decrease in cell motility (Breuzard et al., 2019). Future experiments will help to determine if Tau is an active or passive actor on these phenotypes.

Appart for the control of the microtubule dynamics, Tau has been implicated in other functions like maintenance of the RNA/DNA integrity and the nuclear structure. In addition, Tau contains several domains with a broad pattern of binding partners, including other cytoskeletal molecules that could participate in the regulation of protein transport (Medina et al., 2016; Wang and Mandelkow, 2016). Besides, Tau interacts with a plethora of kinases, phosphatases, chaperones and membrane proteins (Mandelkow and Mandelkow, 2012) and many of those could be Tau partners in cancer. Indeed, it has been shown that in prostate cancer cells, Tau binds to PI3K (phosphatidylinositol 3-kinase) (Souter and Lee, 2009). Furthermore, it has been shown to activate MAPK (Mitogen-activated protein kinase) in response to NGF (nerve growth factor) and EGF (epidermal growth factor) (Leugers and Lee, 2010). Both, PI3K and MAPK are important regulators of glioma growth and survival (Ceccarelli et al., 2016). More recently, Tau deletion has been linked to defects in the insulin signaling pathway in the brain (Marciniak et al., 2017). This could explain why patients with AD appear to be insulin resistant (Talbot et al., 2012). Moreover, it could be the cause of the repression of the orthotopic growth and vascularization of gliomas in genetic mouse models of AD (Paris et al., 2010). Alternatively, we could hypothesize that the decrease in Tau function could participate in the brain neuroinflammation observed in AD models and that this phenomena could favor glioma growth (Sanchez-Valle et al., 2017; Laurent et al., 2018). Indeed, higher levels of inflammatory markers have been observed in the brains of AD mice, which are more prone to develop tumors in the presence of carcinogens (Serrano et al., 2010). Future experiments will help to solve these apparent discrepancies in the frequency of cancer in AD mouse models.

Another important corollary of our study is the possibility that microtubules-stabilizing compounds could imitate Tau and hinder glioma growth. Among these molecules the most commonly used are the taxanes, including paclitaxel and docetaxel, which serve as chemotherapy agents in different cancers. Although they can reduce glioma growth *in vitro*, the clinical trials were not successful due to limitations in their ability to cross the blood brain barrier (Glantz et al., 1999). However, there have been promising results with the next-generation of taxanes like epothilone D and cabazitaxel, which can penetrate the brain and have good anti-tumor activity in mouse glioma models (Semiond et al., 2013). Cabazitaxel has been evaluated with a limited success in a phase II study for temozolomide refractory gliomas (NCT01740570 and NCT01866449) and now is being investigated clinically in combination with cisplatin.

High tau mRNA expression has been associated with a more favorable prognosis in breast cancer (Shao et al., 2010; Baquero et al., 2011). These results were confirmed in the present study (**Table 2**). Moreover, we have extended these results to other unreported cancers, like Kidney Clear Cell Carcinoma. Interestingly, it has been proven that Tau expression has a predictive value for estrogen receptor (ER)-positive breast cancer. In those tumors high levels of Tau are considered a surrogate marker for endocrine-sensitive but otherwise chemotherapy-resistant samples (Pentheroudakis et al., 2009; Shao et al., 2010; Bonneau et al., 2015). By contrast, low Tau expression identifies a subset of ER-positive breast cancers that have poor prognosis when treated with tamoxifen alone, although they may benefit from chemotherapy with taxanes (Rouzier et al., 2005; Andre et al., 2007; Pentheroudakis et al., 2009; Tanaka et al., 2009; Shao et al., 2010; Bonneau et al., 2015). Similarly, Tau-negative expression has been related to a favorable response to Paclitaxel treatment in gastric (Mimori et al., 2006; Wang et al., 2013; He et al., 2014; Yu et al., 2014) and bladder cancer (Wosnitzer et al., 2011). Translating these results into gliomas, our findings suggest that Tau-positive expression could identify a subset of tumors with slowest progression (including those with a higher sensitivity to the standard chemo-radiation therapy). By contrast, low-Tau expression could be a marker of a subset of gliomas that has a poorer prognosis. However, those tumors might benefit from chemotherapies with taxane-derivatives, like cabazitaxel. Therefore, it will be interesting to quantify the value of Tau expression as a surrogate marker in the clinical trials with this compound.

Increasing efforts have focused on the physiological vs. the pathological properties of Tau, investigating mechanisms of neuronal dysfunction attributed to loss-of-normal or gain-of-toxic Tau function in AD and other neurodegenerative pathologies. However, despite the evidences that support a novel role for Tau in cancer, we know very little about the mechanisms that control the expression and/or the function of this protein in tumor cells or in their microenvironment. The results presented here underlines the relevance of Tau in cancer, beyond its capacity to compete with chemotherapy compounds. We propose that this protein might serve as a brake in the evolution of the pathology of several tumors, especially in gliomas and certain breast and kidney cancers, where it is highly expressed. We believe that a profound characterization of the expression and function of Tau in normal and tumorigenic glial cells is needed. These studies will probably uncover novel aspects of the biology of this protein that could help to unravel the etiology of several cancers and neurodegenerative diseases.

AUTHOR CONTRIBUTIONS

RG and PS-G conceived the study. All authors developed the data analysis, wrote and criticized the manuscript, reviewed the literature, and revised and approved the manuscript. RG and BS-C performed the *in vivo* analysis of glioma growth.

ACKNOWLEDGMENTS

The authors would like to acknowledge Teresa Cejalvo and Ramón García-Escudero for their critical comments on the manuscript and Jacqueline Gutiérrez-Guamán for her help in the preparation of the histological sections and to the confocal microscopy service of ISCIII Majadahonda.

REFERENCES

Andre, F., Hatzis, C., Anderson, K., Sotiriou, C., Mazouni, C., Mejia, J., et al. (2007). Microtubule-associated protein-tau is a bifunctional predictor of endocrine sensitivity and chemotherapy resistance in estrogen receptor-positive breast cancer. *Clin. Cancer Res.* 13, 2061–2067. doi: 10.1158/1078-0432.ccr-06-2078

Avila, J., Jimenez, J. S., Sayas, C. L., Bolos, M., Zabala, J. C., Rivas, G., et al. (2016). Tau structures. *Front. Aging Neurosci.* 8:262. doi: 10.3389/fnagi.2016.00262

Baquero, M. T., Lostritto, K., Gustavson, M. D., Bassi, K. A., Appia, F., Camp, R. L., et al. (2011). Evaluation of prognostic and predictive value of microtubule associated protein tau in two independent cohorts. *Breast Cancer Res.* 13:R85. doi: 10.1186/bcr2937

Behrens, M. I., Lendon, C., and Roe, C. M. (2009). A common biological mechanism in cancer and Alzheimer's disease? *Curr. Alzheimer Res.* 6, 196–204. doi: 10.2174/156720509788486608

Bhat, K. P. L., Balasubramaniyan, V., Vaillant, B., Ezhilarasan, R., Hummelink, K., Hollingsworth, F., et al. (2013). Mesenchymal differentiation mediated by NF-kappaB promotes radiation resistance in glioblastoma. *Cancer Cell* 24, 331–346. doi: 10.1016/j.ccr.2013.08.001

Blalock, E. M., Geddes, J. W., Chen, K. C., Porter, N. M., Markesbery, W. R., and Landfield, P. W. (2004). Incipient Alzheimer's disease: microarray correlation analyses reveal major transcriptional and tumor suppressor responses. *Proc. Natl. Acad. Sci. U.S.A.* 101, 2173–2178. doi: 10.1073/pnas.0308512100

Bonneau, C., Gurard-Levin, Z. A., Andre, F., Pusztai, L., and Rouzier, R. (2015). Predictive and prognostic value of the tauprotein in breast cancer. *Anticancer. Res.* 35, 5179–5184.

Breuzard, G., Pagano, A., Bastonero, S., Malesinski, S., Parat, F., Barbier, P., et al. (2019). Tau regulates the microtubule-dependent migration of glioblastoma cells via the Rho-ROCK signaling pathway. *J. Cell Sci.* 132:jcs222851. doi: 10.1242/jcs.222851

Caillet-Boudin, M. L., Buee, L., Sergeant, N., and Lefebvre, B. (2015). Regulation of human MAPT gene expression. *Mol. Neurodegener.* 10:28. doi: 10.1186/s13024-015-0025-28

Catala-Lopez, F., Crespo-Facorro, B., Vieta, E., Valderas, J. M., Valencia, A., and Tabares-Seisdedos, R. (2014). Alzheimer's disease and cancer: current epidemiological evidence for a mutual protection. *Neuroepidemiology* 42, 121–122. doi: 10.1159/000355899

Ceccarelli, M., Barthel, F. P., Malta, T. M., Sabedot, T. S., Salama, S. R., Murray, B. A., et al. (2016). Molecular profiling reveals biologically discrete subsets and pathways of progression in diffuse glioma. *Cell* 164, 550–563. doi: 10.1016/j.cell.2015.12.028

Driver, J. A., Beiser, A., Au, R., Kreger, B. E., Splansky, G. L., Kurth, T., et al. (2012). Inverse association between cancer and Alzheimer's disease: results from the framingham heart study. *BMJ* 344:e1442. doi: 10.1136/bmj.e1442

Ebneth, A., Godemann, R., Stamer, K., Illenberger, S., Trinczek, B., and Mandelkow, E. (1998). Overexpression of tau protein inhibits kinesin-dependent trafficking of vesicles, mitochondria, and endoplasmic reticulum: implications for Alzheimer's disease. *J. Cell Biol.* 143, 777–794. doi: 10.1083/jcb.143.3.777

Fang, F., Al-Chalabi, A., Ronnevi, L. O., Turner, M. R., Wirdefeldt, K., Kamel, F., et al. (2013). Amyotrophic lateral sclerosis and cancer: a register-based study in Sweden. *Amyotroph. Lateral Scler. Frontotemporal Degener.* 14, 362–368. doi: 10.3109/21678421.2013.775309

Freedman, D. M., Wu, J., Daugherty, S. E., Kuncl, R. W., Enewold, L. R., and Pfeiffer, R. M. (2014). The risk of amyotrophic lateral sclerosis after cancer in U.S. elderly adults: a population-based prospective study. *Int. J. Cancer* 135, 1745–1750. doi: 10.1002/ijc.28795

Garcia-Romero, N., Gonzalez-Tejedo, C., Carrion-Navarro, J., Esteban-Rubio, S., Rackov, G., Rodriguez-Fanjul, V., et al. (2016). Cancer stem cells from human glioblastoma resemble but do not mimic original tumors after in vitro passaging in serum-free media. *Oncotarget* 7, 65888–65901. doi: 10.18632/oncotarget.11676

Gibson, S. B., Abbott, D., Farnham, J. M., Thai, K. K., McLean, H., Figueroa, K. P., et al. (2016). Population-based risks for cancer in patients with ALS. *Neurology* 87, 289–294. doi: 10.1212/wnl.0000000000002757

Glantz, M. J., Chamberlain, M. C., Chang, S. M., Prados, M. D., and Cole, B. F. (1999). The role of paclitaxel in the treatment of primary and metastatic brain tumors. *Semin. Radiat. Oncol.* 9(2 Suppl. 1), 27–33.

Gupta, A., Anjomani-Virmouni, S., Koundouros, N., Dimitriadi, M., Choo-Wing, R., Valle, A., et al. (2017). ARK2 depletion connects energy and oxidative stress to PI3K/Akt activation via PTEN S-nitrosylation. *Mol. Cell.* 65, 999-1013.e. doi: 10.1016/j.molcel.2017.02.019

He, W., Zhang, D., Jiang, J., Liu, P., and Wu, C. (2014). The relationships between the chemosensitivity of human gastric cancer to paclitaxel and the expressions of class III beta-tubulin, MAPT, and survivin. *Med. Oncol.* 31:950. doi: 10.1007/s12032-014-0950-953

Ibanez, K., Boullosa, C., Tabares-Seisdedos, R., Baudot, A., and Valencia, A. (2014). Molecular evidence for the inverse comorbidity between central nervous system disorders and cancers detected by transcriptomic meta-analyses. *PLoS Genet.* 10:e1004173. doi: 10.1371/journal.pgen.1004173

Inzelberg, R., and Jankovic, J. (2007). Are Parkinson disease patients protected from some but not all cancers? *Neurology* 69, 1542–1550. doi: 10.1212/01.wnl.0000277638.63767.b8

Kar, S., Fan, J., Smith, M. J., Goedert, M., and Amos, L. A. (2003). Repeat motifs of tau bind to the insides of microtubules in the absence of taxol. *EMBO J.* 22, 70–77. doi: 10.1093/emboj/cdg001

Kareus, S. A., Figueroa, K. P., Cannon-Albright, L. A., and Pulst, S. M. (2012). Shared predispositions of parkinsonism and cancer: a population-based pedigree-linked study. *Arch. Neurol.* 69, 1572–1577. doi: 10.1001/archneurol.2012.2261

Laurent, C., Buee, L., and Blum, D. (2018). Tau and neuroinflammation: what impact for alzheimer's disease and tauopathies? *Biomed. J.* 41, 21–33. doi: 10.1016/j.bj.2018.01.003

Lehrer, S. (2010). Glioblastoma and dementia may share a common cause. *Med. Hypotheses* 75, 67–68. doi: 10.1016/j.mehy.2010.01.031

Lehrer, S. (2018). Glioma and alzheimer's disease. *J. Alzheimers Dis. Rep.* 2, 213–218. doi: 10.3233/adr-180084

Leugers, C. J., and Lee, G. (2010). Tau potentiates nerve growth factor-induced mitogen-activated protein kinase signaling and neurite initiation without a requirement for microtubule binding. *J. Biol. Chem.* 285, 19125–19134. doi: 10.1074/jbc.M110.105387

Lim, S., Kim, D., Ju, S., Shin, S., Cho, I. J., Park, S. H., et al. (2018). Glioblastoma-secreted soluble CD44 activates tau pathology in the brain. *Exp. Mol. Med.* 50:5. doi: 10.1038/s12276-017-0008-7

Liu, R., Gao, X., Lu, Y., and Chen, H. (2011). Meta-analysis of the relationship between parkinson disease and melanoma. *Neurology* 76, 2002–2009. doi: 10.1212/WNL.0b013e31821e554e

Liu, T., Ren, D., Zhu, X., Yin, Z., Jin, G., Zhao, Z., et al. (2013). Transcriptional signaling pathways inversely regulated in Alzheimer's disease and glioblastoma multiform. *Sci. Rep.* 3:3467. doi: 10.1038/srep03467

Loong, H. H., and Yeo, W. (2014). Microtubule-targeting agents in oncology and therapeutic potential in hepatocellular carcinoma. *Onco Targets Ther.* 7, 575–585. doi: 10.2147/ott.s46019

Lopes, M. B., Frankfurter, A., Zientek, G. M., and Herman, M. M. (1992). The presence of neuron-associated microtubule proteins in the human U-251 MG cell line. a comparative immunoblot and immunohistochemical study. *Mol. Chem. Neuropathol.* 17, 273–287. doi: 10.1007/bf03160016

LoPresti, P., Szuchet, S., Papasozomenos, S. C., Zinkowski, R. P., and Binder, L. I. (1995). Functional implications for the microtubule-associated protein tau: localization in oligodendrocytes. *Proc. Natl. Acad. Sci. U.S.A.* 92, 10369–10373. doi: 10.1073/pnas.92.22.10369

Ma, L. L., Yu, J. T., Wang, H. F., Meng, X. F., Tan, C. C., Wang, C., et al. (2014). Association between cancer and Alzheimer's disease: systematic review and meta-analysis. *J. Alzheimers. Dis.* 42, 565–573. doi: 10.3233/jad-140168

Mandelkow, E. M., and Mandelkow, E. (2012). Biochemistry and cell biology of tau protein in neurofibrillary degeneration. *Cold Spring Harb. Perspect. Med.* 2:a006247. doi: 10.1101/cshperspect.a006247

Marciniak, E., Leboucher, A., Caron, E., Ahmed, T., Tailleux, A., Dumont, J., et al. (2017). Tau deletion promotes brain insulin resistance. *J. Exp. Med.* 214, 2257–2269. doi: 10.1084/jem.20161731

Medina, M., Hernandez, F., and Avila, J. (2016). New features about tau function and dysfunction. *Biomolecules* 6:E21. doi: 10.3390/biom6020021

Mimori, K., Sadanaga, N., Yoshikawa, Y., Ishikawa, K., Hashimoto, M., Tanaka, F., et al. (2006). Reduced tau expression in gastric cancer can identify candidates for successful paclitaxel treatment. *Br. J. Cancer* 94, 1894–1897. doi: 10.1038/sj.bjc.6603182

Miyazono, M., Iwaki, T., Kitamoto, T., Shin, R. W., Fukui, M., and Tateishi, J. (1993). Widespread distribution of tau in the astrocytic elements of glial tumors. *Acta Neuropathol.* 86, 236–241. doi: 10.1007/bf00304137

Moller, H., Mellemkjaer, L., McLaughlin, J. K., and Olsen, J. H. (1995). Occurrence of different cancers in patients with Parkinson's disease. *BMJ* 310, 1500–1501. doi: 10.1136/bmj.310.6993.1500

Musicco, M., Adorni, F., Di Santo, S., Prinelli, F., Pettenati, C., Caltagirone, C., et al. (2013). Inverse occurrence of cancer and Alzheimer disease: a population-based incidence study. *Neurology* 81, 322–328. doi: 10.1212/WNL.0b013e31829c5ec1

Ou, S. M., Lee, Y. J., Hu, Y. W., Liu, C. J., Chen, T. J., Fuh, J. L., et al. (2013). Does Alzheimer's disease protect against cancers? a nationwide population-based study. *Neuroepidemiology* 40, 42–49. doi: 10.1159/000341411

Pallas-Bazarra, N., Jurado-Arjona, J., Navarrete, M., Esteban, J. A., Hernandez, F., Avila, J., et al. (2016). Novel function of Tau in regulating the effects of external stimuli on adult hippocampal neurogenesis. *EMBO J.* 35, 1417–1436. doi: 10.15252/embj.201593518

Paris, D., Ganey, N., Banasiak, M., Laporte, V., Patel, N., Mullan, M., et al. (2010). Impaired orthotopic glioma growth and vascularization in transgenic mouse models of Alzheimer's disease. *J. Neurosci.* 30, 11251–11258. doi: 10.1523/jneurosci.2586-10.2010

Pentheroudakis, G., Kalogeras, K. T., Wirtz, R. M., Grimani, I., Zografos, G., Gogas, H., et al. (2009). Gene expression of estrogen receptor, progesterone receptor and microtubule-associated protein Tau in high-risk early breast cancer: a quest for molecular predictors of treatment benefit in the context of a hellenic cooperative oncology group trial. *Breast Cancer Res. Treat.* 116, 131–143. doi: 10.1007/s10549-008-0144-149

Roe, C. M., Behrens, M. I., Xiong, C., Miller, J. P., and Morris, J. C. (2005). Alzheimer disease and cancer. *Neurology* 64, 895–898. doi: 10.1212/01.wnl.0000152889.94785.51

Roe, C. M., Mintun, M. A., Ghoshal, N., Williams, M. M., Grant, E. A., Marcus, D. S., et al. (2010). Alzheimer disease identification using amyloid imaging and reserve variables: proof of concept. *Neurology* 75, 42–48. doi: 10.1212/WNL.0b013e3181e620f4

Rossi, G., Redaelli, V., Contiero, P., Fabiano, S., Tagliabue, G., Perego, P., et al. (2018). Tau mutations serve as a novel risk factor for cancer. *Cancer Res.* 78, 3731–3739. doi: 10.1158/0008-5472.can-17-3175

Rouzier, R., Rajan, R., Wagner, P., Hess, K. R., Gold, D. L., Stec, J., et al. (2005). Microtubule-associated protein tau: a marker of paclitaxel sensitivity in breast cancer. *Proc. Natl. Acad. Sci. U.S.A.* 102, 8315–8320. doi: 10.1073/pnas.0408974102

Sanchez-Valle, J., Tejero, H., Ibanez, K., Portero, J. L., Krallinger, M., Al-Shahrour, F., et al. (2017). A molecular hypothesis to explain direct and inverse co-morbidities between Alzheimer's Disease. Glioblastoma and Lung cancer. *Sci. Rep.* 7:4474. doi: 10.1038/s41598-017-04400-4406

Semiond, D., Sidhu, S. S., Bissery, M. C., and Vrignaud, P. (2013). Can taxanes provide benefit in patients with CNS tumors and in pediatric patients with tumors? An update on the preclinical development of cabazitaxel. *Cancer Chemother. Pharmacol.* 72, 515–528. doi: 10.1007/s00280-013-2214-x

Serrano, J., Fernandez, A. P., Martinez-Murillo, R., and Martinez, A. (2010). High sensitivity to carcinogens in the brain of a mouse model of Alzheimer's disease. *Oncogene* 29, 2165–2171. doi: 10.1038/onc.2009.503

Shao, Y. Y., Kuo, K. T., Hu, F. C., Lu, Y. S., Huang, C. S., Liau, J. Y., et al. (2010). Predictive and prognostic values of tau and ERCC1 in advanced breast cancer patients treated with paclitaxel and cisplatin. *Jpn. J. Clin. Oncol.* 40, 286–293. doi: 10.1093/jjco/hyp184

Sorensen, S. A., Fenger, K., and Olsen, J. H. (1999). Significantly lower incidence of cancer among patients with Huntington disease: an apoptotic effect of an expanded polyglutamine tract? *Cancer* 86, 1342–1346. doi: 10.1002/(sici)1097-0142(19991001)86:7<1342::aid-cncr33>3.0.co;2-3

Souter, S., and Lee, G. (2009). Microtubule-associated protein tau in human prostate cancer cells: isoforms, phosphorylation, and interactions. *J. Cell. Biochem.* 108, 555–564. doi: 10.1002/jcb.22287

Talbot, K., Wang, H. Y., Kazi, H., Han, L. Y., Bakshi, K. P., Stucky, A., et al. (2012). Demonstrated brain insulin resistance in Alzheimer's disease patients is associated with IGF-1 resistance, IRS-1 dysregulation, and cognitive decline. *J. Clin. Invest.* 122, 1316–1338. doi: 10.1172/jci59903

Tanaka, S., Nohara, T., Iwamoto, M., Sumiyoshi, K., Kimura, K., Takahashi, Y., et al. (2009). Tau expression and efficacy of paclitaxel treatment in metastatic breast cancer. *Cancer Chemother. Pharmacol.* 64, 341–346. doi: 10.1007/s00280-008-0877-875

Veeriah, S., Taylor, B. S., Meng, S., Fang, F., Yilmaz, E., Vivanco, I., et al. (2010). Somatic mutations of the Parkinson's disease-associated gene PARK2 in glioblastoma and other human malignancies. *Nat. Genet.* 42, 77–82. doi: 10.1038/ng.491

Viotti, J., Duplan, E., Caillava, C., Condat, J., Goiran, T., Giordano, C., et al. (2014). Glioma tumor grade correlates with parkin depletion in mutant p53-linked tumors and results from loss of function of p53 transcriptional activity. *Oncogene* 33, 1764–1775. doi: 10.1038/onc.2013.124

Wang, Q., Wang, N., Shao, G., Qian, J., Shen, D., Fei, Y., et al. (2013). Relationship between gastric cancer tau protein expression and paclitaxel sensitivity. *Pathol. Oncol. Res.* 19, 429–435. doi: 10.1007/s12253-012-9598-9595

Wang, Y., and Mandelkow, E. (2016). Tau in physiology and pathology. *Nat. Rev. Neurosci.* 17, 5–21. doi: 10.1038/nrn.2015.1

Wosnitzer, M. S., Domingo-Domenech, J., Castillo-Martin, M., Ritch, C., Mansukhani, M., Petrylack, D. P., et al. (2011). Predictive value of microtubule associated proteins tau and stathmin in patients with nonmuscle invasive bladder cancer receiving adjuvant intravesical taxane therapy. *J. Urol.* 186, 2094–2100. doi: 10.1016/j.juro.2011.06.051

Yeo, C. W., Ng, F. S., Chai, C., Tan, J. M., Koh, G. R., Chong, Y. K., et al. (2012). Parkin pathway activation mitigates glioma cell proliferation and predicts patient survival. *Cancer Res.* 72, 2543–2553. doi: 10.1158/0008-5472.can-11-3060

Yu, J., Gao, J., Lu, Z., Gong, J., Li, Y., Dong, B., et al. (2014). Combination of microtubule associated protein-tau and beta-tubulin III predicts chemosensitivity of paclitaxel in patients with advanced gastric cancer. *Eur. J. Cancer* 50, 2328–2335. doi: 10.1016/j.ejca.2014.06.017

Zaman, S., Chobrutskiy, B. I., Sikaria, D., and Blanck, G. (2019). MAPT (Tau) expression is a biomarker for an increased rate of survival for lowgrade glioma. *Oncol. Rep.* 41, 1359–1366. doi: 10.3892/or.2018.6896

20

Alzheimer's Disease Associated Genes Ankyrin and Tau Cause Shortened Lifespan and Memory Loss in *Drosophila*

James P. Higham[1†], Bilal R. Malik[1†], Edgar Buhl[1], Jennifer M. Dawson[1], Anna S. Ogier[1], Katie Lunnon[2] and James J. L. Hodge[1*]

[1] School of Physiology, Pharmacology and Neuroscience, University of Bristol, Bristol, United Kingdom, [2] University of Exeter Medical School, University of Exeter, Exeter, United Kingdom

****Correspondence:***
James J. L. Hodge
james.hodge@bristol.ac.uk

† These authors have contributed equally to this work

Alzheimer's disease (AD) is the most common form of dementia and is characterized by intracellular neurofibrillary tangles of hyperphosphorylated Tau, including the 0N4R isoform and accumulation of extracellular amyloid beta (Aβ) plaques. However, less than 5% of AD cases are familial, with many additional risk factors contributing to AD including aging, lifestyle, the environment and epigenetics. Recent epigenome-wide association studies (EWAS) of AD have identified a number of loci that are differentially methylated in the AD cortex. Indeed, hypermethylation and reduced expression of the *Ankyrin 1* (*ANK1*) gene in AD has been reported in the cortex in numerous different post-mortem brain cohorts. Little is known about the normal function of ANK1 in the healthy brain, nor the role it may play in AD. We have generated *Drosophila* models to allow us to functionally characterize *Drosophila Ank2*, the ortholog of human *ANK1* and to determine its interaction with human Tau and Aβ. We show expression of human Tau 0N4R or the oligomerizing Aβ 42 amino acid peptide caused shortened lifespan, degeneration, disrupted movement, memory loss, and decreased excitability of memory neurons with co-expression tending to make the pathology worse. We find that *Drosophila* with reduced neuronal *Ank2* expression have shortened lifespan, reduced locomotion, reduced memory and reduced neuronal excitability similar to flies overexpressing either human Tau 0N4R or Aβ42. Therefore, we show that the mis-expression of *Ank2* can drive disease relevant processes and phenocopy some features of AD. Therefore, we propose targeting human ANK1 may have therapeutic potential. This represents the first study to characterize an AD-relevant gene nominated from EWAS.

Keywords: Alzheimer's disease, *Drosophila*, memory, lifespan, locomotion, neurodegeneration, Tau, Ankyrin

INTRODUCTION

Alzheimer's disease (AD) is the most common form of dementia, with patients suffering from premature death and accelerated cognitive decline including memory loss. Post-mortem examination of AD brain samples reveals the accumulation of extracellular amyloid-beta (Aβ) plaques and intracellular neurofibrillary tangles (NFTs) of hyperphosphorylated microtubule associated protein Tau (MAPT), which is accompanied by gliosis, neuronal cell loss, and brain atrophy. Aβ is produced by the amyloidogenic cleavage of the amyloid precursor protein (APP) by β and γ secretases resulting in the formation of neurotoxic aggregating Aβ peptides with the 42 amino acid (aa) peptide (Aβ42) being more toxic than Aβ40 (Selkoe and Hardy, 2016). Tau exists in six different isoforms, which vary with the number of N-terminal domains (0N, 1N or 2N) and the number of C-terminal aggregating tubulin binding repeats (3R or 4R) (Arendt et al., 2016). The 4R isoforms are upregulated in AD brain and show stronger tubulin binding and aggregation than the 3R isoforms (Arendt et al., 2016). Another contributing factor to Tau aggregation is its hyperphosphorylation by a number of different kinases including glycogen synthase kinase-3β, cyclin-dependent kinase 5, JNK, microtubule-associated regulatory kinase, DYRK1a and CaMKII (Hanger et al., 1992; Ferrer et al., 2005; Plattner et al., 2006; Wang et al., 2007; Dolan and Johnson, 2010; Ghosh and Giese, 2015). It is not currently known how Aβ and Tau pathology are linked, however, the amyloid cascade hypothesis suggests that Aβ pathology leads to the other hallmarks of AD, including the spread of NFTs (Selkoe and Hardy, 2016) and recent work suggests changes in neuronal excitability and calcium (Ca^{2+}) signaling may be important for their connection and disease progression (Spires-Jones and Hyman, 2014; Wu et al., 2016), but exactly how remains unknown.

Less than 5% of AD cases are due to autosomal dominant mutations in the *APP*, presenilin 1 (*PSEN1*) or *PSEN2* genes. The remainder of AD cases are sporadic, with incidence attributed to both genetic and environmental risk factors. Genome-wide association studies (GWAS) have identified a number of genes where common genetic variation is associated with increased risk of sporadic AD, including *APOE* (ε4 allele), *BIN1* and *PICALM* genes amongst others (Lambert et al., 2013) with many additional risk factors for AD being associated with lifestyle and/or the environment.

Epigenetics refers to the mitotically and meiotically heritable changes in gene expression without alterations in the underlying DNA sequence for instance by DNA methylation and downregulation of genes (Gräff and Sanchez-Mut, 2015). This also potentially allows for alterations in gene expression in response to environmental variation, such as stress, diet or exposure to environmental chemicals. In order to characterize the contribution of epigenetic mechanisms to AD etiology, recent epigenome-wide association studies (EWAS) of AD have been performed and have identified a number of genetic loci that are associated with increased risk of AD (De Jager et al., 2014; Lunnon et al., 2014; Smith et al., 2018). One locus that showed consistent cortical AD-associated hypermethylation in five independent cohorts resided in the *Ankyrin 1* (*ANK1*) gene (De Jager et al., 2014; Lunnon et al., 2014; Smith and Lunnon, 2017). A recent publication has demonstrated that *ANK1* DNA methylation in the entorhinal cortex is observed in only certain neurodegenerative diseases (Smith et al., 2019). This study reported disease-associated hypermethylation in AD, Huntington's disease and to a lesser extent Parkinson's disease (PD). The authors showed that disease-associated hypermethylation was only seen in donors with vascular dementia (VaD) and dementia with Lewy bodies (DLB) when individuals had co-existing AD pathology; in individuals with "pure" VaD or DLB, no *ANK1* hypermethylation was observed. ANK1 is an integral membrane and adaptor protein, that mediates the attachment of membrane proteins such as ion channels, cell adhesion proteins and receptors with the spectrin-actin cytoskeleton and is important for cell proliferation, mobility, activation, and maintenance of specialized membrane domains (Smith and Penzes, 2018).

Most of our understanding of the molecular changes that cause AD pathology comes largely from experiments using rodents to model genetic variation; however, these are models of familial AD, and do not recapitulate sporadic disease. As such, new drugs effective in these rodents have not translated to any new successful treatments for AD highlighting the need to generate and characterize new models of sporadic AD (McGowan et al., 2006; Crews and Masliah, 2010; Van Dam and De Deyn, 2011; Gama Sosa et al., 2012; Guo et al., 2012; De Jager et al., 2014). In *Drosophila*, neuronal overexpression of different human APP products (including Aβ42) and mutants has been reported to cause degeneration of the photoreceptor neurons of the fly eye, shortened lifespan, change in neuronal excitability as well as movement, circadian, sleep, and learning defects in a number of different studies (Iijima et al., 2004; Chiang et al., 2010; Speretta et al., 2012; Chen et al., 2014; Blake et al., 2015; Ping et al., 2015; Tabuchi et al., 2015). Likewise, neuronal overexpression of human Tau isoforms associated with AD have been shown to result in degeneration of the photoreceptor neurons of the fly eye, shortened lifespan, movement and learning defects in many different studies (Wittmann et al., 2001; Folwell et al., 2010; Iijima-Ando and Iijima, 2010; Kosmidis et al., 2010; Beharry et al., 2013; Papanikolopoulou and Skoulakis, 2015; Sealey et al., 2017). Fewer animal models have determined the effect of expression of human Aβ and Tau quantifying the effect on lifespan, axonal transport, synaptic morphology, degeneration of the eye and climbing (Folwell et al., 2010; Iijima et al., 2010; Lee et al., 2012; Shulman et al., 2014). Co-expression more accurately reflects the progression of AD in humans (Guerreiro and Hardy, 2011; Selkoe, 2012; Spires-Jones and Hyman, 2014; Bouleau and Tricoire, 2015; Arendt et al., 2016; Selkoe and Hardy, 2016). Furthermore, fewer studies have compared the effect of common variants nominated from GWAS for AD (Shulman et al., 2011, 2014; Gotz et al., 2012; Chapuis et al., 2013; Dourlen et al., 2016) and to our knowledge none from EWAS for AD. Thus, many genomic and epigenomic loci nominated in these studies remain uncharacterized in any living organism, with many of these genes or loci having a completely unknown function in the brain (Guerreiro and Hardy, 2011; Shulman et al., 2011; Gotz et al., 2012; De Jager et al., 2014; Del-Aguila et al., 2015; Devall et al., 2016).

In order to address these issues, we have characterized the first animal model to investigate the function of a locus nominated from EWAS in AD. We have investigated *ANK* mis-expression and compared its AD relevant phenotypes to *Drosophila* models expressing either (a) human mutant *APP* (which results in an aggregating form of oligomerized Aβ42), (b) MAPT (resulting in 0N4R Tau), (c) *APP* (Aβ42) with *MAPT* (0N4R Tau), and (d) *APP* (Aβ42) or *MAPT* (0N4R Tau) with *Ank* mis-expression, finding that mis-expression of these AD associated genes cause similar reduction in lifespan, movement, memory and neuronal excitability. We also report for the first time the effect of human Aβ42, 0N4R Tau and co-expression on 1 h memory and determine how Aβ42 and 0N4R Tau change mushroom body (MB) memory neuron excitability prior to neurodegeneration.

MATERIALS AND METHODS

Drosophila Genetics

Flies were raised at a standard density with a 12 h:12 h light dark (LD) cycle with lights on at ZT 0 (Zeitgeber time) on standard *Drosophila* medium (0.7% agar, 1.0% soya flour, 8.0% polenta/maize, 1.8% yeast, 8.0% malt extract, 4.0% molasses, 0.8% propionic acid, and 2.3% nipagen) at 25°C. The following flies used in this study were previously described or obtained from the Bloomington and Vienna fly stock centers: wild type control was *Canton S w-* (*CSw-*) (gift from Dr. Scott Waddell, University of Oxford). Experimental genotypes were *elav-Gal4* (Bloomington stock center line number BL8760), *OK107-Gal4* (BL854), *GMR-Gal4* (BL9146), *uas-human MAPT (TAU 0N4R) wild type* (gift from Dr. Linda Partridge, University College London) (Wittmann et al., 2001; Kerr et al., 2011), *uas-human tandem Aβ42-22 amino acid linker-Aβ42* (gift from Dr. Damian Crowther, University of Cambridge) (Speretta et al., 2012), *uas-GFP* (gift from Dr. Mark Wu, Johns Hopkins University), *uas-GCaMP6f* [BL42747 (Shaw et al., 2018)], *uas-Ank2-RNAi* line A (BL29438), *uas-Ank2 RNAi* (Vienna *Drosophila RNAi* Center stock number VDRC107238 and KK10497) and *uas-Ank2* (gift from Dr. Ron R. Dubreuil, University of Illinois) (Mazock et al., 2010).

Survival Assay

Approximately 2 days after eclosion 10 mated females were transferred to a vial containing standard food and maintained at 25°C throughout. Deaths were scored every 2 days and then transferred to a fresh food vial (Kerr et al., 2011). Data was presented as Kaplan–Meier survival curves with statistical analysis performed using log-rank tests to compare survival between genotypes. All statistical tests were performed using Prism (GraphPad Software Inc., La Jolla, CA, United States).

Eye Degeneration Assay

Two to five day old adult flies were anesthetized by CO_2 prior to immersion in ethanol in order to euthanize the fly to prevent any further movement during image capture (Folwell et al., 2010). The eyes were imaged with a Zeiss AxioCam MRm camera attached to a stereomicroscope (Zeiss SteREO Discovery.V8, up to 8× magnification). Surface area was quantified using Zeiss Zen software and normalized to the mean size of the wild type control. One-way ANOVA with Dunnett's multiple comparisons was used to analyze data.

Climbing Assay

Ten 2–5 day old flies were collected and given 1 h to acclimatize to the test vial in an environmentally controlled room at 25°C and 70% humidity. Using the negative geotaxis reflex of *Drosophila*, flies were gently tapped to the bottom of a 7.5 cm plastic vial and the number of flies that crossed a line drawn 2 cm from the top of the tube in 10 s was counted, and then expressed as a % which was referred to as the climbing performance or climbing index (Iijima et al., 2004; Sun et al., 2018). One-way ANOVA with Dunnett's multiple comparisons was used to analyze data.

Memory

One hour memory and sensory controls were performed as previously described using the olfactory-shock aversive conditioning assay (Cavaliere et al., 2013; Malik et al., 2013; Malik and Hodge, 2014). Experiments were performed with groups of 30–50 flies aged between 2 and 5 days old of a given genotype, in a T-maze apparatus housed in an environmentally controlled room at 25°C and 70% humidity under dim red light. Flies were exposed to either 4-methylcyclohexanol (MCH, Sigma, ~1:200) or 3-octanol (OCT, Sigma, ~1:100) diluted in mineral oil (Sigma) paired with 1.5 s pulses of 60 V electric shock interspersed with 3.5 s pauses from shock for a minute. After 30 s of fresh air the flies were exposed to the reciprocal order without shock for another minute. After a 1 h rest, memory was assessed by transferring the flies to a choice point of the T maze, with one arm containing the shock paired odor and the other the non-shock paired odor, flies showed learning by avoiding the shock paired odor (i.e., correct flies).

$$\text{Performance index (PI)} = (\text{number of correct flies} - \text{number of incorrect flies}) / \text{total number of flies}$$

To eliminate odor bias, the assay was performed with two groups of flies (30–50 flies in each), one shocked with MCH and then the other shocked with OCT. The average of the two groups was taken to give an $n = 1$ PI value. Control experiments were performed to show that the different genotypes of flies could respond to MCH, OCT and shock alone. One-way ANOVA with Dunnett's multiple comparisons was used to analyze data.

Calcium Imaging and Microscopy

Calcium imaging and imaging of the MB structure was performed using a genetically encoded GCaMP Ca^{2+} reporter and adapting previously published protocols (Cavaliere et al., 2012; Gillespie and Hodge, 2013; Malik et al., 2013; Schlichting et al., 2016; Shaw et al., 2018). Adult flies of the indicated genotypes using *OK107-Gal4* and *uas-GCaMP6f* were collected between 2 and 5 days post-eclosion, decapitated and the brain dissected in extracellular saline solution containing (in mM): 101 NaCl, 1 $CaCl_2$, 4 $MgCl_2$, 3 KCl, 5 glucose, 1.25 NaH_2PO_4, 20.7 $NaHCO_3$, pH adjusted to 7.2. Brains were placed ventral side up in the recording chamber, secured with a custom-made anchor and continuously perfused with aerated saline. Images of the whole MB of each genotype was captured in the resting state. To activate

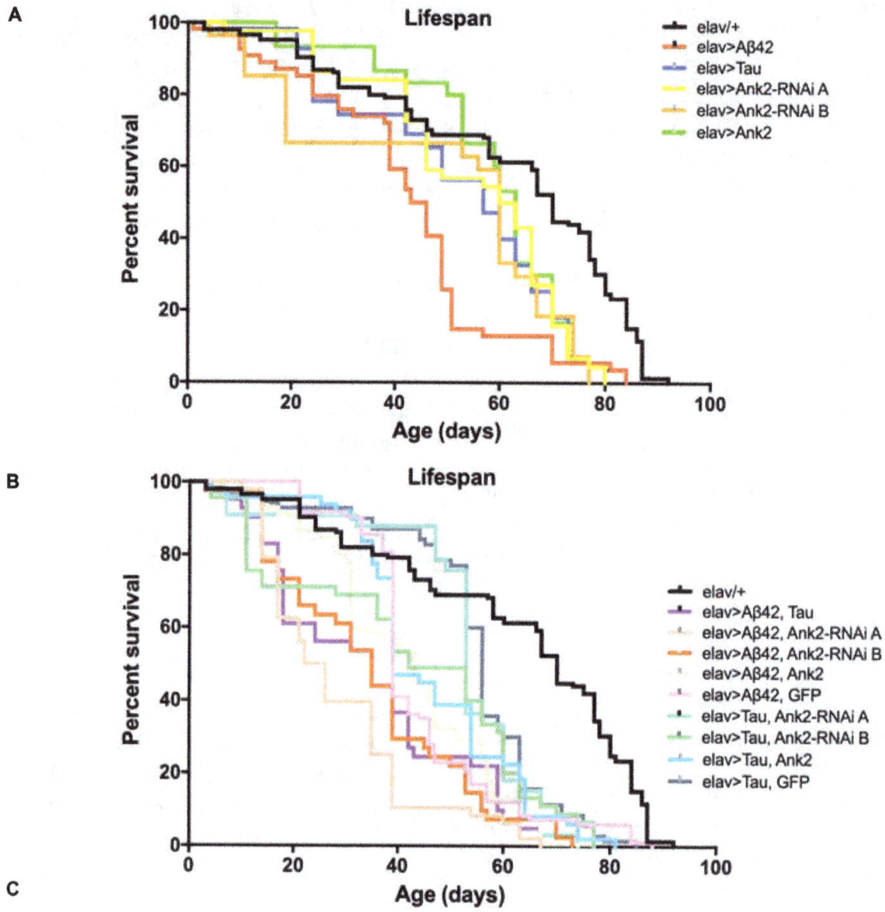

C

Genotype	Median survival (days)	Significance level
elav/+	70	
elav>Aβ42	44.5	****
elav>Tau	57	****
elav>Ank2-RNAi A	61.5	****
elav>Ank2-RNAi B	60	****
elav>Ank2	63	***
elav>Aβ42, Tau	35	****
elav>Aβ42, Ank2-RNAi A	24	****
elav>Aβ42, Ank2-RNAi B	35	****
elav>Aβ42, Ank2	43	****
elav>Aβ42, GFP	39	****
elav>Tau, Ank2-RNAi A	53	****
elav>Tau, Ank2-RNAi B	42	****
elav>Tau, Ank2	39	****
elav>Tau, GFP	56	****

FIGURE 1 | The effect of expression of human mutant *APP* (Aβ42), *MAPT* (Tau 0N4R) and *Drosophila Ank2* on *Drosophila* lifespan. **(A)** Survival curves of pan-neuronal expressing Aβ42 (*elav > Aβ42*), Tau (*elav > Tau*), *Ank2-RNAi* (*elav > Ank2-RNAi line A or B*), Ank2 (*elav > Ank2*), **(B)** Tau with Aβ42 (*elav > Tau, Aβ42*), Aβ42 with *Ank2-RNAi* (*elav > Aβ42, Ank2-RNAi line A or B*), Aβ42 with Ank2 (*elav > Aβ42, Ank2*), Aβ42 with Ank2 (*elav > Aβ42, Ank2*), Aβ42 with Ank2 (*elav > Aβ42, GFP*), Tau with *Ank2-RNAi* (*elav > Tau, Ank2-RNAi line A or B*), Tau with Ank2 (*elav > Tau, Ank2*), Tau with GFP (*elav > Aβ42, GFP*) compared to wild type control (*elav/+*) flies kept at 25°C. Misexpression of all Alzheimer's disease (AD) genes caused a significant reduction in lifespan compared to control using the Kaplan–Meier and log rank test ($n > 100$ per genotype of flies). **(C)** Table listing all genotypes characterized with median lifespan (days) and significant reductions in lifespan as determined by Kaplan–Meier and log rank test and indicated as $*p < 0.05$, $**p < 0.01$, $***p < 0.001$, $****p < 0.0001$ and used in all subsequent figures.

neurons, high concentration KCl (100 mM in saline) was bath applied through the perfusion system for 4 min and then washed out. The calcium fluorescence signal was acquired using a CCD camera (Zeiss Axiocam) and a 470 nm LED light source (Colibri, Zeiss) on an upright Zeiss Examiner microscope with a 20× water immersion lens, recorded with ZEN (Zeiss, 4 frames/sec) and plotted with Microsoft Excel. One-way ANOVA with Dunnett's multiple comparisons was used to analyze data.

RESULTS

Mis-Expression of Human Mutant APP, MAPT or Ank2 Shortens Lifespan

Increased neuronal levels of Aβ or Tau lead to AD pathology and early death (Selkoe, 2012; Selkoe and Hardy, 2016). We therefore overexpressed in all neurons either an aggregating form of human mutant *APP* that encodes oligomerized human Aβ42 [tandem Aβ42 (Speretta et al., 2012)] or human MAPT [0N4R Tau (Papanikolopoulou and Skoulakis, 2015; Sealey et al., 2017)] both of which caused premature death reducing the flies' lifespan by about 25% (**Figures 1A,C**). In order to test for a genetic interaction between the two neurotoxic genes, we overexpressed both mutant *APP* (Aβ42) and *MAPT* (0N4R) together in all neurons and got a further reduction to exactly half the lifespan of a normal fly. The reduction in median lifespan due to co-expression was equivalent to an additive effect of the shortening of life due to mutant *APP* (Aβ42) and *MAPT* (0N4R) alone, this suggests that Aβ42 and Tau pathology may act in separate pathways to cause neurotoxicity and early death.

Recently, human *ANK1* gene has been shown to be differentially methylated in AD (Lunnon et al., 2014). There are two other *ANK* genes in the human genome, *ANK2*, and *ANK3*. In *Drosophila*, there are two *Ank* genes, the ubiquitously expressed *Ank1*, and neuron specific *Ank2* (Koch et al., 2008; Pielage et al., 2008; Mazock et al., 2010; Keller et al., 2011; Siegenthaler et al., 2015). The closest ortholog to *Drosophila Ank1* is human *ANK3* with 51% total amino acid identity while the closest ortholog of *Drosophila Ank2* is human *ANK1* with 43% amino acid identity. Human *ANK2* is more similar to *Drosophila Ank1* (49% identity) than *Drosophila Ank2* (33% identity). Because hypermethylation of human *ANK1* has been reported in AD cortex (Lunnon et al., 2014), we used *RNAi* to knock-down expression of *Ank1* and *Ank2* comparing the effect of reducing these genes in all *Drosophila* neurons using two different *RNAi* transgenes designed to non-overlapping regions of each gene. Pan-neural reduction in expression of *Drosophila Ank1* did not cause any AD relevant behavioral deficits (**Figures 2A,B**), while reduction in *Ank2* using the same promoter and assay did cause a reduction in 1 h memory (**Figure 2B**). Therefore, we conclude, that *Drosophila Ank2* is the closest functional ortholog of human *ANK1*, which we characterized in subsequent experiments.

We found that pan-neural reduction of *Ank2* resulted in a shortening of lifespan by 15% compared to control (**Figures 1B,C**). We verified our results by using two independent

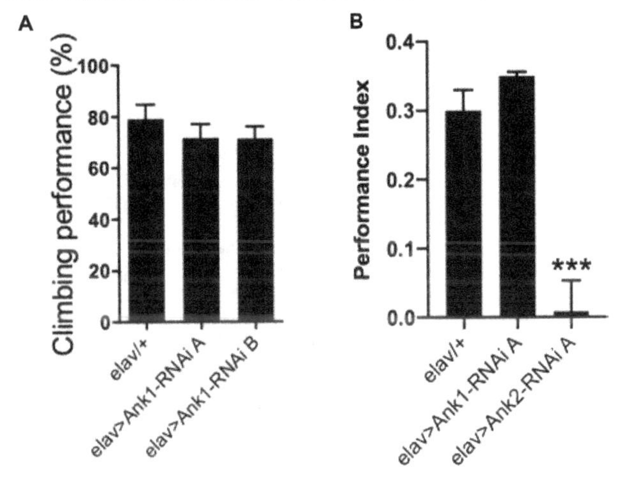

FIGURE 2 | The effect of pan-neuronal expression of *Drosophila Ank1* and *Ank2* on behavior. **(A)** The negative geotaxis-climbing reflex was used to quantify motor deficits of 2–5 day old flies. Pan-neuronal reduction of *Ank1* (*elav-Gal4 > Ank1-RNAi line A or B*) was compared to control using one-way ANOVA with Dunnett's multiple comparison and showed no significant difference. $n \geq 6$ groups of 10 flies. **(B)** One hour memory of 2–5 day old flies was assessed using the olfactory shock-conditioning assay. Pan-neuronal reduction in Ank2 (*elav > Ank2-RNAi line A*) as opposed to Ank1 (*elav > Ank1-RNAi line A*) caused a significant reduction in memory compared to control using one-way ANOVA with Dunnett's multiple comparisons. Error bars are standard error of the mean (SEM). $n \geq 4$ groups of ~50 flies.

RNAi lines (A and B) to non-overlapping sequences in *Ank2*, both lines gave similar results in all assays. Depending on the genomic location of DNA methylation, it can result in either increased or decreased expression of the target gene (Suzuki and Bird, 2008); we therefore tested if neuronal *Ank2* overexpression affected longevity and found that it also shortened lifespan (~10%), but at a lower significance level to all other genotypes. In order to test if there was a genetic interaction between mutant *APP* (Aβ42) or *MAPT* (0N4R) and *Ank2* we generated flies that co-expressed mutant *APP* (Aβ42) or *MAPT* (0N4R) with the *Ank2* transgenes. We found that the detrimental effect of each gene on lifespan remained (**Figures 1B,C**), suggesting changing the level of fly Ank2 could not rescue the shortened lifespan caused by overexpression of human mutant *APP* (Aβ42) or *MAPT* (0N4R) to a level similar to wild type control (*elav/+*). One potential cause of a reduction or suppression of toxicity of a gene product is dilution of Gal4. This is due to a single Gal4 transcription factor driving expression by binding to a single UAS transgene [e.g., mutant *APP* (Aβ42) or *MAPT* (0N4R)] which may get diluted when adding a second UAS site of a gene (e.g., *Ank2*). This results in a reduction in the amount of the AD toxic gene product being made, giving a false positive of a suppression phenotype. To control for such a dilution effect, we generated flies that co-expressed a second unrelated neutral gene product (GFP) with either human mutant *APP* (Aβ42) or *MAPT* (0N4R Tau). There was no significant change in neurotoxicity of the mutant *APP* (Aβ42) or *MAPT* (0N4R Tau) when expressed alone or with GFP.

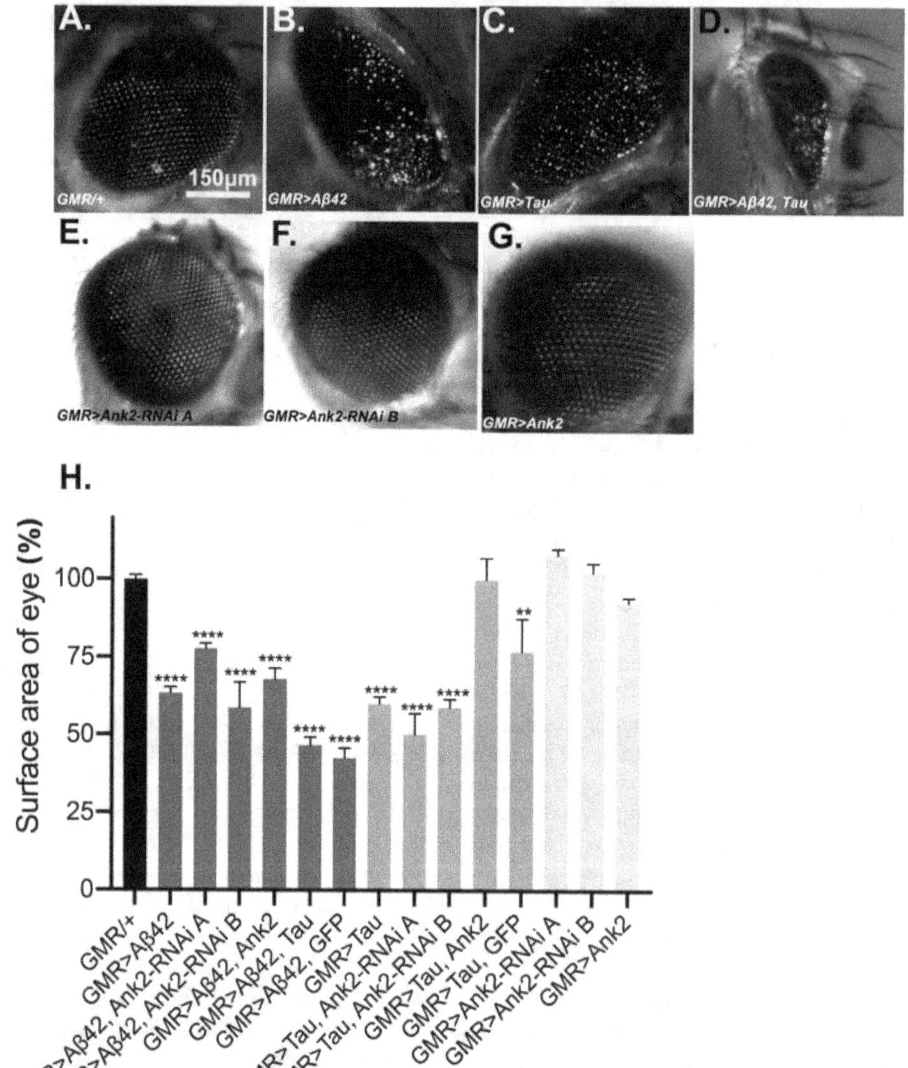

FIGURE 3 | The effect of expression of human mutant *APP* (Aβ42), *MAPT* (Tau 0N4R), and *Drosophila Ank2* on degeneration of photoreceptor neurons. Images of 2–5 day old compound eyes of **(A)** control fly (*GMR-Gal4/+*) showing the regular alignment of ommatidia compared to photoreceptors neurons overexpressing, **(B)** Aβ42 (*GMR-Gal4 > Aβ42*), **(C)** Tau (*GMR-Gal4 > Tau*), and **(D)** Tau with Aβ42 (*GMR-Gal4 > Tau, Aβ42*) which were smaller and displayed a "rough eye" phenotype. **(E,F)** photoreceptors expressing *Ank2-RNAi* (*GMR > Ank2-RNAi line A or B*) or **(G)** Ank2 (*GMR > Ank2*) appeared normal. **(H)** Degeneration of photoreceptor neurons was quantified as normalized percentage surface area of the eye of genotypes compared to the mean of the control (*GMR/+*) which was set at 100%, comparisons were made between to mutant genotypes compared to control using one-way ANOVA with Dunnett's multiple comparisons. Genotypes that included expression of *APP* (Aβ42) or *MAPT* (Tau 0N4R) in the eye showed a significantly reduced size of eye, while those mis-expressing *Drosophila Ank2* did not. Co-expression of *MAPT* (Tau 0N4R) and *Ank2* rescued eye size to a level indistinguishable from wild type. Error bars are SEM. $n \geq 7$ eyes per genotype.

Overexpression of Human Mutant APP or Mutant MAPT but Not Mis-Expression of Ank2 Caused Degeneration of Photoreceptor Neurons

Increased levels of aggregating toxic Aβ and Tau lead to neurodegeneration and AD. In order to model this neurotoxicity in *Drosophila*, human mutant *APP* causing Aβ42 production (**Figure 3B**) or mutant MAPT (0N4R Tau) (**Figure 3C**) was expressed throughout development and adulthood in the photoreceptor neurons of the eye, resulting in a so called "rough eye" phenotype, where the degeneration and loss of the normally regularly arrayed ommatidia of the compound eye of wild type flies (**Figure 3A**) gives rise to a disorganized and smaller eye. The loss of photoreceptors could be quantified by measuring the total surface area of the eye, which showed that expression of human mutant *APP* (Aβ42) and *MAPT* (0N4R Tau) reduced the size of the eye by 37% and 40%, respectively (**Figure 3H**). Co-expression of human mutant *APP* (Aβ42) and *MAPT* (0N4R Tau) (**Figures 3D,H**), resulted in a 53%

reduction in eye size, suggesting that Aβ42 and Tau act in partially overlapping pathways to cause neurotoxicity in the fly eye. Reduction of *Ank2* (**Figures 3E,F**), overexpression of *Ank2* (**Figure 3G**) and co-expression of *Ank2* and *Tau* did not cause degeneration or reduction in size of the eye (**Figure 3H**), although the latter cannot be considered a rescue as although the eye was significantly larger ($p < 0.01$) than eyes expressing Tau it was not significantly bigger than those expressing Tau and GFP suggesting any suppression maybe due to a Gal4 dilution effect.

Overexpression of Human Mutant APP and MAPT Genes and Reduction in Ank2 Expression Caused Locomotor Deficits

Flies exhibit a negative geotaxis reflex, such that after tapping on a surface ~80% of 2–5 day old wild type flies will climb to the top of a tube in 10 s. This startle-induced reflex requires the co-ordinated activity of dopaminergic neurons afferent to the MB, and of MB Kenyon cells, in addition to MB efferent neurons which communicate with central motor centers (Sun et al., 2018). In order to quantify any detrimental effect of *human mutant APP* (Aβ42) and *MAPT* (0N4R Tau) on this behavior, we pan-neuronally (*elav-Gal4* expressed *human mutant APP* (Aβ42) and *MAPT* (0N4R Tau), which resulted in a 20% and 40% reduction in climbing ability, respectively. Likewise, reduction in Ank2 expression caused a 15% reduction in climbing, while Ank2 overexpression had no effect. All other gene combinations were found to significantly reduce gross climbing performance (**Figure 4**).

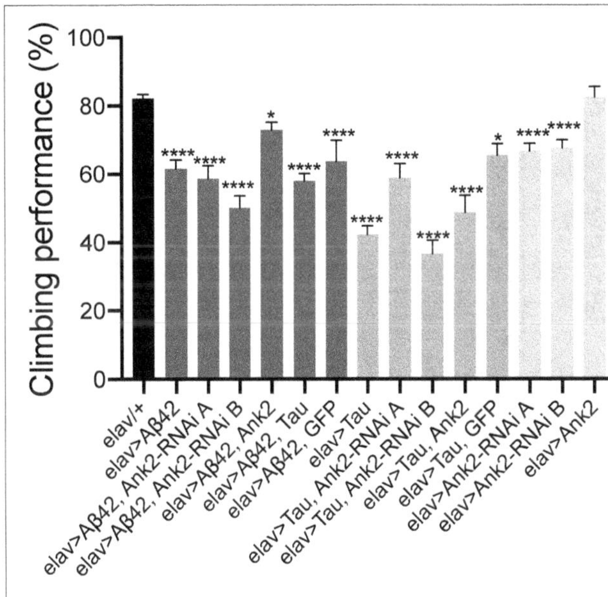

FIGURE 4 | The effect of expression of human mutant *APP* (Aβ42), *MAPT* (Tau 0N4R) or *Drosophila Ank2* on locomotor behavior. The negative geotaxis-climbing reflex was used to quantify locomotor behavior of 2–5 day old flies. About 80% of control (*elav-Gal4/+*) flies were able to climb to the top of test vial within 10 s; this compared to experimental genotypes expressing AD transgenes throughout their nervous system. Mis-expression of all AD associated genes except for overexpression of *Ank2* alone, resulted in a significant reduction in climbing performance using one-way ANOVA with Dunnett's multiple comparisons. Error bars are SEM. $n \geq 15$ groups of 10 flies.

Overexpression of Human Mutant APP and MAPT Genes and Reduced Ank2 Causes Memory Deficits

As multiple forms and phases of memory, including anterograde memory, are affected by AD (Walsh and Selkoe, 2004), therefore we measured the effect of the human mutant *APP* (Aβ42), *MAPT* (0N4R Tau) and *Drosophila Ank2* on memory. We performed the olfactory shock assay on 2–5 day old flies (Cavaliere et al., 2013; Malik et al., 2013; Malik and Hodge, 2014) assessing associative memory at the 1 h time point, which is considered to be intermediate memory in *Drosophila*. Olfactory shock memory is mediated by MB neurons and we therefore drove expression of the genes using a promoter (*OK107-Gal4*) with broad expression in these neurons (Cavaliere et al., 2013; Malik et al., 2013). We found MB expression of human mutant *APP* (Aβ42) or *MAPT* (0N4R Tau) caused a large reduction in memory (**Figure 5**). *Ank2* is highly expressed in the adult MB as shown by *Ank2* reporter line (*R54H11-Gal4*) expression (Pfeiffer et al., 2008) and previous studies (Siegenthaler et al., 2015). Reduction, as opposed to overexpression, of *Ank2* also caused a reduction in memory (**Figure 5**). Co-expression of human mutant *APP* (Aβ42) and *MAPT* (0N4R Tau; **Figure 5**) or either AD gene with *Ank2-RNAi* caused a similar reduction in memory, suggesting that all three genes may act in the same pathway in MB neurons. Overexpression of *Ank2*, or co-expression of *Ank2* with either human mutant *APP* (Aβ42) or *MAPT* (0N4R Tau) did not cause a significant reduction in memory. The latter cannot be considered rescue of the memory deficit caused by expression of Aβ42 or Tau alone, as the memory of *Ank2* co-expressed with either human mutant *APP* (Aβ42) or *MAPT* (0N4R Tau) was not significantly greater than that of human mutant *APP* (Aβ42) or *MAPT* (0N4R Tau) co-expressed with GFP, again suggesting a Gal4 dilution effect was contributing to the rescue of the mutant phenotype.

For flies to be able to perform the olfactory shock assay, the fly must be able to respond normally to shock and the odors used in the memory task. Therefore, we performed behavioral controls on 2–5 day old flies that showed that there was no significant difference between mutant genotypes and wild type in terms of avoidance of electric shock (**Figure 6A**), octanol (**Figure 6B**) and methylcyclohexanol (MCH; **Figure 6C**) odors (Cavaliere et al., 2013; Malik et al., 2013; Malik and Hodge, 2014). Therefore, any mutant genotype showing a significant reduction in memory in **Figure 5** was a bona fide memory mutant.

Mis-Expression of Human Mutant APP (Aβ42), MAPT (0N4R Tau), and Ank2 Decreased the Neural Excitability of Memory Neurons Prior to Any Observable Neurodegeneration

Changes in neuronal excitability and Ca^{2+} signaling are thought to occur early in disease progression prior to neurodegeneration and are proposed to mediate early changes in behavior in AD, such as memory loss (Spires-Jones and Hyman, 2014;

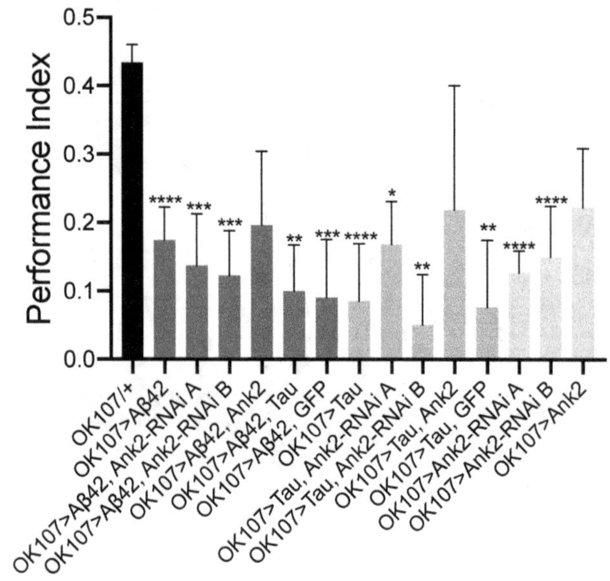

FIGURE 5 | The effect of expression of human mutant *APP* (Aβ42), *MAPT* (Tau 0N4R) and *Drosophila Ank2* on memory. One hour memory of 2–5 day old flies was assessed using the olfactory shock-conditioning assay. The performance index of flies expressing AD transgenes throughout their mushroom body (MB) was compared to control (*OK107-Gal4/+*) and were found to show a significant reduction in memory using one-way ANOVA with Dunnett's multiple comparisons, except genotypes overexpressing *Ank2*. Error bars are SEM. $n \geq 4$ groups of ∼100 flies.

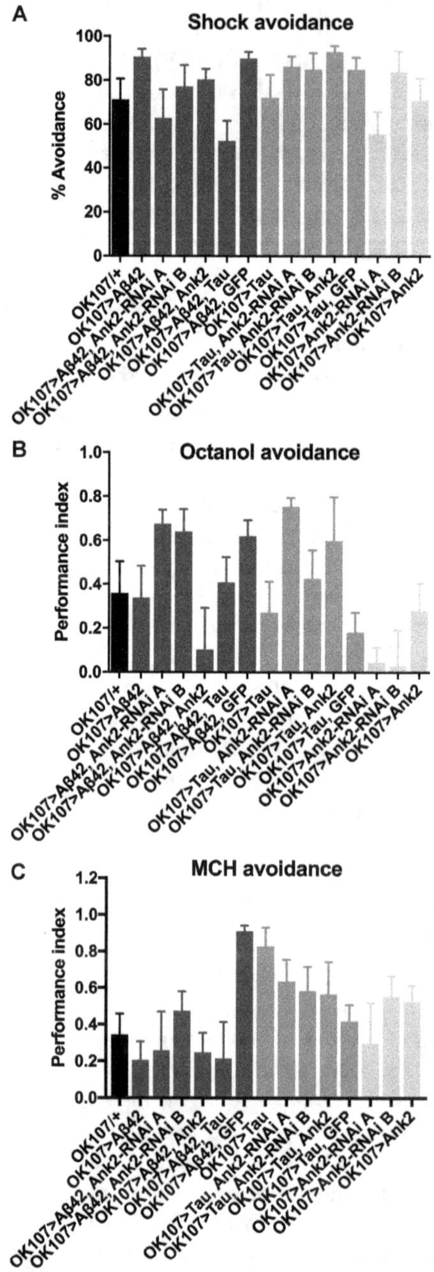

FIGURE 6 | The effect of expression of human mutant *APP* (Aβ42), *MAPT* (Tau 0N4R) and *Drosophila Ank2* on response to negative reinforcement (shock) and olfaction. **(A)** The response of 2–5 day old flies to negative reinforcement was quantified as % avoidance of shock, with experimental genotypes with AD genes expressed throughout their MB compared to control (*OK107/+*). The avoidance of these genotypes of flies to 3-octanol **(B)** and methylcyclohexanol (MCH) **(C)** odors was expressed as a performance index. All genotypes responded to odors and shock in a manner not significantly different from wild type using one-way ANOVA with Dunnett's multiple comparisons. $n \geq 4$ groups of ∼50 flies.

Wu et al., 2016). Therefore, in order to determine how mis-expression of human mutant *APP* (Aβ42), *MAPT* (0N4R Tau), and *Ank2* may lead to changes in neuronal function and AD relevant phenotypes, we expressed the genetically encoded Ca^{2+} reporter, GCaMP6f using the same *OK107*-Gal4 MB promoter as for the memory experiments and then measuring peak intracellular Ca^{2+} in response to high $[K^+]$ solution that non-specifically depolarizes neurons (Malik et al., 2013). The axons and synaptic terminals of MB neurons form a pair of bilaterally arranged and symmetrically lobed structures which show low basal Ca^{2+} fluorescence levels (**Figure 7A** left panel) which, in response to depolarizing high $[K^+]$ saline, show a large peak in Ca^{2+} fluorescence levels (**Figure 7A** right panel). The increase in neuronal activity can be expressed as the relative fluorescence change ($\Delta F/F0$) over time (**Figure 7B**) showing that high K^+ causes a rapid peak Ca^{2+} influx that returns to baseline after washing. MB wide overexpression of human mutant *APP* (Aβ42), *MAPT* (0N4R Tau) or mis-expression of *Ank2* all caused a similar decrease in peak Ca^{2+} influx of memory neurons (**Figure 7C**), suggesting a reduction in neuronal excitability. A previous study showed human 0N4R tau expression in γ MB neurons reduced learning and 1.5 h memory in 3–5 day old young flies which were demonstrated to still have their γ neurons intact. However, by day 45, the 0N4R expressing γ neurons had started to neurodegenerate (Mershin et al., 2004). In order to verify the MB were intact in our 2–5 day old flies overexpressing human mutant *APP* (Aβ42), *MAPT* (0N4R Tau) or mis-expressing fly *Ank2* throughout the MB we imaged the MB with GCaMP6f and saw that all the genotypes had intact MB α, β, γ, α′, and β′ lobes (**Figure 8**).

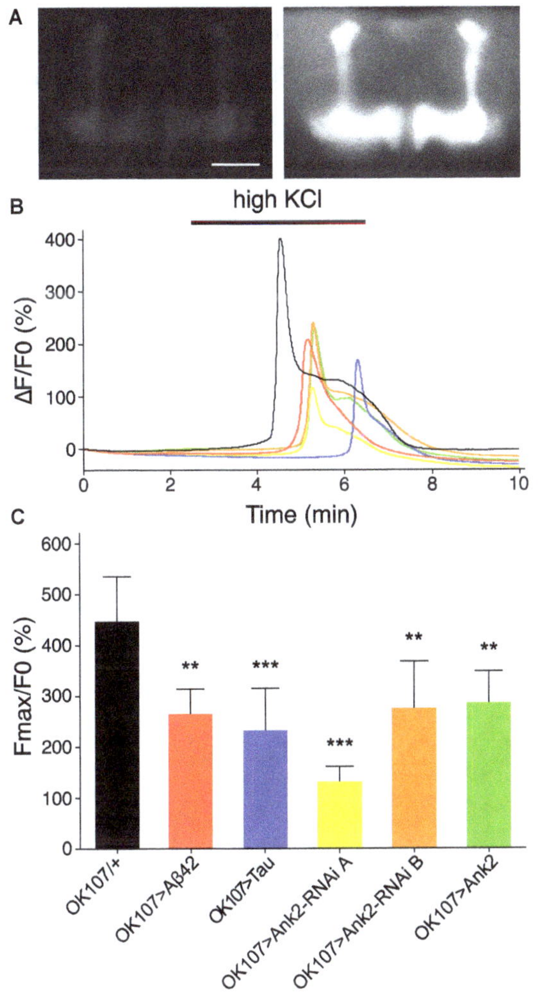

FIGURE 7 | The effect of expression of human mutant *APP* (Aβ42), *MAPT* (Tau 0N4R), and *Drosophila Ank2* on activation of mushroom body neurons. **(A)** Exemplary control 2–5 day old fly MB expressing the calcium reporter GCaMP6f shows a big increase in relative fluorescence in response to elevated KCl (100 mM, bath-applied). Images show the same brain before (left) and during (right) KCl application; scale bar 50 μm. **(B)** The increase in neuronal activity is expressed as the relative change in fluorescence (ΔF/F0) over time showing that high KCl (indicated by bar) causes peak Ca^{2+} influx that returns to baseline after washing. **(C)** Quantitative analysis of the maximal response for the indicated genotypes shows a reduced responsiveness of all mutants. Data was analyzed with one-way ANOVA with Tukey's *post hoc* and error bars are standard deviation, $n \geq 5$ brains.

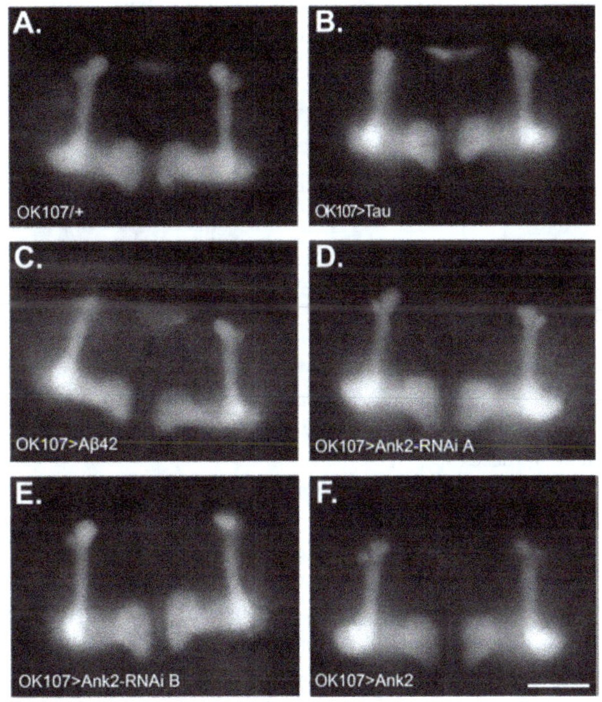

FIGURE 8 | Mushroom body morphology is not affected by expression of human mutant *APP* (Aβ42), *MAPT* (Tau 0N4R), and *Drosophila Ank2* in young flies. Images show representative mushroom bodies of 2–5 day old flies visualized by expression of the Ca^{2+} reporter GCaMP6f of **(A)** a control fly (*OK107/+*), **(B)** *OK107 > Tau*, **(C)** *OK107 > Aβ42*, **(D)** *OK107 > Ank2-RNAi line A*, **(E)** *OK107 > Ank2-RNAi line B*, and **(F)** *OK107 > Ank2* which all show the regular organization of α, β, γ, α′ and β′ lobes. Scale bar is 50 μm.

DISCUSSION

In this study, we have characterized the first animal model based on mis-expression of the AD EWAS nominated *ANK1* gene ortholog in *Drosophila*. Altered DNA methylation of human *ANK1* occurs in AD brains, especially in regions that show gross AD pathology, such as the entorhinal cortex (De Jager et al., 2014; Lunnon et al., 2014). Here, we found reduction in expression of the fly ortholog of human *ANK1*, which is *Drosophila Ank2*, in areas of the brain responsible for memory (the MB), caused memory impairment similar in magnitude to that caused by overexpression of human mutant *APP* resulting in an oligomerizing form of Aβ42 or *MAPT* producing the 0N4R isoform of Tau, both of which are particularly associated with the disease. In flies, overexpression of fly *Ank2*, did not result in degeneration of the eye, locomotor or memory defects but did lead to mild shortening of lifespan (by ~10%) and reduced MB excitability.

In addition to memory loss, animals with reduced neuronal *Ank2* also recapitulated the shortening of lifespan seen in those with AD, again a phenotype seen in flies overexpressing human mutant *APP* (Aβ42) or *MAPT* (0N4R Tau). Co-expression of human mutant *APP* (Aβ42) and *MAPT* (0N4R Tau) caused a further reduction in lifespan, suggesting that the two molecules may act in partially non-overlapping and therefore additive pathways that lead to the pathology causing the flies to die early. A similar effect on lifespan has been reported previously for another form of *APP* that resulted in a non-oligomerizing version of Aβ42 and another form of *MAPT*, resulting in the 1N4R isoform of Tau, however, the longevity assays were only run for roughly half the lifespan of the flies (Folwell et al., 2010). We also found a reduction in locomotion in flies expressing human mutant *APP* (Aβ42), *MAPT* (0N4R Tau) and reduced *Ank2*. Interestingly, a recent study has shown that *ANK1* hypermethylation is observed in PD, a movement disorder, that can also be associated with dementia (Smith et al., 2019). In the eye, overexpression of human mutant *APP* (Aβ42) or *MAPT* (0N4R Tau) were both neurotoxic causing degeneration of the fly eye photoreceptor neurons. Co-expression caused a further reduction implying the two act in separate and additive pathways to cause neurotoxicity and neuronal death. Reduction in *Ank2* did not cause degeneration of the eye suggesting that *Ank2* may affect neuronal function independent of degeneration. This is likely to be via changes in neuronal excitability, as we saw when the gene was misexpressed in MB neurons (Smith and Penzes, 2018). We found misexpression of human mutant *APP* (Aβ42), *MAPT* (0N4R Tau) and *Ank2* all reduced the peak Ca^{2+} response of MB neurons, a decrease in excitability likely to contribute to the memory deficits of these flies.

In *Drosophila*, *Ank2* has been shown to be important for synaptic plasticity and stability (Koch et al., 2008; Pielage et al., 2008; Massaro et al., 2009; Keller et al., 2011; Bulat et al., 2014) and is involved in a glia mediated pathway that causes degeneration of motor neurons (Keller et al., 2011). Therefore, it is possible that reduction of *Ank2* may only cause degeneration in certain types of neurons. Furthermore, because human *ANK1* has also been shown to be misexpressed in glia in the AD brain (Mastroeni et al., 2017), it is also possible that neurodegeneration results from misexpression of *Ank2* in glia.

We do not know how Ankyrin interacts with Tau and what changes in Tau protein level, location or phosphorylation result from *Ankyrin* misexpression. We know that Ankyrins are adaptor proteins that attach to integral membrane proteins such as the Na^+/K^+ ATPase, voltage-gated Na^+ (Na_V1), voltage-gated K^+ (KCNQ) and TrpA1 channels, and then link them to the actin-spectrin based membrane cytoskeleton, with some of these molecules having been associated with AD (Bennett and Baines, 2001; Yamamoto et al., 2007; Smith and Penzes, 2018). Therefore the loss of Ankyrin might be predicted to disrupt the proper clustering of these ion channels, some of which are involved in MB-memory and calcium signaling (Cavaliere et al., 2013), and hence may result in the decreased neuronal excitability detected by our MB calcium imaging experiments and which might be required for proper memory formation. The changes in calcium influx may also cause dysregulation of calcium dependent phosphorylation of Tau, also known to disrupt MB dependent memory and shorten lifespan (Papanikolopoulou and Skoulakis, 2015). Finally, the loss of Ankyrin may distrupt the actin-spectrin cytoskeleton, which may result in pathological changes in microtubules exacerbated by their association with Tau. More experiments are required to investigate the nature of the interaction between Ankyrin and Tau in AD.

In summary, we have characterized the first animal model of a gene implicated in AD that was nominated from EWAS. We found that mis-expression of the fly ortholog of this gene, *Ank2*, in central neurons caused a range of AD-relevant phenotypes such as shortened lifespan, memory loss, and changes in neuronal excitability similar to those resulting from human Aβ42 and 0N4R Tau. In alignment with previous AD studies, we conclude that *Ank2* – or, in humans, *ANK1* – likely plays a role in AD neuropathology.

AUTHOR CONTRIBUTIONS

JH, BM, EB, JD, AO, and JJLH performed the experiments. JH devised the experiments and wrote the manuscript. JJLH and KL secured the funding. JH, BM, EB, and KL edited the drafts of the manuscript.

ACKNOWLEDGMENTS

We thank Drs. Damian Crowther, Ronald Dubreuil, Linda Partridge, Scott Waddell, and Mark Wu for *Drosophila* stocks and Dr. Owen Peters for helpful comments on the manuscript.

REFERENCES

Arendt, T., Stieler, J. T., and Holzer, M. (2016). Tau and tauopathies. *Brain Res. Bull.* 126, 238–292. doi: 10.1016/j.brainresbull.2016.08.018

Beharry, C., Alaniz, M. E., and Alonso Adel, C. (2013). Expression of Alzheimer-like pathological human tau induces a behavioral motor and olfactory learning deficit in *Drosophila melanogaster*. *J. Alzheimer's Dis.* 37, 539–550. doi: 10.3233/JAD-130617

Bennett, V., and Baines, A. J. (2001). Spectrin and ankyrin-based pathways: metazoan inventions for integrating cells into tissues. *Physiol. Rev.* 81, 1353–1392. doi: 10.1152/physrev.2001.81.3.1353

Blake, M. R., Holbrook, S. D., Kotwica-Rolinska, J., Chow, E. S., Kretzschmar, D., and Giebultowicz, J. M. (2015). Manipulations of amyloid precursor protein cleavage disrupt the circadian clock in aging *Drosophila*. *Neurobiol. Dis.* 77, 117–126. doi: 10.1016/j.nbd.2015.02.012

Bouleau, S., and Tricoire, H. (2015). *Drosophila* models of Alzheimer's disease: advances, limits, and perspectives. *J. Alzheimer's Dis.* 45, 1015–1038. doi: 10.3233/JAD-142802

Bulat, V., Rast, M., and Pielage, J. (2014). Presynaptic CK2 promotes synapse organization and stability by targeting Ankyrin2. *J Cell Biol* 204, 77–94. doi: 10.1083/jcb.201305134

Cavaliere, S., Gillespie, J. M., and Hodge, J. J. (2012). KCNQ channels show conserved ethanol block and function in ethanol behaviour. *PLoS One* 7:e50279. doi: 10.1371/journal.pone.0050279

Cavaliere, S., Malik, B. R., and Hodge, J. J. (2013). KCNQ channels regulate age-related memory impairment. *PLoS One* 8:e62445. doi: 10.1371/journal.pone.0062445

Chapuis, J., Hansmannel, F., Gistelinck, M., Mounier, A., Van Cauwenberghe, C., Kolen, K. V., et al. (2013). Increased expression of BIN1 mediates Alzheimer genetic risk by modulating tau pathology. *Mol. Psychiatry* 18, 1225–1234. doi: 10.1038/mp.2013.1

Chen, K. F., Possidente, B., Lomas, D. A., and Crowther, D. C. (2014). The central molecular clock is robust in the face of behavioural arrhythmia in a *Drosophila* model of Alzheimer's disease. *Dis. Models Mech.* 7, 445–458. doi: 10.1242/dmm.014134

Chiang, H. C., Wang, L., Xie, Z., Yau, A., and Zhong, Y. (2010). PI3 kinase signaling is involved in Abeta-induced memory loss in *Drosophila*. *Proc. Natl. Acad. Sci. U.S.A.* 107, 7060–7065. doi: 10.1073/pnas.0909314107

Crews, L., and Masliah, E. (2010). Molecular mechanisms of neurodegeneration in Alzheimer's disease. *Hum. Mol. Genet.* 19:R12–R20. doi: 10.1093/hmg/ddq160

De Jager, P. L., Srivastava, G., Lunnon, K., Burgess, J., Schalkwyk, L. C., Yu, L., et al. (2014). Alzheimer's disease: early alterations in brain DNA methylation at ANK1. BIN1, RHBDF2 and other loci. *Nat. Neurosci.* 17, 1156–1163. doi: 10.1038/nn.3786

Del-Aguila, J. L., Koboldt, D. C., Black, K., Chasse, R., Norton, J., Wilson, R. K., et al. (2015). Alzheimer's disease: rare variants with large effect sizes. *Curr. Opin. Genet. Dev.* 33, 49–55. doi: 10.1016/j.gde.2015.07.008

Devall, M., Roubroeks, J., Mill, J., Weedon, M., and Lunnon, K. (2016). Epigenetic regulation of mitochondrial function in neurodegenerative disease: new insights from advances in genomic technologies. *Neurosci. Lett.* 625, 47–55. doi: 10.1016/j.neulet.2016.02.013

Dolan, P. J., and Johnson, G. V. (2010). The role of tau kinases in Alzheimer's disease. *Curr. Opin. Drug Dis. Dev.* 13, 595–603.

Dourlen, P., Fernandez-Gomez, F. J., Dupont, C., Grenier-Boley, B., Bellenguez, C., Obriot, H., et al. (2016). Functional screening of Alzheimer risk loci identifies PTK2B as an in vivo modulator and early marker of tau pathology. *Mol. Psychiatry* 22, 874–883. doi: 10.1038/mp.2016.59

Ferrer, I., Barrachina, M., Puig, B., Martinez de Lagran, M., Marti, E., Avila, J., et al. (2005). Constitutive Dyrk1A is abnormally expressed in Alzheimer disease. Down syndrome, Pick disease, and related transgenic models. *Neurobiol. Dis.* 20, 392–400. doi: 10.1016/j.nbd.2005.03.020

Folwell, J., Cowan, C. M., Ubhi, K. K., Shiabh, H., Newman, T. A., Shepherd, D., et al. (2010). Abeta exacerbates the neuronal dysfunction caused by human tau expression in a *Drosophila* model of Alzheimer's disease. *Exp. Neurol.* 223, 401–409. doi: 10.1016/j.expneurol.2009.09.014

Gama Sosa, M. A., De Gasperi, R., and Elder, G. A. (2012). Modeling human neurodegenerative diseases in transgenic systems. *Hum. Genet.* 131, 535–563. doi: 10.1007/s00439-011-1119-1

Ghosh, A., and Giese, K. P. (2015). Calcium/calmodulin-dependent kinase II and Alzheimer's disease. *Mol. Brain* 8:78. doi: 10.1016/j.yjmcc.2013.03.005

Gillespie, J. M., and Hodge, J. J. (2013). CASK regulates CaMKII autophosphorylation in neuronal growth, calcium signaling, and learning. *Front. Mol. Neurosci.* 6:27. doi: 10.3389/fnmol.2013.00027

Gotz, J., Matamales, M., Gotz, N. N., Ittner, L. M., and Eckert, A. (2012). Alzheimer's disease models and functional genomics-How many needles are there in the haystack? *Front. Physiol.* 3:320. doi: 10.3389/fphys.2012.00320

Gräff, J., and Sanchez-Mut, J. V. (2015). Epigenetic alterations in Alzheimer's Disease. *Front. Behav. Neurosci.* 9:347. doi: 10.3389/fnbeh.2015.00347

Guerreiro, R. J., and Hardy, J. (2011). Alzheimer's disease genetics: lessons to improve disease modelling. *Biochem. Soc. Trans.* 39, 910–916. doi: 10.1042/BST0390910

Guo, Q., Wang, Z., Li, H., Wiese, M., and Zheng, H. (2012). APP physiological and pathophysiological functions: insights from animal models. *Cell Res.* 22, 78–89. doi: 10.1038/cr.2011.116

Hanger, D. P., Hughes, K., Woodgett, J. R., Brion, J. P., and Anderton, B. H. (1992). Glycogen synthase kinase-3 induces Alzheimer's disease-like phosphorylation of tau: generation of paired helical filament epitopes and neuronal localisation of the kinase. *Neurosci. Lett.* 147, 58–62. doi: 10.1016/0304-3940(92)90774-2

Higham, J. P., Malik, B. R., Buhl, E., Dawson, J., Ogier, A. S., Lunnon, K., et al. (2018). Mis-expression of the Alzheimer's disease associated gene Ankyrin causes memory loss and shortened lifespan in *Drosophila*. *bioRxiv*

Iijima, K., Gatt, A., and Iijima-Ando, K. (2010). Tau Ser262 phosphorylation is critical for Abeta42-induced tau toxicity in a transgenic *Drosophila* model of Alzheimer's disease. *Hum. Mol. Genet.* 19, 2947–2957. doi: 10.1093/hmg/ddq200

Iijima, K., Liu, H. P., Chiang, A. S., Hearn, S. A., Konsolaki, M., and Zhong, Y. (2004). Dissecting the pathological effects of human Abeta40 and Abeta42 in *Drosophila*: a potential model for Alzheimer's disease. *Proc. Natl. Acad. Sci. U.S.A.* 101, 6623–6628. doi: 10.1073/pnas.0400895101

Iijima-Ando, K., and Iijima, K. (2010). Transgenic *Drosophila* models of Alzheimer's disease and tauopathies. *Brain Struc. Func.* 214, 245–262. doi: 10.1007/s00429-009-0234-4

Keller, L. C., Cheng, L., Locke, C. J., Muller, M., Fetter, R. D., and Davis, G. W. (2011). Glial-derived prodegenerative signaling in the *Drosophila* neuromuscular system. *Neuron* 72, 760–775. doi: 10.1016/j.neuron.2011.09.031

Kerr, F., Augustin, H., Piper, M. D., Gandy, C., Allen, M. J., Lovestone, S., et al. (2011). Dietary restriction delays aging, but not neuronal dysfunction, in *Drosophila* models of Alzheimer's disease. *Neurobiol. Aging* 32, 1977–1989. doi: 10.1016/j.neurobiolaging.2009.10.015

Koch, I., Schwarz, H., Beuchle, D., Goellner, B., Langegger, M., and Aberle, H. (2008). *Drosophila* ankyrin 2 is required for synaptic stability. *Neuron* 58, 210–222. doi: 10.1016/j.neuron.2008.03.019

Kosmidis, S., Grammenoudi, S., Papanikolopoulou, K., and Skoulakis, E. M. (2010). Differential effects of Tau on the integrity and function of neurons essential for learning in *Drosophila*. *J. Neurosci.* 30, 464–477. doi: 10.1523/JNEUROSCI.1490-09.2010

Lambert, J. C., Ibrahim-Verbaas, C. A., Harold, D., Naj, A. C., Sims, R., Bellenguez, C., et al. (2013). Meta-analysis of 74,046 individuals identifies 11 new susceptibility loci for Alzheimer's disease. *Nat. Genet.* 45, 1452–1458. doi: 10.1038/ng.2802

Lee, S., Wang, J. W., Yu, W., and Lu, B. (2012). Phospho-dependent ubiquitination and degradation of PAR-1 regulates synaptic morphology and tau-mediated Abeta toxicity in *Drosophila*. *Nat. Commun.* 3:1312. doi: 10.1038/ncomms2278

Lunnon, K., Smith, R., Hannon, E., De Jager, P. L., Srivastava, G., Volta, M., et al. (2014). Methylomic profiling implicates cortical deregulation of ANK1 in Alzheimer's disease. *Nat. Neurosci.* 17, 1164–1170. doi: 10.1038/nn.3782

Malik, B. R., Gillespie, J. M., and Hodge, J. J. (2013). CASK and CaMKII function in the mushroom body α'/β' neurons during *Drosophila* memory formation. *Front. Neural Cir.* 7:52. doi: 10.3389/fncir.2013.00052

Malik, B. R., and Hodge, J. J. (2014). *Drosophila* adult olfactory shock learning. *J. Visual. Exp.* 90:e50107.

Massaro, C. M., Pielage, J., and Davis, G. W. (2009). Molecular mechanisms that enhance synapse stability despite persistent disruption of the spectrin/ankyrin/microtubule cytoskeleton. *J. Cell Biol.* 187, 101–117. doi: 10.1083/jcb.200903166

Mastroeni, D., Sekar, S., Nolz, J., Delvaux, E., Lunnon, K., Mill, J., et al. (2017). ANK1 is up-regulated in laser captured microglia in Alzheimer's brain; the importance of addressing cellular heterogeneity. *PLoS One* 12:e0177814. doi: 10.1371/journal.pone.0177814

Mazock, G. H., Das, A., Base, C., and Dubreuil, R. R. (2010). Transgene rescue identifies an essential function for *Drosophila* beta spectrin in the nervous system and a selective requirement for ankyrin-2-binding activity. *Mol. Biol. Cell* 21, 2860–2868. doi: 10.1091/mbc.E10-03-0180

McGowan, E., Eriksen, J., and Hutton, M. (2006). A decade of modeling Alzheimer's disease in transgenic mice. *Trends Genet.* 22, 281–289. doi: 10.1016/j.tig.2006.03.007

Mershin, A., Pavlopoulos, E., Fitch, O., Braden, B. C., Nanopoulos, D. V., and Skoulakis, E. M. (2004). Learning and memory deficits upon TAU accumulation in *Drosophila* mushroom body neurons. *Learn. Mem.* 11, 277–287. doi: 10.1101/lm.70804

Papanikolopoulou, K., and Skoulakis, E. M. (2015). Temporally distinct phosphorylations differentiate Tau-dependent learning deficits and premature mortality in *Drosophila*. *Hum. Mol. Genet.* 24, 2065–2077. doi: 10.1093/hmg/ddu726

Pfeiffer, B. D., Jenett, A., Hammonds, A. S., Ngo, T. T., Misra, S., Murphy, C., et al. (2008). Tools for neuroanatomy and neurogenetics in *Drosophila*. *Proc. Natl. Acad. Sci. U.S.A.* 105, 9715–9720. doi: 10.1073/pnas.0803697105

Pielage, J., Cheng, L., Fetter, R. D., Carlton, P. M., Sedat, J. W., and Davis, G. W. (2008). A Presynaptic giant ankyrin stabilizes the NMJ through regulation of presynaptic microtubules and transsynaptic cell adhesion. *Neuron* 58, 195–209. doi: 10.1016/j.neuron.2008.02.017

Ping, Y., Hahm, E. T., Waro, G., Song, Q., Vo-Ba, D. A., Licursi, A., et al. (2015). Linking abeta42-induced hyperexcitability to neurodegeneration, learning and motor deficits, and a shorter lifespan in an Alzheimer's model. *PLoS Genet.* 11:e1005025. doi: 10.1371/journal.pgen.1005025

Plattner, F., Angelo, M., and Giese, K. P. (2006). The roles of cyclin-dependent kinase 5 and glycogen synthase kinase 3 in tau hyperphosphorylation. *J. Biol. Chem.* 281, 25457–25465. doi: 10.1074/jbc.m603469200

Schlichting, M., Menegazzi, P., Lelito, K. R., Yao, Z., Buhl, E., Dalla Benetta, E., et al. (2016). A neural network underlying circadian entrainment and photoperiodic adjustment of sleep and activity in *Drosophila. J. Neurosci.* 36, 9084–9096. doi: 10.1523/JNEUROSCI.0992-16.2016

Sealey, M. A., Vourkou, E., Cowan, C. M., Bossing, T., Quraishe, S., Grammenoudi, S., et al. (2017). Distinct phenotypes of three-repeat and four-repeat human tau in a transgenic model of tauopathy. *Neurobiol. Dis.* 105, 74–83. doi: 10.1016/j.nbd.2017.05.003

Selkoe, D. J. (2012). Preventing Alzheimer's disease. *Science* 337, 1488–1492.

Selkoe, D. J., and Hardy, J. (2016). The amyloid hypothesis of Alzheimer's disease at 25 years. *EMBO Mol. Med.* 8, 595–608. doi: 10.15252/emmm.201606210

Shaw, R. E., Kottler, B., Ludlow, Z. N., Buhl, E., Kim, D., Morais da Silva, S., et al. (2018). In vivo expansion of functionally integrated GABAergic interneurons by targeted increase in neural progenitors. *EMBO J.* 37:e98163. doi: 10.15252/embj.201798163

Shulman, J. M., Chipendo, P., Chibnik, L. B., Aubin, C., Tran, D., Keenan, B. T., et al. (2011). Functional screening of Alzheimer pathology genome-wide association signals in *Drosophila. Am. J. Hum. Genet.* 88, 232–238. doi: 10.1016/j.ajhg.2011.01.006

Shulman, J. M., Imboywa, S., Giagtzoglou, N., Powers, M. P., Hu, Y., Devenport, D., et al. (2014). Functional screening in *Drosophila* identifies Alzheimer's disease susceptibility genes and implicates Tau-mediated mechanisms. *Hum. Mol. Genet.* 23, 870–877. doi: 10.1093/hmg/ddt478

Siegenthaler, D., Enneking, E. M., Moreno, E., and Pielage, J. (2015). L1CAM/Neuroglian controls the axon-axon interactions establishing layered and lobular mushroom body architecture. *J. Cell Biol.* 208, 1003–1018. doi: 10.1083/jcb.201407131

Smith, A. R., Smith, R. G., Burrage, J., Troakes, C., Al-Sarraj, S., Kalaria, R. N., et al. (2019). A cross-brain regions study of ANK1 DNA methylation in different neurodegenerative diseases. *Neurobiol. Aging* 74, 70–76. doi: 10.1016/j.neurobiolaging.2018.09.024

Smith, K. R., and Penzes, P. (2018). Ankyrins: roles in synaptic biology and pathology. *Mol. Cell Neurosci.* 91, 131–139. doi: 10.1016/j.mcn.2018.04.010

Smith, R. G., Hannon, E., De Jager, P. L., Chibnik, L., Lott, S. J., Condliffe, D., et al. (2018). Elevated DNA methylation across a 48-kb region spanning the HOXA gene cluster is associated with Alzheimer's disease neuropathology. *Alzheimer's Dementia* 14, 1580–1588. doi: 10.1016/j.jalz.2018.01.017

Smith, R. G., and Lunnon, K. (2017). DNA Modifications and Alzheimer's Disease. *Adv. Exp. Med. Biol.* 978, 303–319.

Speretta, E., Jahn, T. R., Tartaglia, G. G., Favrin, G., Barros, T. P., Imarisio, S., et al. (2012). Expression in *Drosophila* of tandem amyloid beta peptides provides insights into links between aggregation and neurotoxicity. *J. Biol. Chem.* 287, 20748–20754. doi: 10.1074/jbc.M112.350124

Spires-Jones, T. L., and Hyman, B. T. (2014). The intersection of amyloid beta and tau at synapses in Alzheimer's disease. *Neuron* 82, 756–771. doi: 10.1016/j.neuron.2014.05.004

Sun, J., Xu, A. Q., Giraud, J., Poppinga, H., Riemensperger, T., Fiala, A., et al. (2018). Neural control of startle-induced locomotion by the mushroom bodies and associated neurons in *Drosophila. Front. Sys. Neurosci.* 12:6. doi: 10.3389/fnsys.2018.00006

Suzuki, M. M., and Bird, A. (2008). DNA methylation landscapes: provocative insights from epigenomics. *Nat. Rev. Genet.* 9, 465–476. doi: 10.1038/nrg2341

Tabuchi, M., Lone, S. R., Liu, S., Liu, Q., Zhang, J., Spira, A. P., et al. (2015). Sleep interacts with abeta to modulate intrinsic neuronal excitability. *Curr. Biol.* 25, 702–712. doi: 10.1016/j.cub.2015.01.016

Van Dam, D., and De Deyn, P. P. (2011). Animal models in the drug discovery pipeline for Alzheimer's disease. *Br. J. Pharmacol.* 164, 1285–1300. doi: 10.1111/j.1476-5381.2011.01299.x

Walsh, D. M., and Selkoe, D. J. (2004). Deciphering the molecular basis of memory failure in Alzheimer's disease. *Neuron* 44, 181–193. doi: 10.1016/j.neuron.2004.09.010

Wang, J. Z., Grundke-Iqbal, I., and Iqbal, K. (2007). Kinases and phosphatases and tau sites involved in Alzheimer neurofibrillary degeneration. *Eur. J. Neurosci.* 25, 59–68. doi: 10.1111/j.1460-9568.2006.05226.x

Wittmann, C. W., Wszolek, M. F., Shulman, J. M., Salvaterra, P. M., Lewis, J., Hutton, M., et al. (2001). Tauopathy in *Drosophila*: neurodegeneration without neurofibrillary tangles. *Science* 293, 711–714. doi: 10.1126/science.1062382

Wu, J. W., Hussaini, S. A., Bastille, I. M., Rodriguez, G. A., Mrejeru, A., Rilett, K., et al. (2016). Neuronal activity enhances tau propagation and tau pathology in vivo. *Nat. Neurosci.* 19, 1085–1092. doi: 10.1038/nn.4328

Yamamoto, S., Wajima, T., Hara, Y., Nishida, M., and Mori, Y. (2007). Transient receptor potential channels in Alzheimer's disease. *Biochim. Biophys. Acta* 1772, 958–967.

Permissions

All chapters in this book were first published by Frontiers; hereby published with permission under the Creative Commons Attribution License or equivalent. Every chapter published in this book has been scrutinized by our experts. Their significance has been extensively debated. The topics covered herein carry significant findings which will fuel the growth of the discipline. They may even be implemented as practical applications or may be referred to as a beginning point for another development.

The contributors of this book come from diverse backgrounds, making this book a truly international effort. This book will bring forth new frontiers with its revolutionizing research information and detailed analysis of the nascent developments around the world.

We would like to thank all the contributing authors for lending their expertise to make the book truly unique. They have played a crucial role in the development of this book. Without their invaluable contributions this book wouldn't have been possible. They have made vital efforts to compile up to date information on the varied aspects of this subject to make this book a valuable addition to the collection of many professionals and students.

This book was conceptualized with the vision of imparting up-to-date information and advanced data in this field. To ensure the same, a matchless editorial board was set up. Every individual on the board went through rigorous rounds of assessment to prove their worth. After which they invested a large part of their time researching and compiling the most relevant data for our readers.

The editorial board has been involved in producing this book since its inception. They have spent rigorous hours researching and exploring the diverse topics which have resulted in the successful publishing of this book. They have passed on their knowledge of decades through this book. To expedite this challenging task, the publisher supported the team at every step. A small team of assistant editors was also appointed to further simplify the editing procedure and attain best results for the readers.

Apart from the editorial board, the designing team has also invested a significant amount of their time in understanding the subject and creating the most relevant covers. They scrutinized every image to scout for the most suitable representation of the subject and create an appropriate cover for the book.

The publishing team has been an ardent support to the editorial, designing and production team. Their endless efforts to recruit the best for this project, has resulted in the accomplishment of this book. They are a veteran in the field of academics and their pool of knowledge is as vast as their experience in printing. Their expertise and guidance has proved useful at every step. Their uncompromising quality standards have made this book an exceptional effort. Their encouragement from time to time has been an inspiration for everyone.

The publisher and the editorial board hope that this book will prove to be a valuable piece of knowledge for researchers, students, practitioners and scholars across the globe.

List of Contributors

Marianna Alves, Aidan Kenny, Gioacchino de Leo, Edward H. Beamer and Tobias Engel
Department of Physiology and Medical Physics, Royal College of Surgeons in Ireland, Dublin, Ireland

Laura Montrreal and Adelina Orellana
Center for Networked Biomedical Research on Neurodegenerative Diseases, National Institute of Health Carlos III, Ministry of Economy and Competitiveness, Madrid, Spain

Pascual Sánchez-Juan, Carmen Lage, Sara López-García and Eloy Rodrííguez-Rodríguez
Center for Networked Biomedical Research on Neurodegenerative Diseases, National Institute of Health Carlos III, Ministry of Economy and Competitiveness, Madrid, Spain
Service of Neurology, University Hospital Marqués de Valdecilla, IDIVAL, University of Cantabria, Santander, Spain

Sonia Moreno, Itziar de Rojas, Isabel Hernández, Sergi Valero, Montse Alegret, Pablo García González, Lluís Tárraga, Mercè Boada and Agustín Ruiz
Center for Networked Biomedical Research on Neurodegenerative Diseases, National Institute of Health Carlos III, Ministry of Economy and Competitiveness, Madrid, Spain
Research Center and Memory Clinic, Fundació ACE, Institut Català de Neurociències Aplicades, Universitat Internacional de Catalunya, Barcelona, Spain

Andrew Umstead
Department of Translational Science and Molecular Medicine, College of Human Medicine, Grand Rapids, MI, United States

Irving E. Vega
Department of Translational Science and Molecular Medicine, College of Human Medicine, Grand Rapids, MI, United States
Neuroscience Program, Michigan State University, Grand Rapids, MI, United States
Department of Neurology, University of Michigan, Ann Arbor, MI, United States

Nicholas M. Kanaan
Department of Translational Science and Molecular Medicine, College of Human Medicine, Grand Rapids, MI, United States
Neuroscience Program, Michigan State University, Grand Rapids, MI, United States
Hauenstein Neuroscience Center, Mercy Health Saint Mary's, Grand Rapids, MI, United States

Bernadeta Valachova
Axon Neuroscience R&D Services SE, Bratislava, Slovakia

Veronika Brezovakova
Institute of Neuroimmunology, Slovak Academy of Sciences, Bratislava, Slovakia

Tomas Smolek, Veronika Cubinkova, Peter Szalay, Norbert Zilka and Santosh Jadhav
Institute of Neuroimmunology, Slovak Academy of Sciences, Bratislava, Slovakia
Axon Neuroscience R&D Services SE, Bratislava, Slovakia

James P. Higham, Sergio Hidalgo, Edgar Buhl and James J. L. Hodge
School of Physiology, Pharmacology and Neuroscience, University of Bristol, Bristol, United Kingdom

Yan Lin, Hameetha B. Rajamohamedsait, Leslie A. Sandusky-Beltran, Begona Gamallo-Lana and Adam Mar
Department of Neuroscience and Physiology, Neuroscience Institute, New York University School of Medicine, New York, NY, United States

Einar M. Sigurdsson
Department of Neuroscience and Physiology, Neuroscience Institute, New York University School of Medicine, New York, NY, United States
Department of Psychiatry, New York University School of Medicine, New York, NY, United States

Mercedes Arnes, Maria E. Alaniz, Joshua D. Cho and Ismael Santa-Maria
Taub Institute for Research on Alzheimer's Disease and the Aging Brain, Columbia University, New York, NY, United States
Department of Pathology and Cell Biology, Columbia University, New York, NY, United States

Caline S. Karam
Department of Psychiatry, Vagelos College of Physicians and Surgeons, Columbia University, New York, NY, United States

Gonzalo Lopez
Department of Genetics and Genomic Sciences, Icahn School of Medicine at Mount Sinai, New York, NY, United States

Jonathan A. Javitch
Department of Psychiatry, Vagelos College of Physicians and Surgeons, Columbia University, New York, NY, United States
Division of Molecular Therapeutics, New York State Psychiatric Institute, New York, NY, United States
Department of Pharmacology, Vagelos College of Physicians and Surgeons, Columbia University, New York, NY, United States

Pascale Barbier, Philipp O. Tsvetkov and François Devred
Fac Pharm, Aix Marseille Univ., Centre National de la Recherche Scientifique (CNRS), Inst Neurophysiopathol (INP), Fac Pharm, Marseille, France

Alessia Lasorsa, Caroline Smet-Nocca and Isabelle Landrieu
Univ. Lille, Centre National de la Recherche Scientifique (CNRS), UMR 8576, Unité de Glycobiologie Structurale et Fonctionnelle (UGSF), Lille, France

Orgeta Zejneli
Univ. Lille, Centre National de la Recherche Scientifique (CNRS), UMR 8576, Unité de Glycobiologie Structurale et Fonctionnelle (UGSF), Lille, France
Univ. Lille, Institut National de la Santé et de la Recherche Médicale (INSERM), CHU-Lille, UMR-S 1172, Centre de Recherche Jean-Pierre AUBERT (JPArc), Lille, France

Marlène Martinho and Valérie Belle
Aix Marseille Univ., Centre National de la Recherche Scientifique (CNRS), UMR 7281, Bioénergétique et Ingénierie des Protéines (BIP), Marseille, France

Félix Hernández and Jesús Avila
Network Center for Biomedical Research in Neurodegenerative Diseases (CIBERNED), Carlos III Institute of Health, Madrid, Spain
Centro de Biología Molecular Severo Ochoa, Consejo Superior de Investigaciones Científicas (CSIC), Universidad Autonoma de Madrid (UAM), Madrid, Spain

Jesús Merchán-Rubira, Laura Vallés-Saiz and Alberto Rodríguez-Matellán
Centro de Biología Molecular Severo Ochoa, Consejo Superior de Investigaciones Científicas (CSIC), Universidad Autonoma de Madrid (UAM), Madrid, Spain

Yanina Ivashko-Pachima and Illana Gozes
Dr. Diana and Zelman Elton (Elbaum) Laboratory for Molecular Neuroendocrinology, Department of Human Molecular Genetics and Biochemistry, Sackler Faculty of Medicine, Sagol School of Neuroscience, Adams Super Center for Brain Studies, Tel Aviv University, Tel Aviv, Israel

Shunsuke Kobayashi and Toru Tanaka
Department of Biochemistry, School of Pharmacy, Nihon University, Funabashi, Japan

Yoshiyuki Soeda and Akihiko Takashima
Laboratory for Alzheimer's Disease, Department of Life Science, Faculty of Science, Gakushuin University, Tokyo, Japan

Thomas K. Karikari
School of Life Sciences, University of Warwick, Coventry, United Kingdom
Midlands Integrative Biosciences Training Partnership, University of Warwick, Coventry, United Kingdom

Kevin G. Moffat
School of Life Sciences, University of Warwick, Coventry, United Kingdom

David A. Nagel, Alastair Grainger, Charlotte Clarke-Bland, James Crowe and Eric J. Hill
School of Life and Health Sciences, Aston University, Birmingham, United Kingdom

Marta Fernández-Nogales
Instituto Neurociencias Alicante (CSIC-UMH), San Juan de Alicante, Spain

José J. Lucas
Centro de Biología Molecular Severo Ochoa (CBMSO) (CSIC-UAM), Madrid, Spain
Networking Research Center on Neurodegenerative Diseases (CIBERNED), Instituto de Salud Carlos III, Madrid, Spain

Nataliya I. Trushina and Lidia Bakota
Department of Neurobiology, University of Osnabrück, Osnabrück, Germany

Armen Y. Mulkidjanian
Department of Physics, University of Osnabrück, Osnabrück, Germany
School of Bioengineering and Bioinformatics, Lomonosov Moscow State University, Moscow, Russia
A.N. Belozersky Institute of Physico-Chemical Biology, Lomonosov Moscow State University, Moscow, Russia

Roland Brandt
Department of Neurobiology, University of Osnabrück, Osnabrück, Germany
Center for Cellular Nanoanalytics, University of Osnabrück, Osnabrück, Germany
Institute of Cognitive Science, University of Osnabrück, Osnabrück, Germany

Gabor G. Kovacs
Tanz Centre for Research in Neurodegenerative Disease, University of Toronto, Toronto, ON, Canada
Department of Laboratory Medicine and Pathobiology, University of Toronto, Toronto, ON, Canada
Laboratory Medicine Program, University Health Network, Toronto, ON, Canada

Ena Španić, Lea Langer Horvat and Goran Šimić
Laboratory for Developmental Neuropathology, Department of Neuroscience, Croatian Institute for Brain Research, University of Zagreb School of Medicine, Zagreb, Croatia

Patrick R. Hof
Nash Family Department of Neuroscience, Ronald M. Loeb Center for Alzheimer's Disease, Friedman Brain Institute, Icahn School of Medicine at Mount Sinai, New York, NY, United States

Isidro Ferrer
Department of Pathology and Experimental Therapeutics, University of Barcelona, Barcelona, Spain
Senior Consultant, Bellvitge University Hospital, IDIBELL (Bellvitge Biomedical Research Centre), Barcelona, Spain
CIBERNED (Network Centre of Biomedical Research of Neurodegenerative Diseases), Institute of Health Carlos III, Ministry of Economy and Competitiveness, Madrid, Spain
Institute of Neurosciences, University of Barcelona, Barcelona, Spain

Meritxell Aguiló García
Department of Pathology and Experimental Therapeutics, University of Barcelona, Barcelona, Spain

Margarita Carmona, Pol Andrés-Benito and Paula Garcia-Esparcia
Department of Pathology and Experimental Therapeutics, University of Barcelona, Barcelona, Spain
CIBERNED (Network Centre of Biomedical Research of Neurodegenerative Diseases), Institute of Health Carlos III, Ministry of Economy and Competitiveness, Madrid, Spain

Benjamin Torrejón-Escribano
Biology Unit, Scientific and Technical Services, Hospitalet de Llobregat, University of Barcelona, Barcelona, Spain

José Antonio del Rio
CIBERNED (Network Centre of Biomedical Research of Neurodegenerative Diseases), Institute of Health Carlos III, Ministry of Economy and Competitiveness, Madrid, Spain
Institute of Neurosciences, University of Barcelona, Barcelona, Spain
Molecular and Cellular Neurobiotechnology, Institute of Bioengineering of Catalonia (IBEC), Barcelona Institute for Science and Technology, Parc Científic de Barcelona, Barcelona, Spain
Department of Cell Biology, Physiology and Immunology, Faculty of Biology, University of Barcelona, Barcelona, Spain

Yann Fichou, Zachary R. Oberholtzer, Hoang Ngo, Chi-Yuan Cheng, Timothy J. Keller and Neil A. Eschmann
Department of Chemistry and Biochemistry, University of California, Santa Barbara, Santa Barbara, CA, United States

Songi Han
Department of Chemistry and Biochemistry, University of California, Santa Barbara, Santa Barbara, CA, United States
Department of Chemical Engineering, University of California, Santa Barbara, Santa Barbara, CA, United States

Ricardo Gargini
Centro de Biología Molecular, CSIC, Madrid, Spain

Berta Segura-Collar and Pilar Sánchez-Gómez
Neurooncology Unit, Instituto de Salud Carlos IIIUFIEC, Madrid, Spain

Bilal R. Malik, Jennifer M. Dawson and Anna S. Ogier
School of Physiology, Pharmacology and Neuroscience, University of Bristol, Bristol, United Kingdom

Katie Lunnon
School of Physiology, Pharmacology and Neuroscience, University of Bristol, Bristol, United Kingdom
University of Exeter Medical School, University of Exeter, Exeter, United Kingdom

Index

www.ingramcontent.com/pod-product-compliance
Lightning Source LLC
LaVergne TN
LVHW060057220926
848484LV00008BA/2098
9798887404011